The Oxford Handbook
of Auditory Science
The Ear

The Oxford Handbook of Auditory Science
The Ear

VOLUME 1

Edited by

Paul A Fuchs
Center for Hearing and Balance
Johns Hopkins University School of Medicine
Baltimore
USA

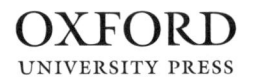

OXFORD
UNIVERSITY PRESS

OXFORD
UNIVERSITY PRESS

Great Clarendon Street, Oxford OX2 6DP

Oxford University Press is a department of the University of Oxford.
It furthers the University's objective of excellence in research, scholarship,
and education by publishing worldwide in

Oxford New York

Auckland Cape Town Dar es Salaam Hong Kong Karachi
Kuala Lumpur Madrid Melbourne Mexico City Nairobi
New Delhi Shanghai Taipei Toronto

With offices in

Argentina Austria Brazil Chile Czech Republic France Greece Guatemala
Hungary Italy Japan Poland Portugal Singapore South
Korea Switzerland Thailand Turkey Ukraine Vietnam

Oxford is a registered trade mark of Oxford University Press
in the UK and in certain other countries

Published in the United States
by Oxford University Press Inc., New York

British Library Cataloguing in Publication Data
Data available

Library of Congress Cataloging in Publication Data
Oxford handbook of auditory science. The ear / edited by Paul Fuchs.
    p. cm.
    Includes bibliographical references and index.
    ISBN 978-0-19-923339-7 (pbk. : alk. paper)
1. Ear—Physiology. 2. Hearing—Physiological aspects. 3. Deafness.
I. Fuchs, Paul, 1951- II. Title: Ear.
    [DNLM: 1. Ear—physiology. 2. Hearing—physiology. 3. Hearing Loss.
WV 200 O98 2010]
    QP461.O94 2010
    612.8'5—dc22   2009032940

Typeset in Minion by Glyph International, Bangalore, India
Printed in China
on acid-free paper
through Asia Pacific Offset

ISBN 978–0–19–923339–7

10 9 8 7 6 5 4 3 2 1

Series Preface

Auditory science has been, over the past three decades, one of the fastest growing areas of biomedical research. Worldwide there are now perhaps 10 000 researchers whose primary job is auditory research, and ten times that number working in allied, mainly clinical, hearing professions. This rapid growth is attributable to and, in turn, fuelled by several major developments in our understanding. While this Handbook focuses on fundamental research and underlying mechanisms, it does so from the perspective of understanding the impact of auditory science on the quality of our life. That impact has been realized through the explosive growth of digital technology and microelectronics, and delivered by devices as diverse as MP3 compression for music listening (based on models of perceptual coding) to the latest instruments for the management of hearing loss, including digital hearing aids and multichannel cochlear implants. The discovery of otoacoustic emissions (OAEs) – sounds produced by the cochlea – has enabled a step change both in our understanding of ear function and in the development of a clinical tool for deafness screening in newborn infants.

Fundamental research on the inner ear has shown that an elaborate system of sound-induced active processes, acting through the outer hair cells, serves to improve sensitivity, sharpen frequency tuning, dynamically modulate the mechanical response of the ear to sound, and create sound energy that passes back out of the ear. Each of these processes is also influenced by descending neural input to the hair cells. Most recently, the molecular machinery underlying these incredible phenomena has been explored and described in detail. The development, maintenance, and repair of the ear are also subjects of contemporary interest at the molecular level, as is the genetics of hearing disorders due to cochlear malfunctions. The auditory brain is responsible for sound (including speech) identification and localization. Through functional neuroimaging in humans, and the application of novel methods in animals, such as multichannel recordings of single unit activity, multiple cortical and subcortical areas necessarily involved in hearing and listening have now been identified and characterized. These areas occupy the superior (dorsal) temporal cortex, and extend into non-classical cortical regions, including the more rostral and ventral temporal lobe, the limbic system, and elsewhere in the frontal and parietal lobes. Understanding of subcortical processing has expanded through the use of molecular and cellular techniques *in vitro* and recordings in awake and behaving humans and animals *in vivo*. Increasingly, the widespread descending pathways are being shown to have profound functional importance, and to influence the coding of both simple and complex sounds. Recent studies of hearing (auditory perception) have shown how our perceptions relate to the underlying physiological mechanisms. For example, behavioural measures of peripheral auditory function have led to the development of sophisticated models of cochlear processing in humans. These models are having widespread influence in understanding both normal and pathological hearing. At the same time, there has been an increasing focus on auditory 'ecology', on complex sound perception in real (or virtual) environments. Traditional distinctions between spectral, temporal, and binaural processing have evolved into more functional concerns, including auditory scene analysis and auditory object perception.

Here, then, are the three major domains of auditory science – the ear, the brain, and hearing – and I am proud to present a corresponding three-volume Handbook. However, as the volume editors and I started sifting through all the areas we wished to cover, a number of recent developments in our science became apparent that made us question the way in which we had decided to partition the field. Spurred on by ever-increasing knowledge, the availability of enabling technology, and cultural shifts in attitudes towards 'relevance' and 'interdisciplinary' research, the three domains have begun to blur into one. Several instances of this are hinted at above: a transition from more segmented to more holistic approaches to audition; a shift in focus from more simple to more complex and, hence, more realistic sounds; and a drilling down across traditional disciplinary boundaries from the phenomenological to the mechanistic and generic. Dynamic properties of hearing are becoming more prominent across all three domains, and beyond, as lifespan development, adaptation, and learning receive increasing recognition. Reciprocal influences of hearing on and from cognition (attention, memory, and emotion), action, and vision add to a picture of a powerful, working, integrated sense that is arguably the most important we possess for what makes us distinctly human – our social interaction with our world. Organizationally, researchers at all levels (peripheral, central, and perceptual) now work increasingly together, with many major and several new interdisciplinary centres of auditory science dotted across the globe.

Our ambitious aim has been to deliver a working Handbook that would fill an unmet need for a single reference work spanning all of auditory science. We wanted it to offer a basic background for all those interested in the subject, from the curious undergraduate to the professional researcher and clinician, while also capturing the excitement, and some of the detail, of the most recent developments in this rapidly evolving discipline. Consequently, we set out with the conflicting aims of producing a comprehensive, even definitive work, but of completing it within the minimum time possible. We optimistically targeted this at one year, recognizing that the finished product would have a finite lifespan. In fact, the preparation of the chapters, from commissioning to collection of the final versions of the final chapters, has taken about two years. Although disappointing to us, Martin Baum, our very helpful and ever patient senior commissioning editor at Oxford University Press, has tried to console us, suggesting that even this effort has been something of a world record.

I knew at the outset of this project that its success would be completely dependent on the recruitment of the right volume editors. I feel incredibly lucky and humbled to have retained the services of four colleagues whose insight, experience, determination, interpersonal skills, and sheer hard work have managed to get this Handbook together more quickly than some of my own previous book chapters have taken to be read by the book's editors, and more professionally than I had dreamed possible. Many, many thanks to all four – my dedication is to you.

David R Moore
MRC Institute of Hearing Research
Nottingham
April 2009

Contents

Contributors

Jonathan Ashmore
Department of Neuroscience,
Physiology and Pharmacology
University College London
Gower Street
London
UK

Lynne M Bianchi
Oberlin College
Neuroscience Department
Oberlin, Ohio
USA

Egbert de Boer
Academic Medical Center
Amsterdam
The Netherlands

Douglas A Cotanche
Lab for Cellular and Molecular
Hearing Research
Boston University School of Medicine
Boston, Massachusetts
USA

A Belén Elgoyhen
Institute for Research in
Genetic Engineering
INGEBI-CONICET
Buenos Aires
Argentina

Paul A Fuchs
Center for Hearing and Balance
Johns Hopkins University
School of Medicine
Baltimore, Maryland
USA

David N Furness
Institute for Science and Technology
in Medicine
Keele University School of Life Sciences
Keele, Staffordshire
UK

Jonathan Gale
UCL Ear Institute
University College London
London
UK

Anne BS Giersch
Department of Pathology
Brigham and Women's Hospital
Harvard Medical School
Boston, Massachusetts
USA

Carole M Hackney
Department of Biomedical Science
Addison Building
Western Bank
Sheffield, Yorkshire
UK

Kuni H Iwasa
National Institute on Deafness and Other
Communication Disorders
National Institutes of Health
Rockville, Maryland
USA

Daniel Jagger
UCL Ear Institute
University College London
London
UK

David T Kemp
UCL Ear Institute
Centre for Auditory Research
University College London
London
UK

Lawrence R Lustig
Department of Otolaryngology-HNS
University of California at
San Francisco
San Francisco, California
USA

Daniel C Marcus
Anatomy and Physiology Department
Cellular Biophysics Laboratory
Kansas State University
Manhattan, Kansas
USA

Andrea Marlowe
Department of Otolaryngology-HNS
Johns Hopkins School of Medicine
Baltimore, Maryland
USA

Cynthia C Morton
Departments of Pathology and Obstetrics,
Gynecology and Reproductive Biology
Brigham and Women's Hospital
Harvard Medical School
Boston, Massachusetts
USA

John K Niparko
Department of Otolaryngology-HNS
Johns Hopkins School of Medicine
Baltimore, Maryland
USA

Alfred L Nuttall
Oregon Health and Sciences University
Oregon Hearing Research Center
Portland, Oregon
USA

John J Rosowski
Massachusetts Eye and Ear Infirmary
Eaton-Peabody Laboratory
Boston, Massachusetts
USA

Philine Wangemann
Anatomy/Physiology Department
Cell Physiology Lab
College of Veterinary Medicine
Kansas State University
Manhattan, Kansas
USA

Chapter 1

Introduction and overview

Paul A Fuchs

1.1 Introduction

This volume of the Oxford University Press *Handbook of Auditory Sciences* (OUPHAS) has a simple title. *The Ear* expresses the intention of providing a handbook of fundamental material that can serve both as an introduction and as a reference work for anyone interested in the auditory periphery. Thus, each chapter aims for a mix of tutorial and advanced information. The focus throughout is on mechanistic, functional evidence, and many chapters concentrate on cellular and molecular explanations. Before continuing it is essential to acknowledge the diligent and generous efforts of the authors who contributed to this volume. Obviously, scientific resources such as this exist only through such dedication and every reader should appreciate the thoughtful explanations and insights these authors have provided. As an overview and introduction, this chapter will be only lightly referenced, but rather will, in the main, refer to those chapters that cover each topic in depth.

It seems almost unnecessary to address the motivation for a volume titled *The Ear*. Even the briefest exposure to the structure and function of this sensory organ causes a sense of wonder in the observer. The more we probe its inner workings, the more wondrous seem to be its capacities, and the biological mechanisms underlying them. This volume is aimed at describing those mechanisms in some detail. Of course the additional motivation for understanding the auditory periphery is to understand central processing of peripherally derived information that becomes our perception of sound. The process of mechanotransduction leads to altered activity of auditory nerve fibers. The responses of auditory nerve fibers and their onward transmission will be covered in the second volume of this Handbook, *The Auditory Brain*. Still higher levels of analysis are examined in the third volume, *Hearing*.

Two tasks are central to peripheral auditory function: conversion of the mechanical energy carried by airborne sounds into bioelectrical signals, and coding the information content of those sounds by frequency filtering. We will see that multiple elements combine to meet these challenges, ranging from middle-ear mechanics (Chapter 3) to the specialized ionic environment of the inner ear (Chapter 7). In a remarkable example of biological adaptation, the differentiated mechanics of the cochlea map stimulus frequency onto a neurosensory epithelium. Many aspects of peripheral auditory function have become better understood. For example, we have a clear appreciation of the fact that the mechanosensory hair cells themselves empower the cochlear amplifier (Chapter 6). We now know some of the proteins that contribute to inner ear development and function, raising the hope for repair (Chapter 13) or improved protection of hearing in the clinical setting. This volume describes not only basic physiological mechanisms, but also clinical aspects (Chapters 2 and 15), development (Chapter 12), and genetics of the inner ear (Chapter 14). This opening chapter briefly outlines the structure and function of the auditory periphery to preview and motivate the following chapters.

1.2 **The external and middle ear**

The auditory periphery has three anatomical divisions: the *external ear*, which includes the pinna and concha on the surface and the external auditory canal bounded by the tympanum or eardrum, the *middle ear* cavity, which contains the ossicular chain that couples airborne vibration to the third part, the *inner ear*, the cochlea (Fig. 1.1).

The propagation of acoustic energy through the external and middle ears is covered thoroughly in Chapter 3, and earlier reviews (Merchant *et al.*, 1998). Here we provide a brief summary. The visible external ear collects sound and funnels it toward the opening of the auditory canal, thus providing some amplification. Because the human ear canal is a nearly straight tube about 2.5 cm long, it is broadly resonant at 4 kHz. Thus, frequencies near 4 kHz tend to be enhanced by the resonant quality of the external ear, accounting in part for our best sensitivity in that frequency range. More importantly, the external ear (and head) provides important 'sound shadows' so that sounds originating from different positions in space can be recognized by their intensity profile and characteristic frequency signatures.

Sound waves traveling down the canal cause motion of the tympanic membrane, lower pressure (rarefaction) causing it to bulge out, higher pressure (compression) to move in. At this point, the airborne pressure wave is transmitted to the attached ossicular chain of the middle ear. The middle ear bones or ossicles, the *malleus, incus,* and *stapes* (Figs 1.2 and 1.3) have the essential task of transferring the airborne pressure waves into motion of the fluid of the inner ear. Since the cochlear fluids are incompressible compared with air, there is an impedance mismatch that must be overcome. The middle ear alleviates this problem in two ways. First, the area of the tympanic

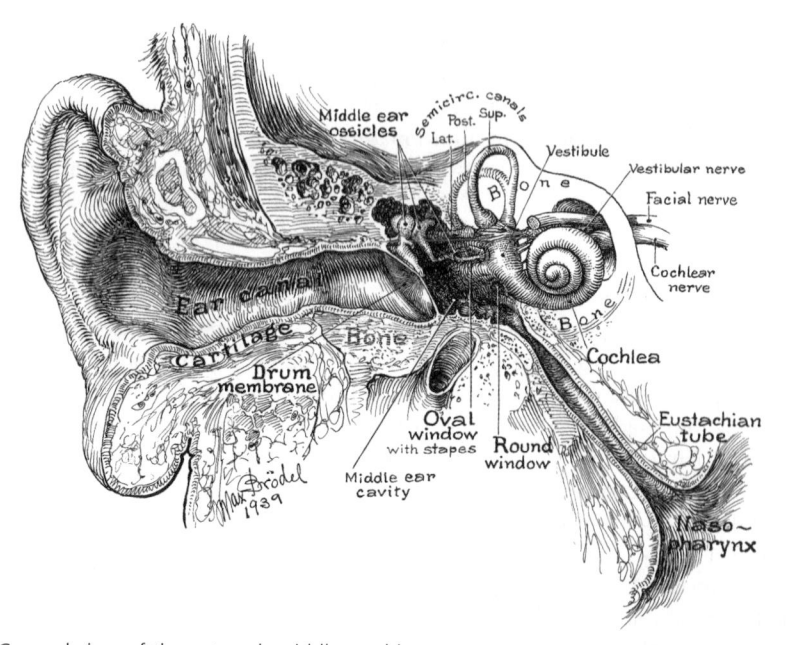

Fig. 1.1 Coronal view of the external, middle, and inner ear.
Drawing (1939) by M Brödel, assisted by PD Malone, SR Guild, and SJ Crowe. Reproduced with permission from 'Three Unpublished Drawings of The Anatomy of the Human Ear', 1946. Original art in the Max Brödel Archives, Walters Collection #980, Department of Art as Applied to Medicine, Johns Hopkins University School of Medicine, Baltimore, Maryland, USA.

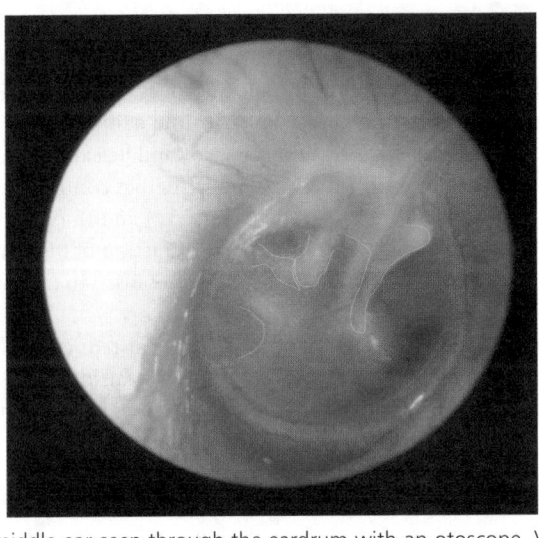

Fig. 1.2 The normal middle ear seen through the eardrum with an otoscope. Visible portions of the ossicular chain are emphasized with a thin white line.
Image courtesy of Dr Howard Francis, Otolaryngology – Head and Neck Surgery, Johns Hopkins University School of Medicine, Baltimore, Maryland, USA.

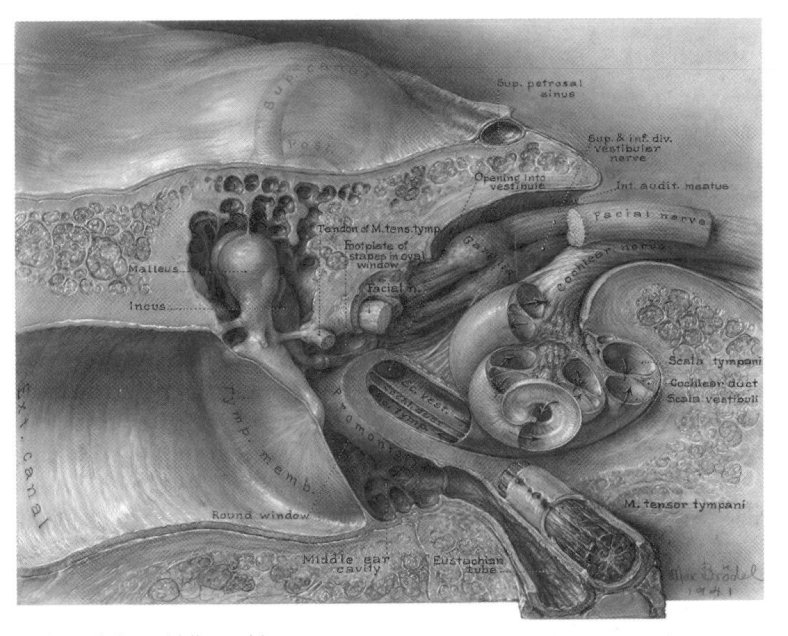

Fig. 1.3 Drawing of the middle and inner ear.
Drawing by M Brödel (1941), assisted by PD Malone, SR Guild, and SJ Crowe. Reproduced with permission from 'Three Unpublished Drawings of The Anatomy of the Human Ear', 1946. Original art in the Max Brödel Archives, Walters Collection #989, Department of Art as Applied to Medicine, Johns Hopkins University School of Medicine, Baltimore, Maryland, USA.

membrane is about 25 times that of the stapes footplate. Thus, airborne vibrations falling onto the larger tympanic area are concentrated into more energetic motions of the much smaller stapes footplate. In addition, the orientation of the middle ear bones confers a slight mechanical advantage, about 1.3 to 1. These factors together (about 30-fold gain) serve to lessen the otherwise severe acoustic impedance mismatch. The importance of middle ear transmission is emphasized by the fact of efferent feedback in the form of small muscles that control the motion of the stapes (stapedius muscle innervated from the VIIth, facial, nerve) and the eardrum (tensor tympani innervated from the Vth, trigeminal, motor branch). Contraction of these muscles limits motion of the ossicular chain, and can reduce the trauma otherwise caused to the inner ear by excessively loud sound.

Thus, it should be obvious that disruption of the middle ear reduces acoustic sensitivity, producing a 'conductive' hearing loss. This can be temporary, as during middle ear infection (otitis media), or permanent when bony scarring (otosclerosis) impedes motion of the ossicles (although this can be corrected surgically). In some cases middle ear loss requires some functional measure. For example, a tuning fork might be inaudible to a person with conductive hearing loss, but can be heard when the stem is pressed to the skull and transmits to the inner ear by bone conduction, bypassing the middle ear. In contrast, damage to the inner ear causes 'sensorineural' hearing loss that does not benefit in this test. The origins and assessment of sensorineural hearing loss are described in Chapter 2. An important addition to these methods is the use of distortion product otoacoustic emissions (DPOAEs) to assess cochlear viability and middle ear patency, especially in infants (Chapter 4). These 'ear sounds' also occur spontaneously and are thought to result from the active mechanical amplification arising from outer hair cell electromotility (Chapter 6).

1.3 The inner ear

The cochlear duct of mammals consists of a coiled tube formed by three parallel membranous compartments. Movement of the stapes footplate in the oval window sets up waves within the fluid of the scala vestibuli. These deflect the cochlear partition to propagate through the scala tympani to the distensible membrane covering the round window. Static displacements of the stapes are relieved by fluid movement through the helicotrema at the apical end of the cochlea. However, stimulation by sound is not static but periodic, and the pattern of motion of the cochlear partition depends on the stimulation frequency (Fig. 1.4). The basilar membrane is narrower and stiffer near the oval window (the cochlear base) and so vibrates maximally for higher frequency tones. The basilar membrane becomes progressively broader and more flexible toward the cochlear apex, where lower frequency tones cause maximal vibration. Afferent neurons carrying acoustic information to the brain usually innervate a single hair cell at only one point along the cochlear spiral (Ginzberg & Morest, 1984). Thus, as explained in Chapter 5, the frequency-dependent motion of the cochlear partition (the basilar membrane and cellular elements of the organ of Corti) lies at the heart of auditory perception. The inner ear can distinguish the frequency content of sounds because of the selective innervation of a mechanically tuned sensory epithelium, the organ of Corti in the cochlea.

1.3.1 The cochlear partition

Viewed in cross-section (Fig. 1.5), the cochlear partition consists of the basilar membrane and the hair cells and supporting cells (the organ of Corti) lying upon it. These all lie beneath the *scala media*, the central membranous tube that is flanked on top and bottom by the *scala vestibuli* and the *scala tympani*, respectively. Within the scala media is the tectorial membrane, an acellular gelatinous sheet that is mechanically coupled to the stereociliary bundles of hair cells (as seen in

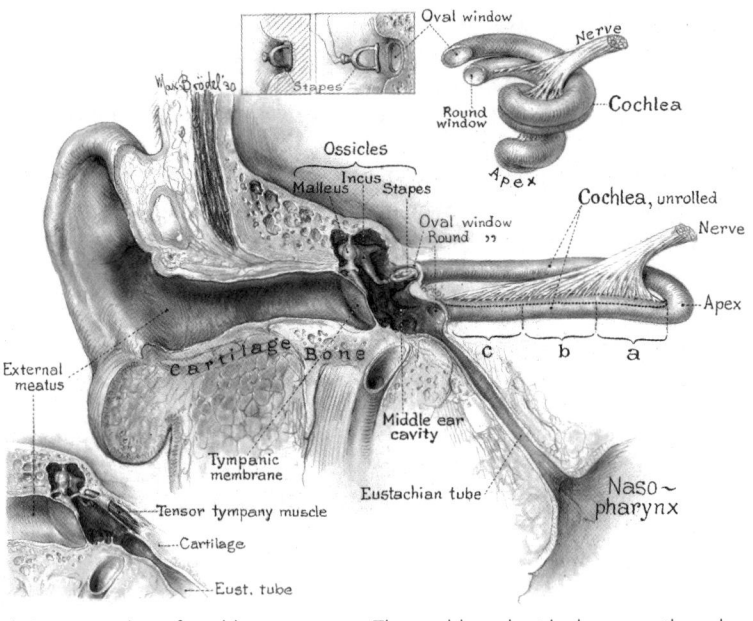

Fig. 1.4 Artist's conception of cochlear tonotopy. The cochlear duct is drawn as though unrolled from its original spiral. Segments 'c', 'b', and 'a' indicate high, to middle, to low frequency regions. Reproduced with permission from unpublished illustration by M Brödel for Dr Samuel J Crowe in 1930. Original art in the Max Brödel Archives, Walters collection #879, Department of Art as Applied to Medicine, Johns Hopkins University School of Medicine, Baltimore, Maryland, USA.

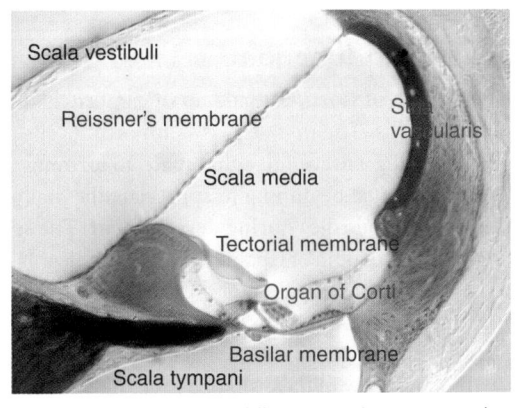

Fig. 1.5 Cross-section of the mouse cochlea, middle turn. Reissner's membrane separates the perilymph in the scala vestibuli from the endolymph produced in the scala media by the stria vascularis. The organ of Corti is subject to differential motion of the overlying tectorial membrane (retracted during fixation in this image) and the underlying basilar membrane.
Modified from original micrograph, osmium-stained plastic section, courtesy of J Taranda, University of Buenos Aires, Buenos Aires, Argentina.

Fig. 2.5, this often retracts and lifts away from the hair cells during fixation). The scala media is bounded by Reissner's membrane on the top, and is delimited by the reticular lamina that forms the apical surface of the hair cell epithelium, and not by the basilar membrane. This distinction is important because the scala media is filled with *endolymph*, a high potassium, low sodium, and low calcium fluid similar in ionic makeup to cytoplasm. The endolymph is produced by a secreting epithelium called the *stria vascularis*, which lines the outer wall of the scala media. The scala vestibuli and scala tympani contain perilymph, which has the low potassium, high sodium, and millimolar calcium concentrations of normal extracellular fluid. Since the basilar membrane itself does not present a diffusion barrier, the basal surface of the hair cells is bathed by low-potassium *perilymph*, while their apical, hair-bearing surface faces high-potassium endolymph. At their apical surface, the hair cells and supporting cells are joined by intercellular junctions (*zona occludens*) that provide a tight seal against fluid exchange across that surface. As we will see, this unique disposition of ionic media is important for hair cell function (Wangemann, 2006). One important result is that a voltage difference exists between endolymph and perilymph, with the endolymph being 80–90 mV positive to perilymph. The *endolymphatic potential* provides additional driving force for potassium ions to flow into the cochlear hair cells. The topic of inner ear ionic homeostasis is covered in Chapter 7.

Disruption of inner ear fluid balance is often cited as a possible basis for Ménière's disease that can include sensorineural hearing loss but more notably vestibular dysfunction, including dizziness, nausea, and inappropriate eye movements. In some cases it seems that the normal circulation of endolymphatic fluid is blocked or otherwise altered, leading to distension of the scala media – a condition called endolymphatic hydrops. The pathogenic mechanisms remain unknown but may relate to the complex ionic homeostasis of the cochlea. In this respect it is of some interest that the most common non-syndromic 'deafness' genes in some human populations are mutations in connexin proteins that form gap junctions among cochlear supporting cells (Chapter 14). One hypothesis suggests that endolymphatic potassium is recycled through the interconnected supporting cells of the organ of Corti (Chapter 11), perhaps by way of gap junctions.

1.3.2 Hair cell structure and function

The sensory epithelium, the organ of Corti, is made up of exquisitely differentiated supporting cells and mechanosensory hair cells. The *non*-sensory supporting cells play important roles in cochlear function, from sequestering extracellular glutamate, to forming rigid 'beams' that stiffen the cochlear partition. We are only just beginning to appreciate the many capabilities of the supporting cells, including their potential roles during development. The specialized structure and function of the supporting cells is the topic of Chapter 11. The cochlear hair cells in mammals are divided into two types, inner and outer, based on their position relative to the center of the cochlear spiral. Inner hair cell function is detailed in Chapter 9. Chapter 6 examines outer hair cell electromotility, while efferent inhibition of these cells is covered in Chapter 10. In a cochlear cross-section, one can see the single row of flask-shaped inner hair cells and three rows of columnar outer hair cells (Fig. 1.6). The hair bundle of each cell is coupled to the overlying tectorial membrane (either by direct contact (outer hair cells), or through fluid viscosity (inner hair cells)) and is subject to lateral shear by the differential motion of the tectorial and basilar membranes.

How is this motion of the cochlear membranes converted into bioelectrical receptor potentials? The answer begins by noting the structure of the staggered stereociliary array atop each hair cell (Fig. 1.7). This staircase-like arrangement of modified microvilli is oriented similarly in all cochlear hair cells, with the tallest hairs furthest from the center of the cochlear spiral (the modiolus). This specific orientation is essential to mechanotransduction. Deflection toward the tallest hairs depolarizes the cell and opposite motion hyperpolarizes. Thus, the relative motion between the

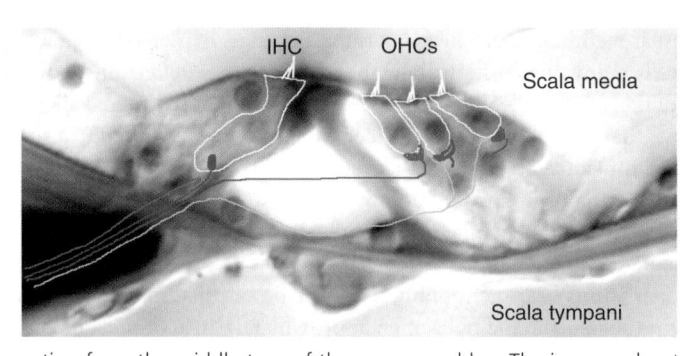

Fig. 1.6 Cross-section from the middle turn of the mouse cochlea. The inner and outer cells (IHCs and OHCs) are outlined in white, and the hair bundles have been drawn exaggerated to emphasize their functional polarity. Blue: type I afferent neuron to an IHC; turquoise: type II afferent to an OHC; red: medial olivocochlear efferent; fuchsia: lateral olivocochlear efferent.
Original micrograph courtesy of J Taranda, University of Buenos Aires, Buenos Aires, Argentina.

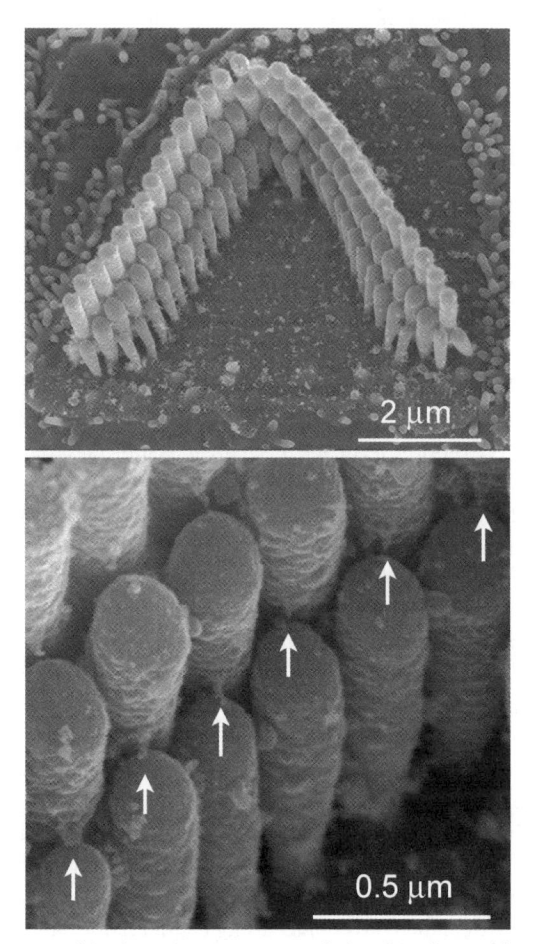

Fig. 1.7 (A) Stereocilia arranged in three tiers on an outer hair cell in the cochlea of an adult rat. (B) Tip links (indicated by arrows) connecting shorter stereocilia to their taller neighbors on a rat outer hair cell. Images courtesy of Drs D Furness and C Hackney, Keele University, Staffordshire, UK.

tectorial and basilar membranes produces coordinate changes in membrane potential in the inner and outer hair cells at any one position along the cochlear duct. Deflection along the axis of bilateral symmetry of the hair bundle pulls on molecular tethers that link stereocilia in adjacent rows. Evidence suggests that tension on these so-called 'tip links' is transmitted to a spring-like gate of mechanosensitive transducer channels (Ricci et al., 2006). While the molecular identity of the transducer channel remains unknown, biophysical measurements classify it as a very large conductance, non-selective cation channel. Further details of hair bundle structure and function are provided in Chapter 8.

Three additional points bear mentioning here. The first is that, in the absence of stimulation, resting tension in the hair bundle pulls open approximately 10% of the hair cell's transduction channels. Thus, sinusoidal deflection of the hair bundle results in a sinusoidal change of tension on the transducer channel gates (i.e. open probability) to alternately depolarize and hyperpolarize the hair cell's membrane potential. The second and third points are related to the first. The resting tension in the hair bundle is calcium sensitive, so that the low level of calcium in endolymph plays an important role in setting the resting level and dynamic range for hair cell stimulation (Farris et al., 2006). Third, the calcium-dependent tensioning results from active molecular motors, composed of non-muscle myosin that pulls against the actin core of the stereocilium (Gillespie, 2004). Since the actin–myosin interaction is calcium dependent, calcium influx through open transduction channels provides a feedback mechanism that helps to set the hair cell's dynamic range. A second, very rapid feedback of calcium onto channel gating underlies a mechanical resonance that contributes to frequency tuning in some non-mammalian hair cells. Active hair bundle mechanics may combine with outer hair cell electromotility in the overall scheme of cochlear signaling (Fettiplace & Hackney, 2006; Hudspeth, 2008).

1.3.3 Hair cell innervation and functional differentiation

Sound-induced changes in membrane potential trigger subsequent voltage-dependent processes in cochlear hair cells, whose functional significance is related to the differential innervation pattern of inner and outer hair cells (Figs 1.6 and 1.8). As will be detailed later, outer hair cells possess a voltage-driven molecular motor that returns mechanical energy to the cochlear vibration pattern (Chapter 6). This electromotile feedback mechanism is subject to central control through the predominant efferent cholinergic innervation of the outer hair cells (Chapter 10). In contrast, the inner hair cells receive the great majority of afferent contacts from spiral ganglion neurons. Thus their receptor potentials encode transmitter (glutamate-like) release onto afferent dendrites by altering the open probability of voltage-gated calcium channels clustered near to transmitter release sites, or ribbons (Chapter 9). Electromotility, and transmitter release, are strongly modulated by voltage-gated potassium channels that make up the bulk of the membrane conductance in both the outer and inner hair cells. It is worth noting that potassium channels in the basolateral membranes of hair cells face a perilymph-like solution with a low level of potassium. Consequently, potassium flux through these channels is outward and hyperpolarizing. Conveniently then, potassium flux *in* through apical transducer channels and *out* across the basolateral membrane of hair cells can be 'downhill' in both directions, off-loading the energy demands of ionic pumping to the stria vascularis that generates the potassium-rich endolymph (Chapter 7).

Cochlear afferent neurons have their cell bodies within the central core, or modiolus of the cochlear spiral (hence 'spiral ganglion neurons (SGNs)'). Type I afferents make up 95% of SGNs and project a single dendrite radially to contact a single inner hair cell. In fact, in most inner hair cells, a single presynaptic density, or 'ribbon', provides the sole synaptic input to a single type I afferent (Nouvian et al., 2006). This uniquely specialized arrangement means that type I afferent

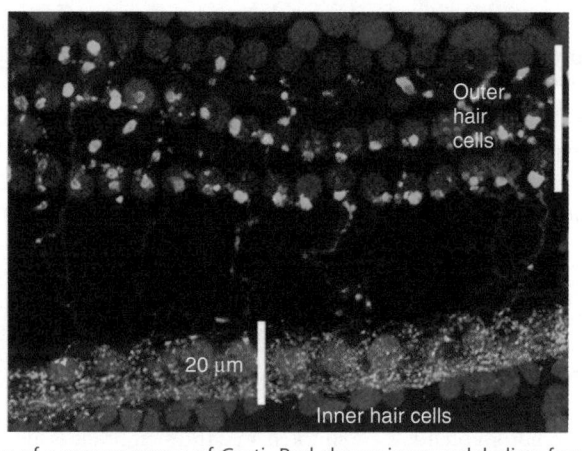

Fig. 1.8 Surface view of a mouse organ of Corti. Red shows immunolabeling for CTBP2 ('ribeye'), a protein found in the nucleus and at ribbon synapses. Green is the immunolabel for synapsin 2, a marker of efferent nerve terminals found on outer hair cells, and on afferent dendrites below inner hair cells. Scale bar: 20 μm.
Micrograph courtesy of S Pyott, University of North Carolina, Wilmington, North Carolina, USA.

signaling reflects the transmission capacities of a single ribbon synapse. This is all the more remarkable when one observes that single ribbons possess a few hundred synaptic vesicles at most, and depend on the gating of a cluster of ~100 voltage-gated calcium channels. Nonetheless, this limited arsenal can support spontaneous activity up to 100 Hz in some SGNs, and encodes the timing and intensity of acoustic signals throughout the lifetime of the organism. To help overcome these limitations, dozens of type I afferents contact a single inner hair cell, providing multiple parallel channels. Hair cell synaptic function is covered in Chapter 9.

There are many fewer type II afferents and these smaller neurons send a dendrite into the region of the outer hair cells, where it turns basally to extend hundreds of micrometers, appearing to contact large numbers of outer hair cells and supporting cells (Perkins & Morest, 1975; Fechner *et al.*, 2001). The functional consequence of this innervation pattern, and indeed the function of type II afferents overall, remains enigmatic since there is essentially no information about their adequate stimulus. The other neuronal contacts of the outer hair cells are better understood. Efferent cholinergic neurons project from somata in the superior olivary complex to synapse on the basal pole of outer hair cells. These larger medial-olivocochlear neurons (MOCs) are distinct from a population of lateral olivocochlear neurons (LOCs) that synapse onto type I afferent neurons beneath inner hair cells in the mature cochlea (Guinan, 2006). Reminiscent of the situation for type I and type II afferents, the larger MOC efferents have revealed important details of their function, while the smaller LOC efferents remain unresolved with respect to function, pharmacology, and activation pattern. Release of acetylcholine (ACh) from MOC efferents causes outer hair cells to hyperpolarize. This effect has several unusual features, among them that the hair cell's ACh receptor (composed of $\alpha9$ and $\alpha10$ subunits) is a ligand-gated cation channel genetically related to nicotinic receptors of nerve and muscle (Chapter 10). Calcium entry through this receptor activates calcium-dependent potassium channels to hyperpolarize and inhibit the hair cell (Fuchs & Murrow, 1992; Glowatzki & Fuchs, 2000; Oliver *et al.*, 2000).

Electrical activation of the MOC efferent axons reduces the amplitude of the compound cochlear action potential evoked by a brief tone burst (Galambos, 1956). Recordings from single type

I SGNs showed that sensitivity is reduced most at the best frequency for that neuron, corresponding to a loss of tuning by the cochlea (Wiederhold & Kiang, 1970). Given that MOC efferents contact outer hair cells, and that type I SGNs innervate inner hair cells, the logical conclusion is that outer hair cells must somehow contribute to the acoustic sensitivity and tuning of inner hair cells and their postsynaptic type I SGNs. We now know that this contribution occurs through the mechanism of electromotility, the ability of outer hair cells to generate mechanical force in response to a change in their membrane potential (Chapter 6). This mechanical contribution from outer hair cells confers high sensitivity, enhanced tuning, and non-linearity to the cochlear vibration pattern (Chapter 5). Although many aspects remain to be detailed, the central core of this hypothesis is well established (Oghalai, 2004). Outer hair cells most definitely can generate movement in response to a voltage signal (the chorus line of 'dancing hair cell' videos on the internet attest to this fact). Thus, it is presumed that sound-evoked receptor potentials drive outer hair cell mechanical output, which enhances the cochlear motion stimulating the inner hair cell. During efferent inhibition, receptor potentials are shunted, and the membrane is hyperpolarized, shifting and diminishing the voltage-to-force relation of the outer hair cell and so reducing this positive feedback. Electromotility is produced by a 'piezoelectric protein' called prestin, a modified organic anion transporter highly expressed in the basolateral membranes of outer hair cells (Zheng *et al.*, 2000). Charge-coupled conformational changes in thousands of prestin molecules sum to alter cellular shape and stiffness. Targeted disruption of the prestin gene causes hearing loss in mice (Cheatham *et al.*, 2004), and a prestin mutation is associated with a form of inherited deafness in humans (Liu *et al.*, 2003).

Remarkably then, the exquisite sensitivity and tuning of the cochlea result in part from the fact that cochlear hair cells themselves can generate movement. A perhaps even more remarkable consequence is that the resulting motion of the cochlear partition produces fluid motions that can propagate backward through the middle ear to be detected in the external ear canal! Such otoacoustic emissions are, in fact, a normal property of the healthy inner ear, and they have become an important diagnostic tool (Chapter 4). 'Ear sounds' can be spontaneous, or evoked by clicks, or as distortion products resulting from the presentation of combination tones. Otoacoustic emissions report on the health of the cochlea (especially the outer hair cells), independent of deficits that may affect signal propagation from inner hair cell to afferent neuron, and further upstream (Kemp, 2002).

1.4 **Development and repair**

The structural and functional complexity of the inner ear inspires one to ask: how does it get this way? What morphogenetic patterns and molecular cues can produce the intricately coiled and differentiated cochlear duct (Chapter 12)? Beyond a desire to understand this process lies the hope of finding cues to trigger the regeneration of sensory hair cells, whose irretrievable loss deafens the mammalian cochlea. Hair cell regeneration does occur in non-mammalian vertebrates, inspiring studies to find the molecular determinants that distinguish these epithelia from those of mammals (Chapter 13).

The inner ear begins as an ectodermal invagination to form the otocyst adjacent to the hindbrain. With limited exceptions, nearly all the sensory cells, supporting cells, and neurons of the inner ear will develop from this apparently featureless hollow sphere. The requisite sequence of induction/specification, proliferation, and differentiation begins in the second embryonic week in rodents, and can continue into postnatal life for some aspects of functional maturation (Kelley, 2007). A succession of extrinsic growth factors and intrinsic transcription factors concatenate to direct the developmental stages (Chapter 12). For example, fibroblast growth factors released from the hindbrain or periotic mesenchyme direct otocyst induction. Anteroposterior and dorsoventral axes of development are influenced by bone morphogenetic proteins (BMPs), whereas auditory epithelial specification is directed in part by *Six1* and sonic hedgehog genes. The coordinated orientation of hair cells within a sensory sheet depends in part on so-called 'planar-cell-polarity' factors (Deans *et al.*, 2007). In some ways the most intriguing questions arise when one considers these later steps of hair cell and supporting cell differentiation. It is here that mammalian and non-mammalian inner ears diverge, since supporting cells in birds, for example, are able to re-differentiate into sensory hair cells after loss (Chapter 13). It is thought that specific transcription factors (Hes1, Hes5) act to prevent hair cell formation by presumptive supporting cells in the mammalian inner ear (Chapter 12) (White *et al.*, 2006).

Even after the cochlea is morphologically complete, development continues as hair cells and associated neurons gradually reach functional maturity. Altricial rodents such as mice and rats respond to sound in the second postnatal week. Even at the day of birth, however, cochlear hair cells can mechanotransduce, and excitation of afferent neurons is quickly established. Days before the onset of hearing, afferent SGNs display 'spontaneous' action potentials that are driven by hair cell transmitter release. These occur at low frequencies (~1 Hz) and are patterned into bursts. Evidence now exists that this behavior is driven by slow oscillations in cochlear supporting cells, exciting hair cells by release of adenosine triphosphate (ATP) (Tritsch *et al.*, 2007). Although they are electrically active, cochlear hair cells at this stage are not yet mature. In particular, they generate calcium action potentials that cease to occur about the onset of hearing. This change from excitable to more 'linear' behavior results from a reduction in the number of voltage-gated calcium channels, and an increase in voltage-gated potassium conductance through the appearance of novel channel types (Kros, 2007). Afferent synaptic transmitter release also becomes more efficient at this same time. Indeed, these coordinate changes in hair cell functionality within a 24-hour period around the onset of hearing suggest that this late maturational stage is as critical as earlier, more visible phases of morphogenesis.

1.5 The genetics of hearing and deafness

As in all aspects of biology and medicine, the genetic revolution has enhanced our understanding of the inner ear, and emphatically changed the way we study it (Chapter 14) (Steel & Kros, 2001). Linkage analysis of inherited hearing loss in isolated human populations has identified proteins involved in ionic homeostasis, intercellular integrity, hair bundle structure, and synaptic transmission, to name but a few (Petit, 2006). Human 'deafness genes' have been incorporated into transgenic mouse models for detailed studies of structure and function (Friedman *et al.*, 2007). Still further insights have arisen from the study of spontaneously arising mutations in mice that affect balance and hearing. At the same time, it is important to recognize that 'hearing loss' is an extremely complex and generic concept. The potential causes range from genetic mutation through environmental toxins, to overuse via loud sound exposure. Furthermore, these all can be interacting partners in pathogenesis. It is likely, for example, that genetic variance, as well as the history of sound exposure contributes to age-related hearing loss – 'presbycusis'. Consequently, presbycusis is being investigated through genome-wide association studies in which a large number of markers (small nucleotide polymorphisms, 'snips') are correlated with hearing status to identify multiple genetic loci (Van Laer *et al.*, 2008).

All these methods are generating an ever-growing list of gene products whose mutation leads to inner ear dysfunction. Some of these mutations produce syndromes in which hearing loss is just one symptom. Usher's syndrome, for example, is characterized by hearing loss and blindness due to retinitis pigmentosa. To date, 11 different genetic loci, including nine identified genes have been associated with variants of Usher's syndrome (Chapter 14). Remarkably, of the known 'Usher proteins' virtually all are involved in some aspect of stereociliary formation or function

(El-Amraoui & Petit, 2005). 'Non-syndromic' hearing loss, as the name implies, has no other (apparent) associated deficits and accounts for the majority of inherited deafness, including more than 100 genetic loci to date. As mentioned above, the range of involved proteins is wide. A striking number of these involve the gap junction protein connexin, attesting to the fundamental importance of epithelial integrity and signaling for inner ear function (Nickel & Forge, 2008). Likewise, numerous mutations of potassium channels are causal to hearing loss in humans or mouse models (Yan & Liu, 2008), as expected from the unique potassium homeostasis of the inner ear, as well as the predominance of potassium conductances in the hair cell's basolateral membranes.

1.6 From fundamentals to therapies

This volume intends to introduce the fundamental mechanisms that underlie the function of the auditory periphery. Of course no such effort can remain tutorial, as this volume aims to be, without leaving out interesting and important topics. These omissions become more obvious when considering the array of problems that are presented to the practicing clinician. For example, one would like also to consider blood flow to the inner ear when concerned with pathogenesis. A survey of some of the clinical problems that confront the otolaryngologist is presented in Chapter 2. The challenge lies in determining the underlying pathogenic mechanisms at a molecular level, with the hope of translating that knowledge into effective therapies. Unfortunately, we have a long way to go in treating almost every aspect of inner ear disease, with hair cell regeneration as perhaps the highest peak in that mountain range of challenges. Thus the enormous benefit provided by cochlear implants more than justifies their expanded utilization and further development (Chapter 15). The extraordinary growth of nanotechnology and tissue engineering promises still further progress in implant utility, and may provide methods for enhanced integration with cochlear nerve fibers, or stimulation within the central nervous system.

Of equal importance to repairing hearing is improved prevention of damage. A variety of necessary drugs from antibiotics to cancer therapeutics are ototoxic (Chapter 2). Obviously, exposure to excessively loud sound also is a major source of inner ear damage. The efforts to avoid any such risks will be better motivated with improved understanding of how the damage occurs, that is, through continued investigation of the fundamental mechanisms of inner ear function described in these chapters. Further, this knowledge of molecular mechanisms will combine with the identification of genetic variations that predispose to some types of cochlear damage (Chapter 14). Consequently, the risk–benefit calculations for ototoxic antibiotics can be sharpened if genetic predispositions to that type of damage are known in advance. Likewise for persuasive recommendations to protect against sound damage – when genetic variants that increase risk are understood, and can inform each individual's choices of occupational and recreational loud sound exposure.

Finally, this volume aims to give every reader a better understanding of the intricate machinery of the auditory periphery. Whether that reader is a student entering the field, a clinical practitioner, or a worker in an allied field of study, the hope is that they will find this volume a resource of basic information, and perhaps a catalyst to make their own contributions to the ongoing challenge, and adventure, of understanding the beautiful mysteries of the ear.

References

Cheatham MA, Huynh KH, Gao J, Zuo J & Dallos P. (2004) Cochlear function in Prestin knockout mice. *J Physiol* **560**: 821–30.

Deans MR, Antic D, Suyama K, Scott MP, Axelrod JD & Goodrich LV. (2007) Asymmetric distribution of prickle-like 2 reveals an early underlying polarization of vestibular sensory epithelia in the inner ear. *J Neurosci* **27**: 3139–47.

El-Amraoui A & Petit C. (2005) Usher I syndrome: unravelling the mechanisms that underlie the cohesion of the growing hair bundle in inner ear sensory cells. *J Cell Sci* **118**: 4593–603.

Farris HE, Wells GB & Ricci AJ. (2006) Steady-state adaptation of mechanotransduction modulates the resting potential of auditory hair cells, providing an assay for endolymph [Ca2+]. *J Neurosci* **26**: 12526–12536.

Fechner FP, Nadol JJ, Burgess BJ & Brown MC. (2001) Innervation of supporting cells in the apical turns of the guinea pig cochlea is from type II afferent fibers. *J Comp Neurol* **429**: 289–98.

Fettiplace R & Hackney CM. (2006) The sensory and motor roles of auditory hair cells. *Nat Rev* **7**: 19–29.

Friedman LM, Dror AA & Avraham KB. (2007) Mouse models to study inner ear development and hereditary hearing loss. *Int J Dev Biol* **51**: 609–31.

Fuchs PA & Murrow BW. (1992) Cholinergic inhibition of short (outer) hair cells of the chick's cochlea. *J Neurosci* **12**: 800–9.

Galambos R. (1956) Suppression of auditory nerve activity by stimulation of efferent fibers to the cochlea. *J Neurophysiol* **19**: 424–37.

Gillespie PG. (2004) Myosin I and adaptation of mechanical transduction by the inner ear. *Philos Trans R Soc Lond* **359**: 1945–51.

Ginzberg RD & Morest DK. (1984) Fine structure of cochlear innervation in the cat. *Hear Res* **14**: 109–27.

Glowatzki E & Fuchs PA. (2000) Cholinergic synaptic inhibition of inner hair cells in the neonatal mammalian cochlea. *Science* **288**: 2366–8.

Guinan JJ Jr. (2006) Olivocochlear efferents: anatomy, physiology, function, and the measurement of efferent effects in humans. *Ear Hear* **27**: 589–607.

Hudspeth AJ. (2008) Making an effort to listen: mechanical amplification in the ear. *Neuron* **59**: 530–45.

Kelley MW. (2007) Cellular commitment and differentiation in the organ of Corti. *Int J Dev Biol* **51**: 571–83.

Kemp DT. (2002) Otoacoustic emissions, their origin in cochlear function, and use. *Br Med Bull* **63**: 223–41.

Kros CJ. (2007) How to build an inner hair cell: challenges for regeneration. *Hear Res* **227**: 3–10.

Liu XZ, Ouyang XM, Xia XJ, Zheng J, Pandya A, Li F, Du LL, Welch KO, Petit C, Smith RJ, Webb BT, Yan D, Arnos KS, Corey D, Dallos P, Nance WE & Chen ZY. (2003) Prestin, a cochlear motor protein, is defective in non-syndromic hearing loss. *Hum Mol Genet* **12**: 1155–62.

Merchant SN, Ravicz ME, Voss SE, Peake WT & Rosowski JJ. (1998) Toynbee Memorial Lecture 1997. Middle ear mechanics in normal, diseased and reconstructed ears. *J Laryngol Otol* **112**: 715–31.

Nickel R & Forge A. (2008) Gap junctions and connexins in the inner ear: their roles in homeostasis and deafness. *Curr Opin Otolaryngol Head Neck Surg* **16**: 452–7.

Nouvian R, Beutner D, Parsons TD & Moser T. (2006) Structure and function of the hair cell ribbon synapse. *J Membr Biol* **209**: 153–65.

Oghalai JS. (2004) The cochlear amplifier: augmentation of the traveling wave within the inner ear. *Curr Opin Otolaryngol Head Neck Surg* **12**: 431–8.

Oliver D, Klocker N, Schuck J, Baukrowitz T, Ruppersberg JP & Fakler B. (2000) Gating of Ca2+-activated K+ channels controls fast inhibitory synaptic transmission at auditory outer hair cells. *Neuron* **26**: 595–601.

Perkins RE & Morest DK. (1975) A study of cochlear innervation patterns in cats and rats with the Golgi method and Nomarkski Optics. *J Comp Neurol* **163**: 129–58.

Petit C. (2006) From deafness genes to hearing mechanisms: harmony and counterpoint. *Trends Mol Med* **12**: 57–64.

Ricci AJ, Kachar B, Gale J & Van Netten SM. (2006) Mechano-electrical transduction: new insights into old ideas. *J Membr Biol* **209**: 71–88.

Steel KP & Kros CJ. (2001) A genetic approach to understanding auditory function. *Nat Genet* **27**: 143–9.

Tritsch NX, Yi E, Gale JE, Glowatzki E & Bergles DE. (2007) The origin of spontaneous activity in the developing auditory system. *Nature* **450**: 50–5.

Van Laer L, Van Eyken E, Fransen E, Huyghe JR, Topsakal V, Hendrickx JJ, Hannula S, Maki-Torkko E, Jensen M, Demeester K, Baur M, Bonaconsa A, Mazzoli M, Espeso A, Verbruggen K, Huyghe J, Huygen P, Kunst S, Manninen M, Konings A, Diaz-Lacava AN, Steffens M, Wienker TF, Pyykko I, Cremers CW, Kremer H, Dhooge I, Stephens D, Orzan E, Pfister M, Bille M, Parving A, Sorri M, Van de Heyning PH & Van Camp G. (2008) The grainyhead like 2 gene (GRHL2), alias TFCP2L3, is associated with age-related hearing impairment. *Hum Mol Genet* 17: 159–69.

Wangemann P. (2006) Supporting sensory transduction: cochlear fluid homeostasis and the endocochlear potential. *J Physiol* 576: 11–21.

White PM, Doetzlhofer A, Lee YS, Groves AK & Segil N. (2006) Mammalian cochlear supporting cells can divide and trans-differentiate into hair cells. *Nature* 441: 984–7.

Wiederhold ML & Kiang NY. (1970) Effects of electric stimulation of the crossed olivocochlear bundle on single auditory-nerve fibers in the cat. *J Acoust Soc Am* 48: 950–65.

Yan D & Liu XZ. (2008) Cochlear molecules and hereditary deafness. *Front Biosci* 13: 4972–83.

Zheng J, Shen W, He DZ, Long KB, Madison LD & Dallos P. (2000) Prestin is the motor protein of cochlear outer hair cells. *Nature* 405: 149–55.

Chapter 2

The clinical cochlea

Lawrence R Lustig

2.1 Introduction

The cochlea is a highly complex, tightly regulated sensory end-organ responsible for the conversion of environmental sound into a meaningful auditory neuronal response. Like all such highly ordered systems, with this complexity comes a vulnerability to many intrinsic and extrinsic phenomena leading to temporary or permanent injury. More simply stated, there are many things that can lead to hearing loss. This chapter will provide a basic foundation of how the clinician approaches the cochlea and the various pathologies that can affect it and lead to hearing loss.

2.2 Clinical hearing assessment

Critical to evaluating cochlear pathology is an accurate measure of the ability to hear. Hearing loss can occur at any stage of the auditory pathway, from the ear canal to the auditory cortex. Although simple otoscopy can identify obvious pathology in the external and middle ear, the ability to determine the cause and nature of hearing loss is often limited by physical exam alone. Thus, subjective and objective measures of hearing have become paramount in the clinical evaluation of the cochlea. With contemporary techniques, it is now possible to evaluate the functional integrity of the entire auditory pathway, from the tympanic membrane to cerebral cortex. Such testing, including tympanometry, pure-tone threshold and speech testing, immitance testing, and auditory brainstem response testing, allow clinicians to characterize and localize the nature of hearing loss in most cases. An additional important electrical measure of auditory function, otoacoustic emissions, also has important and useful clinical applications, and this is discussed separately in another chapter.

2.2.1 Pure-tone audiometry

Pure-tone threshold audiometry, the most fundamental of all diagnostic hearing tests, is a behaviorally based measure of hearing that is used to distinguish between sensorineural (cochlear and central auditory pathways) and conductive (external and middle ear) types of hearing loss, representing a critical clinical distinction. The primary goal of pure-tone testing is to obtain a representation of the softest sound intensities one can hear across the frequency spectrum. These data can then be compared with well-established normative population-based standards to determine the nature and degree of the hearing loss.

To obtain pure-tone thresholds, auditory stimuli are presented in a soundproof chamber to eliminate confounding background noise. In general, air conduction thresholds are obtained to determine actual levels of hearing and bone conduction thresholds are also obtained to determine true cochlear function; differences between these values represent conductive forms of hearing loss, caused by pathological processes impeding sound transduction to the cochlea. With air conduction, stimuli consist of pure tones at octave levels presented most commonly from 25 Hz to

8000 Hz while patients wear either an earphone or headphone. In some special circumstances (e.g. ototoxicity screens), higher frequencies are tested (Gordon *et al.*, 2005). The patient indicates whenever a stimulus is heard, allowing the audiologist to record the softest intensity the patient is able to hear for each frequency. Bone conduction testing is identical, except that instead of headphones, a bone oscillator is placed on the mastoid of the test ear (immediately behind the auricle) and results are recorded at only 500 Hz, 1000 Hz, 2000 Hz, and 4000 Hz (ANSI, 1978). Various methods have been developed for systematic tone presentations, such as the modified Hughson–Westlake technique, allowing an accurate and efficient recording of pure-tone thresholds (Carhart & Jerger, 1959; Beiter & Talley, 1976).

For widespread clinical consistency, the results of an audiological evaluation are commonly plotted on an audiogram, which depicts *frequencies* (represented in Hertz, Hz) on the x-axis and *intensities* (represented in decibels, dB) on the y-axis (Fig. 2.1). This visual representation of an individual's hearing allows a rapid assessment of a pattern of hearing loss and ability to readily compare one audiogram to another, or monitor changes over time. To aid in standardization, graphic representation and symbols were recommended in 1974 by the American Speech and Hearing Association and later revised by the American National Standards Institute (ANSI, 1978). Hearing loss is also commonly described by degree of severity and in relation to the intensity or decibel level of the threshold response (Table 2.1), allowing terms such as 'severe' or 'moderate' hearing loss to have consistent meanings across clinical settings (Goodman, 1965; Clark, 1981).

Another useful recorded value is the pure-tone average (PTA), which is simply the average of threshold responses obtained at 500 Hz, 1000 Hz, and 2000 Hz, key frequencies within the speech range (Fletcher, 1950; Carhart, 1971). This measure provides a rapid way of imparting, in a single number, a basic score of hearing.

2.2.2 Patterns of hearing loss

Hearing loss is grouped under two broad categories: *conductive* and *sensorineural*, determined by comparison of the air and bone conduction threshold results. The difference in thresholds between air and bone conduction is termed the *air–bone gap* and determines the degree of conductive hearing loss. Conductive hearing loss occurs when a pathological process impedes sound transmission to the cochlea. In contrast, a sensorineural hearing loss is due to pathological processes within the cochlea or central auditory pathways. A *mixed* hearing loss results when both air and bone conduction thresholds are elevated in the presence of an air–bone gap. There are some clinical conditions where these classic definitions break down, such as in cochlear otosclerosis, whereby a bony pathology results in a mixed or sensorineural hearing loss (Ramsden *et al.*, 2007).

In addition to the type of hearing loss, there are several classic audiometric configurations that are commonly seen, essentially describing the shape or slope of the pure-tone thresholds (Fig. 2.2). A *downsloping* pattern implies worse high-frequency than low-frequency thresholds, and is commonly seen with such conditions as presbycusis, noise-induced hearing loss, and ototoxicity. A *rising*, or up-sloping, pattern denote poorer thresholds in the low-frequency range, and is commonly seen in such pathologies as sudden sensorineural hearing loss, cochlear hydrops, and Ménière's disease. Flat losses are indicative of equal threshold drops across the frequency range. Lastly, the 'cookie-bite' deformity demonstrates better preservation of low- and high-frequency thresholds with a greater drop in the mid-frequencies. The 'cookie-bite' pattern is a classically seen in patients with congenital forms of hearing loss (Wong & Bance, 2004).

2.2.3 Speech audiometry

While pure-tone thresholds give an indication of the cochlea's ability to detect sounds and at what intensity levels, they do not provide qualitative information regarding sound perception. A common

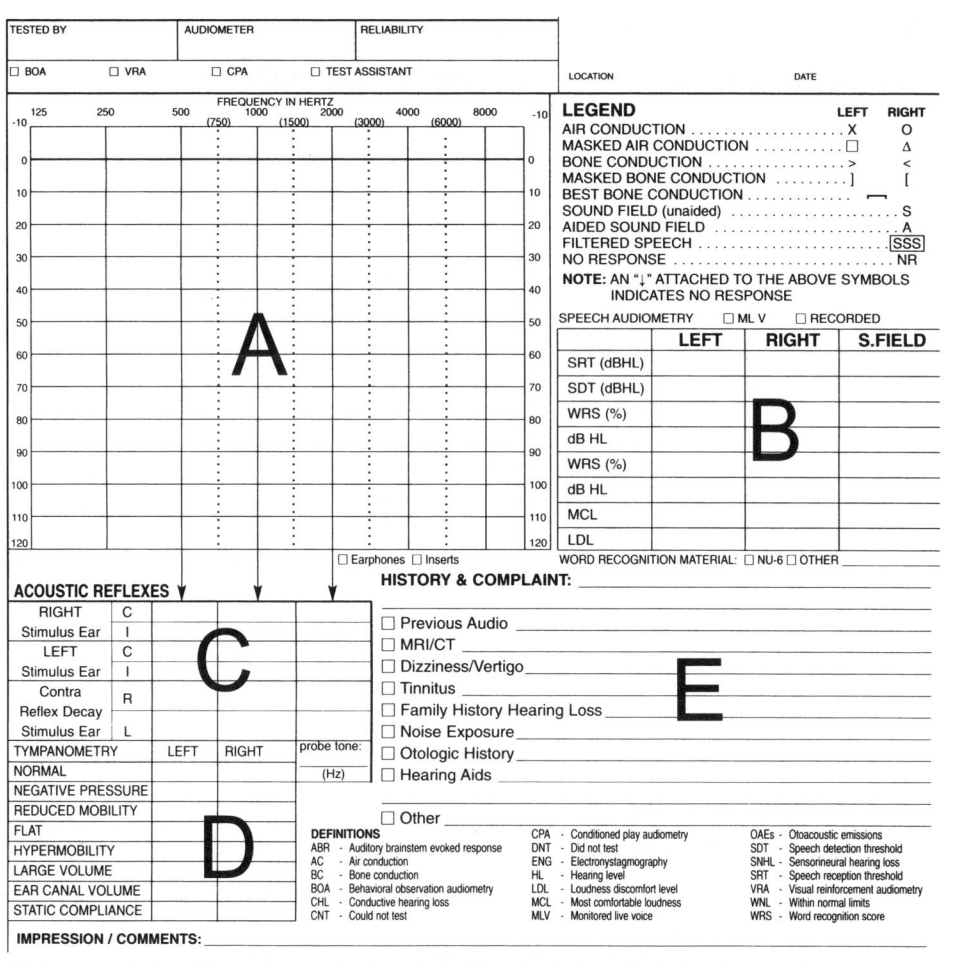

Fig. 2.1 A typical audiometric examination sheet. The single sheet includes the pure-tone audiogram (region 'A'), a standardized measure of hearing based on pure-tone thresholds. Hearing is charted for each frequency, between 250 Hz and 8000 Hz at the lowest intensity (in dB) heard by the listener. Universally accepted symbols to document the pure-tone scores are noted in the upper right corner (marked 'Legend'). Speech and word understanding scores are charted alongside the audiogram (region 'B'). Acoustic reflexes and tympanometry results are documented in regions C and D, respectively. Many examination sheets also contain an area for clinical information ('E'). Commonly used definitions and abbreviations are also commonly included, and here noted in the lower right corner ('Definitions'). By plotting all data on a single sheet, the clinician can rapidly assess a patient's degree of hearing loss and the nature of the hearing loss.

refrain of patients with hearing loss is that, 'I can hear, but I cannot understand…' Speech audiometry provides this additional qualitative hearing assessment, and offering a better view of how a patient with hearing loss is functioning (Penrod, 1994).

The speech reception threshold (SRT) is defined as the softest level at which a patient can repeat a word. Since this measure typically correlates closely with pure-tone thresholds, it is one objective way to determine the accuracy of the pure-tone audiometry results (Penrod, 1994). In this test, words are presented either by live voice or a recording. The presented words are called spondees, two-syllable words with an equal stress on each syllable (e.g. 'baseball'). After the patient is

Table 2.1 Severity of hearing loss by pure-tone threshold*

Average threshold level (db)	Suggested description
−10 to 15	Normal hearing
16 to 25	Slight hearing loss
26 to 40	Mild hearing loss
41 to 55	Moderately severe hearing loss
56 to 70	Severe hearing loss
>71	Profound hearing loss

* Goodman (1965) and Clark (1981).

familiarized with the words at an audible intensity level, the test proceeds as with decreasing intensity level, until the words are no longer audible and a threshold is determined. Differences between the SRT and the PTA (average of pure-tone thresholds at 500 Hz, 1000 Hz, and 2000 Hz) of more than 6 dB might suggest patient malingering or inaccurate measures of either score (Carhart, 1971).

After determining the SRT, the next test is the speech discrimination score (SDS), calculated as the percentage of words a patient can repeat at a comfortable listening level. In contrast to spondees used in SRT, phonemes, phonetically balanced single-syllable words, are used for SDS. The more challenging word list provides additional insight into patient functioning and is perhaps the best prognostic indicator of successful use of hearing aids (Dillon, 1982; Festen & Plomp, 1983).

2.2.4 Immitance testing

Acoustic immitance testing in the most broad sense objectively measures the ease with which sound is transmitted through the tympanic membrane and middle ear. The two principal tests used in immitance measurements are *tympanometry* and the *acoustic reflex*. The objective nature of immitance measures makes it a particularly valuable tool when testing those unable to give accurate responses, such as in infants and toddlers, and the medically infirm.

Tympanometry measures the changes that occur in the tympanic membrane and ossicles as a result of a change in air pressure in the ear canal. The test allows the measure of canal volume as well as peak compliance and middle ear pressure. Canal volume measures are useful for determining obstruction or tympanic membrane perforation. In contrast, peak compliance and middle ear air pressure are used to assess the status of the middle ear. Three widely recognized patterns of middle ear compliance or peak pressure are recognized, types A–C (Fig. 2.3) (Jerger, 1970). A type A tympanogram is characterized by a relatively sharp maximum at or near 0 mm, and is commonly seen in ears with normal middle ear pressure. A subtype of the type A tympanogram, termed As (s indicates 'stiff') can be seen in patients with otosclerosis. The type B tympanogram shows little or no maximum, with a flat peak. Type B tympanograms are typically found in ears with serous otitis media. In the type C tympanogram the maximum is shifted to the left of zero by negative pressure in the middle ear, and is commonly seen in eustachian tube dysfunction (Onusko, 2004).

The stapedius muscle reflex, or acoustic reflex, is another important component of immitance testing, and represents stapedius muscle contraction in response to a loud auditory signal. This reflex is tested with both ipsilateral and contralateral stimulation, and the reflex measured when the stapedial muscle contracts (measured by sensing the altered compliance of the tympanic membrane).

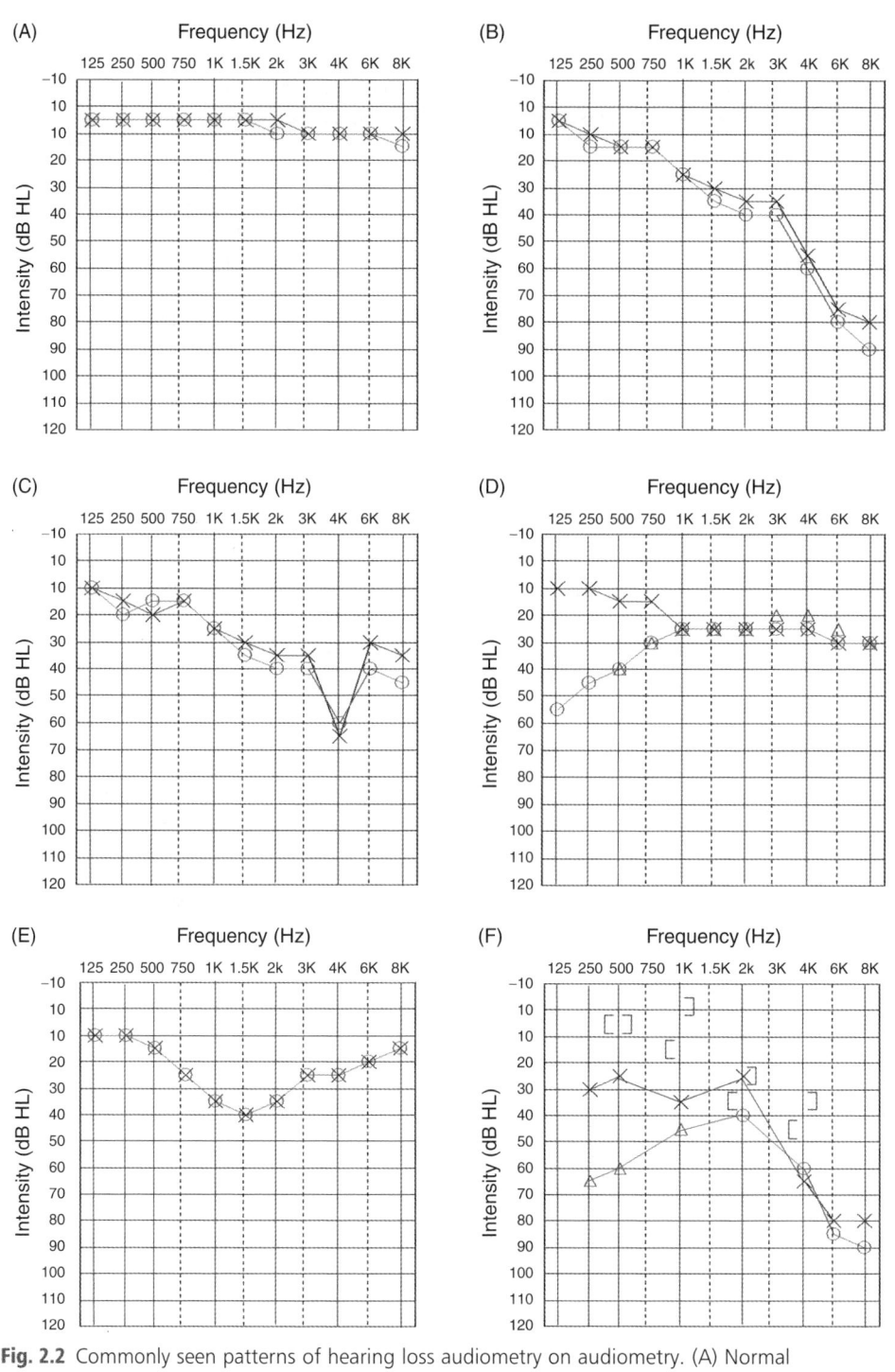

Fig. 2.2 Commonly seen patterns of hearing loss audiometry on audiometry. (A) Normal hearing. With pure-tone air conduction thresholds under 25 db for all frequencies tested, this would be considered hearing within the normal range. By convention, the left ear is represented by an 'X' at each frequency while the right ear is represented by an 'O'. In this case, both the left and right ear hear nearly identically, and thus overlapping patterns are seen.

(continued)

Fig. 2.2 *(Continued)* (B) Downsloping sensorineural hearing loss is the most common pattern of hearing loss seen, and is typically seen in age-related hearing loss. (C) A 'notch' at 4 kHz is commonly seen in cases of noise-induced hearing loss, due to the susceptibility of this range of hearing to noise damage. (D) An up-sloping pattern of hearing loss, here seen in the right ear, is commonly seen in cases of endolymphatic hydrops or sudden sensorineural hearing loss. (E) A 'cookie-bite' deformity is commonly seen in cases of congenital hearing loss, whereby the mid-frequencies demonstrate a greater threshold shift than both the low and high frequencies. (F) An example of 'mixed' hearing loss, that is both sensorineural and conductive hearing losses in the same ear. The bone conduction thresholds are represented by the open boxes while the air conduction thresholds are represented by the standard 'X' and 'O' markings. Differences between the air and bone conduction thresholds represents the air–bone gap and the degree of conductive hearing loss. This patient exhibits a moderate low-frequency conductive hearing loss with a moderate to severe high-frequency sensorineural loss.

The acoustic reflex threshold is the lowest intensity level presented where a change in compliance can be observed. Testing is typically performed at 500 Hz, 1000 Hz, 2000 Hz, and 4000 Hz, with thresholds in the 70–100 dB range. Pathologies that reduce or abolish the acoustic reflex include any form of conductive hearing loss, severe sensorineural hearing loss, or retrocochlear lesions such as tumors of the auditory nerve or pathway (Jerger, 1970). One example in which the acoustic reflex has gained contemporary relevance is the recently described entity of superior semicircular

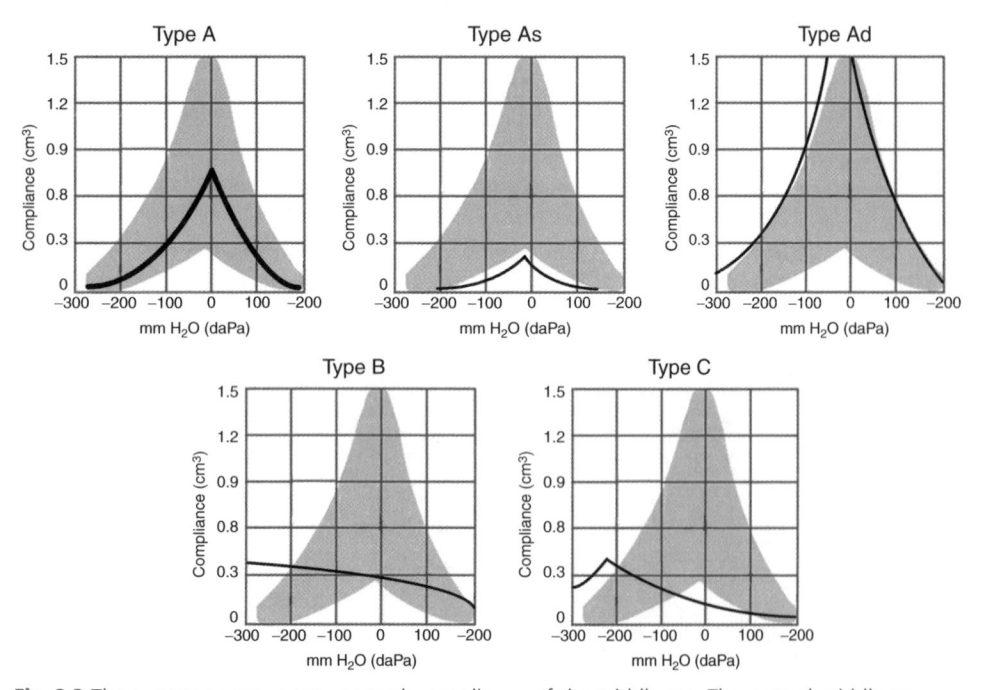

Fig. 2.3 The tympanogram measures peak compliance of the middle ear. The normal middle ear produces a sharp compliance peak at zero pressure (type A). Otosclerosis increases stiffness (reduces compliance), producing the type As tympanogram. Type Ad indicates reduced stiffness associated with atelectasis ('breathlessness'). The flat type B tympanogram is associated with serous otitis media (middle ear infection), while the left-shifted type C response results from negative middle ear pressure and can indicate eustachian-type malfunction.

canal dehiscence (Minor *et al.*, 2003). A common presenting finding in this condition is a conductive hearing loss; however it is not a true conductive hearing loss but likely the presence of a third mobile window from the dehiscence that leads to an *apparent* CHL. The acoustic reflex can thus readily distinguish this entity (with intact responses) versus a true conductive hearing loss (absent acoustic reflex) (Halmagyi *et al.*, 2003; Minor *et al.*, 2003; Merchant *et al.*, 2007).

2.2.5 Acoustic brainstem response testing

Auditory brain response testing (ABR; also referred to by terms such as BAER, brainstem auditory evoked response, or BAEP, brainstem auditory evoked potential) is an important electrical test to measure cochlear and retrocochlear function. The ABR is an averaged surface recording of the sound-activated auditory pathway beginning in the cochlea. The objective nature of this test, independent of a patient's ability to respond, has made it an integral component of auditory testing in newborns, infants and,toddlers, as well any patient who might not be able to respond accurately to pure-tone testing.

   The ABR is measured with surface electrodes on the skull (usually mastoid process and vertex). Clicks or tone-pips are presented while neural electrical potentials are measured. Responses are averaged over large numbers of presentations to eliminate background noise. Normally, the first five positive measured peaks that can be recorded (termed waves I–V) (Fig. 2.4), occurring within a 10 ms timeframe, are used for clinical analysis. Waves I and II are felt to represent synchronized activity with the cochlea and cochlear nerve (Moller *et al.*, 1995). Wave III is believed to be due to activity within the cochlear nucleus, while wave IV represents activation of the superior olivary complex. Wave V is thought to represent activity within the lateral lemniscus of the brainstem

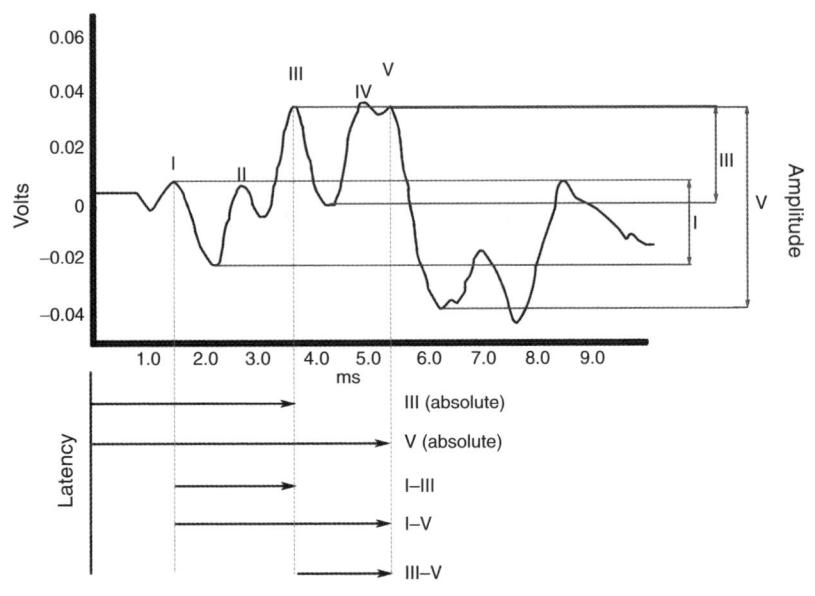

Fig. 2.4 The acoustic brainstem response (ABR) test. Five repeatable waves are present in the normal ABR, waves I–V. Standard measures of ABR include amplitude of waves I, III, and V (demonstrated graphically on the right of the ABR waveform), absolute latency of waves III and V, and latencies between waves I and III, waves I and V, and waves III and V (shown graphically below the waveform).

(Moller *et al.*, 1995). It is wave V that seems to be the most susceptible to hearing loss; wave V latency has been shown to increase with increasing hearing loss, becoming absent in severe cases (Coats, 1978; Bauch & Olsen, 1986). In contrast, wave I tends to be the most stable in sensorineural hearing loss (Galambos & Hecox, 1978; Jerger & Johnson, 1988).

Because of its consistency across patients and its ability to measure the retrocochlear auditory pathways, the ABR has become an important tool in clinical diagnosis. The two principal electrical abnormalities that are analyzed on the ABR are wave amplitude and latency changes (Jewett & Williston, 1971). Changes in peak amplitudes (as measured from the baseline to the wave peak), as well as changes in time interval between the similar contralateral wave (*relative* latency) or beyond accepted normative data (*absolute* latency) may indicate a form of retrocochlear (between the cochlea and auditory cortex) pathology, triggering the need for further evaluation with magnetic resonance imaging (MRI). However, ABR abnormalities are not absolutely indicative of central pathology, since a variety of other factors can influence ABR results (Hood, 1988; Hall, 1992).

Screening newborns and infants for hearing loss is the most common application of ABR testing, which is now universally applied in varying algorithms along with otoacoustic emissions (Kaye *et al.*, 2006). The next most common application of ABR is its use in the diagnosis of vestibular schwannomas, the most common tumor affecting the auditory nerve. ABR has been cited as a highly sensitive (>90%) tool in the identification of tumors of the VIIIth nerve pathway (Eggermont *et al.*, 1980; Musiek, 1982; Josey *et al.*, 1988; Montaguti *et al.*, 2007). The presence of a wave I and absence of waves II–V is the most specific finding for acoustic neuroma, though one must be wary for both false positive (>80%) and false negative (12–18%) results (Weiss *et al.*, 1990; Wilson *et al.*, 1992). With the ubiquity of magnetic resonance imaging and its clearly superior diagnostic capabilities, the utility of ABR has thus been questioned by many clinicians. Since an abnormal ABR warrants further evaluation with an MRI, many have suggested to simply avoid the ABR altogether and obtain an MRI in all cases of concern for retrocochlear lesions (such as with asymmetrical sensorineural hearing loss). The primary rationale for ABR has been its favorable cost-utility as part of the clinical workup for vestibular schwannoma (Chandrasekhar *et al.*, 1995).

2.2.6 Radiographic evaluation of the ear

Computed tomography (CT) and MRI give the clinical an extraordinary ability to localize pathology within the inner ear and auditory pathway. The decision to pursue one or both of these imaging modalities in patients with hearing loss depends on a number of factors, including type of hearing loss (conductive or sensorineural), age, and symmetry of hearing loss.

CT imaging of the temporal bones remains an important clinical tool for evaluating several pathological processes. The strengths of the CT scan include its superior bone detail, and its ability to detect bony erosive processes (e.g. cholesteatoma, tumor), spongiotic changes in the otic capsule (otosclerosis) and congenital abnormalities (e.g. aural atresia, congenital ossicular fixation). High-resolution CT detail is sufficient to evaluate the status of the ossicles and general morphology of the cochlea and vestibular organs (Fig. 2.5). With the addition of contrast, CT can also identify some inflammatory processes within the inner ear and mastoid, as well as tumors of the facial or auditory nerves as small as 5 mm (Jackler & Dillon, 1988). However, CT is inferior to MRI at identifying soft tissue lesions such as tumors of the ear or brainstem. It remains useful for these purposes, however, in cases where an implanted device would contraindicate the use of MRI, or when someone cannot physically sit still for the 30-minute exam because of such issues as anxiety or claustrophobia.

MRI is one of the most important modalities clinicians have to evaluate otological and retrocochlear pathology (Fig. 2.6). The image itself, in contrast to an x-ray-based modality such as CT, is

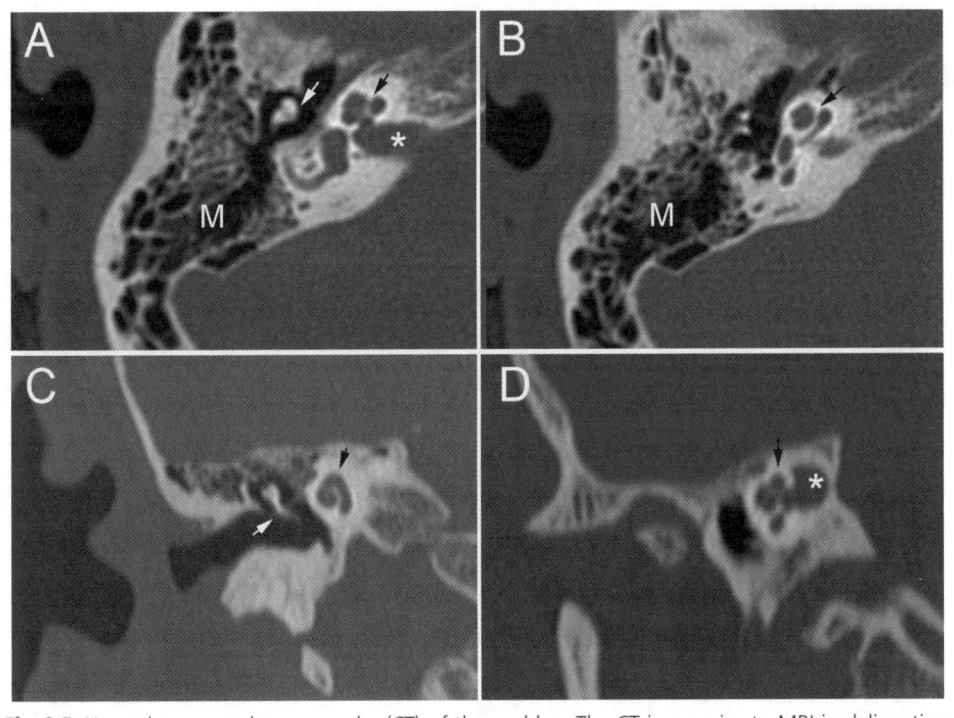

Fig. 2.5 Normal computed tomography (CT) of the cochlea. The CT is superior to MRI in delineating the anatomy of the temporal bone. There are two axial (A, B), a coronal (C), and an oblique (D) view. In these images, the cochlea (black arrows) can be seen, including the basal, mid, and apical turns. The ossicles can also be visualized (white arrows), as can the internal auditory canal (*). The mastoid air cell system (M) is also clearly visualized by CT imaging.

based on mobile proton density and the time required for proton reorientation within a magnetic field. Varying degrees of water content and vascularity thus account for differences in signal (Jackler & Dillon, 1988). As a result, bony structures do not produce a signal on MRI, limiting its usefulness within the temporal bone where most clinically relevant structures are osseous. However, due to its superior detail of all soft tissue structures, MRI with contrast material such as gadolinium-DTA is clearly superior than CT in identifying inflammatory processes (e.g. labyrinthitis) or neoplasms (e.g. vestibular schwannoma) within the temporal bone or along the central auditory pathways (Fig. 2.7) (Jackler & Dillon, 1988). Newer imaging modalities and stronger magnets have also led to improving resolution of the cochlea itself. Most contemporary scanners can adequately visualize the turns of the cochlea, the presence of fluid within the cochlea, and the presence or absence of the auditory nerve. These improvements have made MRI an invaluable tool in the evaluation of patients with severe to profound hearing for the suitability of cochlear implantation (Papsin, 2005; Trimble *et al.*, 2007).

2.3 Clinical disorders of the cochlea

2.3.1 The epidemiology of sensorineural hearing loss

Hearing loss is widely recognized as one of the most common disorders experienced by humans. Estimates of the prevalence of hearing loss are fraught with inaccuracies for a number of reasons

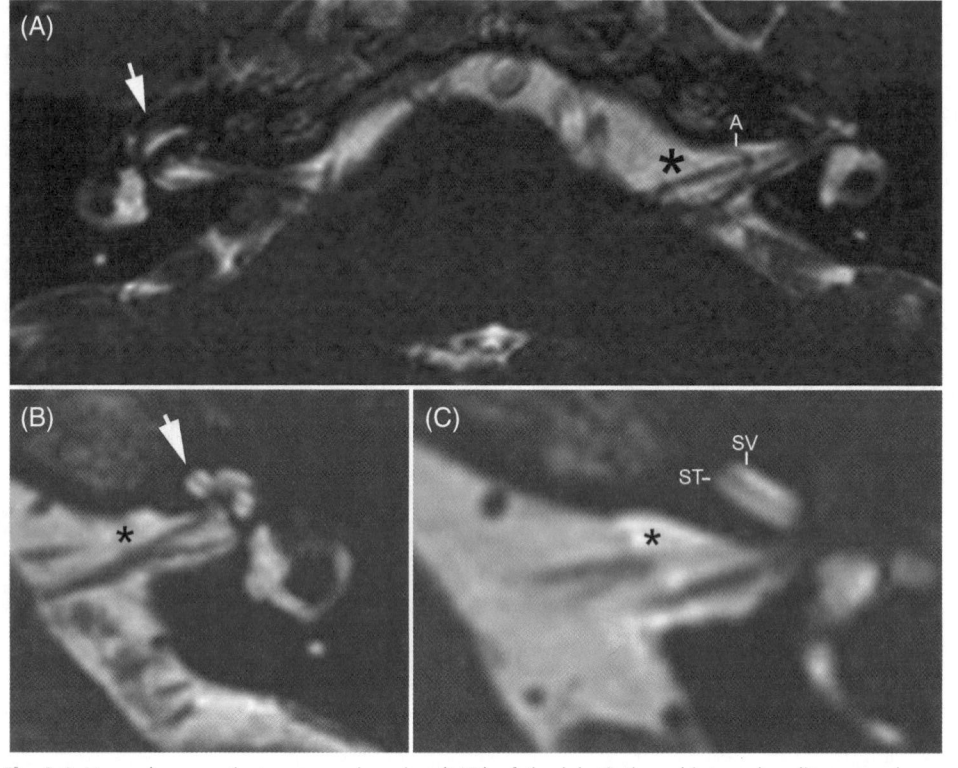

Fig. 2.6 Normal magnetic resonance imaging (MRI) of the labyrinth and internal auditory canal. Images such as these, using a three-dimensional Fiesta protocol, highlight fluid-filled structures such as the cochlea, while bone generates no signal (black). In this image, there is a view of the basal (A, arrow) and mid and apical (B, white arrow) regions of the fluid-filled cochlear scalae. The left cochleovestibular and facial nerves traveling within the internal auditory canal (IAC) can be seen in relief against the cerebrospinal fluid (*), along with a loop of the anterior inferior cerebellar artery ('A' in (A)) coursing through the IAC. In part (B), one can differentiate between the scala tympani (ST) and scala vestibule (SV) within the basal turn of the cochlea.

however, including patient denial of a hearing loss and the difficulty of getting population-based audiometric data on a sufficient scale (Gates *et al.*, 1990). There is also a wide variability in hearing loss across different populations, varying by socioeconomic status (for example noise exposure in factory workers), making generalizations difficult (Davis *et al.*, 1992).

Universal newborn infant hearing screening has facilitated data collection in this population, providing better estimates than in adults. Data indicate that congenital or prelingual severe to profound losses occur in approximately 0.5–3/1000 livebirths (Fortnum *et al.*, 1995; Riko *et al.*, 1985; Prager *et al.*, 1987; Augustsson *et al.*, 1990; Morgan & Canalis, 1991; Smith *et al.*, 1992). In an older pediatric population of 3–10-year olds, estimates of serious hearing impairment was 1.1 cases per 1000 children, with 90% of cases being sensorineural (Van Naarden *et al.*, 1999; Wake *et al.*, 2006). Data suggest that prevalence rates are higher in boys than girls (1.23 vs. 0.95/1000 individuals) (Van Naarden *et al.*, 1999). Factors that increase the risk for congenital or delayed-onset sensorineural hearing loss include a family history of hearing loss, congenital or central nervous system infections, ototoxic drug exposure, congenital deformities involving the head and

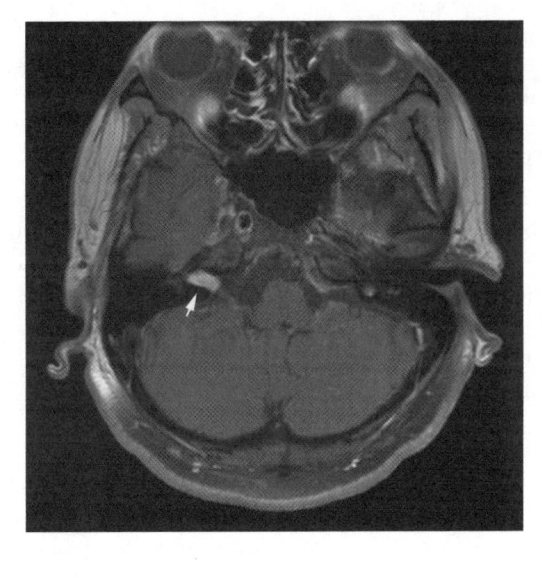

Fig. 2.7 Vestibular Schwannoma. Various retrocochlear pathologies can present with asymmetrical sensorineural hearing loss. In most such cases, an MRI can definitively diagnose such a disorder. In this case, a patient with a right-sided sensorineural hearing loss underwent an MRI with contrast dye enhancement (Gadolinium), leading to a diagnosis of a vestibular schwannoma located within the internal auditory canal (arrow).

neck, birth trauma, minority ethnicity, lower socioeconomic status, and other conditions often related to prematurity that prompt admission to an intensive care nursery (Davis *et al.*, 1992).

Hearing loss in adults is widespread, being the third-most self-reported health problem in individuals over the age of 65 (arthritis and high blood pressure being first and second, respectively) (Havlik, 1986). New-onset hearing loss in patients between adolescence and their fifties is predominantly due to pathological disorders such as loud noise exposure, trauma, otosclerosis, Ménière's disease, ototoxicity, idiopathic sudden sensorineural loss, and tumors (predominantly vestibular schwannomas). Noise exposure appears to be one of the most common causes of sensorineural hearing loss in this age group, predominantly due to occupational exposure to hazardous noise levels in such fields as farming, trucking, and heavy industry (Department of Labor, 1981; Green, 2002; Mrena *et al.*, 2007). Farming, trucking, and heavy industry are also the most common ear-damaging vocations. Most of the workers in these professions are men. This observation helps to explain why men of working age constitute the fastest growing population of hearing-impaired individuals.

After 50, however, the prevalence of hearing loss accelerates dramatically, with age-related hearing loss and presbycusis contributing the most to this increase. Approximately 25% of patients between ages 51 and 65 years have hearing thresholds greater than 30 dB (normal range being 0–20 dB) in at least one ear (Davis *et al.*, 1992). Patients in this age group cannot be relied on for accurate self-reported diagnosis of hearing loss, whereas about a third of people over 65 and half of those over 85 will admit to a hearing loss; rigorous audiometric screening would identify an additional 15% of individuals with marked hearing loss in these age groups (Havlik, 1986; Gates *et al.*, 1990; Mulrow & Lichtenstein, 1991).

A 1996 population study by the National Institutes of Health (NIH) identified over 28 million Americans who are deaf or hearing impaired (NIH Consensus Statement Online 1990). Additional studies have demonstrated a greater than 50% increase in the number of patients with hearing loss between 1971 and 1991 (Dobie, 1993). As our population continues to age, these rates of incidence and prevalence of hearing loss will also continue to grow, with estimates as high as 14% (Department of Labor, 1981; Dobie *et al.*, 1989; Dobie, 1993).

Combining these data, one can estimate that approximately one in ten Americans has a signifi-cant enough impairment to have a deficit in hearing conversational speech, and one in 100 have a loss severe enough to prevent the use of conventional hearing aids.

2.3.2 Ototoxicity and drug-induced hearing loss

Modern medicines have greatly added to our overall quality of life, longevity, and ability to posi-tively affect the course of numerous diseases. The 'flipside' to this benefit, however, is the potential side effects and complications inherent in nearly all drugs. Ototoxicity refers to the ability of a drug or substance to damage the inner ear, causing a functional impairment such as tinnitus, or loss of hearing or balance. Currently several classes of drug are known to cause ototoxicity: salicylates, aminoglycoside antibiotics, macrolide antibiotics, vancomycin, loop diuretics, and certain classes of chemotherapeutic agents (Box 2.1).

Salicylates

Salicylates such as acetylsalicylic acid (ASA), more commonly referred to as aspirin, are some of the earliest known ototoxic agents. In high doses, ASA can cause sensorineural hearing loss, tin-nitus, and vertigo. In fact, it was precisely these side effects that were instrumental in determining appropriate dosages of ASA for rheumatic fever and gout in the beginning of the twentieth cen-tury (Myers & Bernstein, 1965; Marchese-Ragona et al., 2007). While early studies showed that serum ASA concentrations of 20–50 mg/dL result in hearing losses of up to 30 dB, concentrations as low as 11 mg/dL have also been shown to be ototoxic in some individuals, with reversible tin-nitus occurring at dosages much lower than this (Day et al., 1989). Clinically, patients with oto-toxicity due to salicylates will experience 'supra-threshold' changes in hearing such as decreased temporal integration and resolution and impaired frequency selectivity (Boettcher & Salvi, 1991). These changes are generally reversible within 72 hours of drug cessation, however.

The exact mechanism of salicylate ototoxicity remains in questions. Some theories of ASA-induced ototoxicity include altered levels of prostaglandins (Jung et al., 1988), inhibition of ace-tylcholinesterase activity of the efferent nerve endings in the organ of Corti (Ishii et al., 1967), alterations in adenosine triphosphate levels in Reissner's membrane (Krzanowski & Matschinsky, 1971), and alterations in some transaminase and dehydrogenase systems (Silverstein et al., 1967). The exact anatomical portion of the inner that is effected by salicylates also remains in question. To date, histological studies have shown that the stria vascularis, organ of Corti (including hair cells), and cochlear blood vessels all appear normal in animal models subjected to high doses of salicylates (Deer & Hunter-Duvar, 1982).

Physiologic studies of salicylate-induced effects on hearing have shown that the drug mimics the effects of efferent neuronal stimulation. By studying endocochlear potentials after high-dose ASA administration in adult cats, it has been shown that the compound action potential and summating potential were reduced, the endocochlear potential was unaffected, and the cochlear microphonic was increased (Stypulowski, 1990). It is inferred from these studies that salicylates may cause tinnitus by its direct effect on outer hair cells (controlled by the efferent neuronal pathways) and by selectively sparing the inner hair cells (afferent neuronal pathway). Other physiological studies have implicated alterations in cochlear blood flow as a potential mechanism of salicylate-induced ototoxicity (Cazals et al., 1988). Interestingly, salicylates, perhaps through their antioxidant properties, provides some degree of protection against cisplatin ototoxicity (Hyppolito et al., 2006).

Aminoglycosides

Because of the frequency of use, aminoglycosides are probably one of the most common causes of drug-induced ototoxicity. Because this class of antibiotics continues to remain highly effective

Box 2.1 Drugs with reported ototoxic and vestibulotoxic potential

Antibiotics
- ◆ Aminoglycosides
  - Amikacin
  - Dibekacin
  - Gentamicin
  - Kanamycin
  - Neomycin
  - Netilmicin
  - Sisomicin
  - Streptomycin
  - Tobramycin
- ◆ Macrolides
  - Erythromycin
  - Clarithromycin
  - Azithromycin
  - Vancomycin

Loop diuretics
- ◆ Azosemide
- ◆ Bumetanide
- ◆ Ethacrynic acid
- ◆ Furosemide
- ◆ Indapamide
- ◆ Piretanide
- ◆ Triflocin

Salicylates
- ◆ Acetylsalicylic acid (aspirin)

Quinine

Antineoplastic drugs

Platinum compounds
- ◆ Cisplatin
- ◆ Carboplatin

Difluoromethylornithine (DFMO)

against infection by Gram-negative bacteria, knowledge about the presenting features of aminoglycoside ototoxicity is extremely important.

Aminoglycosides act by inhibition of bacterial ribosomal protein synthesis. Drugs within this class include streptomycin, neomycin, kanamycin, gentamicin, amikacin, tobramycin, netilmicin, dibekacin, and sisomicin. Of these, the most commonly used today in a form (intravenous) and dosage that may cause ototoxicity are gentamicin and tobramycin. Neomycin, used commonly in topical antibiotic ointments and oral bowel preparations, rarely achieves sufficient serum blood levels via these routes that would induce inner ear injury. The prevalence of ototoxicity differs for each antibiotic, although it ranges from 2% to 15% (Kahlmeter & Kahlager, 1984; Matz, 1993). An interesting feature of this class of drugs is that some tend to preferentially injure the balance organs (vestibulotoxic – streptomycin, gentamicin, and tobramycin), while others tend to have their most damaging effects on the organ of Corti (ototoxic – neomycin, kanamycin, amikacin, sisomicin). Both subclasses of medications, however, are able to injure either organ with a high enough dosage.

The mechanism of aminoglycoside-induced ototoxicity has been thoroughly studied, although many important details remain to be worked out (Williams *et al.*, 1987; Rizzi & Hirose, 2007). Initially, the antibiotic enters the apical region of the hair cell, likely via receptor-mediated endocytosis (Hashino & Shero, 1995). Because of the highly polar biochemical nature of antibiotics, the drug must be actively transported into the cell in an energy-dependent manner, partially dependent on the structural protein myosin VIIa (Richardson *et al.*, 1999). Within the hair cell, after being initially incorporated into lysosomes, the antibiotic will then lead to apoptosis via a mechanism that still remains to be worked out (Rizzi & Hirose, 2007). Studies of patients with genetic mitochondrial disorders and aminoglycoside ototoxic sensitivity has also shed light on its potential mechanism of inner ear injury (Fischel-Ghodsian, 1999). Studies have shown that aminoglycosides may exert their detrimental effect through an alteration of mitochondrial protein synthesis. This exacerbates the inherent defect caused by the mutation, reducing the overall mitochondrial translation rate down to and below the minimal level required for normal cellular function (Guan *et al.*, 2000).

As only approximately 3% of an orally administered dose of an aminoglycoside is absorbed through the gastrointestinal tract, the preferred route of delivery for infections is intravenous. The half-life of the drug ranges from 3 to 15 hours under normal circumstances, but factors such as kidney disease can markedly alter the half life (Lerner & Matz, 1980). As a result, whenever administering these drugs, serum peak and trough levels need to be monitored. However, the impact of an altered half-life or increased serum concentrations on the ototoxic potential is unclear. Although aminoglycosides are clearly ototoxic, a variety of studies have not shown a direct correlation between its ototoxicity and concentrations of the drug in serum or cochlear fluids (Lerner & Matz, 1980; Kahlmeter & Kahlager, 1984; Tran Ba Huy *et al.*, 1986; Henley & Schacht, 1988; Huang & Schacht, 1988; Matz, 1993). A consistent feature of aminoglycoside ototoxicity is the delayed onset between drug administration and onset of the hearing loss (Beaubien *et al.*, 1990). This may be in part explained by the finding that a cytotoxic metabolite of the drug has been shown to cause death in hair cells (Huang & Schacht, 1988).

The histopathology of aminoglycoside-induced ototoxicity has been well documented. Gentamicin, tobramycin, and streptomycin preferentially act on the balance organs, though in higher dosages, they will also injure the organ of Corti. These drugs have a predilection for type I hair cells of the crista ampullaris, though later stages may also see destruction of type II hair cells. Similarly, those drugs preferentially acting upon the organ of Corti (neomycin, kanamycin, amikacin) will selectively injure outer hair cells, while sparing inner hair cells. Further, outer hair cells at the base appear to more susceptible than those at the apex. Inner hair cells are not completely spared and have been shown to be injured in several animal studies, along with other supporting structures (Hawkins & Engstrom, 1964; Hawkins, 1976; Rybak & Matz, 1986). Long-term effects of aminoglycoside ototoxicity include delayed secondary degeneration of spiral ganglion neurons (Kiang *et al.*, 1976). While most of these findings have been shown in animal models, similar changes have been seen in human temporal bone specimens.

The clinical effects of aminoglycoside ototoxicity are variable. As previously stated, although drug levels of antibiotic do not clearly correlate with ototoxicity, patients with renal insufficiency are more susceptible. Initial auditory effects of ototoxicity are tinnitus and high-frequency sensorineural hearing loss. The lower frequencies become involved as the ototoxicity progresses. Because most audiograms will only test for hearing up through 8 kHz, if ototoxicity is suspected, special equipment or testing procedures at ultra-high-frequencies may be required to detect early damage induced by the suspected antibiotic. Early identification of aminoglycoside ototoxicity is important, since stopping the antibiotic might halt further sensorineural hearing loss, though hearing loss can progress even after withdrawal of the medication (Lerner & Matz, 1980). Though the hearing loss sustained is sometimes partially reversible, once a loss has been present for three weeks, it is likely permanent (Rybak & Matz, 1986).

Vestibulotoxicity is common with the antibiotics gentamicin and streptomycin. For reasons that are not entirely known, these drugs preferentially act upon vestibular hair cells, and only in more advanced cases will the organ of Corti become involved. As in the cochlea, the obvious histological deficit is loss of vestibular hair cells in the utricle, saccule, and semicircular canal ampullae (Koegel, 1985). Clinically, patients with vestibulotoxicity will experience vertigo, dysequilibrium, and oscillopsia. While in some cases the injury resulting from vestibulotoxicity can be compensated for, more often bilateral vestibular hypofunction as a result of aminoglyco-side ototoxicity can be partially or completely disabling. As an aside, the vestibulotoxic potential of gentamicin is used *advantageously* to treat Ménière's disease by inducing a 'chemical laby-rinthectomy' through transtympanic application of the antibiotic (Nedzelski *et al.*, 1992).

Frequent assessment of vestibular function in patients undergoing intravenous gentamicin therapy is important to identify early vestibulotoxicity. The head thrust maneuver, a useful bedside clinical test that can accurately pick up early vestibulotoxicity, employs brief, high-acceleration horizontal head thrusts applied while instructing the patient to look carefully at the examiner's nose (Brock *et al.*, 1991; Halmagyi *et al.*, 1997; Goebel, 2001; Halmagyi *et al.*, 2005). Damage to the vestibular-ocular reflex from aminoglycoside vestibulotoxicity will manifest as catch-up saccades of the patient's eyes as they try to maintain a fixed eye position during the rapid head rotation. Another useful test of vestibulotoxicity involves dynamic visual acuity testing. In this test, the results of a Snellen eye chart exam (with both eyes open) are compared with the exam while the patient's head is undergoing back and forth head turns (Herdman *et al.*, 2007). If there is sufficient damage to the vestibulo-ocular reflex as a result of vestibulotoxicity, there will be a degradation of at least two lines on the eye exam. These highly sensitive tests can be an extremely useful part of the clinical armamentarium of physicians who administer aminogly-coside antibiotics.

As a result of these potentially serious complications resulting from oto- and vestibulotoxicity, predisposing factors to their development have been sought. Duration of therapy more than ten days, decreased pure-tone sensitivity, the presence of a severe underlying illness, a high total dose of drug, and high drug peak and trough levels have all been associated with an increased risk of ototoxicity (Jackson & Arcieri, 1971; Brummett & Fox, 1989). Thus despite no clear correlation with serum levels of antibiotic, clinicians and pharmacists are strongly encouraged to closely monitor aminoglycoside peak and trough levels. Additionally, the patient's underlying renal con-dition needs to be taken into account by factoring in the creatinine clearance and adjusting the dosage appropriately.

As with most disorders, the best treatment of ototoxicity is prevention. A variety of compounds are currently being evaluated for the ability to ameliorate the effects of gentamicin-induced oto-toxicity. To date, antioxidants have shown the greatest promise. Salicylates (aspirin), vitamin E, *N*-acetylcysteine, desferrioxamine, oleandrin, and minocycline, are a few of the compounds that have been tried (Wei *et al.*, 2005; Chen *et al.*, 2007a; Emanuele *et al.*, 2007; Kharkheli *et al.*, 2007; Mostafa *et al.*, 2007; Saxena, 2007).

Macrolide antibiotics

Macrolide antibiotics, most notably erythromycin, have been reported to be ototoxic. Though not nearly as common as aminoglycoside-induced ototoxicity, high-dose erythromycin (oral and intravenous) has been reported to be associated with high-frequency sensorineural hearing loss in at least 35 cases (Schweitzer & Olson, 1984; Brummett & Fox, 1989). The newer macrolides, including azithromycin and clarithromycin, also have been reported to cause ototoxicity (Wallace *et al.*, 1994; Bizjak *et al.*, 1999). Those most susceptible include elderly individuals with liver or kidney disease. There also appears to be an association with legionnaire disease, most likely because the treatment for this disorder is high-dose erythromycin. Patients with erythromycin ototoxicity may also have central nervous system findings, including diplopia, dysarthria, and psychiatric alterations. Fortunately, in most cases, the ototoxicity and associated central findings are reversible once the drug is stopped. Guidelines for the prevention of erythromycin-induced ototoxicity have been put forth by Schweitzer and Olson. These include a maximum daily dosage of 1.5 g if there is associated elevation in the serum creatinine above 180 mol/L, pre- and post-treatment audiograms in all elderly patients with kidney and liver disease, and the exercise of great caution when administered along with other drugs with known ototoxic potential.

Vancomycin

The ototoxic potential of vancomycin, a powerful antibiotic used to treat aggressive staphylococcus infections such as methicillin-resistant *Staphylococcus aureus* (MRSA), is controversial (Brummett & Fox, 1989; Brummett, 1993; Klibanov *et al.*, 2003). One problem in evaluating its ototoxic potential is that nearly all of the patients who have been reported to have hearing problems following vancomycin therapy have also been given an aminoglycoside during the course of treatment. Further, animal studies have failed to demonstrate the ototoxic potential of vancomycin when given alone, while co-administration with gentamicin does cause increased inner ear damage as compared with aminoglycosides alone (Brummett *et al.*, 1990). Lastly, a newborn hearing loss study in 2003 showed no association of vancomycin with sensorineural hearing loss (de Hoog *et al.*, 2003). Thus the data for vancomycin as a sole causative agent of ototoxicity are not strong. However, vancomycin may augment the ototoxic potential of aminoglycosides, though the precise mechanism for this potentiation is not clear.

Loop diuretics

The loop diuretics are a family of drugs used for the treatment of kidney disease. These include the drugs azosemide, bumetanide, ethacrynic acid, furosemide, indacrinone, piretanide, and torasemide. Of these, by far the most commonly used is furosemide, also known by its trade name Lasix, while ethacrynic acid is rarely used. They are named loop diuretics because they act on the loop of Henle in the kidney to inhibit the reabsorption of sodium and chloride. This allows water to osmotically follow the salts as they are excreted, leading to diuresis. Ethacrynic acid is a more potent inhibitor of the ion transport than furosemide. With a half-life of approximately 30 minutes, furosemide is entirely eliminated by the kidney. Thus, individuals with renal insufficiency may have a markedly prolonged drug half-life in serum, increasing its ototoxic potential.

The precise mechanism of ototoxicity for loop diuretics has not been completely elucidated, though a variety of studies have implicated the stria vascularis of the inner ear as the principal site of injury (Bates *et al.*, 2002; de Hoog *et al.*, 2003; Shine & Coates, 2005).The loop diuretics are direct inhibitors of the $Na^{(+)}$-$K^{(+)}$- $2Cl^-$ co-transport system, that also exists in the marginal and dark cells of the stria vascularis and is responsible for endolymph secretion (Marks & Schacht, 1983; Humes, 1999). This similarity may also explain the link between agents with known ototoxicity and nephrotoxicity. In rodents, furosemide has been shown to inhibit several enzymatic pathways important for ion transport, one of the primary presumed functions of the stria vascularis (Rybak, 1982). This site of action has been bolstered by several histopathological studies as well, demonstrating a variety of degenerative changes in the stria vascularis following high-dose loop diuretic administration (Arnold *et al.*, 1981; Rybak, 1982). Some less severe alterations have also been observed in the outer hair cells in the basal turn of the cochlea, but no injury has been identified in the cochlear nerve or spiral ganglion cells (Quick & Duvall, 1970). Within the balance organs, hair cells have shown mitochondrial abnormalities and increased granularity (Arnold *et al.*, 1981).

Clinically, ototoxicity induced by loop diuretics may be transient or irreversible. Further, hearing loss has been seen with both oral and intravenous dosages of the drugs. Fortunately, transient hearing loss appears to be more common, with hearing recovery taking place within two days of stopping the medication (Arnold *et al.*, 1981). There are, however, clearly cases of irreversible hearing loss with loop diuretics (Rybak, 1982). The infusion of loop diuretics has also been shown to suppress otoacoustic emissions and affect frequency selectivity (Martin *et al.*, 1998). Rapid intravenous infusion of furosemide has been shown to increase the risk of the development of ototoxicity (Bosher, 1979) Other risk factors include administering the drug in those with renal insufficiency or premature infants (Gallagher & Jones, 1979; Bates *et al.*, 2002; Shine & Coates, 2005).

Platinum chemotherapeutic compounds

Cisplatin (*cis*-diamminedichloroplatinum II) and carboplatin (*cis*-diammin-1, 1-cyclobutane decarboxylate platinum II) are potent antineoplastic drugs that have been used to successfully treat a variety of malignancies. An unfortunate side effect of these potentially life-saving medications, however, is ototoxicity in approximately 7% of recipients. The hearing loss is generally high-frequency (>4000 Hz), bilateral, permanent, and accompanied by tinnitus (Schweitzer, 1993). The inner ear injury from platinum compounds is generally more severe in children, and has been reported as high as 82% in those undergoing autologous bone marrow transplantation (Brock *et al.*, 1991; Parsons *et al.*, 1998). Other risk factors for cisplatin ototoxicity include high cumulative dose of cisplatin, a history of noise exposure, a concomitant high doses of vincristine, another chemotherapeutic agent, and decreased serum albumin level, hemoglobin level, red blood cell count, and hematocrit (Blakley *et al.*, 1994; Bokemeyer *et al.*, 1998; Chen *et al.*, 2006). There also appears to be a genetic predisposition to cisplatin-induced ototoxicity (Huang *et al.*, 2007; Rybak, 2007). Patients undergoing cisplatin or carboplatin therapy therefore require audiometry prior to the onset of therapy, and at any suggestion of hearing loss or tinnitus.

It has been postulated that a possible mechanism of cisplatin ototoxicity is through the production of reactive oxygen species, which in turn leads to hair cell apoptosis. Inhibition of adenylate cyclase is one of the cellular effects that has been implicated (Bagger-Sjoback *et al.*, 1980). Cisplatin has also been shown to cause a rise in perilymph prostaglandins (Rybak & Matz, 1986). Other studies have concluded that blockage of outer hair cell ion transduction channels is responsible for the ototoxicity (McAlpine & Johnstone, 1990). Lastly, recent studies have implicated the inflammatory cytokines tumor necrosis factor-alpha (TNF-α) and interleukin-1-beta (IL-1β) and IL-6β (So *et al.*, 2007).

The histopathological changes in the inner ear as a result of cisplatin ototoxicity have been well described (Hinojosa *et al.*, 1995). These include loss of inner and outer hair cells in the basal turn of the cochlea, degeneration of the stria vascularis, and a considerable decrease in spiral ganglion cells, predominantly in the upper turns.

There has been some success in limiting the ototoxic potential of platinum agents by co-administration of a variety of compounds, including antioxidants, caspase inhibitors, and inhibitors of apoptosis (Rybak, 2007). There has also been some success using sulfur- or sulfhydryl-containing compounds (thio compounds), which are thought to provide protection from cisplatin toxicity either by direct interaction between the cisplatin and the thio moiety, by displacing platinum from its site of toxic action, by preventing platinum from interfering with superoxide dismutase, or by scavenging of cisplatin-induced free radicals (Smoorenburg *et al.*, 1999).

DFMO

DFMO is an irreversible inhibitor of ornithine decarboxylase (ODC), the essential enzyme in mammalian polyamine biosynthesis, and is another chemotherapeutic agent with considerable ototoxic potential (Pasic *et al.*, 1997; McWilliams *et al.*, 2000; Lao *et al.*, 2004). DFMO has the potential to cause a *reversible*, dose-dependent vertigo-like syndrome and hearing loss (Meyskens & Gerner, 1995; Pasic *et al.*, 1997). In rare cases, a permanent hearing loss has been reported with its use (Lao *et al.*, 2004). A history of prior hearing loss appears to increase the ototoxic susceptibility of DFMO (Croghan *et al.*, 1991). Histological studies in animal models has shown that both outer and inner hair cells in the cochlea are damaged by DFMO exposure, with inner more affected than outer hair cells, particularly in the basal turn (McWilliams *et al.*, 2000). The mechanism of DFMO ototoxicity is currently unknown, but has been postulated to be due to alterations in polyamine levels in the cochlea (McWilliams *et al.*, 2000).

2.3.3 Autoimmune causes of hearing loss

Autoimmune inner ear disorders are a poorly understood group of disorders that can lead to loss of both hearing and balance. The rapid onset and resulting potentially severe disabilities of deafness and vertigo can be devastating to patients. However, prompt recognition and the institution of appropriate treatment can often reverse, or at least stabilize the hearing and balance deficit.

Like the barrier that exists between the brain and the blood, a similar 'blood–labyrinthine' barrier also exists to maintain the ionic gradients of the inner ear (Harris & Ryan, 1995; Juhn *et al.*, 2001). Both organs also lack an established lymphatic drainage pathway. The ear appears to be less immunoresponsive than the brain, however (Harris *et al.*, 1997). When the ear does respond immunologically, the endolymphatic sac, which contains a majority of the immune cells of the inner ear, has been shown to have a major role in this response (Rask-Andersen & Stahle, 1980; Tomiyama & Harris, 1987). It is the inflammation associated with immune response that can produce a considerable amount of cochlear injury, damage than can be partially mitigated by administering immunosuppressive agents (Darmstadt *et al.*, 1990).

While there are clearly systemic autoimmune diseases that can also involve the ear, there are also autoimmune processes that solely affect the inner ear. The principal challenge for the clinician in either case is prompt diagnosis (Box 2.2). The first report on an immune-mediated hearing loss was by McCabe in 1979. Since this seminal report, the diagnosis of autoimmune inner ear disorders has been aided by the availability of a western blot assay towards a 68 kD antigen that was associated with a positive response to steroid treatment for the disorder (Harris & Sharp, 1990). Although the 68 kD protein has not been conclusively identified, evidence points to heat-shock protein (Billings *et al.*, 1995). In a study of 279 patients with suspected autoimmune hearing loss, 90 (32%) were positive by western blot, and there was a distinct female predominance in

---

Box 2.2 Diagnostic evaluation of a patient with suspected autoimmune hearing loss

Blood work

- Complete blood count with differential (CBC)
- Fluorescent treponemal antibody (FTA-ABS)
- Rheumatoid factor (RF)
- Antinuclear antibody (ANA)
- Anti-double-stranded DNA antibody
- Complement assay
- Immunoglobin analysis by subclass
- Thyroid function tests

Additional testing

- Urinalysis
- Soft tissue biopsy (e.g. minor salivary gland for Sjögren's disease)

the positive group (63%), correlating with the clinical distribution of autoimmune hearing loss (Harris et al., 1997). The clinical utility of the test is questionable, however, since test results will often not dictate treatment, and patients with suspected hearing loss will usually receive the same treatment regardless of the test result (Bonaguri et al., 2007).

Clinically, patients with autoimmune inner ear disease will develop rapidly progressive, bilateral hearing loss over several weeks. There is also a roughly 2:1 female to male preponderance. Fluctuations in hearing are common during the course, as are the symptoms of aural fullness. Vertigo and disequilibrium are present in approximately a third of cases (Hughes et al., 1996; Yehudai et al., 2006). Approximately 30% of patients will also have manifestations of systemic autoimmune dysfunction (Hughes et al., 1988). Autoimmune diseases commonly associated with sensorineural hearing loss include rheumatoid arthritis, polyarteritis nodosa, Wegener's granulomatosis, Cogan's syndrome, Behçet's syndrome, relapsing polychondritis, and systemic lupus erythematosus ('lupus'). If one of these disorders is suspected, consultation with a rheumatologist is warranted.

Owing to the potentially devastating effects of loss of hearing and balance, treatment of autoimmune inner ear disease consists of high-dose steroids. Although there is no consensus dosage of steroids, a common treatment regimen is 1–2 mg/kg/day (approximately 60 mg/day) of prednisone for four weeks (Harris et al., 1997). Patients whose hearing loss returns following withdrawal of steroids can be considered for a longer course of prednisone with a slow taper. For patients in whom autoimmune inner ear disease is strongly suspected and who either receive no benefit from steroids or develop side effects from steroid usage, or require long-term steroids to maintain hearing (>3 months), consideration should be given to the use of cytotoxic medications such as methotrexate or cyclophosphamide (Berrettini et al., 1998; Matteson et al., 2000). In one of the only well-designed, controlled trials to date of autoimmune hearing loss, methotrexate was tested for its efficacy in this condition. The results, however, suggested that following an initial good response to steroids, methotrexate provided no benefit over placebo in maintaining hearing (Harris et al., 2003). However, the use of such medications requires close clinical monitoring of blood counts, liver enzymes, and renal function to detect the potential complications of liver and pulmonary interstitial fibrosis. For severe cases not responding to the above treatment regimens, the use of plasmapheresis has also been described, although cost and reimbursement factors are major obstacles in the use of this therapy (Luetje & Berliner, 1997).

2.3.4 Idiopathic sudden sensorineural hearing loss

Perhaps one of the most frightening conditions for patients in otology is idiopathic sudden sensorineural hearing (ISSHL). In contrast to autoimmune inner ear disorders where hearing may be lost over the course of several months, patients with ISSHL may develop a partial or complete sensorineural hearing loss over the course of several hours, or may simply wake up one morning without warning with a 'dead ear'. The name (idiopathic) as well as the numerous theories of its etiology underscores how little is known about this condition (Jaffe, 1973; Finger & Gostian, 2006).

The incidence of ISSHL has been estimated to range from 5 to 20/100 000 persons per year, most commonly occurring in the sixth decade of life (Byl, 1984). This accounts for approximately 15 000 cases worldwide annually, or roughly 1% of all cases of sensorineural hearing loss (Byl, 1977). The disorder affects men and women equally. Unlike autoimmune inner ear disorders, bilateral involvement is rare, and simultaneous bilateral involvement is even rarer (Shaia & Sheehy, 1976; Mattox & Simmons, 1977). Patients most commonly present with a rapidly progressive unilateral sudden sensorineural hearing loss, often upon awakening (Mattox & Simmons, 1977). This is often accompanied by a sensation of aural fullness and tinnitus. Vertigo is seen in fewer than half of cases (Mattox & Simmons, 1977).

As the name implies, the etiology of ISSHL remains a mystery. The most commonly believed etiology for ISSHL is viral, despite no clearly established link between the two (Nosrati-Zarenoe *et al.*, 2007). This association comes from several lines of evidence: nearly a of patients presenting with sudden sensorineural hearing loss report a viral-like upper respiratory infection prior to the onset of their hearing loss (Mattox & Lyles, 1989). Further, temporal bone histopathological studies have implicated a viral etiology for ISSHL based on postmortem findings (Beal *et al.*, 1967; Vasama & Linthicum, 2000). Despite these associations however, no study has ever shown a clear relationship between viral titers and degree of hearing loss, and antiviral medication has not been shown to impact on the hearing outcome in patients with ISSHL (Wilson *et al.*, 1980; Norris, 1988; Stokroos *et al.*, 1998; Haberkamp & Tanyeri, 1999).

A vascular etiology has also been proposed for ISSHL. Vascular disorders such as leukemia and sickle cell disease have been shown to cause hearing loss, while cardiac bypass surgery also has a low risk of causing sensorineural hearing loss presumably due to embolic events intra operatively (Millen *et al.*, 1982; De la Cruz & Bance, 1998; Walsted *et al.*, 2000; Van Prooyen-Keyzer *et al.*, 2005). Further, vasospasm of the internal auditory artery during cerebellopontine angle surgery has also been shown to cause hearing loss (Mom *et al.*, 2000). However, vasodilatory medications have not been shown to be clearly efficacious with regard to ISSHL, although they are still frequently used for lack of a better alternative in many cases (Mattox, 1980; Fisch, 1983; Norris, 1988; Fetterman *et al.*, 1996; Haberkamp & Tanyeri, 1999). Additional etiologies proposed for ISSHL include diabetes mellitus, autoimmune, perilymphatic fistula, and cochlear hydrops (Wilson *et al.*, 1982; Adkisson & Meredith, 1990).

A number of other potentially treatable disorders can mimic ISSHL, and these should be sought in the initial diagnostic evaluation of patients who present with a rapid onset hearing loss. In approximately one in eight patients with vestibular schwannoma, for example, patients will present with a sudden hearing loss mimicking ISSHL, and will often initially respond favorably to steroids (Berg *et al.*, 1986; Berenholz *et al.*, 1992). Occasionally, patients with autoimmune hearing loss will also present with a rapidly progressive hearing loss. Thus, it is important to exclude such potentially treatable diseases.

A complete evaluation of patients presenting with a sudden sensorineural hearing loss should proceed forthright, to establish a diagnosis as rapidly as possible. Laboratory screening should include a CBC, electrolyte panel, liver function tests, syphilis screening (FTA-ABS), thyroid function tests, C-reactive protein, c-antineutrophilic cytoplasmic antibodies (ANCA), sedimentation rate, and ANA (Nosrati-Zarenoe *et al.*, 2007). An MRI is also indicated to exclude a retrocochlear or central pathology such as a vestibular schwannoma. Audiometry is also a requisite portion of the evaluation, as are serial audiograms during the treatment course to monitor treatment response.

In a majority of cases, the laboratory and radiological evaluation will be entirely normal in patients presenting with a sudden hearing loss. However, treatment should begin promptly at the first indication of a hearing loss, even while the evaluation is progressing and no clear diagnosis has been reached. Currently, the most commonly agreed treatment for this condition is steroids (prednisone), in dosages that are similar to those used for autoimmune inner ear disease: 1 mg/kg/day (typically 60 mg/day) for a total of one to three weeks. If a favorable response to steroids is noted by improvement on audiometry, then the treatment can be extended for an additional one to two months. Intratympanic steroid injections (dexamethasone) are also currently being used for ISSHL, though this route of delivery has not yet been conclusively proven effective, despite many positive anecdotal reports (Silverstein *et al.*, 1996; Chandrasekhar *et al.*, 2000; Shulman & Goldstein, 2000; Banerjee & Parnes, 2005; Battista, 2005; Gouveris *et al.*, 2005; Selivanova *et al.*,

2005; Haynes *et al.*, 2007). An ongoing NIH-sponsored multicenter trial of intratympanic steroids for ISSHL, led by Rauch and colleagues, will hopefully answer the question of the utility of oral versus intratympanic routes of steroid administration for this condition within the next several years. Beyond steroids, there has been no proven treatment for ISSHL, despite the numerous medications and treatments that have been tried. These include vasodilators, antiviral medications, carbogen (95% oxygen + 5% carbon dioxide) inhalation, and low-salt diet and diuretics (as in endolymphatic hydrops) (Mattox, 1980; Wilson *et al.*, 1980; Moskowitz *et al.*, 1984; Norris, 1988; Veldman *et al.*, 1993; Fetterman *et al.*, 1996; Hughes *et al.*, 1996; Stokroos *et al.*, 1998; Haberkamp & Tanyeri, 1999). One of the difficulties in assessing the efficacy of these treatment regimens is lack of well -controlled studies, since without any treatment 30–65% of patients will experience partial or complete recovery (Mattox & Simmons, 1977; Wilson *et al.*, 1980).

The prognosis of patients with ISSHL is variable, and depends on several factors (Xenellis *et al.*, 2006). Studies have shown that the more severe the initial hearing loss, the less likely hearing will recover, regardless of treatment modality used. In addition, patients who show a predominantly low-frequency hearing loss, or an up-sloping and mid-frequency losses recover more frequently than do patients with a downsloping or flat hearing loss. Other poor prognostic factors include the presence of vertigo, reduced speech discrimination, and a sudden hearing loss in both children and adults over the age of 40 (Byl, 1977; Mattox & Simmons, 1977; Wilson *et al.*, 1980; Byl, 1984).

2.3.5 Tinnitus

Tinnitus is defined as the sensation of sound in the absence of an exogenous sound source. Tinnitus can accompany any form of hearing loss and its presence provides no diagnostic value in determining the cause of a hearing loss. Approximately 15% of the general population experience some type of tinnitus (Coles, 1984), with prevalence beyond 20% in aging populations (Axelsson & Ringdahl, 1987). Simple forms of tinnitus include the low-pitch tinnitus that results from the accumulation of cerumen in the external ear canal, or that due to tympanic membrane perforation. Eustachian tube insufficiency manifesting a middle ear effusion can produce tinnitus, as can an abnormally patent eustachian tube that produces a 'blowing' tinnitus that coincides with respiration. More complex presentations of tinnitus are categorized as either objective (heard or recordable by others) or subjective (reported by the patient and not heard or recordable by others). The most common presentation of tinnitus however, is in the setting of sensorineural hearing loss. Sensorineural hearing loss has several psychophysical correlates (Pickles, 1988). In addition to diminished hearing sensitivity, reduced frequency resolution, loudness recruitment, and tinnitus commonly associate with many forms of sensorineural hearing loss. Indeed, the vast majority of cases of clinical tinnitus are subjective and are associated with sensorineural hearing loss.

Objective tinnitus

Objective tinnitus can be recorded objectively with a microphone or heard by another listener. Classic descriptions place the site of lesion of objective tinnitus peripheral to the cochlea. Contractions of soft palate and middle ear muscles can produce a clicking-like objective tinnitus. The presence of pulsatile tinnitus should prompt an evaluation of the skull base and major vessels of the head and neck, as this represents a vascular etiology. Arterial causes for pulsatile tinnitus include arteriovenous shunts (as seen with malformations, fistulae, and in Paget's disease), arterio-arterial anastomoses including rare congenital anomalies and intraluminal irregularities of the carotid system (such as atherosclerotic plaques or fibromuscular dysplasia) (Hafeez *et al.*, 1999;

Baumgartner & Bogousslavsky, 2005; Arganbright & Friedland, 2008; Chen *et al.*, 2007b; Lerut *et al.*, 2007; Magliulo *et al.*, 2007; Sonmez *et al.*, 2007; Topal *et al.*, 2008). As a result, modalities employed in the evaluation of the patient with pulsatile tinnitus should include an MRI and MR angiography, and venography of the intracranial vessels or an angiogram. For arteriovenous malformations or fistulae, these can often be treated during the angiography by the interventional radiologist (Shownkeen *et al.*, 2001). Additional modalities can include a carotid ultrasound if vascular disease in the neck is suspected.

Subjective tinnitus

Subjective tinnitus is a common clinical disorder characterized by auditory sensations without external stimulation. The sensation can last anywhere from several seconds to a lifelong affliction. The sensation itself can be one of a high-tone ring (most commonly), buzzing, humming, crickets, whistle, hissing, or roaring. In rare cases, patients can sometimes perceive actual musical melodies. Tinnitus can affect patients in many ways, ranging from mild annoyance to severe depression and suicide (Dobie, 2003; Kaltenbach, 2006a,b).

Perhaps one of the most frustrating aspects of tinnitus is our own ignorance regarding its etiology and anatomical origin. The best argument for a peripheral contribution from the cochlea comes from the well-documented association of tinnitus with various forms of hearing loss, including noise-exposure, presbycusis, and drug-induced ototoxicity (Konig *et al.*, 2006). While it is widely agreed that such triggers can generate tinnitus, whether pure cochlear causes are enough to sustain tinnitus over the long term remains controversial (Baguley, 2002; Saunders, 2007). Spontaneous otoacoustic emissions are one means by which the cochlea can physically generate sound, which can be objectively recorded (Kemp, 1978). This process, representing active outer hair cell motion, has been shown to be a rare form of objective tinnitus (Plinkert *et al.*, 1990). However, most who have studied the phenomenon believe this is an unlikely cause of tinnitus in most patients (Penner, 1989). Loss of cochlear hair cells has also been hypothesized to contribute to tinnitus by altering the afferent auditory signal from abnormal motion of the basilar membrane (Jastreboff, 1990; Saunders, 2007). Other theories of the peripheral origin of tinnitus include loss of efferent connectivity to the outer hair cells (Chery-Croze *et al.*, 1994), excessive release of the neurotransmitter glutamate by the inner hair cells, and reduced hair cell stiffness in response to change in its cytoskeletal structure (Saunders, 2007). Yet, if tinnitus were purely a peripheral phenomenon, then ablating cochlear function should reduce, if not abolish tinnitus. In fact, the opposite is true: tinnitus persists following cochlear destruction or sectioning of the auditory nerve, as clinicians have know for many years (House & Brackmann, 1981). Compounding the difficulty of identifying the source of chronic, subjective tinnitus is the lack of a robust animal model for study. To date, animal models for tinnitus have been based on predominantly behavioral, psychophysical paradigms (Bauer, 2003).

In the absence of compelling data that the cochlea is the site of origin of chronic tinnitus, researchers have focused on the central auditory system and maladaptive central neuroplastic changes as underlying factor in many, if not all forms of chronic tinnitus (Eggermont, 2005). Though the initial damage may be peripheral (i.e. cochlear), a variety of evidence implicates that there are ensuing changes throughout the central auditory system, including new axonal growth, synaptogenesis and synapse degeneration, and changes in the structural properties of neurons (Saunders, 2007). Increased spontaneous neuronal activity in the dorsal cochlear nucleus (DCN) is one theory for chronic tinnitus, backed by data demonstrating cochlear damage altering outer hair cell afferent type II fibers, which in turn leads to reduced inhibition of fusiform cells within the cochlear nucleus (Kaltenbach, 2006b). Within the DCN, increased spontaneous neuronal activation has also been attributed to bursting discharges and neuronal synchrony following oto-toxic drug exposure (Baguley, 2002; Saunders, 2007).

Beyond the DCN, the auditory cortex has also been implicated in chronic tinnitus. As with the DCN, hyperactive spontaneous neuronal activity has been implicated along with neuronal synchronization (Saunders, 2007). These theories of tinnitus mirror those changes seen in the somatosensory system in response to loss of sensory input due to amputation (Rauschecker, 1999). Newer imaging modalities, including positron emission tomography (PET) and functional magnetic resonance imaging (fMRI) will hopefully shed new light onto some of the potential central causes of chronic tinnitus (Langguth *et al.*, 2006; Saunders, 2007; Smits *et al.*, 2007).

Treatment

Though tinnitus is commonly associated with hearing loss, tinnitus severity correlates poorly with the degree of hearing loss (Chung *et al.*, 1984). Studies have shown that approximately one in seven tinnitus sufferers experience severe annoyance while 4% are severely disabled (Evered & Lawrenson, 1981). To date, both pharmacological and surgical approaches have shown little to no efficacy towards tinnitus. Those treatments that have demonstrated benefit relate to the use of masking external inputs, in the form of an external masking (Vernon *et al.*, 1990) or cochlear implantation (Miyamoto *et al.*, 1997). Behavioral adaptive methods offer benefit in enhancing tolerance of the symptom and alleviating associated anxiety.

The potential concurrence of tinnitus and depression should be assessed in all patients with subjective tinnitus. Dobie and co-workers (1989) have examined the simple notion that 'tinnitus causes depression', and noted that many patients believe this to be the case. However, Sullivan and co-workers (1988) observed that depressed subjects noted having had episodes of major depression prior to the onset of their tinnitus. In 32 patients with tinnitus and current or past major depression, depression preceded tinnitus in 15, and five patients noted simultaneous onset. Mathew and co-workers (1981) evaluated the physical symptoms of depressed patients and found that roughly half of a cohort of depressed patients complained of tinnitus, compared to 12% of controls. Does this suggest that depression causes tinnitus? Dobie notes that this seems implausible, but it is certainly likely that depression erodes the coping process that probably develops for most patients with tinnitus, thus changing a normally insignificant symptom into one with high life-impact. Depression can certainly amplify disability associated with chronic medical illness (Wells & Sherbourne, 1999). For example, not all individuals with irritable bowel syndrome seek medical advice; and those who do seek medical advice differ from those who do not. Those who do seek advice demonstrate greater levels anxiety and depression after controlling for severity of gastrointestinal symptoms (Olden & Drossman, 2000).

Treatment results using antidepressants in tinnitus sufferers are encouraging. Nortriptyline, a tricyclic antidepressant administered with careful dosing adjustments, appears to improve symptoms in several domains in depressed tinnitus patients (Dobie *et al.*, 1993). Clearly, the largest treatment effect is a reduction in depressive symptoms. Further, however, not only did patients' estimates of tinnitus severity (i.e. 'How much does it bother you?') decline as depression improved, but many patients also reported quieter tinnitus. Nonetheless, the authors of this study indicate that the major therapeutic benefit was in mood and coping ability, with less change in tinnitus, *per se*.

Transcranial magnetic stimulation, or TMS, is newer modality being directed towards tinnitus and has shown early promise (De Ridder *et al.*, 2007; Dornhoffer & Mennemeier, 2007; Langguth *et al.*, 2007). Already in trials for such disorders as depression (Loo *et al.*, 2007), TMS may offer people with tinnitus a non-pharmacological, non-surgical treatment.

References

American National Standards Institute (1978) *Methods for Manual Pure-tone Threshold Audiometry*, Vol. S3.21–1978 (R1986). American National Standards Institute, New York.

Adkisson GH, Meredith AP. (1990) Inner ear decompression sickness combined with a fistula of the round window. Case report [see comments]. *Ann Otol Rhinol Laryngol* **99**: 733–7.

Arganbright J & Friedland DR. (2008) Pulsatile tinnitus. *Otol Neurotol* **29**: 416.

Arnold W, Nadol JB Jr & Weidauer H. (1981) Ultrastructural histopathology in a case of human ototoxicity due to loop diuretics. *Acta Otolaryngol* **91**: 399–414.

Augustsson I, Nilson C & Engstrand I. (1990) The preventive value of audiometric screening of preschool and young school-children. *Int J Pediatr Otorhinolaryngol* **20**: 51–62.

Axelsson A & Ringdahl A. (1987) The occurrence and severity of tinnitus: A prevalence study. In: Harsch Verlag, ed. *Proceedings of the Third International Tinnitus Seminar*. Karlsruhe, Germany.

Bagger-Sjoback D, Filipek C & Schacht J. (1980) Characteristics and drug responses of cochlear and vestibular adenylate cyclase. *Arch Otorhinolaryngol* **228**: 217–22.

Baguley DM. (2002) Mechanisms of tinnitus. *Br Med Bull* **63**: 195–212.

Banerjee A & Parnes LS. (2005) Intratympanic corticosteroids for sudden idiopathic sensorineural hearing loss. *Otol Neurotol* **26**: 878–81.

Bates DE, Beaumont SJ & Baylis BW. (2002) Ototoxicity induced by gentamicin and furosemide. *Ann Pharmacother* **36**: 446–51.

Battista RA. (2005) Intratympanic dexamethasone for profound idiopathic sudden sensorineural hearing loss. *Otolaryngol Head Neck Surg* **132**: 902–5.

Bauch CD & Olsen WO. (1986) The effect of 2000–4000 Hz hearing sensitivity on ABR results. *Ear Hear* **7**: 314–17.

Bauer CA. (2003) Animal models of tinnitus. *Otolaryngol Clin North Am* **36**: 267–285, vi.

Baumgartner RW & Bogousslavsky J. (2005) Clinical manifestations of carotid dissection. *Front Neurol Neurosci* **20**: 70–6.

Beal DD, Hemenway WG & Lindsay JR. (1967) Inner ear pathology of sudden deafness. Histopathology of acquired deafness in the adult coincident with viral infection. *Arch Otolaryngol* **85**: 591–8.

Beaubien AR, Desjardins S, Ormsby E, Bayne A, Carrier K, Cauchy MJ, Henri R, Hodgen M, Salley J & St Pierre A. (1990) Delay in hearing loss following drug administration: a consistent feature of amikacin ototoxicity. *Acta Otolaryngol* **109**: 345–1.

Beiter RC & Talley JN. (1976) High-frequency audiometry above 8,000 Hz. *Audiology* **15**: 207–14.

Berenholz LP, Eriksen C & Hirsh FA. (1992) Recovery from repeated sudden hearing loss with corticosteroid use in the presence of an acoustic neuroma. *Ann Otol Rhinol Laryngol* **101**: 827–31.

Berg HM, Cohen NL, Hammerschlag PE & Waltzman SB. (1986) Acoustic neuroma presenting as sudden hearing loss with recovery. *Otolaryngol Head Neck Surg* **94**: 15–22.

Berrettini S, Ferri C, Ravecca F, LaCivita L, Bruschini L, Riente L, Mosca M & Sellari-Franceschini S. (1998) Progressive sensorineural hearing impairment in systemic vasculitides. *Semin Arthritis Rheum* **27**: 301–18.

Billings PB, Keithley EM & Harris JP. (1995) Evidence linking the 68 kilodalton antigen identified in progressive sensorineural hearing loss patient sera with heat shock protein 70. *Ann Otol Rhinol Laryngol* **104**: 181–8.

Bizjak ED, Haug MT 3rd, Schilz RJ, Sarodia BD & Dresing JM. (1999) Intravenous azithromycin-induced ototoxicity. *Pharmacotherapy* **19**: 245–8.

Blakley BW, Gupta AK, Myers SF & Schwan S. (1994) Risk factors for ototoxicity due to cisplatin. *Arch Otolaryngol Head Neck Surg* **120**: 541–6.

Boettcher FA & Salvi RJ. (1991) Salicylate ototoxicity: review and synthesis. *Am J Otolaryngol* **12**: 33–47.

Bokemeyer C, Berger CC, Hartmann JT, Kollmannsberger C, Schmoll HJ, Kuczyk MA & Kanz L. (1998) Analysis of risk factors for cisplatin-induced ototoxicity in patients with testicular cancer. *Br J Cancer* **77**: 1355–62.

Bonaguri C, Orsoni JG, Zavota L, Monica C, Russo A, Pellistri I, Rubino P, Giovannelli L, Manzotti F & Piazza F. (2007) Anti-68kDa antibodies in autoimmune sensorineural hearing loss: are these autoantibodies really a diagnostic tool?. *Autoimmunity* **40**: 73–8.

Bosher S. (1979) Ethacrynic acid ototoxicity as a general model in cochlear pathology. *Adv Otorhinolaryngol* **22**: 81–9.

Brock PR, Bellman SC, Yeomans EC, Pinkerton CR & Pritchard J. (1991) Cisplatin ototoxicity in children: a practical grading system. *Med Pediatr Oncol* **19**: 295–300.

Brummett RE. (1993) Ototoxicity of vancomycin and analogues. *Otolaryngol Clin North Am* **26**: 821–8.

Brummett RE & Fox KE. (1989) Vancomycin and erythromycin induced hearing loss in humans. *Antimicrob Agents Chemother* **33**: 791–6.

Brummett RE, Fox KE, Jacobs F, Kempton JB, Stokes Z & Richmond AB. (1990) Augmented gentamicin ototoxicity induced by vancomycin in guinea pigs. *Arch Otolaryngol Head Neck Surg* **116**: 61–4.

Byl FM. (1977) Seventy-six cases of presumed sudden hearing loss occurring in 1973: prognosis and incidence. *Laryngoscope* **87**: 817–25.

Byl FM Jr. (1984) Sudden hearing loss: eight years' experience and suggested prognostic table. *Laryngoscope* **94**: 647–61.

Carhart R. (1971) Observations on relations between thresholds for pure tones and for speech. *J Speech Hear Disord* **36**: 476–83.

Carhart R & Jerger JF. (1959) Preferred method for clinical determination of pure-tone thresholds. *J Speech Hear Disord* **24**: 330–45.

Cazals Y, Li X, Aurousseau C & Didier A. (1988) Acute effects of noradrenalin-related vasoactive agents on the ototoxicity of aspirin: an experimental study in the guinea pig. *Hear Res* **36**: 89–94.

Chandrasekhar SS, Brackmann DE & Devgan KK. (1995) Utility of auditory brainstem response audiometry in diagnosis of acoustic neuromas. *Am J Otol* **16**: 63–7.

Chandrasekhar SS, Rubinstein RY, Kwartler JA, Gatz M, Connelly PE, Huang E & Baredes S. (2000) Dexamethasone pharmacokinetics in the inner ear: comparison of route of administration and use of facilitating agents. *Otolaryngol Head Neck Surg* **122**: 521–8.

Chen WC, Jackson A, Budnick AS, Pfister DG, Kraus DH, Hunt MA, Stambuk H, Levegrun S & Wolden SL. (2006) Sensorineural hearing loss in combined modality treatment of nasopharyngeal carcinoma. *Cancer* **106**: 820–9.

Chen Y, Huang WG, Zha DJ, Qiu JH, Wang JL, Sha SH & Schacht J. (2007a) Aspirin attenuates gentamicin ototoxicity: from the laboratory to the clinic. *Hear Res* **226**: 178–82.

Chen Y, How CK & Chern CH. (2007b) Cerebral dural arteriovenous fistulas presenting as pulsatile tinnitus. *Intern Med J* **37**: 503.

Chery-Croze S, Truy E & Morgon A. (1994) Contralateral suppression of transiently evoked otoacoustic emissions and tinnitus. *Br J Audiol* **28**: 255–66.

Chung DY, Gannon RP & Mason K. (1984) Factors affecting the prevalence of tinnitus. *Audiology* **23**: 441–52.

Clark JG. (1981) Uses and abuses of hearing loss classification. *ASHA* **23**: 493–500.

Coats AC. (1978) Human auditory nerve action potentials and brain stem evoked responses. *Arch Otolaryngol* **104**: 709–17.

Coles RR. (1984) Epidemiology of tinnitus: (1) prevalence. *J Laryngol Otol Suppl* **9**: 7–15.

Croghan MK, Aickin MG & Meyskens FL. (1991) Dose-related alpha-difluoromethylornithine ototoxicity. *Am J Clin Oncol* **14**: 331–5.

Darmstadt GL, Keithley EM & Harris JP. (1990) Effects of cyclophosphamide on the pathogenesis of cytomegalovirus - induced labyrinthitis. *Ann Otol Rhinol Laryngol* **99**: 960–8.

Davis A, Stephens D, Rayment A & Thomas K. (1992) Hearing impairments in middle age: the acceptability, benefit and cost of detection (ABCD). *Br J Audiol* **26**: 1–14.

Day R *et al.* (1989) Concentration-response relationships for salicylate-induced ototoxicity in normal volunteers. *Br J Clin Pharmacol* **28**: 295–701.

Deer B & Hunter-Duvar I. (1982) Salicylate ototoxicity in the chinchilla: a behavioral and electron microscope study. *J Otolaryngol* 11: 260–71.

de Hoog M, van Zanten BA, Hop WC, Overbosch E, Weisglas-Kuperus N & van den Anker JN. (2003) Newborn hearing screening: tobramycin and vancomycin are not risk factors for hearing loss. *J Pediatr* 142: 41–6.

De la Cruz M & Bance M. (1998) Bilateral sudden sensorineural hearing loss following non-otologic surgery [see comments]. *J Laryngol Otol* 112: 769–71.

Department of Labor OSaHA. (1981) Occupational noise exposure: hearing conservation amendment. *Fed Reg* 46: 4078–180.

De Ridder D, De Mulder G, Verstraeten E, Seidman M, Elisevich K, Sunaert S, Kovacs S, Van der Kelen K, Van de Heyning P & Moller A. (2007) Auditory cortex stimulation for tinnitus. *Acta Neurochir Suppl* 97: 451–62.

Dillon H. (1982) A quantitative examination of the sources of speech discrimination test score variability. *Ear Hear* 3: 51–8.

Dobie R. (1993) *Medical-Legal Evaluation of Hearing Loss*. Van Nostrand Reinhold, New York.

Dobie R, Katon W, Sulliva nM & Sakai C. (1989) Tinnitus Depression and Aging. In: Goldstein J, Kashima H & Koopmann C, eds. *Geriatric Otolaryngology*. BC Decker, Toronto, pp. 45–49.

Dobie RA. (2003) Depression and tinnitus. *Otolaryngol Clin North Am* 36: 383–8.

Dornhoffer JL & Mennemeier M. (2007) Transcranial magnetic stimulation and tinnitus: implications for theory and practice. *J Neurol Neurosurg Psychiatry* 78: 113.

Eggermont JJ. (2005) Tinnitus: neurobiological substrates. *Drug Discov Today* 10: 1283–90.

Eggermont JJ, Don M & Brackmann DE. (1980) Electrocochleography and auditory brainstem electric responses in patients with pontine angle tumors. *Ann Otol Rhinol Laryngol Suppl* 89: 1–19.

Emanuele E, Olivieri V, Aldeghi A & Minoretti P. (2007) Topical administration of oleandrin could protect against gentamicin ototoxicity via inhibition of activator protein-1 and c-Jun N-terminal kinase. *Med Hypotheses* 68: 711.

Evered D & Lawrenson G. (1981) *Tinnitus, CIBA Symposium #85*. Pitman Medical, London.

Festen JM & Plomp R. (1983) Relations between auditory functions in impaired hearing. *J Acoust Soc Am* 73: 652–62.

Fetterman BL, Saunders JE & Luxford WM. (1996) Prognosis and treatment of sudden sensorineural hearing loss. *Am J Otol* 17: 529–36.

Finger RP & Gostian AO. (2006) Idiopathic sudden hearing loss: contradictory clinical evidence, placebo effects and high spontaneous recovery rate–where do we stand in assessing treatment outcomes?. *Acta Otolaryngol* 126: 1124–7.

Fisch U. (1983) Management of sudden deafness. *Otolaryngol Head Neck Surg* 91: 3–8.

Fischel-Ghodsian N. (1999) Genetic factors in aminoglycoside toxicity. *Ann N Y Acad Sci* 884: 99–109.

Fletcher H. (1950) A method of calculating hearing loss for speech from an audiogram. *Acta Otolaryngol Suppl* 90: 26–37.

Fortnum H, Davis A, Butler A & Stevens J (1995). *Health Service Implications of Changes in Aetiology and Referral Patterns of Hearing Impaired Children in Trent 1985–1993. Report to Trent Health*. MRC Institute of Hearing Research and Trent Health, Nottingham/Sheffield.

Galambos R & Hecox KE. (1978) Clinical applications of the auditory brain stem response. *Otolaryngol Clin North Am* 11: 709–22.

Gallagher KL & Jones JK. (1979) Furosemide-induced ototoxicity. *Ann Intern Med* 91: 744–5.

Gates GA, Cooper JC, Kannel WB & Miller NJ. (1990) Hearing in the elderly: the Framingham cohort, 1983–1985. Part I. Basic audiometric test results. *Ear Hear* 11: 247–56.

Goebel JA. (2001) The ten-minute examination of the dizzy patient. *Semin Neurol* 21: 391–8.

Goodman A. (1965) Reference zero levels for pure tone audiometer. *ASHA* 7: 262–3.

Gordon JS, Phillips DS, Helt WJ, Konrad-Martin D & Fausti SA. (2005) Evaluation of insert earphones for high-frequency bedside ototoxicity monitoring. *J Rehabil Res Dev* **42**: 353–61.

Gouveris H, Selivanova O & Mann W. (2005) Intratympanic dexamethasone with hyaluronic acid in the treatment of idiopathic sudden sensorineural hearing loss after failure of intravenous steroid and vasoactive therapy. *Eur Arch Otorhinolaryngol* **262**: 131–4.

Green J. (2002) Noise-induced hearing loss. *Pediatrics* **109**: 987–8.

Guan MX, Fischel-Ghodsian N & Attardi G. (2000) A biochemical basis for the inherited susceptibility to aminoglycoside ototoxicity [in process citation]. *Hum Mol Genet* **9**: 1787–93.

Haberkamp TJ & Tanyeri HM. (1999) Management of idiopathic sudden sensorineural hearing loss [see comments]. *Am J Otol* **20**: 587–92; discussion 593–5.

Hafeez F, Levine RL & Dulli DA. (1999) Pulsatile tinnitus in cerebrovascular arterial diseases. *J Stroke Cerebrovasc Dis* **8**: 217–23.

Hall JW. (1992) *Handbook of Auditory Evoked Responses*. Allyn & Bacon, Needham Heights, MA, USA.

Halmagyi GM, Yavor RA & McGarvie LA. (1997) Testing the vestibulo-ocular reflex. *Adv Otorhinolaryngol* **53**: 132–54.

Halmagyi GM, Aw ST, McGarvie LA, Todd MJ, Bradshaw A, Yavor RA & Fagan PA. (2003) Superior semicircular canal dehiscence simulating otosclerosis. *J Laryngol Otol* **117**: 553–7.

Halmagyi GM, Curthoys IS, Colebatch JG & Aw ST. (2005) Vestibular responses to sound. *Ann N Y Acad Sci* **1039**: 54–67.

Harris JP & Ryan AF. (1995) Fundamental immune mechanisms of the brain and inner ear. *Otolaryngol Head Neck Surg* **112**: 639–53.

Harris JP & Sharp PA. (1990) Inner ear autoantibodies in patients with rapidly progressive sensorineural hearing loss. *Laryngoscope* **100**: 516–24.

Harris JP, Moscicki RA & Ryan AF. (1997) Immunologic disorders of the inner ear. In: Hughes GB & Pensak ML, eds. *Clinical Otology*. Thieme Medical Publishers, New York, pp. 381–91.

Harris JP, Weisman MH, Derebery JM, Espeland MA, Gantz BJ, Gulya AJ, Hammerschlag PE, Hannley M, Hughes GB, Moscicki R, Nelson RA, Niparko JK, Rauch SD, Telian SA & Brookhouser PE. (2003) Treatment of corticosteroid-responsive autoimmune inner ear disease with methotrexate: a randomized controlled trial. *JAMA* **290**: 1875–83.

Hashino E & Shero M. (1995) Endocytosis of aminoglycoside antibiotics in sensory hair cells. *Brain Res* **704**: 135–40.

Havlik R. (1986) Aging in the eighties: impaired senses for sound and light in persons age 65 years and over. Preliminary data from the supplement on aging to the National Health Interview Survey: United States January–June 1984. Advance data from vital and health statistics, #125. National Center for Health Statistics Publication, Hyattsville, MD, USA. No. DHHS (PHS) 86–1250.

Hawkins J. (1976) Drug ototoxicity. In: Keidel W & Neff W, eds. *Handbook of Sensory Physiology, Vol 5: Auditory System*. Springer-Verlag, Berlin.

Hawkins J & Engstrom H. (1964) Effect of kanamycin on cochlear cytoarchitecture. *Acta otolaryngol Suppl (Stockh)* **188**: 100–12.

Haynes DS, O'Malley M, Cohen S, Watford K & Labadie RF. (2007) Intratympanic dexamethasone for sudden sensorineural hearing loss after failure of systemic therapy. *Laryngoscope* **117**: 3–15.

Henley C & Schacht J. (1988) Pharmacokinetics of aminoglycoside antibiotics in inner ear fluids and their relationship to ototoxicity. *Audiology* **27**: 137–46.

Herdman SJ, Hall CD, Schubert MC, Das VE & Tusa RJ. (2007) Recovery of dynamic visual acuity in bilateral vestibular hypofunction. *Arch Otolaryngol Head Neck Surg* **133**: 383–9.

Hinojosa R, Riggs LC, Strauss M & Matz GJ. (1995) Temporal bone histopathology of cisplatin ototoxicity. *Am J Otol* **16**: 731–40.

Hood LJ. (1988) *Clinical Applications of the Auditory Brainstem Response*. Singular Publishing Group, San Diego, CA, pp. 49–63.

House JW & Brackmann DE. (1981) Tinnitus: surgical treatment. *Ciba Found Symp* **85**: 204–16.

Huang M & Schacht J. (1988) Formation of a cytotoxic metabolite from gentamicin by liver. *Biochem Pharmacol* **40**: 11–21.

Huang RS, Duan S, Shukla SJ, Kistner EO, Clark TA, Chen TX, Schweitzer AC, Blume JE & Dolan ME. (2007) Identification of genetic variants contributing to cisplatin-induced cytotoxicity by use of a genomewide approach. *Am J Hum Genet* **81**: 427–37.

Hughes GB, Barna BP, Kinney SE, Calabrese LH & Nalepa NJ. (1988) Clinical diagnosis of immune inner-ear disease. *Laryngoscope* **98**: 251–3.

Hughes GB, Freedman MA, Haberkamp TJ & Guay ME. (1996) Sudden sensorineural hearing loss. *Otolaryngol Clin North Am* **29**: 393–405.

Humes HD. (1999) Insights into ototoxicity. Analogies to nephrotoxicity. *Ann N Y Acad Sci* **884**: 15–18.

Hyppolito MA, de Oliveira JA & Rossato M. (2006) Cisplatin ototoxicity and otoprotection with sodium salicylate. *Eur Arch Otorhinolaryngol* **263**: 798–803.

Ishii T, Bernstein J & Bulogh K. (1967) Distribution of tritium-labelled salicylate in the cochlea. *Ann Otol Rhinol Laryngol* **76**: 368–72.

Jackler RK & Dillon WP. (1988) Computed tomography and magnetic resonance imaging of the inner ear. *Otolaryngol Head Neck Surg* **99**: 494–504.

Jackson G & Arcieri G. (1971) Ototoxicity of gentamicin in man: a survey and controlled analysis of clinical experience in the United States. *J Infect Dis* **124** (**Suppl**): 130–7.

Jaffe BF. (1973) Clinical studies in sudden deafness. *Adv Otorhinolaryngol* **20**: 221–8.

Jastreboff PJ. (1990) Phantom auditory perception (tinnitus): mechanisms of generation and perception. *Neurosci Res* **8**: 221–54.

Jerger J & Johnson K. (1988) Interactions of age, gender, and sensorineural hearing loss on ABR latency. *Ear Hear* **9**: 168–76.

Jerger JF. (1970) Clinical experience with impedance audiometry. *Arch Otolaryngol* **92**: 311–24.

Jewett DL & Williston JS. (1971) Auditory-evoked far fields averaged from the scalp of humans. *Brain* **94**: 681–96.

Josey AF, Glasscock ME 3rd & Musiek FE. (1988) Correlation of ABR and medical imaging in patients with cerebellopontine angle tumors. *Am J Otol* **9** (**Suppl**): 12–16.

Juhn SK, Hunter BA & Odland RM. (2001) Blood-labyrinth barrier and fluid dynamics of the inner ear. *Int Tinnitus J* **7**: 72–83.

Jung TT, Hunter LL, Alper CM, Paradise JL, Roberts JE, Park SK, Casselbrant ML, Spratley J, Eriksson PO, Tos M, Gravel JS, Wallace I & Hellström SO. (2005) Recent advances in otitis media. 9. Complications and sequelae. *Ann Otol Rhinol Laryngol Suppl* **194**: 140–60.

Kahlmeter G & Kahlager J. (1984) Aminoglycoside toxicity and review of medical studies published between 1975 and 1982. *J Antimicrob Chemother* **13** (**Suppl**): 9–22.

Kaltenbach JA. (2006a) The dorsal cochlear nucleus as a participant in the auditory, attentional and emotional components of tinnitus. *Hear Res* **216–217**: 224–34.

Kaltenbach JA. (2006b) Summary of evidence pointing to a role of the dorsal cochlear nucleus in the etiology of tinnitus. *Acta Otolaryngol Suppl* 20–26.

Kaye CI, Accurso F, La Franchi S, Lane PA, Northrup H, Pang S & Schaefer GB. (2006) Introduction to the newborn screening fact sheets. *Pediatrics* **118**: 1304–12.

Kemp DT. (1978) Stimulated acoustic emissions from within the human auditory system. *J Acoust Soc Am* **64**: 1386–91.

Kharkheli E, Kevanishvili Z, Maglakelidze T, Davitashvili O & Schacht J. (2007) Does vitamin E prevent gentamicin-induced ototoxicity?. *Georgian Med News* 14–17.

Kiang N, Liberman M & Levine R. (1976) Auditory nerve activity in cats exposed to ototoxic drugs and high-intensity sounds. *Ann Otol Rhinol Laryngol* **85**: 752–61.

Klibanov OM, Filicko JE, DeSimone JA Jr & Tice DS. (2003) Sensorineural hearing loss associated with intrathecal vancomycin. *Ann Pharmacother* 37: 61–5.

Koegel L Jr. (1985) Ototoxicity: a contemporary review of aminoglycosides, loop diuretics, acetylsalicylic acid, quinine, erythromycin, and cisplatinum. *Am J Otol* 6: 190–9.

Konig O, Schaette R, Kempter R & Gross M. (2006) Course of hearing loss and occurrence of tinnitus. *Hear Res* 221: 59–64.

Krzanowski J & Matschinsky F. (1971) Phosphocreatine gradient opposite to that of glycogen in the organ of Corti and the effect of salicylate on adenosine triphosphate and P-creatine in cochlear structures. *J Histochem* 19: 321–6.

Langguth B, Eichhammer P, Kreutzer A, Maenner P, Marienhagen J, Kleinjung T, Sand P & Hajak G. (2006) The impact of auditory cortex activity on characterizing and treating patients with chronic tinnitus–first results from a PET study. *Acta Otolaryngol Suppl* 84–88.

Langguth B, Kleinjung T, Marienhagen J, Binder H, Sand PG, Hajak G & Eichhammer P. (2007) Transcranial magnetic stimulation for the treatment of tinnitus: effects on cortical excitability. *BMC Neurosci* 8: 45.

Lao CD, Backoff P, Shotland LI, McCarty D, Eaton T, Ondrey FG, Viner JL, Spechler SJ, Hawk ET & Brenner DE. (2004) Irreversible ototoxicity associated with difluoromethylornithine. *Cancer Epidemiol Biomarkers Prev* 13: 1250–2.

Lerner S & Matz G. (1980) Aminoglycoside ototoxicity. *Am J Otol* 1: 169–79.

Lerut B, De Vuyst C, Ghekiere J, Vanopdenbosch L & Kuhweide R. (2007) Post-traumatic pulsatile tinnitus: the hallmark of a direct carotico-cavernous fistula. *J Laryngol Otol* 121: 1103–7.

Loo CK, McFarquhar TF & Mitchell PB. (2007) A review of the safety of repetitive transcranial magnetic stimulation as a clinical treatment for depression. *Int J Neuropsychopharmacol* 11: 131–47.

Luetje CM & Berliner KI. (1997) Plasmapheresis in autoimmune inner ear disease: long-term follow-up. *Am J Otol* 18: 572–6.

Magliulo G, Parrotto D, Sardella B, Della Rocca C & Re M. (2007) Cavernous hemangioma of the tympanic membrane and external ear canal. *Am J Otolaryngol* 28: 180–3.

Marchese-Ragona R, Marioni G, Marson P, Martini A & Staffieri A. (2007) The Discovery of Salicylate Ototoxicity. *Audiol Neurootol* 13: 34–6.

Marks S & Schacht J. (1983) Effects of ototoxic diuretics on cochlear Na-K-ATPase and adenylate cyclase. *Scand Audiol Suppl* 14: 131–6.

Martin GK, Jassir D, Stagner BB & Lonsbury-Martin BL. (1998) Effects of loop diuretics on the suppression tuning of distortion- product otoacoustic emissions in rabbits. *J Acoust Soc Am* 104: 972–83.

Mathew RJ, Weinman ML & Mirabi M. (1981) Physical symptoms of depression. *Br J Psychiatry* 139: 293–6.

Matteson EL, Tirzaman O, Facer GW, Fabry DA, Kasperbauer J, Beatty CW & McDonald TJ. (2000) Use of methotrexate for autoimmune hearing loss. *Ann Otol Rhinol Laryngol* 109: 710–14.

Mattox DE. (1980) Medical management of sudden hearing loss. *Otolaryngol Head Neck Surg* 88: 111–13.

Mattox DE & Lyles CA. (1989) Idiopathic sudden sensorineural hearing loss. *Am J Otol* 10: 242–7.

Mattox DE & Simmons FB. (1977) Natural history of sudden sensorineural hearing loss. *Ann Otol Rhinol Laryngol* 86: 463–80.

Matz G. (1993) Aminoglycoside cochlear ototoxicity. *Otolaryngol Clin North Am* 26: 705–12.

McAlpine D & Johnstone B. (1990) The ototoxic mechanisms of cisplatin. *Hear Res* 47: 191–203.

McCabe BF. (1979) Autoimmune sensorineural hearing loss. *Ann Otol Rhinol Laryngol* 88: 585–9.

McWilliams ML, Chen GD & Fechter LD. (2000) Characterization of the ototoxicity of difluoromethylornithine and its enantiomers. *Toxicol Sci* 56: 124–32.

Merchant SN, Rosowski JJ & McKenna MJ. (2007) Superior semicircular canal dehiscence mimicking otosclerotic hearing loss. *Adv Otorhinolaryngol* 65: 137–45.

Meyskens FL Jr & Gerner EW. (1995) Development of difluoromethylornithine as a chemoprevention agent for the management of colon cancer. *J Cell Biochem Suppl* 22: 126–31.

Millen SJ, Toohill RJ & Lehman RH. (1982) Sudden sensorineural hearing loss: operative complication in non-otologic surgery. *Laryngoscope* 92: 613–17.

Minor LB, Carey JP, Cremer PD, Lustig LR, Streubel SO & Ruckenstein MJ. (2003) Dehiscence of bone overlying the superior canal as a cause of apparent conductive hearing loss. *Otol Neurotol* 24: 270–8.

Miyamoto RT, Wynne MK, McKnight C & Bichey B. (1997) Electrical Suppression of Tinnitus via Cochlear Implants. *Int Tinnitus J* 3: 35–8.

Moller AR, Jho HD, Yokota M & Jannetta PJ. (1995) Contribution from crossed and uncrossed brainstem structures to the brainstem auditory evoked potentials: a study in humans. *Laryngoscope* 105: 596–605.

Mom T, Telischi FF, Martin GK, Stagner BB & Lonsbury-Martin BL. (2000) Vasospasm of the internal auditory artery: significance in cerebellopontine angle surgery [in process citation]. *Am J Otol* 21: 735–42.

Montaguti M, Bergonzoni C, Zanetti MA & Rinaldi Ceroni A. (2007) Comparative evaluation of ABR abnormalities in patients with and without neurinoma of VIII cranial nerve. *Acta Otorhinolaryngol Ital* 27: 68–72.

Morgan DE & Canalis RF. (1991) Auditory screening of infants. *Otolaryngol Clin North Am* 24: 277–84.

Moskowitz D, Lee KJ & Smith HW. (1984) Steroid use in idiopathic sudden sensorineural hearing loss. *Laryngoscope* 94: 664–6.

Mostafa BE, Tawfik S, Hefnawi NG, Hassan MA & Ismail FA. (2007) The role of deferoxamine in the prevention of gentamicin ototoxicity: a histological and audiological study in guinea pigs. *Acta Otolaryngol* 127: 234–9.

Mrena R, Ylikoski M, Makitie A, Pirvola U & Ylikoski J. (2007) Occupational noise-induced hearing loss reports and tinnitus in Finland. *Acta Otolaryngol* 127: 729–35.

Mulrow CD & Lichtenstein MJ. (1991) Screening for hearing impairment in the elderly: rationale and strategy. *J Gen Intern Med* 6: 249–58.

Musiek FE. (1982) ABR in eighth-nerve and brain-stem disorders. *Am J Otol* 3: 243–8.

Myers E & Bernstein J. (1965) Salicylate ototoxicity. *Arch Otolaryngol* 82: 483–93.

National Institutes of Health (1990) Noise and Hearing Loss. *NIH Consens Statement Online 1990.* Jan 22–24; 8(1):1–24.

Nedzelski J, Schessel D, Bryce G & Pfleiderer A. (1992) Chemical labyrinthectomy: local application of gentamicin for the treatment of unilateral Meniere's disease. *Am J Otol* 13: 18–22.

Norris CH. (1988) Drugs affecting the inner ear. A review of their clinical efficacy, mechanisms of action, toxicity, and place in therapy. *Drugs* 36: 754–72.

Nosrati-Zarenoe R, Arlinger S & Hultcrantz E. (2007) Idiopathic sudden sensorineural hearing loss: results drawn from the Swedish national database. *Acta Otolaryngol* 127: 1168–75.

Olden KW & Drossman DA. (2000) Psychologic and psychiatric aspects of gastrointestinal disease. *Med Clin North Am* 84: 1313–27.

Onusko E. (2004) Tympanometry. *Am Fam Physician* 70: 1713–20.

Papsin BC. (2005) Cochlear implantation in children with anomalous cochleovestibular anatomy. *Laryngoscope* 115: 1–26.

Parsons SK, Neault MW, Lehmann LE, Brennan LL, Eickhoff CE, Kretschmar CS & Diller LR. (1998) Severe ototoxicity following carboplatin-containing conditioning regimen for autologous marrow transplantation for neuroblastoma. *Bone Marrow Transplant* 22: 669–74.

Pasic TR, Heisey D & Love RR. (1997) alpha-difluoromethylornithine ototoxicity. Chemoprevention clinical trial results. *Arch Otolaryngol Head Neck Surg* 123: 1281–6.

Penner MJ. (1989) Empirical tests demonstrating two coexisting sources of tinnitus: a case study. *J Speech Hear Res* 32: 458–62.

Penrod JP. (1994) Speech threshold and word recognition/discrimination testing. In: Katz J, ed. *Handbook of Clinical Audiology*. Williams & Wilkins, Baltimore MD, p. 174.

Pickles J. (1988) *An Introduction to the Physiology of Hearing*. Academic Press, London.

Plinkert PK, Gitter AH & Zenner HP. (1990) Tinnitus associated spontaneous otoacoustic emissions. Active outer hair cell movements as common origin? *Acta Otolaryngol* 110: 342–7.

Prager DA, Stone DA & Rose DN. (1987) Hearing loss screening in the neonatal intensive care unit: auditory brain stem response versus Crib-O-Gram; a cost-effectiveness analysis. *Ear Hear* 8: 213–16.

Quick C & Duvall A. (1970) Early changes in the cochlear duct from ethacrynic acid: an electron-microscopic evaluation. *Laryngoscope* 80: 954–63.

Ramsden R, Rotteveel L, Proops D, Saeed S, van Olphen A & Mylanus E. (2007) Cochlear implantation in otosclerotic deafness. *Adv Otorhinolaryngol* 65: 328–34.

Rask-Andersen H & Stahle J. (1980) Immunodefence of the inner ear? Lymphocyte-macrophage interaction in the endolymphatic sac. *Acta Otolaryngol* 89: 283–94.

Rauschecker JP. (1999) Auditory cortical plasticity: a comparison with other sensory systems. *Trends Neurosci* 22: 74–80.

Richardson GP, Forge A, Kros CJ, Marcotti W, Becker D, Williams DS, Thorpe J, Fleming J, Brown SD & Steel KP. (1999) A missense mutation in myosin VIIA prevents aminoglycoside accumulation in early postnatal cochlear hair cells. *Ann N Y Acad Sci* 884: 110–24.

Riko K, Hyde ML & Alberti PW. (1985) Hearing loss in early infancy: incidence, detection and assessment. *Laryngoscope* 95: 137–45.

Rizzi MD & Hirose K. (2007) Aminoglycoside ototoxicity. *Curr Opin Otolaryngol Head Neck Surg* 15: 352–7.

Rybak L & Matz G. (1986) Effect of Toxic Agents. In: Cummings C, Fredrickson J, Harker L, Krause C & Schuller D, eds. *Otolaryngology-Head and Neck Surgery*, 2nd edn. Mosby Year Book, St Louis, pp. 2943–64.

Rybak LP. (1982) Pathophysiology of furosemide ototoxicity. *J Otolaryngol* 11: 127–33.

Rybak LP. (2007) Mechanisms of cisplatin ototoxicity and progress in otoprotection. *Curr Opin Otolaryngol Head Neck Surg* 15: 364–9.

Saunders JC. (2007) The role of central nervous system plasticity in tinnitus. *J Commun Disord* 40: 313–34.

Saxena AK. (2007) N-acetylcysteine for preventing ototoxicity in hemodialysis patients receiving gentamicin. *Nat Clin Pract Nephrol* 3: 478–9.

Schweitzer V & Olson N. (1984) Ototoxic effect of erythromycin therapy. *Arch Otolaryngol* 110: 258–63.

Schweitzer VG. (1993) Ototoxicity of chemotherapeutic agents. *Otolaryngol Clin North Am* 26: 759–89.

Selivanova OA, Gouveris H, Victor A, Amedee RG & Mann W. (2005) Intratympanic dexamethasone and hyaluronic acid in patients with low-frequency and Meniere's-associated sudden sensorineural hearing loss. *Otol Neurotol* 26: 890–5.

Shaia FT & Sheehy JL. (1976) Sudden sensori-neural hearing impairment: a report of 1,220 cases. *Laryngoscope* 86: 389–98.

Shine NP & Coates H. (2005) Systemic ototoxicity: a review. *East Afr Med J* 82: 536–9.

Shownkeen H, Yoo K, Leonetti J & Origitano TC. (2001) Endovascular treatment of transverse-sigmoid sinus dural arteriovenous malformations presenting as pulsatile tinnitus. *Skull Base* 11: 13–23.

Shulman A & Goldstein B. (2000) Intratympanic drug therapy with steroids for tinnitus control: a preliminary report. *Int Tinnitus J* 6: 10–20.

Silverstein H, Choo D, Rosenberg SI, Kuhn J, Seidman M & Stein I. (1996) Intratympanic steroid treatment of inner ear disease and tinnitus (preliminary report). *Ear Nose Throat J* 75: 468–471, 474, 476 passim.

Silverstein J, Bernstein J & Davies D. (1967) Salicylate ototoxicity: a biochemical and electrophysiological study. *Ann Otol Rhinol Larngol* 76: 118–27.

Smith RJ, Zimmerman B, Connolly PK, Jerger SW & Yelich A. (1992) Screening audiometry using the high-risk register in a level III nursery. *Arch Otolaryngol Head Neck Surg* 118: 1306–11.

Smits M, Kovacs S, de Ridder D, Peeters RR, van Hecke P & Sunaert S. (2007) Lateralization of functional magnetic resonance imaging (fMRI) activation in the auditory pathway of patients with lateralized tinnitus. *Neuroradiology* **49**: 669–79.

Smoorenburg GF, De Groot JC, Hamers FP & Klis SF. (1999) Protection and spontaneous recovery from cisplatin-induced hearing loss. *Ann N Y Acad Sci* **884**: 192–210.

So H, Kim H, Lee JH, Park C, Kim Y, Kim E, Kim JK, Yun KJ, Lee KM, Lee HY, Moon SK, Lim DJ & Park R. (2007) Cisplatin cytotoxicity of auditory cells requires secretions of proinflammatory cytokines via activation of ERK and NF-kappaB. *J Assoc Res Otolaryngol* **8**: 338–55.

Sonmez G, Basekim CC, Ozturk E, Gungor A & Kizilkaya E. (2007) Imaging of pulsatile tinnitus: a review of 74 patients. *Clin Imaging* **31**: 102–8.

Stokroos RJ, Albers FW & Tenvergert EM. (1998) Antiviral treatment of idiopathic sudden sensorineural hearing loss: a prospective, randomized, double-blind clinical trial. *Acta Otolaryngol* **118**: 488–95.

Stypulowski P. (1990) Mechanisms of salicylate ototoxicity. *Hear Res* **46**.

Sullivan MD, Katon W, Dobie R, Sakai C, Russo J & Harrop-Griffiths J. (1988) Disabling tinnitus. Association with affective disorder. *Gen Hosp Psychiatry* **10**: 285–91.

Tomiyama S & Harris JP. (1987) The role of the endolymphatic sac in inner ear immunity. *Acta Otolaryngol* **103**: 182–8.

Topal O, Erbek SS, Erbek S & Ozluoglu LN. (2008) Subjective pulsatile tinnitus associated with extensive pneumatization of temporal bone. *Eur Arch Otorhinolaryngol* **265**: 123–5.

Tran Ba Huy P, Bernard P & Schacht J. (1986) Kinetics of gentamicin uptake and release in the rat: comparison of inner ear tissues and fluids with other organs. *J Clin Invest* **77**: 1492–500.

Trimble K, Blaser S, James AL & Papsin BC. (2007) Computed tomography and/or magnetic resonance imaging before pediatric cochlear implantation? Developing an investigative strategy. *Otol Neurotol* **28**: 317–24.

Van Naarden K, Decoufle P & Caldwell K. (1999) Prevalence and characteristics of children with serious hearing impairment in metropolitan Atlanta, 1991–1993. *Pediatrics* **103**: 570–5.

Van Prooyen-Keyzer S, Sadik JC, Ulanovski D, Parmantier M & Ayache D. (2005) Study of the posterior communicating arteries of the circle of Willis in idiopathic sudden sensorineural hearing loss. *Otol Neurotol* **26**: 385–6.

Vasama JP & Linthicum FH Jr. (2000) Idiopathic sudden sensorineural hearing loss: temporal bone histopathologic study. *Ann Otol Rhinol Laryngol* **109**: 527–32.

Veldman JE, Hanada T & Meeuwsen F. (1993) Diagnostic and therapeutic dilemmas in rapidly progressive sensorineural hearing loss and sudden deafness. A reappraisal of immune reactivity in inner ear disorders. *Acta Otolaryngol* **113**: 303–6.

Vernon J, Griest S & Press L. (1990) Attributes of tinnitus and the acceptance of masking. *Am J Otolaryngol* **11**: 44–50.

Wake M, Tobin S, Cone-Wesson B, Dahl HH, Gillam L, McCormick L, Poulakis Z, Rickards FW, Saunders K, Ukoumunne OC & Williams J. (2006) Slight/mild sensorineural hearing loss in children. *Pediatrics* **118**: 1842–51.

Wallace MR, Miller LK, Nguyen MT & Shields AR. (1994) Ototoxicity with azithromycin [letter]. *Lancet* **343**: 241.

Walsted A, Andreassen UK, Berthelsen PG & Olesen A. (2000) Hearing loss after cardiopulmonary bypass surgery. *Eur Arch Otorhinolaryngol* **257**: 124–7.

Wei X, Zhao L, Liu J, Dodel RC, Farlow MR & Du Y. (2005) Minocycline prevents gentamicin-induced ototoxicity by inhibiting p38 MAP kinase phosphorylation and caspase 3 activation. *Neuroscience* **131**: 513–21.

Weiss M, Kisiel D & Bhatia P. (1990) Predictive value of brainstem evoked response in the diagnosis of acoustic neuroma. *Otolaryngol Head Neck Surg* **103**: 583–5.

Wells KB & Sherbourne CD. (1999) Functioning and utility for current health of patients with depression or chronic medical conditions in managed, primary care practices. *Arch Gen Psychiatry* **56**: 897–904.

Williams S, Zenner H & Schacht J. (1987) Three molecular steps of aminoglycoside ototoxicity demonstrated in outer hair cells. *Hear Res* **30**: 11–22.

Wilson D, Hodgson R, Gustafson M, Hogue S & Mills L. (1992) The sensitivity of auditory brainstem response testing in small acoustic neuromas. *Laryngoscope* **102**: 961–4.

Wilson WR, Byl FM & Laird N. (1980) The efficacy of steroids in the treatment of idiopathic sudden hearing loss. A double-blind clinical study. *Arch Otolaryngol* **106**: 772–6.

Wilson WR, Laird N, Moo-Young G, Soeldner JS, Kavesh DA & MacMeel JW. (1982) The relationship of idiopathic sudden hearing loss to diabetes mellitus. *Laryngoscope* **92**: 155–60.

Wong L & Bance M. (2004) Are all cookie-bite audiograms hereditary hearing loss?. *J Otolaryngol* **33**: 390–2.

Xenellis J, Karapatsas I, Papadimitriou N, Nikolopoulos T, Maragoudakis P, Tzagkaroulakis M & Ferekidis E. (2006) Idiopathic sudden sensorineural hearing loss: prognostic factors. *J Laryngol Otol* **120**: 718–24.

Yehudai D, Shoenfeld Y & Toubi E. (2006) The autoimmune characteristics of progressive or sudden sensorineural hearing loss. *Autoimmunity* **39**: 153–8.

Chapter 3

External and middle ear function

John J Rosowski

3.1 Introduction

My objective in writing this chapter is to give a general background to the study of the external and middle ear, as well as to highlight the important advances made in our understanding of the roles of the external and middle ear over the past 15 years. The chapter starts with an overview of the auditory periphery, including a brief discussion of the structure and function of the external and middle ear. Since the primary role of the external and middle ear is to pass the sound stimulus from the environment to the inner ear, the next section discusses the fundamental sound stimulus to the inner ear. This is followed by an overview of how the external and middle ear work together to produce an effective cochlear stimulus. The fourth section of the chapter reviews some of the more recent findings on external and middle ear function. The fifth section discusses the clinical relevance of some of these findings to both our understanding of pathology and the diagnosis of disease. The last section highlights some of the unanswered questions regarding the structure and function of the external and middle ear.

3.2 An overview of the auditory periphery

The primary purpose of the auditory periphery is to gather sound and transduce it into neural impulses in the auditory portion of cranial nerve VIII. This process is summarized in a schematic of the auditory periphery of a mammal in Fig. 3.1. The auditory periphery can be broken into three functionally and anatomically distinct components: the external, middle, and inner ear. Sound from the free-field, here quantified in terms of its sound pressure, P_{PW}, impinges on the head and body. The sound wave is diffracted and scattered by the head, body, and the ear, and some fraction of the incident sound energy is gathered at the entrance to the ear canal, where it produces a sound pressure, P_{EX}. That sound is transformed as it travels down the roughly cylindrical ear canal to the tympanic membrane (TM), where it results in a sound pressure, P_T, and a volume velocity of the TM, U_T. The sound acting on the TM sets the ossicles into motion. The mechanical motion of the ossicles produces a sound pressure, P_V, and volume velocity of the stapes, U_S, in the oval window, OW, at the entrance to the lymph-filled inner ear. As discussed in later chapters, the sound pressure and volume velocity in the lymphs within the vestibule (or entrance) of the inner ear stimulate the cochlear partition, resulting in motion of the partition's basilar membrane and mechanical stimulation of the hair cells within the partition. The hair cells produce graded electrical activity that evokes synaptic stimulation of the auditory portion of the VIIIth cranial nerve.

The external ear is the most peripheral subunit of the auditory periphery; it is made up of the pinna flange or flap, the funnel-shaped concha (the parts of the ear that are most visible to observers), and the more hidden tube-like external ear canal. (As will be discussed later, it can be argued that the functional components of the external ear include the head and body.) Figure 3.2

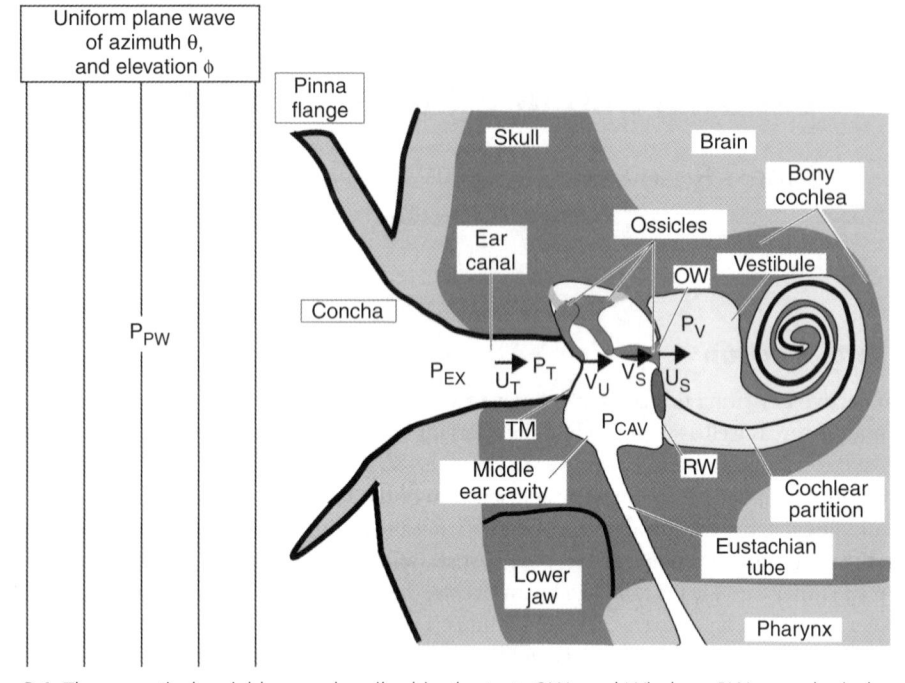

Fig. 3.1 The acoustical variables are described in the text. OW, oval Window; RW, round window; TM, tympanic membrane.
Modified from Rosowski (1994).

illustrates the schematics of these structures in humans based on the illustrations of Shaw (1974b). The medial boundary of the external ear is the tympanic membrane, which serves as the entrance to the air-filled middle ear. A typical human pinna flange is about 7 cm in height and 6 cm in width, while a typical human ear canal is about 0.75 cm in diameter and 2.3 cm long (Shaw, 1974b). However, there is much variation in size and the details of the external ear structure within humans (e.g. Keefe *et al.*, 1993, 1994; Middlebrooks, 1999; Xu & Middlebrooks, 2000). These deviations in size affect the external ear gain, the transformation of sound pressure between the environmental stimulus P_{PW} and the sound pressure at the entrance to the middle ear P_T.

The middle ear (Fig. 3.3) consists of the middle ear air space or tympanum, the tympanic or drum membrane, the ossicles (the malleus, incus, and stapes) and their supports, and the middle ear muscles and tendons (the tensor tympani muscle and the stapedius muscle). The middle ear is connected to the inner ear via the oval and round windows (OW and RW in Fig. 3.3). The aeration of the middle ear air spaces is maintained by periodic opening of the eustachian tube (Ingelstedt & Jonson, 1966), and pathologies that induce temporary or permanent failure of the eustachian tube lead to replacement of the middle ear air by fluid (Sadé & Amos, 1997; Doyle, 2000) as well as atelectasis, a pathological inward displacement of the tympanic membrane that helps compensate for the loss of air within the middle ear (Luntz & Sadé, 1990; Luntz *et al.*, 1997). The middle ear air space is often broken into multiple compartments, whose morphology varies greatly in a species-dependent manner (Hyrtl, 1844; Onchi, 1961; Zwislocki, 1962; Henson, 1974; Novacek, 1977; Browning & Granich, 1978; Huang *et al.*, 1997; see Fig. 3.4B). Indeed, the morphology of the middle ear air spaces, including the particular bones of the skull that surround them (e.g. the petrous, tympanic, and squamosal bones contribute to the middle ear walls in

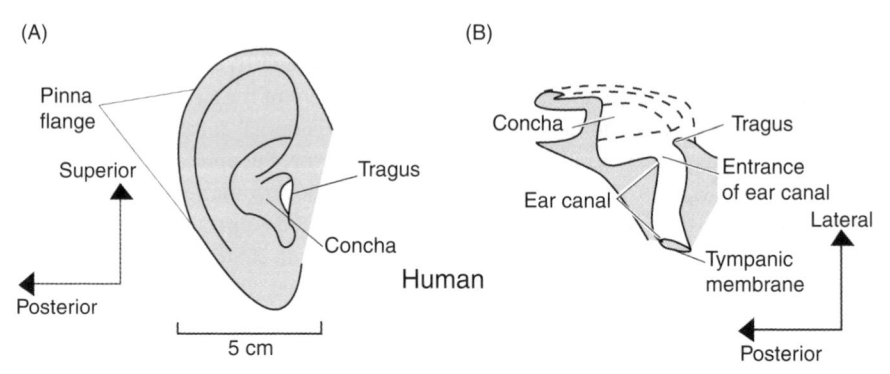

Fig. 3.2 The human external ear. (A) Lateral view of the flap-like pinna flange and the funnel-shaped concha. The tragus, a small projection of skin near the entrance of the ear canal is also visible. (B) A schematic horizontal section through the external ear at the level of the ear canal. The gently curving ear canal is approximately cylindrical in shape. The canal is terminated at its medial end by the tympanic membrane.
Modified from Shaw (1974b).

humans) has been used to decide taxonomic relationships between different mammalian species (Hunt, 1974; Novacek, 1977; Hunt & Korth, 1980; Moore, 1981).

The mammalian tympanic membrane generally is separated into two subunits (Kohllöffel, 1984; Vrettakos *et al.*, 1988). The pars tensa, which is tightly coupled to the handle of the malleus (the manubrium of the malleus; Fig. 3.4A), is usually the larger of the two subunits, though there is wide interspecies variation in the relative sizes of the subunits (Kohllöffel, 1984; Vrettakos *et al.*, 1988; Rosowski *et al.*, 1997). The pars tensa of the mammalian tympanic membrane is usually tent shaped, with a central spine coupled to the malleus handle and a circular or oval-shaped surround. The coupling between the tympanic membrane and malleus handle can be one continuous band or more localized as in humans (Schuknecht, 1974), where the coupling is strongest near the two extremes of the malleus handle. The malleus handle is positioned medially to the supporting tympanic ring with the result that the center of the tympanic membrane is pulled into the middle ear air space relative to the ring. Sound-induced motion of the pars tensa is strongly (but not perfectly) coupled to the motion of the malleus handle. The pars flaccida is generally smaller than

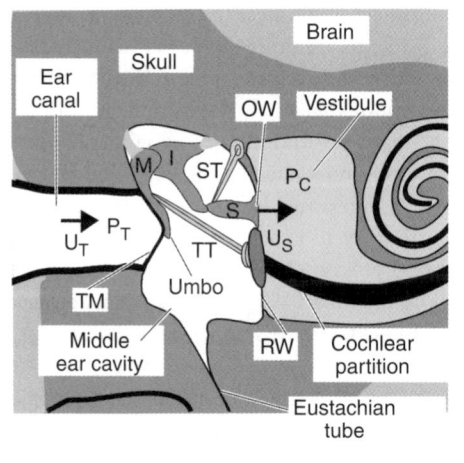

Fig. 3.3 The ossicular chain: malleus (M); incus (I); and stapes (S). ST, tendon of the stapedius muscle; TT, tendon of the tensor tympani muscle. (Three-dimensional reconstructions of the human middle ear are available from http://research.meei.harvard.edu/otopathology/3dmodels/3dviewer.html.)

the tensa and positioned dorsally or posteriorly to the tympanic ring. The flaccida was first described by Shrapnell (1832), and is much looser in form. The difference in tension within the tensa and flaccida may be due to differences in the arrangement of the structural fibers that contribute to the middle ear layer of these trilaminar structures (Funnell & Laszlo, 1982). The fibers have a well-organized circular or radial arrangement in the tensa, but appear randomly organized in flaccida (Lim, 1968a,b, 1970). The flaccida is easily displaced by variations in middle ear static pressure (Decraemer & Dirckx, 1998) and has been suggested to protect the ear from small changes in air volume or pressure (Stenfors et al., 1979; Hellstrom & Stenfors, 1983) although the maximum volume displacement of the flaccida is small compared with the volume of the middle ear (Decraemer & Dirckx, 1998; Dirckx et al., 1998). Others have suggested that the flaccida can serve to decrease the sensitivity of the ear to low sound frequencies (Kohllöffel, 1984; Rosowski et al., 1997; Teoh et al., 1997) by shunting ear canal sound pressure through the relatively low-impedance flaccida into the middle ear air space without displacing the pars tensa. In support of this idea, several studies have demonstrated that the sound-induced motions of the flaccida are not coupled to the motion of the ossicles (Rosowski et al., 1997; Teoh et al., 1997; Rosowski & Lee, 2002).

The three ossicles (Fig. 3.4) – the small bones of the middle ear sound transmission system – are: the malleus (hammer), with its long handle (the manubrium, which is partially embedded in the tympanic membrane), neck and head; the incus with its large body attached to the head of the malleus by a synovial joint in some animals (e.g. primates, carnivores), but in others (many rodents) the joint is very thin and stiff or even ankylosed; and the stirrup-shaped stapes with its nearly flat footplate. (This is another point of variation, where some animals, for example, some moles and kangaroo rats have a bulbous convexity in the surface of the footplate (Henson, 1974; Mason, 2001)). The stapes is attached to the incus by another synovial joint (Funnell et al., 2005), which allows flexing of the joint in some directions but not others (Pang & Peake, 1986; Funnell et al., 2005). Recent findings on the functions of the two ossicular joints will be a point of later discussion.

The three ossicles are supported by the tympanic membrane and three primary ligaments: the anterior ligament of the malleus (AML in Fig. 3.4B), the posterior ligament of the incus (PIL in Fig. 3.4B) and the annular ligament that holds the stapes footplate within the oval window. These three ligaments act to constrain the motion of the ossicles: at low frequencies – frequencies less than 1000 Hz in humans, and less than 10 000 Hz in mouse (Saunders & Summers, 1982) – the ossicles rotate about the axis defined by the AML and PIL, but, as will be discussed later, ossicular motion is more complicated at frequencies above 1000 Hz (Decraemer & Khanna, 2004). Some authors (e.g. Dai et al., 2007; Sim & Puria, 2008) suggest that there are other ossicular ligaments, for example, the superior mallear ligament, but others (e.g. Merchant, 2006, personal communication) suggest that these putative ligaments are simply folds in the mucosal lining that surrounds the ossicles and the inner surface of the middle ear and add no firm support to the ossicles.

The middle ear muscles and their tendons (Figs 3.3, 3.4) are effectors for the efferent control of middle ear sound transmission and static positioning of the tympanic membrane and ossicles. The stapedius muscle (SM in Fig. 3.4B) is innervated by the VIIth (facial) nerve, while the tensor tympani muscle (TTM in Fig. 3.4B) is innervated by the motor branch of the Vth (trigeminal) nerve. Contractions of the stapedius muscle are associated with the 'acoustic reflex', where moderate to loud sounds (60–100 dB sound pressure level (SPL)) in conscious humans and animals (Møller, 1964, 1974; Borg, 1968; Borg & Møller, 1968; Silman, 1984; Feeney & Keefe, 1999) produce reflex contractions that lead to increases in the stapes–annular-ligament impedance (Pang & Peake, 1986) and decreases in middle ear sound transmission (Wever & Lawrence, 1954; Møller, 1974). Louder sounds can also evoke reflex contraction of the tensor tympani. The muscles are also known to contract just prior to vocalization in humans and bats (Henson, 1965; Borg &

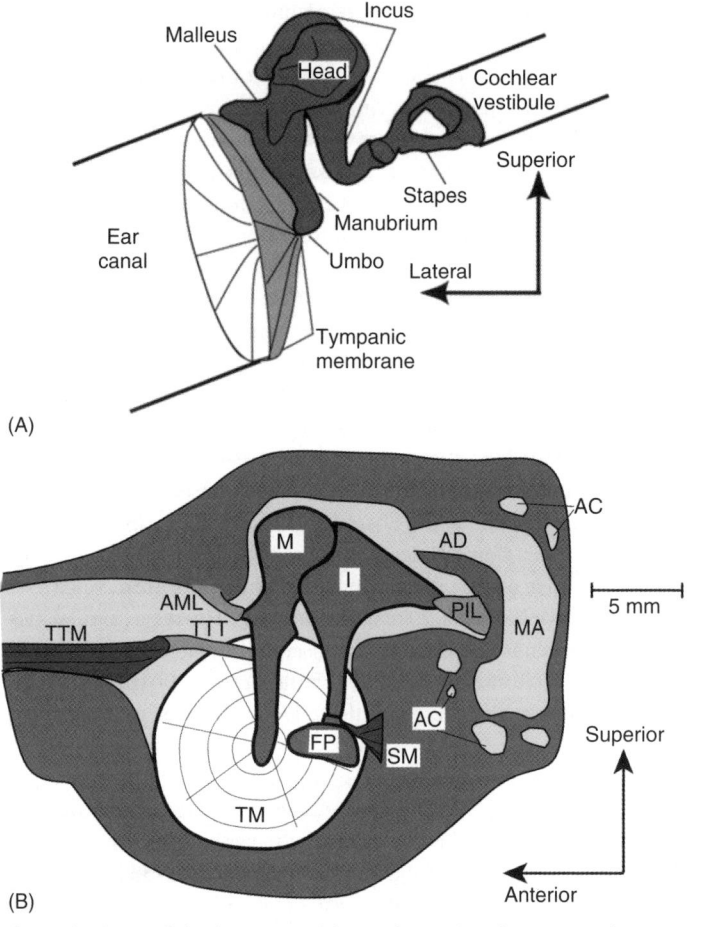

Fig. 3.4 Two schematic views of the human ossicles and associated anatomical structures. (A) Anterolateral view of the ossicles. The malleus and its three components, the head, manubrium, and umbo, are labeled along with the incus and stapes. (B) A medial view of the middle ear. The ossicles: FP, footplate of the stapes; I, incus; M, malleus. The muscles, tendons and ligaments: AML, anterior mallear ligament; PIL, posterior incudal ligament; SM, stapedius muscle and its tendon; TTT, tensor tympani tendon; TTM, tensor tympani muscle. The middle ear spaces are lighter gray in color and include the area behind the tympanic membrane (TM): AD, aditus ad antrum; MA, mastoid antrum; AC, mastoid air cells.
Modified from Henson (1974).

Zakrisson, 1975). The tensor tympani is closely associated with the muscles that control tension in the walls of the eustachian tube and it has been suggested that tensor contraction is an important part of the reflex that opens the eustachian tube (Ingelstedt & Jonson, 1966). The combination of the two muscles and three ossicles allows independent control of different parts of the ossicular chain (Møller, 1983). For example, slippage in the incudostapedial joint permits contractions of the stapedius muscle to produce changes in the position of stapes head of several hundred micrometers in amplitude (Pang & Peake, 1986) without generating similar large movements of the incus. Similarly, the presence of the incudomalleal joint allows the tensor tympani to produce

100–500 μm-sized inward movements of the tympanic membrane without generating similar large-sized motions of the stapes (Marquet, 1981; Hüttenbrink, 1988).

In recent years there has been discussion of a possible third middle ear efferent system. These reports center on findings of putative smooth muscle elements within the tympanic ring that appear closely associated with the radial fibers of the pars tensa (Kuijpers et al., 1999; Henson & Henson, 2000; Henson et al., 2005). Yang & Henson (2002) have also reported small alterations in middle ear sound transmission produced by the application of pharmacological agents that are known to modulate smooth muscle contraction to the tympanic membrane. However, at least one attempt to repeat these observations was not successful (Graves, 2005).

A question that is open to speculation is whether the middle ear muscles produce an active pretension on the middle ear sound transmission system. It has been repeatedly demonstrated that excision of the middle ear muscles produces little change in the sound-induced motion of the ossicles in anesthetized or dead (before the onset or after the relaxation of rigor) animals (Wever & Lawrence, 1954; Guinan & Peake, 1967; Voss et al., 2000a; Chien et al., 2006a; Rosowski et al., 2006). However, in chinchillas anesthetized with pentobarbital and ketamine for several hours, rhythmic or chronic contractions of the muscles have been observed that can reduce middle ear sound transmission by more than 20 dB (Rosowski et al., 2006). (Similar rhythmic contractions have been observed in guinea pigs (Wiggers, 1937).) Whether the relaxed state or the chronic contraction is more evocative of the normal conscious state is not clear, since few measurements of middle ear function have been made in awake animals. However, similarities in middle ear admittance and sound-driven umbo velocity in conscious humans and cadaveric temporal bones (Rosowski et al., 1990; Goode et al., 1993, 1996; Huber et al., 2001b; Whittemore et al., 2004; Chien et al., 2006a,b) suggest that there is little active pretension produced by the middle ear muscles in live humans.

The final topic of this overview deals with the interdependence of the function of the different external and middle ear components. This can be seen at the gross structural level between segments of the ear, where it is known that the external-ear-based transformation between free-field sound and sound pressure and volume velocity at the tympanic membrane depends on the acoustic load of the middle ear at the termination of the ear canal (this load is often called the middle ear input impedance; Shaw, 1974a; Rosowski, 1994). Variations in the impedance of the middle ear can alter the sound pressure and volume-velocity at the tympanic membrane produced by a controlled external stimulus (Bismarck & Pfeiffer, 1967 cited in Shaw, 1974b; Voss et al., 2000b). Similarly the sound-induced motion of the tympanic membrane and the stapes depends on the inner ear's load on the middle ear (the cochlear input impedance; Møller, 1965; Allen, 1986; Peake et al., 1992; Puria & Allen, 1998; Songer & Rosowski, 2007a). These interactions of 'source' and 'load' are also apparent at the level of individual structural components, where the motion of the malleus depends on the mobility of the body of the incus and the rest of the ossicular chain (Willi et al., 2002; Rosowski et al., 2008). This interdependence of the function of components of the auditory periphery is explicit in simple electrical circuits models (Fig. 3.5; Goode et al., 1994), as well as more complicated finite-element and finite-difference models of external and middle ear function (Ladak & Funnell, 1996; Koike et al., 2002; Gan et al., 2006b).

A simple acoustic-electric analog model that clearly specifies the load-dependences of the sound transformations performed by the different model blocks is illustrated in Figure 3.5. Other electric and mechanical analogs have the same feature (Møller, 1961; Zwislocki, 1962; Kringlebotn, 1988; Shera & Zweig, 1992a; Goode et al., 1994; Songer & Rosowski, 2007a,b). The simple network of Figure 3.5 also has the advantage that each of the acoustical variables in the block can be quantified by measurements in real ears (Rosowski et al., 1986; Rosowski, 1991a,b).

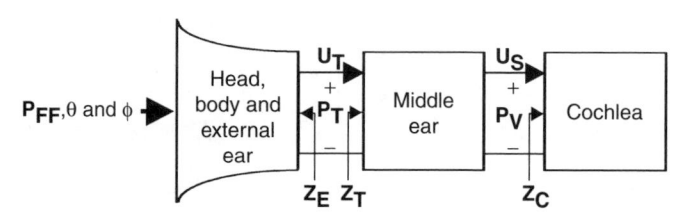

Fig. 3.5 A general acoustic-electric model of external and middle ear function. P_{FF}, free-field sound pressure; Z_E, radiation impedance from the ear; Z_T, middle ear input impedance; U_T, volume velocity of the tympanic membrane; P_T, sound pressure at the tympanic membrane; U_S, stapes volume velocity; Z_C, cochlear input impedance; P_V, sound pressure in the vestibule. After Rosowski (1991a).

3.3 What is the effective stimulus to the inner ear, and how is it produced by the external and middle ear?

3.3.1 The standard model of two cochlear windows looking into an incompressible space

The inner ear of mammals and many terrestrial vertebrates is often described as being made up of incompressible fluid, surrounded by incompressible bone, where 'incompressible' is shorthand for much less compressible than air. The relative incompressibility of the water-like inner ear lymphs and bone can be described more quantitatively by comparing the bulk modulus (a measure of the stiffness of a volume of material) for air (10^5 Pa: Kinsler *et al.*, 1982), water (2×10^9: Kinsler *et al.*, 1982) and bone ($5–10 \times 10^9$: Fung, 1981), where we see that water and bone are 20 000–100 000 times more stiff than air. Because of this great stiffness, an inner ear made up of a simple volume of lymph and soft tissue surrounded by bone would have an extremely high input impedance and would require extremely large ossicularly derived sound pressures acting on the stapes within the oval window in order to induce any motion of cochlear fluids. Nature's solution to this dilemma was the development of a second window into the 'incompressible' inner ear, the round window, which acts as a low-impedance boundary or more colloquially, a pressure release. (Round windows are apparent in fossil vertebrates that pre-date the age of dinosaurs and early mammals (Allin & Hopson, 1992).) The two-window system permits inward and outward motions of the stapes in the oval window to be balanced by displacements of the round window of equal volume but opposite direction (Fig. 3.6; Stenfelt *et al.*, 2004). (This coupling of the window motions is known by clinicians as the 'round window reflex' (Goodhill, 1979).) The two fluid-coupled cochlear windows change the cochlear load on the middle ear from a quantity dependent on the low compressibility of the water-like lymphs to one dependent on the impedance of the cochlear windows as well as the impedance associated with sound transfer through the inner ear (Zwislocki, 1950, 1965; Lynch *et al.*, 1982; Puria & Allen, 1991).

The coupling of the motion of the two cochlear windows by an incompressible fluid requires that sound-induced motion of the cochlea fluids must be accompanied by a difference in sound pressure outside the two cochlear windows, for it is only with such a pressure difference that the 'column' of fluid connecting the windows can be set into motion. (This requirement can be weakened if there are compressible elements within the cochlea (Shera & Zweig, 1992b) or more than the two windows into the cochlea (Ranke, 1953 as cited in Tonndorf, 1972; Peake *et al.*, 1992).) It is generally believed that the alternating motions of the incompressible cochlear fluid, which

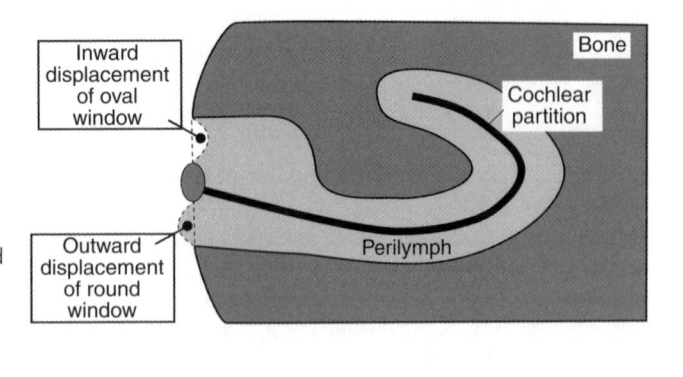

Fig. 3.6 Two cochlear windows bordering a volume of 'incompressible' fluid surrounded by 'incompressible' bone. After Voss *et al.* (1996).

result from the window-pressure difference, produce the transcochlear-partition pressure difference that launches the slow waves of partition motion required for stimulation of the organ of Corti and its hair cells. However, others suggest the hair cells respond directly to the sound pressure within the inner ear, for example, Sohmer and colleagues (Sohmer & Freeman, 2004; Sohmer *et al.*, 2004; Sohmer, 2006).

Wever and Lawrence (1950, 1954) and others (Voss *et al.*, 1996) have performed some simple experiments designed to differentiate between the pressure-difference and direct pressure stimulation hypotheses. The approach used by Voss and colleagues (as well as Wever and others) was to control independently the sound pressure at both the oval window (P_{OW}) and round window (P_{RW}). Tonal sound stimuli of equal magnitude but varied phase were presented to the two windows, while the cochlear microphonic was recorded with an electrode near the round window. The results from one set of stimuli are presented in Figure 3.7, where 90 dB SPL 1000 Hz tones were presented simultaneously at the two cochlear windows; the two stimuli were of varied phase and the difference in phase was defined by Ψ. Figure 3.7 showed that a maximum cochlear microphonic response was obtained when Ψ was about ± 0.5 cycles, and that the response decreased by more than 40 dB, when the two stimuli were in phase and Ψ equaled 0. An inner ear that responds to the absolute sound pressure within the cochlea (rather than the window-pressure difference) would show a pattern of response opposite to that of Figure 3.7, with large response when $\Psi = 0$ (where the two pressures summed within the inner ear) and a minima in response when $\Psi = \pm 0.5$ (where the two pressures cancel). Furthermore, Voss *et al.* (1996) demonstrated that the shape of the measured relationship between the magnitude and phase of the cochlear microphonic and Ψ was consistent with a sensor whose response to a difference in pressure at the two windows was at least 100 times larger than a response to the summed pressures. (Voss *et al.* (1996) pointed out that their estimates of the relative sensitivity to the pressure difference and the pressure sum were noise limited. The 100 times difference in sensitivity to the summed and difference pressures they measured is a minimum estimate of the relative sizes of the response to these different stimuli.)

The deep notches measured by Wever and Lawrence (1950, 1954) and Voss *et al.* (1996) in these cancellation experiments demonstrate the dominance of the window pressure-difference mode of cochlear sensitivity and also place severe limits on the sensitivity of the inner ear to direct-pressure stimulation. The data of Voss *et al.* (1996) also place considerable limits on the importance of any normal 'third-window' paths within the inner ear (the 'third window' is a term applied to the sum of the effects of the multiple small fluid pathways that connect the inner ear to the cranial cavity, and includes the cochlear and vestibular aqueduct as well as the vascular and neural pathways that feed and innervate the inner ear (see e.g. Tonndorf & Khanna, 1970; Ranke, 1953) and on the innate compressibility of cochlear structures (Shera & Zweig, 1992b)).

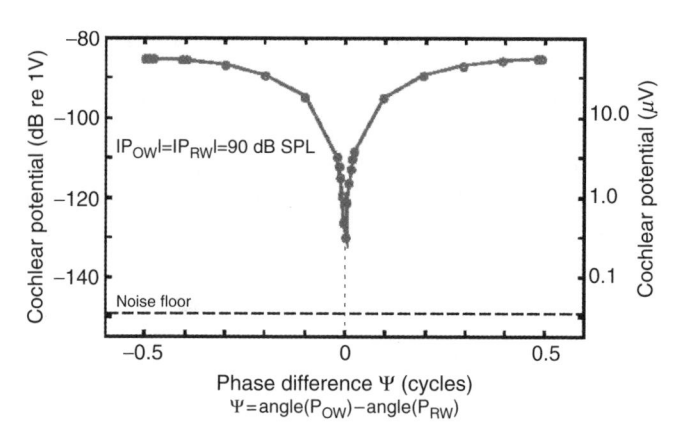

Fig. 3.7 A cat's cochlear response to the simultaneous stimulation of the oval and round window with equal amplitude tonal sound pressures (the magnitudes of P_{OW} and P_{RW} = 90 dB SPL) of varying phase. The sound frequency is 1 kHz. the difference in phase between the two stimuli is defined by the phase difference (Ψ) on the x-axis.
Modified from Voss *et al.* (1996).

Third-window paths or cochlear compressibility, however, may play a role in the ears response to bone-conduction stimulation (Ranke, 1953; Békésy, 1960; Tonndorf & Tabor, 1962; Tonndorf, 1972; Stenfelt *et al.*, 2004; Stenfelt & Goode, 2005a).

One criticism of the Wever and Lawrence type of cancellation measurements (as in Fig. 3.7) is that they were performed using fairly high-level (90–110 dB SPL) sound stimuli to directly stimulate the cochlear windows. It should be noted that because of the approximately 25 dB of amplification of ear canal sound-pressure stimulus produced by the normal cat middle ear (Nedzelnitsky, 1980; Décory *et al.*, 1988), the 90 dB SPL oval window sound pressure used in gathering the data of Figure 3.7 is equivalent to an ear canal sound pressure of only 65 dB SPL, a moderate stimulus level. Furthermore even with a 65 dB SPL ear canal sound pressure equivalent, the deep notch in Figure 3.7 suggests that any pressure-sum component is at least 40 dB smaller than the pressure-difference component.

3.3.2 Clinical support for the window pressure-difference model of cochlear sensitivity to sound

There are several bodies of clinical evidence consistent with the window pressure-difference model of the inner ear's sensitivity to sound. These data include the effects of stapes and round window fixation on air-conducted thresholds in patients (e.g. Harrison *et al.*, 1964; Schuknecht, 1974; Cherukupally *et al.*, 1998; Linder *et al.*, 2003), but more direct evidence can be found in pathologies and surgical interventions that directly affect the window-pressure difference. As will be discussed in the next section, one way in which the tympanic membrane and ossicular chain maximize the window-pressure difference in the normal ear is to couple the sound they gather to a single cochlear window, the oval window, while reducing the sound pressure that reaches the round window. Pathologies that interfere with the ossicularly coupled sound greatly reduce the effective sound pressure at the oval window, resulting in more equal window pressures and a smaller window-pressure difference. A total interruption of the ossicular chain nearly equalizes the sound pressure at the oval and round windows (Békésy, 1947, 1960; Voss *et al.*, 2007), which reduces the window-pressure difference to near 0, and results in a 50–60 dB hearing loss

(Fig. 3.8B; Peake *et al.*, 1992). Otological surgeons attempt to reintroduce the window-pressure difference by using ossicular replacement prostheses to recouple the original tympanic membrane (or a graft tympanic membrane) to the oval window (Wüllstein, 1956; Lee & Schuknecht, 1971; Brackmann *et al.*, 1984; Merchant *et al.*, 2003).

In cases of severe middle ear disease in which the tympanic membrane, malleus, and incus are severely diseased or missing, a simpler middle ear reconstruction might be attempted, where the oval window and much of the original middle ear air space are left externalized to the ear canal, and a grafted 'sound-shield' is placed between the ear canal and the round window. The new air space formed behind the graft (the 'cavum minor') contains the round window and retains a connection to the eustachian tube (Fig. 3.8A). This procedure has been labeled a type IV tympanoplasty by Wüllstein (1956). Patients with successful type IV surgery show a 30–40 dB improvement in their presurgical hearing loss (Fig. 3.8B). This increase in hearing sensitivity is consistent with the grafted sound-shield reducing the sound pressure near the round window and increasing the window-pressure difference by 30–40 dB (Peake *et al.*, 1992). As we shall see later, the residual postsurgical hearing loss of about 20–25 dB after type IV surgery is consistent with the loss of the pressure gain that results from the action of the normal tympanic membrane and ossicles.

(A)

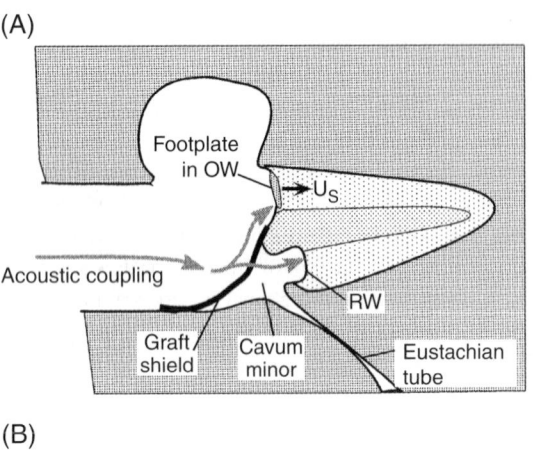

(B)

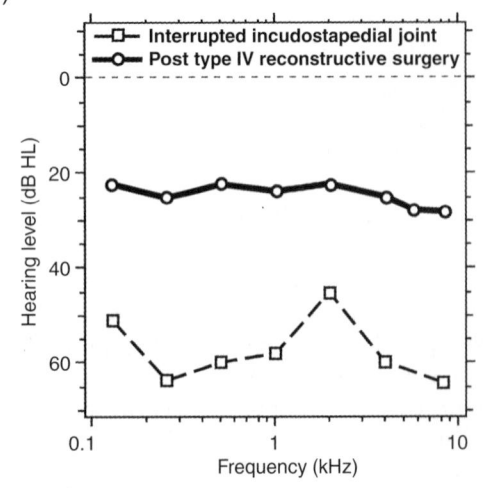

Fig. 3.8 Type IV tympanoplasty. (A) Schematic of the reconstructive surgery where a stiff acoustic graft shield is placed between the ear canal and the round window (RW) to form a 'cavum minor' that is coupled to the functioning eustachian tube. (B) Comparison of the average audiograms of eight patients with total interruption of the incudostapedial joint and four patients after type IV tympanoplasty. U_S, stapes volume velocity. Modified after Peake *et al.* (1992).

In discussing type IV surgery, Wüllstein (1956) clearly described the technique in terms of using the grafted sound-shield to maximize the difference in sound pressure at the two windows. However, surgical case studies since that time (Proctor, 1964; Gotay-Rodriguez & Schuknecht, 1977) point to highly variable postoperative results in patients with type IV surgery. Several factors seem to explain the variability in response, including the use of thin flexible graft shields that inadequately reduce the sound pressure outside the round window (Merchant *et al.*, 1995, 1997). A surgical procedure which minimizes the round window sound pressure and maximizes the mobility of the stapes and round window yields postsurgical hearing results much like those in Figure 3.8B (Merchant *et al.*, 1997).

3.3.3 Sound transmission through the middle ear

The sensitivity of the inner ear to the difference in sound pressure between the oval and round window suggests that there are two acoustic pathways for airborne sound from the environment to stimulate the inner ear (Kobrak, 1959; Peake *et al.*, 1992; Fig. 3.9). (A third potential stimulus path is bone conduction, which will be discussed separately.) One acoustic pathway ('acoustic coupling' in Fig. 3.9) depends on sound directly stimulating the oval and round windows within the middle ear air space, much like the controlled sound stimulus of the Wever and Lawrence (1950) and Voss *et al.* (1996) experiments. Sound conducted down the ear canal sets the tympanic membrane into motion, which condenses and rarifies the air within the closed middle ear air space, creating a sound pressure, P_{ME}. This middle ear sound pressure stimulates the oval and round windows. Since for much of the frequency range of interest, the dimensions of the middle ear spaces are much smaller than the wavelength of sound, the middle ear sound pressures just outside the oval and round windows will be very similar to the pressure within the middle ear: $P_{ME} \cong P_{OW} \cong P_{RW}$. However, because of small non-uniformities in the cavity shape, P_{OW} and P_{RW} are not exactly equal and the difference, $\Delta P = P_{OW} - P_{RW}$, is non-zero but small. Békésy (1947, 1960) and Voss *et al.* (2007, see Fig. 3.10) measured the acoustically coupled P_{OW} and P_{RW} produced by an ear canal sound pressure and found the window-pressure difference (ΔP) to be 30–50 dB smaller in magnitude than the ear canal sound pressure. The small size of the acoustically coupled window-pressure difference relative to the ear canal stimulus points out that acoustic coupling is not an efficient method of stimulating the inner ear, although in cases of ossicular interruption or near-total tympanic membrane perforations the acoustically coupled ΔP can act as the primary stimulus to the inner ear (Peake *et al.*, 1992; Merchant *et al.*, 1997; Voss *et al.*, 2007).

The major pathway by which airborne sound stimulates the inner ear is via ossicular coupling, where the sound-induced motion of the tympanic membrane is directly coupled to the inner ear

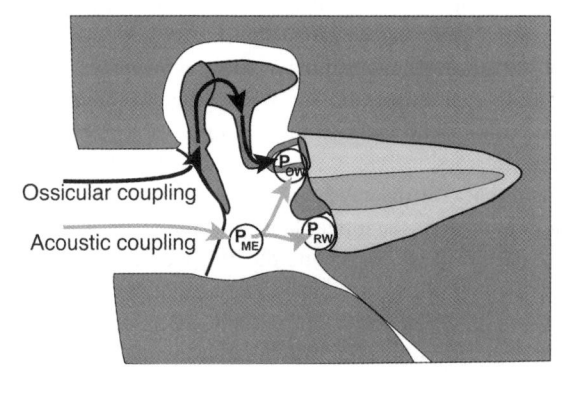

Ossicular coupling

Acoustic coupling

Fig. 3.9 Ossicular and acoustic coupling. The three schematized sound pressures include: the pressure in the middle ear cavity (P_{ME}); the sound pressure outside of the round window (P_{RW}); and the sum of the acoustic and ossicular pressures acting at the oval window (P_{OW}). After Merchant and Rosowski (2002).

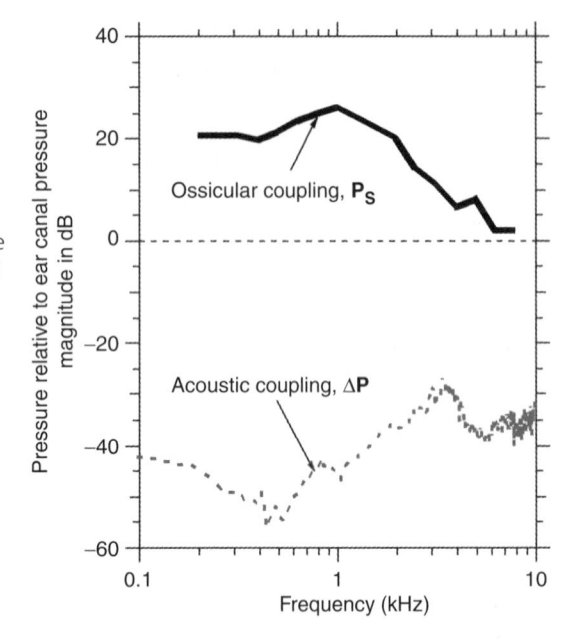

Fig. 3.10 The magnitude of the acoustic- and ossicular-coupled sound stimulus in a normal human ear. Ossicular coupling is plotted as P_S, the effective ossicular-coupled sound pressure acting on the stapes footplate in the oval window measured by Kurokawa and Goode (1995). The acoustic-coupled $\Delta P = P_{OW} - P_{RW}$, is from measurements of Voss et al. (2007).

via the ossicular chain (Fig. 3.9). Measurements of ossicularly coupled sound generally show that the sound pressure that reaches the inner ear via the motion of the tympanic membrane and ossicular chain is greater than the sound pressure in the ear canal (Fig. 3.10). This increase in sound pressure has been called the *middle ear gain*. Figure 3.10 illustrates an estimate of this gain by Kurokawa and Goode (1995) who compared the ear canal sound pressure necessary to move the stapes a criterion amount with the oval window sound pressure needed to meet the same criterion. The middle ear gain produced by ossicularly coupled sound is frequency dependent, with a magnitude of 20–25 dB at frequencies less than 1000 Hz and decreasing magnitude at higher frequencies. Other measurements of this pressure gain in cadaveric human temporal bones (Puria et al., 1997; Aibara et al., 2001) and animals (Nedzelnitsky, 1980; Dancer & Franke, 1980; Décory et al., 1988; Olson, 1998) also show a frequency dependent middle ear gain with a gain maximum of 20–40 dB, which occurs in the middle or upper frequencies. How does this gain arise?

The middle ear gain results from the transformer properties of the middle ear as it attempts to compensate for the difference between the relatively high input impedance of the inner ear (the load on the transformer) and the lower impedance of air within the ear canal (the source impedance) (Helmholtz, 1868; Wever & Lawrence, 1954; Dallos, 1973; Rosowski et al., 1986; Hemilä et al., 1995; Rosowski, 1996). The transformer mechanisms include a hydraulic or acoustic lever related to the ratio of the areas of the tympanic membrane and stapes footplate. This area ratio varies between 15 (chimpanzee) and 48 (the common shrew) in different mammalian species with a mean value of 28 and a standard deviation of 8.2 in 36 mammalian species (Hemilä et al., 1995), and it is about 23 in humans (Rosowski, 1992, 1994; Hemilä et al., 1995).

A second transformer mechanism that contributes to middle ear function is the mechanical lever that results from the coupled rotation of the longer handle of the malleus and the shorter long arm of the incus about an axis defined by the AML and the PIL (Fig. 3.4B; Helmholtz, 1868; Dahmann, 1929; Wever & Lawrence, 1954; Willi et al., 2002). The ratio of the lengths of the lever arms varies between about 1.3 (owl monkey and humans) and 3.9 (house mouse) with a mean value of 2.4 and a standard deviation of 0.77 for the 36 mammalian species studied by

Hemilä *et al.* (1995). Regardless of species, the lever ratio is always markedly smaller than the area ratio. A third transformer mechanism based on the curvature of the tympanic membrane was suggested by Helmholtz (1868) and others (e.g. Tonndorf & Khanna, 1970), although the existence of this mechanism is controversial. Helmholtz based his idea on the transformation between force and displacement that occurs in a catenary, where small displacements at the center of the catenary produce large changes in the force at its supports (Tonndorf & Khanna, 1970). Békésy (1960) and Wever and Lawrence (1954) performed static measurements of the tympanic membrane catenary effect and decided it was not operational in the middle ear. On the other hand, time-average holographic measurements of the sound-induced motion of the surface of the tympanic membrane (Tonndorf & Khanna, 1970, 1972; Khanna & Tonndorf, 1972) and modern models of the tympanic membrane (Funnell *et al.*, 1987; Fay *et al.*, 2005, 2006) that show the largest motions of the tympanic membrane occur at locations away from the malleus arm in the membrane are consistent with the catenary lever theory of tympanic membrane action.

It is important to realize that the transformer mechanisms that operate within the middle ear are not 'ideal'. Therefore, the motion of the tympanic membrane and ossicles that results from the ear canal sound stimulus depend not only on the transformer properties of the middle ear and the input impedance of the inner ear, but also on the impedance of the ossicles, tympanic membrane, and the air-filled middle ear (Zwislocki, 1962, 1963, 1965; Dallos, 1973; Rosowski, 1994, 1996; Hemilä *et al.*, 1995). Furthermore, it is clear that the tympanic membrane does not move as a rigid plate (Khanna & Tonndorf, 1972; Manley & Johnstone, 1974; Decraemer *et al.*, 1989; Fay *et al.*, 2005, 2006; Rosowski *et al.*, 2007): a contradiction of a basic assumption of the area-ratio transformer model. The non-ideal behavior of the tympanic membrane depends on frequency: at low frequencies, the surface of the membrane moves in phase, allowing a description of an effective area of the tympanic membrane by a simple ratio (Békésy, 1960; Shera & Zweig, 1992a; Lynch *et al.*, 1994; Rosowski, 1994, 1996). At high frequencies the pattern of sound-induced TM displacements breaks up showing multiple peaks and varying phases of motion (Decraemer *et al.*, 1989, 1999; Fay *et al.*, 2005, 2006; Rosowski *et al.*, 2007).

There are also frequency-dependent non-idealities in the motion of the ossicles. The ossicular ligaments are known to flex (Zwislocki, 1962, 1963; Guinan & Peake, 1967; Willi *et al.*, 2002; Decraemer & Khanna, 2004); the bony ossicles themselves may bend (Funnell *et al.*, 1992; Decraemer *et al.*, 1995), and the motion of the ossicles may be better described as a complicated summing of rotation and translation in three dimensions rather than simple rotation about a fixed axis (Decraemer *et al.*, 2000; Decraemer & Khanna, 2004), where these more complex motions are most prominent at higher frequencies. Such relative motions within the chain weaken any lever action of the ossicles. The non-rigidities in the TM and ossicular chain, together with the frequency-dependent impedances of the middle ear components, contribute to the frequency dependence of the middle ear. In general, at the lower frequencies to which the ear is sensitive, the stiffness of the tympanic membrane, the annular ligament around the stapes, and the other ossicular supports and ligaments constrain the motion of the different components, where the magnitude of the total middle ear stiffness varies greatly among species (Rosowski, 1992, 1994). Above this low-frequency range, the impedance of the inner ear plays a major role in determining how the tympanic membrane and ossicles move with sound (Zwislocki, 1962; Møller, 1965; Allen, 1986; Peake *et al.*, 1992; Puria & Allen, 1998; Rosowski *et al.*, 2006; Songer & Rosowski, 2007a). Some recent findings regarding the motion of the TM and ossicles will be discussed later.

3.3.4 The role of the external ear

If we define the external ear conceptually as all of the structures that effect sound transfer between the environment and the tympanic membrane, the components of the external ear include the

Fig. 3.11 The contribution of the head, body, and external ear structures to the transformation of sound pressure from the free-field to the medial end of the ear canal just outside the tympanic membrane: P_T/P_{FF}. After Shaw (1974a,b).

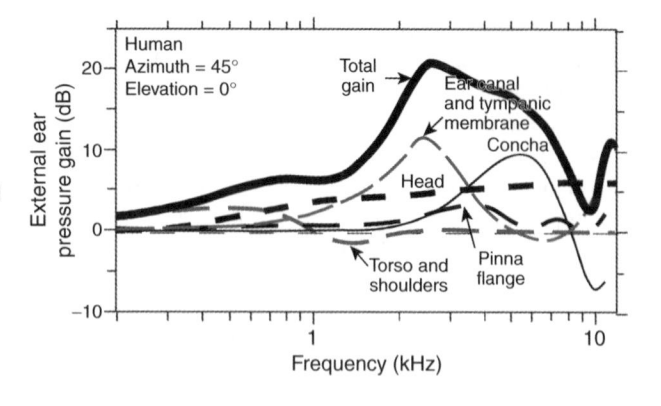

head and body of the animal (Shaw, 1974b; Kuhn, 1977; Algazi et al., 2002), as well as the pinna flange, concha, and external ear canal. These five structures contribute to sound transmission between the environment and the inner ear by gathering and transforming environmental sound and thereby increasing the sound pressure at the tympanic membrane at particular frequencies. Four of these five anatomical components, all but the external ear canal, also impart directionality to the auditory periphery. The contributions of the different peripheral structures to sound capture and transmission depend on the size of the structure relative to the wavelength of sound, where the larger the structure, the lower the sound frequency affected by the structure. Shaw (1974a,b) illustrated this concept by dissecting the contribution of different peripheral structures to the transformation of sound by the entire external ear. The results of his dissection are show in Figure 3.11.

As a baseline in his dissection, Shaw (1974a) computed the external ear gain – the ratio of the magnitude of the pressure at the tympanic membrane, P_{TM}, relative to the free-field sound pressure used as a stimulus, P_{FF} – from a collection of measurements for a source at horizontal azimuth of 45° and elevation of 0°. (The external ear gain is a variant of the head-related transfer function (Wightman & Kistler, 1989; Kulkarni et al., 1999) – the latter usually does not include the transformation of pressure produced by the ear canal.) Shaw then gathered measurements and computations that separated out the contributions of the diffraction of sound by the head, the scattering of sound by the torso, shoulders, and pinna, the resonance of the ear canal when terminated by the middle and inner ear, and the concha resonance (Shaw, 1974a,b). The sum of all of the separate factors (when defined in terms of the dB values of the different pressure ratios) added up to the total gain in decibels (Fig. 3.11). This summing of decibels is equivalent to the external ear gain resulting from the multiplication of the gains of each of these separate processes.

The external ear also imparts directionality to the auditory periphery, in that sound collection by all but one of the components of the external ear gain – the exception is the external ear canal (Wiener et al., 1946, 1965; Hammershøi & Møller, 1996) – varies with the direction of the sound source (Fig. 3.12, also Shaw, 1974a,b; Middlebrooks et al., 1989). The scattering of sound from the torso and shoulders to the ear canal entrance is greatest when the sound comes from the side and the head is straight ahead, whereas when the sound is below the level of the ears, the ear is within the sound shadow of the torso (Algazi et al., 2002). The diffraction of sound around the head produces the largest sound pressure at the entrance to the concha when the sound source points at the entrance to the ear (azimuth = 90°, elevation = 0); a sound source directed to the front of the head (azimuth = 0°, elevation = 0) produces a grazing incidence of sound at the entrance to the ear with little gain, and a sound source directed at the ear on the opposite side of the head

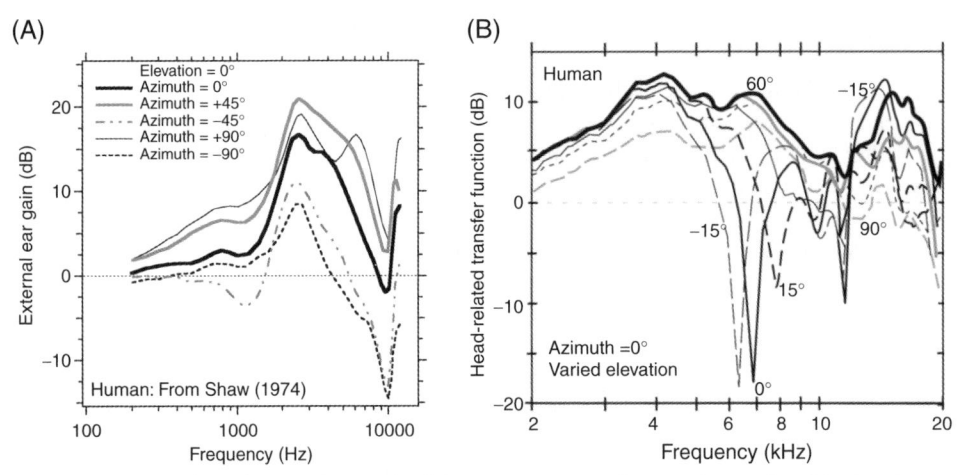

Fig. 3.12 Directionality of external ear gain. (A) Measurements of external ear gain with elevation set to 0° and varied azimuths (data from Shaw 1974a,b). (B) Measurements of head-related transfer function, the ratio of sound pressure at the entrance of the blocked ear canal and the sound pressure in the free-field with azimuth set to 0° and varied elevation. After Shaw (1982).

(azimuth = −90°, elevation = 0) produces a sound shadow at the reference ear. (Sound shadows can result in sound pressures at the entrance to the opposite ear canal that are smaller than the free-field sound pressure, that is, an external ear gain with a negative decibel value (Shaw, 1974b).) At mid and high frequencies the complex additions of direct sound and sound reflected from the various complexities of the conchal structure produce minima and maxima at the entrance to the ear canal that are highly sensitive to changes in the azimuth and elevation of the sound source (Batteau, 1967; Shaw & Teranishi, 1968; Butler & Belendiuk, 1977; Shaw, 1982; Lopez-Poveda & Meddis, 1996). These 'conchal resonances' are responsible for the mid- to high-frequency minima in external ear gain that vary regularly with elevation (Fig. 3.12B) and are thought to act as cues for the elevation of sound sources (Middlebrooks *et al.*, 1989; Rice *et al.*, 1992; Kulkarni & Colburn, 1998).

3.4 Recent findings in external and middle ear function

3.4.1 The directionality of the external ear

Since the late 1980s, much of the work on the external ear has been concerned with its directional response, the so-called head-related transfer function (HRTF), where the driving forces behind this work were the synthesis of three-dimensional listening systems under ear phones (Wightman & Kistler, 1989; Pralong, 1996; Kulkarni & Colburn, 1998; Kulkarni *et al.*, 1999), and the definition of the cues used by listeners in determining the location of a sound source (Middlebrooks *et al.*, 1989; Wightman & Kistler, 1992; Rice *et al.*, 1992; Huang & May, 1996; Algazi *et al.*, 2001; Langendijk & Bronkhorst, 2002). To address these issues, multiple determinations of HRTFs were made in humans and animals (e.g. Wightman & Kistler, 1989; Middlebrooks *et al.*, 1989; Rice *et al.*, 1992; Keller *et al.*, 1998; Spezio *et al.*, 2000; Aytekin *et al.*, 2004; Firzlaff & Schuller, 2004; Maki & Furukawa, 2005). The results of these measurements support the trimodal theory of sound localization, where interaural time differences are used as cues for the location of low-frequency sound sources in the horizontal plane, interaural level differences are useful in localizing high-frequency sound sources in the horizontal plane, and variations in the ear canal sound pressure spectra produced primarily by direction-dependent conchal and pinna resonances give information on vertical position of broad-band high-frequency sound sources.

Other recent work includes studies to test the best way of measuring HRTF, e.g. Hammershøi and Møller (1996) concluded that measuring the sound pressure at the blocked entrance of the ear canal was the method of choice for measuring HRTFs. This conclusion is consistent with other measurements showing that the ear canal's transformation of sound pressure from the ear canal entrance to the tympanic membrane does not vary with sound source direction (Wiener & Ross, 1946; Wiener *et al.*, 1966; Middlebrooks *et al.*, 1989). The results of other work suggests that the large intersubject variability observed in humans and animal HRTFs is reduced by frequency scaling, which acts to normalize the locations of prominent minima and maxima in the HRTF (Middlebrooks *et al.*, 1989; Xu & Middlebrooks, 2000), where some of the observed variability is related to intersubject differences in the size and shape of the pinna and concha. Consistent with the use of scaling to unify the HRTF, detailed analyses of HRTF patterns with varied stimulus direction concluded that the directional dependence of the HRTFs could be described by a few principal components (Kistler & Wightman, 1992) and that smoothing out of all but the most prominent frequency dependences had little effect on the perceived direction of a sound (Kulkarni & Colburn, 1998). Another simplification in the directional dependence of the HRTF can be found in measurements of HRTF in cats with mobile pinnas which demonstrate that the HRTF pattern is simply translated in space as the position of the pinna changes (Young *et al.*, 1996).

3.4.2 Recent findings in middle ear function

Sound-induced motion of the tympanic membrane

A common view of the tympanic membrane's response to sound dates back to the work of Khanna and Tonndorf (Tonndorf & Khanna, 1970, 1972; Khanna & Tonndorf, 1972), who used time-averaged holography to describe patterns of sound-induced tympanic membrane motion. As summarized earlier, those measurements demonstrated:

- in-phase motion of the cat and human tympanic membrane with sounds of frequency less than 1000 Hz, where locations between the mallear arm embedded in the tympanic membrane and its bony support ring moved more than the mallear arm
- an irregular pattern of tympanic membrane surface motions with a multitude of displacement maxima of various phases at frequencies between 1 and 8 kHz.

The 'breakup' of TM motion into multiple, apparently disordered, minima and maxima at frequencies above 1000 Hz was compared with the undesirable breakup of an earphone or microphone diaphragm that is known to limit the high-frequency response of these instruments (Tonndorf & Khanna, 1976). Shaw suggested this irregular behavior was incompatible with an efficient working of the tympanic membrane at high frequencies and hypothesized that the irregular high-frequency motions of the tympanic membrane were essentially uncoupled from the mallear arm embedded within it (Shaw & Stinson, 1983).

Recent measurements and models of tympanic membrane function have led to somewhat different conclusions. In 1998, Puria and Allen, based on measurements of middle ear input admittance and average tympanic membrane motion in cats, advanced a model of tympanic membrane and ossicular motion and hypothesized the propagation of surface displacement waves along the tympanic membrane between its bony support ring and the manubrium. The basis for this hypothesis was the observation of frequency-dependent group delays (of about 40 μs) in the acoustic reflectance computed from the measured admittances (Puria & Allen, 1998). The presence of tympanic membrane surface waves was later supported by newer measurements of its motion. Decraemer and coworkers (1999; also shown in Fay et al., 2005) used a heterodyne laser coupled to a remote-controlled micro-positioning system to measure the sound-induced displacement at many finely spaced points along a line that went through the center of the tympanic membrane in a cat. With a stimulus tone of frequency less than 600 Hz, the motions were in phase at all points along the line. However, with tonal stimuli of 2000–15 000 Hz, the motion at the different points varied regularly in magnitude and phase in a manner consistent with wave motion on the tympanic membrane surface.

More recently, computer-aided, real-time, fiberoptic electro-holographic techniques (Furlong & Pryputniewicz, 1998, 2000) have been used to measure the sound-induced displacement of the tympanic membrane surface of cadaveric cats and chinchillas using tonal sound stimuli of frequencies between 300 Hz and 20 000 Hz (Rosowski et al., 2007). The data taken in response to sound frequencies greater than 8000 Hz clearly demonstrate wave motion on the surface of the tympanic membrane (Fig. 3.13). These data also shed light on the patterns of tympanic membrane motion observed in earlier studies. The earlier holographic studies on cat and human tympanic membranes did not test at frequencies above 8000 Hz and did not observe the highly ordered patterns of high-frequency tympanic membrane motion illustrated in Figure 3.13 which suggest waves of motion flowing between the manubrium and the bony rim of the tympanic membrane. These distinctive ordered patterns are clearly visible at frequencies as low as 2000 Hz in the chinchilla and were also observed at frequencies above 8000 Hz in cat and human temporal bones. The ordered patterns depend on frequency in that the distance between the crests of the displacement waves decreases as frequency increases from 2000 Hz to 20 000 Hz. Such an inverse relationship between frequency and inter-peak distance, is expected for a wave propagating with a roughly constant wave velocity. Interestingly, at frequencies where the tympanic membrane displacement patterns appear irregular (e.g. below 8000 Hz in cat), the extrapolated inter-wave distance is larger than the radius of the tympanic membrane, suggesting that the irregular patterns are really the first few wave fronts of an ordered displacement pattern. This suggestion requires further investigation.

The demonstration of wave motion on the surface of the tympanic membrane has led to another view of its response to high-frequency sound. Contrary to the suggestion of Tonndorf and Khanna (1976) and Shaw and Stinson (1983) that the complex patterns of displacement suggest a breakup of the tympanic membrane which uncouples the motion of its more distant parts from the motions of the malleus, Fay et al. (2006) suggest that these patterns instead indicate a complex series of modal patterns on the TM surface, with each mode representing one of a multitude of natural frequencies of the membrane. In this scenario, the manubrial motion is related to a weighted sum of the different modes, where the large number of modes on the tympanic membrane surface act to smooth the frequency dependence of the sum. While it is an attractive alternative to the old 'breakup' and 'uncoupling' idea, this hypothesis requires further investigation.

Ossicular motion

The common conception of the motion of the ossicles is that the malleoincudal complex rotates about an axis defined by the AML and PIL (Figs 3.4B, 3.14A), and that these motions enable a piston-like, inward and outward translation of the stapes in the oval window (e.g. Guinan & Peake, 1967). Although this picture is a reasonable approximation of the low-frequency behavior of the ossicles, considerable deviations from this behavior have been described. Some of these deviations (e.g. the rocking of the human stapes described by Békésy (1960)) have been attributed to the use of high stimulus levels (levels that were necessary to observe ossicular motion), more sophisticated measurements now exist. The group that has investigated ossicular motion in most

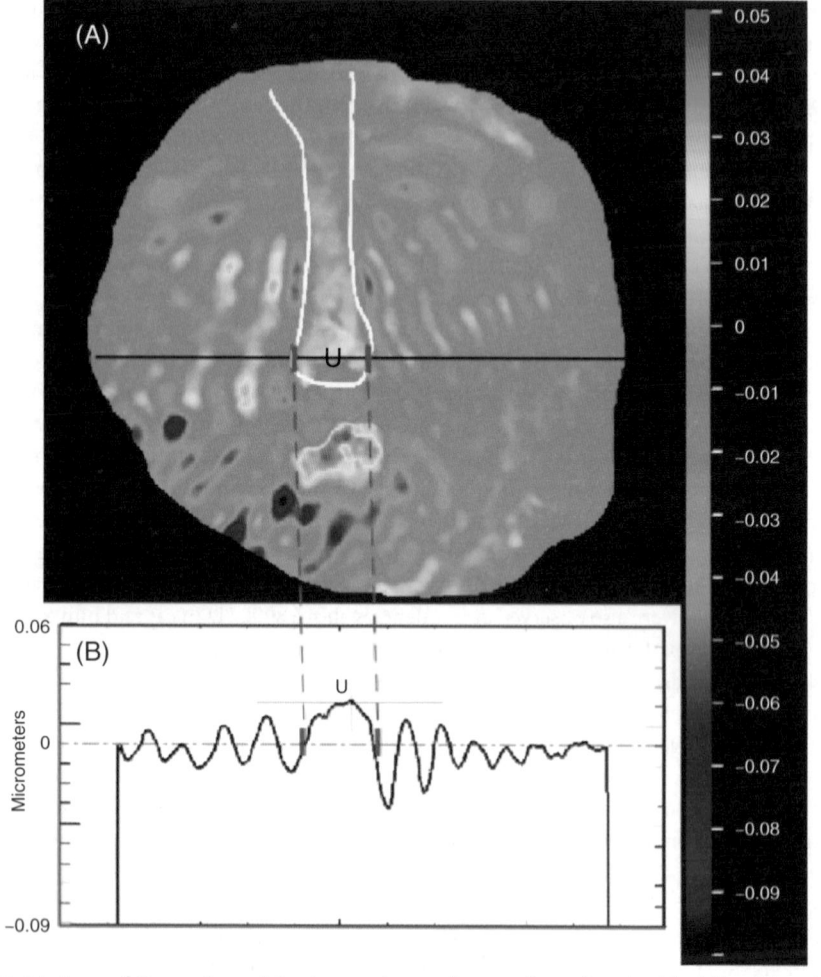

Fig. 3.13 Motions of the surface of the tympanic membrane of a cadaveric chinchilla with a 15.7 kHz tonal stimulus of 106 dB SPL. (A) A 'stop-action' hologram of the sound-induced motion of a cadaveric chinchilla tympanic membrane (Furlong and Pryputniewicz 1998, 2000). The outline of the manubrium is shown in white. U, umbo. The colors between green and red code inward displacements of the tympanic membrane surface; colors varying between green and purple code outward motions. The data for the image were gathered using stroboscopic averages of two short temporal segments of a stimulus period that differed by half a stimulus cycle. (B) The displacement along the black line in (A).
After Rosowski et al. (2007).

detail is Decraemer, Khanna, and Funnell (e.g. Funnell et al., 1992; Decraemer et al., 1995, 2000; Decraemer & Khanna, 2004). Their results in cats, gerbils, and humans describe complex three-dimensional motion of the manubrium of the malleus that are consistent with bending of the manubrium, and frequency-dependent translations in the axis of rotation of the ossicles (Decraemer et al., 1995; Decraemer & Khanna, 2004). Somewhat surprisingly, the large spatial complexities in the motion of the malleus are only mildly echoed in the motion of the stapes, in that the largest component of stapes motion is piston-like translation, even though large rocking motions are superimposed on the simple translation (Decraemer & Khanna, 2004; Decraemer *et al.*, 2000). A similar combination of piston-like translation and rocking of the stapes about the long and short axes of the footplate has been observed by others (notably Goode and co-workers) in human temporal bones (Heiland *et al.*, 1999; Hato *et al.*, 2003). Whether these rocking motions contribute to, detract from, or are of little consequence to sound transfer between the middle and inner ear is a point of current study (Decraemer *et al.*, 2007; Eiber *et al.*, 2007; Sequeira *et al.*, 2007), although they do complicate estimation of stapes motion from measurements made at a single point (Voss *et al.*, 2000a; Chien *et al.*, 2006a).

Another area of noteworthy research recently has been descriptions of the contribution of the ossicular joints to middle ear sound transmission. While all animals have roughly similar synovial incudostapedial joints, there is wide variation in the form of the incudomalleal joint across animals. In a large subset of animals (mostly rodents: Hyrtl, 1844; Henson, 1974) the joint is either ankylosed (e.g. chinchilla, guinea pig, agouti, porcupine) or so stiff as to be considered rigid (mouse, rat, gerbil). In others, notably human, a flexible incudomalleal joint allows a 'gliding' motion between the malleus and the incus (Marquet, 1981; Hüttenbrink, 1988; Willi *et al.*, 2002). This gliding motion helps insulate the incus and attached stapes from large motions of the tympanic membrane related to changes in static pressure (Hüttenbrink, 1988) or contraction of the tensor tympani muscle (Marquet, 1981). Willi *et al.* (2002) clearly demonstrated that this gliding was also an integral part of the human middle ear's response to sound. Using a scanning laser Doppler vibrometer to determine the sound-induced velocity of multiple points on the coupled malleus head and incus body in a human temporal bone, Willi and co-workers quantified the rotary component of the sound-induced motion of the malleal and incus lever arms (ω_α and ω_β in Fig. 4.14A). Figure 4.14B is a plot of Willi *et al.*'s (2002) measurements of the ratio of the angular velocity of the incus and malleus around the ossicular axis ($\omega_\beta/\omega_\alpha$). If the malleus and incus were tightly coupled, we would expect that both would rotate with identical radial velocities and yield a ratio of one. Instead the incus rotates less than the malleus with a rotation ratio magnitude less than one at all frequencies. Furthermore, the rotation ratio is frequency dependent: at frequencies below 1000 Hz, the rotational motion of the incus is about half the motion of the malleus; at frequencies above 3000 Hz the ratio decreases. A similar slippage within the incudomalleal joint of a human temporal bone was described by Decraemer and Khanna (2004). This reduction in incus and stapes motion due to the slipping incudomalleal joint also explains earlier observations that the ratio of stapes velocity to umbo velocity in human temporal bones was smaller than predicted by a simple anatomically based ossicular lever (Gyo *et al.*, 1987; Goode *et al.*, 1994), and may account for observations of a significant high-frequency roll off in the motion of the human stapes.

Another approach to understanding the function of the ossicular joints was taken by Nakajima *et al.* (2005a,b) who made measurements of the effects of glues and cements, used to impede ossicular motion, on the sound-induced velocity of the stapes and malleus in cadaveric human temporal bones. Application of glue to the stapes footplate was shown to greatly reduce the sound-driven motion of the stapes, but produce only a small reduction (factor of two) in the motion of the malleus. Glues applied to the malleus, on the other hand, produced moderate reductions in both sound-driven stapes and malleus velocities. These results are consistent with flexible joints between the stapes and the malleus that allow the malleus to move when the stapes is fixed, and transmit the reduced malleus motion caused by malleus 'fixations' to the stapes. Furthermore, these fixation results are quantitatively consistent with a simple model of ossicular joint flexibility (Ravicz *et al.*, 2004a) based on the results of Willi *et al.* (2002). The temporal bone ossicular fixations of Nakajima *et al.* (2005a,b) produce changes in ossicular mobility that mimic the pathological changes in umbo velocity induced by malleus and stapes fixation in living human

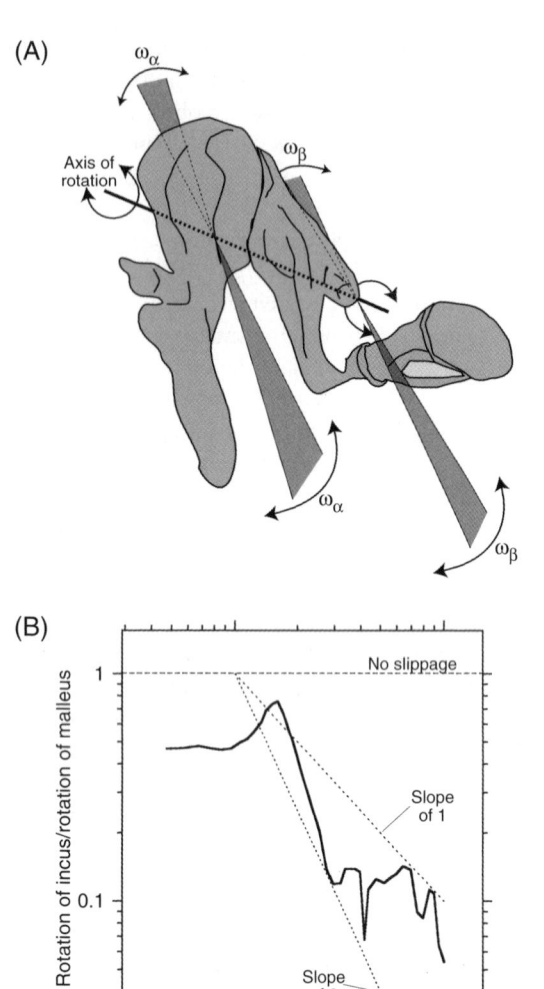

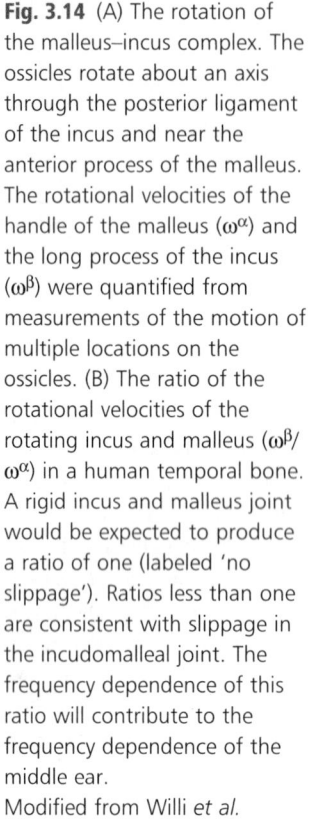

Fig. 3.14 (A) The rotation of the malleus–incus complex. The ossicles rotate about an axis through the posterior ligament of the incus and near the anterior process of the malleus. The rotational velocities of the handle of the malleus (ω^α) and the long process of the incus (ω^β) were quantified from measurements of the motion of multiple locations on the ossicles. (B) The ratio of the rotational velocities of the rotating incus and malleus ($\omega^\beta/\omega^\alpha$) in a human temporal bone. A rigid incus and malleus joint would be expected to produce a ratio of one (labeled 'no slippage'). Ratios less than one are consistent with slippage in the incudomalleal joint. The frequency dependence of this ratio will contribute to the frequency dependence of the middle ear.
Modified from Willi *et al.* (2002).

patients (Rosowski *et al.*, 2003a; Nakajima *et al.*, 2005a,b; Rosowski *et al.*, 2008). This similarity of live ear and temporal bone results supports the utility of temporal bone measurements in understanding middle ear function in live human ears.

High-frequency ossicular motion and ossicular delay

Recently, there has been much interest in the motion of the ossicles produced by high-frequency sound. This interest has been fueled by observations of middle ear output sound pressure and ossicular motion in gerbils by Olson (1998) and Overstreet and Ruggero (2002) at frequencies up to 40 kHz. These new data have several features that were not well described before:

◆ The gerbil middle ear output pressures measured by Olson (1998) and the stapes velocity measurements of Overstreet and Ruggero (2002) have magnitudes that are roughly invariant with sound frequencies between 1 kHz and 40 kHz. This frequency range approaches the high-frequency limit of gerbil hearing (Ryan, 1976), and the data have been used to argue against the simple idea that the range of audibility is determined by the frequency dependence of the middle ear (Ruggero & Temchin, 2002).

♦ Over the same frequency range, the phase of the middle ear output (either vestibule sound pressure or stapes velocity) relative to the phase of the ear-canal sound pressure is well fit by a simple delay of about 20–40 μs depending on the species.

The first feature, the near-constancy of the stapes velocity transfer function magnitude at frequencies between 1000 Hz and 40 000 Hz is a simplification that fits the median of the Overstreet and Ruggero (2002) data but is clearly counter to data gathered with higher-frequency resolution. Figure 3.15A compares the stapes velocity measurements of Overstreet and Ruggero (2002) with others measured by Ravicz et al., 2008). The Ravicz data were taken with a fairly high-frequency density of 50 Hz and covered a broader range of stimulus frequencies (from 100 Hz to 80 kHz). The Ravicz data clearly show a proportional increase in the velocity/pressure as frequency increases from 100 Hz to 1000 Hz, which is a sign of the compliance-dominated middle ear. They also show a clear minimum in velocity near 3000 Hz that has been described in other measurements and determined to result from the presence of the holes placed in the middle ear cavity walls to expose the stapes to view (e.g. Møller, 1965; Guinan & Peake, 1967; Ravicz et al., 1992).

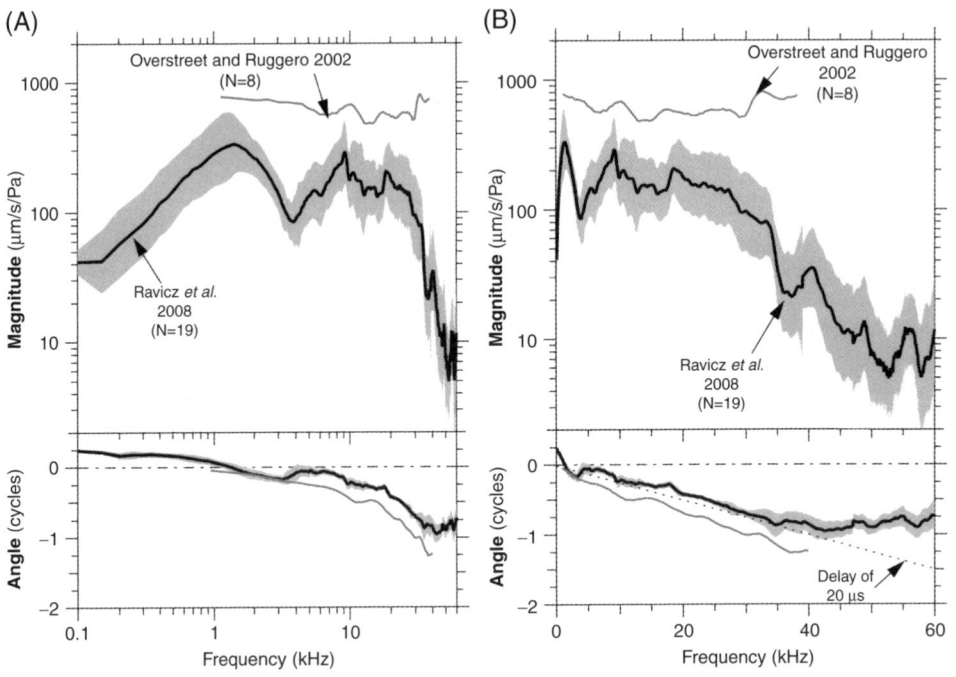

Fig. 3.15 The magnitude and phase angle of stapes velocity transfer functions (stapes velocity normalized by estimates of the sound pressure near the tympanic membrane) in gerbils. The upper plots of each panel describes the ratio of the magnitude of the velocity and sound pressure. The lower plot shows the phase angle, the difference in phase between the stapes velocity and the ear canal sound pressure. The thin gray lines are the median of eight measurements from Overstreet and Ruggero (2002). The solid lines and the shaded region are the mean ± one standard deviation from 19 measurements performed by Ravicz et al. (2008). (A) The data are plotted on a logarithmic frequency scale. (B) The same data are plotted on a linear frequency scale. The phase-angle plot includes the phase of a theoretical 20 μs delay.

The low-frequency increase in velocity is missed by Overstreet and Ruggero because they concentrate on the high-frequency response. The minima near 3000 Hz is missed because of the relatively low-frequency resolution (500 Hz) in those measurements. A third difference is the decrease in stapes velocity that occurs outside the stimulus range of the Overstreet and Ruggero data. The Ravicz data suggest that near-constancy of the magnitude of the stapes velocity transfer function can be observed between 5000 Hz and 40 000 Hz, but at lower and higher frequencies there are marked deviations from a frequency-independent stapes velocity transfer function with a general decrease in measured velocity at frequencies above 40 kHz: the amplitude drops by more than a factor of ten between ~30 kHz and 60 kHz, then levels off at a value roughly a factor of ten beneath its maximum value. Other data by de La Rochefoucauld and Olson (2007) show a similar high-frequency roll-off of gerbil stapes velocity at frequencies above 40 kHz.

The second feature noted above, the ossicular delay, was actually predicted by Puria and Allen's (1998) model of wave motion on the tympanic membrane and ossicular delay, and has been observed in other measurements of ossicular motion (e.g. Olson & Cooper, 2000; de La Rochefoucauld & Olson, 2007; Ravicz et al., 2008). Such a delay is readily apparent when the phase of the measured stapes velocity is plotted versus linear frequency (Fig. 3.15B, where the phase varies linearly with frequency). This linear relationship between phase and frequency is consistent with a delay of 20 μs. The precise origin of this delay is unclear, although candidates include wave motion on the tympanic membrane (Puria & Allen, 1998; Decraemer et al., 1999; Fay et al., 2005, 2006; Rosowski et al., 2007) as well as delay within the ossicular system (Puria & Allen, 1998; de La Rochefoucauld & Olson, 2007) related to the presence of the ossicular joints and bending within the ossicles themselves.

Specification of the input to the middle ear at high frequency

A complication in specifying the motion of the ossicles referenced to the magnitude and phase of a high-frequency sound pressure stimulus is a difficulty in defining the stimulus when the dimensions of the ear canal become a significant fraction of the wavelength of sound. It is well known that variations in sound pressure can occur along the length of the ear canal at sound frequencies where the wavelength is less than ten times the canal length (Wiener & Ross, 1946; Wiener et al., 1966; Shaw, 1974b; Chan & Geisler, 1990). In human ear canals, there are considerable differences between the sound pressures at the entrance of the ear canal and at the tympanic membrane with sound frequencies above 1000 Hz. In gerbils, with their shorter ear canal, these sound pressures are markedly different at frequencies above 25 000 Hz (Fig. 3.16B). Variations in sound pressure across the diameter of the canal are also possible at frequencies where the wavelength approximates or is less than the canal diameter (Siebert, 1973; Stinson, 1986; Stinson & Khanna, 1989).

A common experimental approach to avoid the spatial variation in sound pressure along the canal length is to specify the sound pressure at a position as close to the tympanic membrane as possible; however this is not always practical in animals with small ear canals (e.g. mice or gerbils) in which the probe microphone can be large enough to interfere with the sound stimulus. A potential solution to this problem, put forward by Pearce et al. (2001), is to use a calibration coupler, much like the artificial ear couplers used to determine the output of audiological earphones (Zwislocki, 1980), to estimate the output of the sound source when it is placed in an ear (Pearce et al., 2001; Overstreet & Ruggero, 2002). A second solution is to place a small probe tube into the bony ear canal via a surgically placed hole that reduces the interference between the microphone probe and the sound stimulus (e.g. Olson, 1998; Ravicz et al., 2007). Figure 3.16 shows some of the benefits of and differences between the two approaches.

Starting with the second method, Figure 3.16A shows a comparison of the sound pressure measured at the entrance of the ear canal and near the tympanic membrane in five gerbil ears.

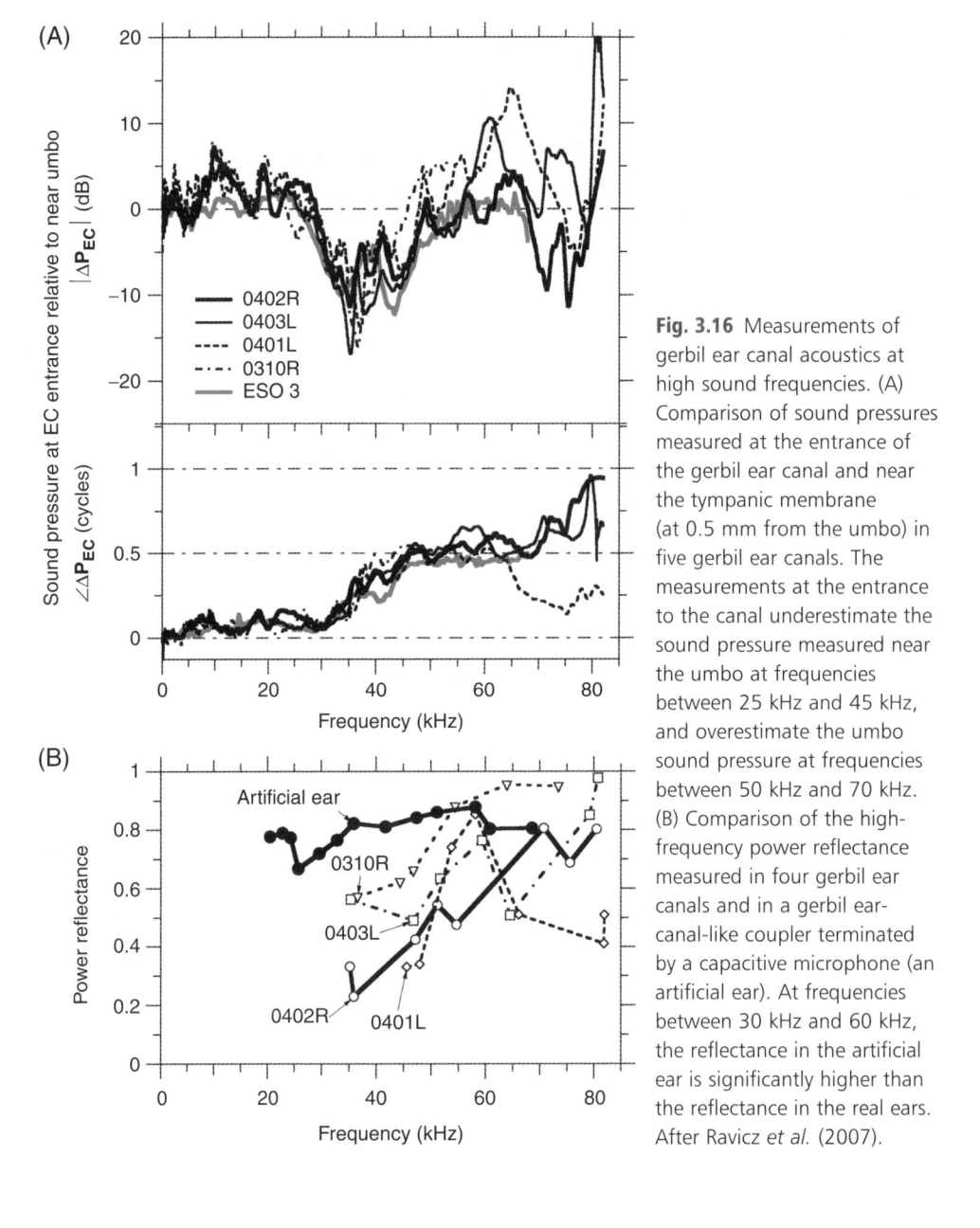

Fig. 3.16 Measurements of gerbil ear canal acoustics at high sound frequencies. (A) Comparison of sound pressures measured at the entrance of the gerbil ear canal and near the tympanic membrane (at 0.5 mm from the umbo) in five gerbil ear canals. The measurements at the entrance to the canal underestimate the sound pressure measured near the umbo at frequencies between 25 kHz and 45 kHz, and overestimate the umbo sound pressure at frequencies between 50 kHz and 70 kHz. (B) Comparison of the high-frequency power reflectance measured in four gerbil ear canals and in a gerbil ear-canal-like coupler terminated by a capacitive microphone (an artificial ear). At frequencies between 30 kHz and 60 kHz, the reflectance in the artificial ear is significantly higher than the reflectance in the real ears. After Ravicz *et al.* (2007).

The plotted ratio suggests that the magnitude of the sound pressure at the entrance of the ear canal underestimates the sound pressure near the umbo in the center of the tympanic membrane by 10–15 dB at frequencies around 30 kHz. The ear canal pressure also tends to overestimate the pressure at the tympanic membrane by as much as 10 dB at frequencies near 60 kHz. Associated with those two frequency ranges are half-cycle shifts in the phase angle between the two pressures. Ravicz *et al.* (2007) argue that the magnitude minima and maxima in this ratio together with the phase shifts are consistent with standing waves in the gerbil ear canal at frequencies above 25 kHz. It should be noted that one can compensate for the spatial variations identified in Figure 3.16A with an adequate model of the gerbil ear canal and middle ear input impedance; the impedance loads the ear canal and determines how much sound is reflected at the ear canal terminus. Such compensation is the goal of the artificial ear canal coupler technique.

Figure 3.16B shows that an overly simple acoustic coupler is a poor substitute for an actual in ear calibration. The problem is one of differences in the impedance of the middle ear and most microphones. In general, calibration microphone diaphragms are of high impedance and highly reflective, whereas the middle ear input impedance is relatively resistive but not well characterized at high frequencies. In order to quantify the difference between in ear and coupler calibrations, Ravicz *et al.* (2007) measured the high-frequency reflectance at the tympanic membrane in gerbils and compared that with the reflectance found with a simple acoustic coupler composed of an artificial gerbil ear canal terminated with a capacitive microphone. The result is shown in Figure 3.16B; the large differences in reflectance between the real and artificial ear observed at frequencies between 30 kHz and 60 kHz suggest an earphone calibration based on a coupler terminated by a high-impedance capacitive microphone will yield considerable errors in estimated sound pressure in this frequency range.

Problems with high-frequency sound specification are still unresolved. It has been demonstrated that earphone calibrations based on artificial animal ear canals terminated by a rigid capacitive microphone yield spurious results in some frequency ranges (Ravicz *et al.*, 2007). While it has also been demonstrated that miniature probe-microphones can be used to estimate sound pressure at positions within 0.5 mm of the center of the tympanic membrane (Ravicz *et al.*, 2007), there is some frequency above which the presence of the probe microphone interferes with the sound stimulus (Ravicz *et al.*, 2007), and it is not always possible or desirable to implant a microphone probe tube within the bony ear canal. Another possible solution to this issue has been put forward by Neely and Gorga (1998); they suggest that measurements of average sound power within the ear canal (the power absorbed at the tympanic membrane) are independent of ear canal geometry, and may be superior estimates of the sound stimulus. This suggestion has yet to be taken up by the hearing-research field: specially calibrated earphones are required, and since the techniques still depends on estimates of sound pressure it will also be affected by spatial variations in sound pressures at frequencies above some high-frequency limit. Until the issue of how to specify the stimulus to the middle ear at high audiometric frequencies is resolved, one should look carefully at any results that depend on measurements of sound pressure either at a point within the ear canal or use ear-like sound couplers to specify the sound stimulus at high (>20 kHz) sound frequencies. Discrepancies between results at high frequency are likely to derive from differences in sound pressure estimation method or location (Dong & Olson, 2006; Ravicz *et al.*, 2007).

Measurements of middle ear function in live humans

During the past 15 years two techniques for understanding the workings of the human middle ear have matured. The first of these is the measurement of acoustic power and pressure reflectance within the ear canal (Stinson *et al.*, 1982; Lawton & Stinson, 1985; Keefe *et al.*, 1993; Voss & Allen, 1994; Neely & Gorga, 1998; Feeney & Keefe, 1999; Margolis *et al.*, 1999; Allen *et al.*, 2005), the second is the use of laser-Doppler vibrometry to measure sound-induced tympanic membrane and ossicular motion in live human ears (Goode *et al.*, 1993, 1996; Rodriguez Jorge *et al.*, 1997; Huber *et al.*, 2001a,b; Rosowski *et al.*, 2003a; Whittemore *et al.*, 2004; Rosowski *et al.*, 2008). Both of these techniques can quickly estimate the status of the middle ear in awake human subjects. Oto-reflectance is based on an acoustic measurements of the sound pressure produced by a calibrated source in the ear canal, whereas laser-Doppler vibrometry in awake humans uses a laser focused on the tympanic membrane near the umbo through a glass-backed sound coupler placed in the ear canal (e.g. Whittemore *et al.*, 2004). Laser-Doppler vibrometry has also been used in anesthetized surgical patients to measure the motion of the human stapes (Huber *et al.*, 2001a; Chien *et al.*, 2006b).

Both reflectometry and laser-Doppler vibrometry are used as clinical research tools to evaluate middle ear function (Feeney & Keefe, 1999; Margolis *et al.*, 1999; Huber *et al.*, 2001b; Rosowski *et al.*, 2003a; Allen *et al.*, 2005; Rosowski *et al.*, 2008). Tests in clinical populations have demonstrated that both techniques are more sensitive to changes in middle ear function than standard tympanometry. In particular both techniques have been shown to have a high specificity and selectivity in the diagnosis of various disorders of the ossicular chain (Feeney *et al.*, 2003; Rosowski *et al.*, 2008). Another topic that both techniques have been used to address is the possible contribution of the middle ear to age-related hearing loss. The reflectometry data of Feeney and Sanford (2004) and the laser-Doppler vibrometry data of Whittemore *et al.* (2004) both suggest that there are changes in middle ear function with age, but that these changes are small relative to the large age-related changes in hearing thresholds observed in the aging human population. Similar small age-related changes in middle ear function have been noted in mice (Doan *et al.*, 1996; Rosowski *et al.*, 2003b).

Reverse middle ear transmission

The use of otoacoustic emissions in the clinic and as a research tool has driven an interest in understanding the reverse transmission of emissions from the inner ear to the external ear. Several measurements of reverse transmission have been made. Two similar studies were performed in the guinea pig (Magnan *et al.*, 1997) and gerbil (Dong & Olson, 2006) in which cochlear distortion pressures, produced in response to two-tone stimulation, were measured simultaneously within the vestibule of the inner ear and the ear canal. A study in cat (Voss & Shera, 2004) used measurements of the velocity of the stapes from 'forward-traveling' ear-canal two-tone stimuli to produce inner ear distortion pressures that evoked 'reverse-traveling' motions of the stapes. Reverse middle ear transfer was also estimated in human temporal bones by Puria (2003) using a preparation in which a sound source was implanted into the vestibule of the inner ear. While a simplistic model of the middle ear might suggest that reverse transmission would have a frequency dependence and magnitude equivalent to one over the forward transmission, all of the measurements cited above show more complicated relationships between the magnitude and frequency dependence of forward and reverse transmission. Such non-simplistic relationships between the two directions of transmission do not imply that the middle ear system fails the engineering constraint of reciprocity (see e.g. Shera & Zweig, 1992a). As a non-active, linear and time-invariant mechanical system, the middle ear is almost certainly reciprocal; however, forward and reverse sound transmission through the middle ear also depends on the load and the source impedances. The differences in frequency dependence and inverse magnitude observed in the above studies all reflect the differences between the cochlear load on the middle ear in forward sound transmission and the external ear load on the middle ear in reverse transmission.

Models of middle ear function

The past 15 years have seen advances in models of the middle ear. These advances include the use of circuit tools to help understand middle ear function (e.g. Peake *et al.*, 1992; Shera & Zweig, 1992a; Puria & Allen, 1998; Songer & Rosowski, 2007a,b) as well as improvements in finite-element models (FEMs) of the middle ear. The largest area of improvement in FEMs has been in the detail of anatomical structure as well as the inclusion of the external ear and middle ear air spaces (e.g. Funnell & Decraemer, 1996; Decraemer *et al.*, 2000; Gan *et al.*, 2002; Koike *et al.*, 2002; Decraemer *et al.*, 2003; Funnell *et al.*, 2005; Gan *et al.*, 2006b; Qi *et al.*, 2006). There have also been new investigations into the physical properties of the middle ear structural components (e.g. Fay *et al.*, 2005; Cheng *et al.*, 2007), as well as novel suggestions regarding models of tympanic membrane structure and function (Fay *et al.*, 2005, 2006).

3.5 **Advances in the understanding of conductive hearing loss**

Pathologies that interfere with the conduction of sound to the auditory sensory cells within the inner ear are classified as conductive hearing losses, where the common diagnostic definition of such a hearing loss is a loss of sensitivity to air-conducted sound relative to the measured sensitivity of the ear to bone-conducted sound. The increase in thresholds in air conduction relative to bone conduction results in an 'air–bone gap', where the presence of such a gap is the primary indicator of conductive hearing loss. In the past 15 years, measurements of middle ear function in temporal bones and animals have been used to address multiple causes of conductive hearing loss.

3.5.1 **Reconstructions of the middle ear**

The cadaveric temporal bone preparation has been used repeatedly to investigate the effects of various middle ear reconstructive surgical techniques, including the choice of ossicular prosthesis, the positioning of the prosthesis and the style of middle ear surgery (e.g. Gyo *et al.*, 1986; Goode & Nishihara, 1994; Merchant *et al.*, 1997; Whittemore *et al.*, 1998; Asai *et al.*, 1999; Mehta *et al.*, 2003; Puria *et al.*, 2005; Morris *et al.*, 2006; Bance *et al.*, 2007a,b). The results of these studies add insight into the techniques used in surgical reconstruction of the middle ear.

3.5.2 **Middle ear fluid**

Ravicz *et al.* (2004b) and Gan *et al.* (2006a) have used cadaveric temporal bones to investigate the effect of fluid in the middle ear on middle ear sound transmission; they concluded that fluid affects tympanic membrane and ossicular motion, first, by adding an additional load to the TM and ossicles, and, second, by reducing the volume and decreasing the compressibility of the middle ear air spaces. The change in volume is generally a small effect that is most marked at low frequencies, while the loading of the tympanic membrane can produce important effects on the motion of the tympanic membrane and ossicles at frequencies above 800 Hz. These middle ear fluid related decreases in tympanic membrane and ossicular motion in temporal bones are comparable to the 30 dB hearing loss observed in cases of middle ear effusion (Ravicz *et al.*, 2004b).

3.5.3 **Mechanisms of ossicular disorders**

Laser-Doppler vibrometry measurements of umbo velocity in live pathological ears, and umbo and stapes velocity in cadaveric temporal bones with artificial ossicular pathologies, have highlighted how the ossicular joints allow motion of the peripheral ossicles after pathological stapes fixation (Huber *et al.*, 2003; Rosowski *et al.*, 2003a, 2008; Nakajima *et al.*, 2005a,b). The action of the slipping incudomalleal joint in cases of stapes fixation described in these studies is a key diagnostic feature for differentiating patients with stapes fixation from those with malleus fixation (Nakajima *et al.*, 2005a,b; Rosowski *et al.*, 2008). Patients with a fixed stapes have a marked conductive hearing loss, with nearly normal sound-induced motion of the umbo, whereas patients with fixed mallei show decreases in umbo motion that are comparable to the size of their conductive hearing loss (Rosowski *et al.*, 2008). The match between temporal bone and live ear results with artificial and natural pathologies (Nakajima *et al.*, 2005a,b) again demonstrates the utility of the temporal bone preparation.

3.5.4 **Perforations of the tympanic membrane**

Measurements of middle ear input impedance and laser-Doppler measurements of stapes velocity in temporal bones before and after controlled tympanic membrane perforations have led to a comprehensive description of the mechanisms of hearing loss in perforation (Voss *et al.*, 2001a–c). These papers demonstrate that the primary effect of a tympanic membrane perforation is on the sound–pressure difference across the tympanic membrane, as previously suggested by Kruger and Tonndorf (1977, 1978). As described in Section 3.2 above, motions of the tympanic membrane are coupled with the compression and rarefaction of the air in the middle ear air spaces. The normal tympanic membrane moves because the middle ear sound pressures produced by these motions are smaller than the sound pressure in the ear canal. The motion of the tympanic membrane is proportional to the difference in sound pressure between the ear canal and the middle ear air spaces. In the case of a perforation, low-frequency sound can flow through the perforation reducing the sound–pressure difference across the tympanic membrane, thereby reducing the drive for motion of the tympanic membrane. Because of physical constraints (Voss et al., 2001c) high-frequency sounds do not flow as efficiently through perforations.

The border between low-frequency loss and near-normal high-frequency response depends on the size of the perforation; larger perforations produce hearing losses over a wider frequency range. This leads to the following predictions:

- perforation-induced hearing losses are largest at lower frequencies
- the larger the perforation the larger the loss and the broader frequency range affected
- the hearing loss does not depend on the location of the perforation – an anterior perforation should produce the same amount of hearing loss as a similarly sized posterior perforation in the same ear
- because of the role of the middle ear sound pressure in producing the loss, the size of the loss depends on the volume of the middle ear air spaces. Similar-sized perforations will produce larger hearing losses in ears with smaller middle ear air spaces.

All of these predictions have been supported in a recent clinical investigation of hearing loss in patients with perforations (Mehta et al., 2006).

3.5.5 Pathological inner ear third windows

The description of superior canal dehiscence (SCD) as a pathological entity (Minor et al., 1998; Minor, 2000) with sound- or pressure-evoked vestibular symptoms and a conductive hearing loss, as determined by an audiologically defined air–bone gap (Minor et al., 2003; Mikulec et al., 2004), renewed interest in what some clinicians had previously described as 'inner ear conductive losses'. An SCD is a break in the bone that separates the superior semicircular canal from the cranial cavity (Fig. 3.17). The paradox in these cases was how an inner ear disorder could lead to an apparent conductive loss as characterized by the audiologically determined air–bone gap. Subsequently, the coupling between the conductive hearing loss and the break in the inner ear bone was strengthened by multiple demonstrations that surgically repairing an SCD can close the air–bone gap (Minor et al., 2003; Mikulec et al., 2005; Limb et al., 2006).

A hypothesis that was put forward to explain both the sound-evoked vestibular symptoms and the conductive hearing loss was that the dehiscence acts as a large pathological 'third window' between the inner ear and the cranial cavity (Fig. 3.17; Minor, 2000; Mikulec et al., 2004). The new open window, in the roof of the superior semicircular canal, allows ossicularly coupled sound energy to flow from the oval window, through the superior semicircular canal and out of the dehiscence into the cranial cavity. The passing sound is thought to stimulate the vestibular organs in its path, thereby producing the sound-evoked dizziness and unsteadiness that is part of the syndrome, while the shunting of sound energy out of the dehiscence and away from the cochlea could explain the loss in sensitivity to air-conducted sound.

The 'third window' model of SCD has been successfully tested by measurements of sound conduction in animals (Rosowski et al., 2004; Songer et al., 2004; Songer & Rosowski, 2005, 2006), human temporal bones (Chien et al., 2007) and live human ears (Rosowski et al., 2008). These tests include measurements of sound-evoked motions of the vestibular lymphs within a dehiscent

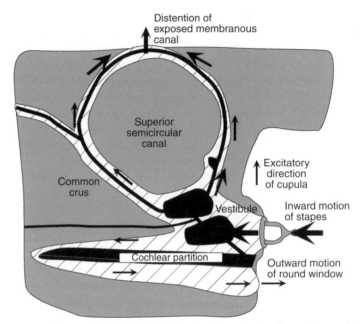

Fig. 3.17 A schematic of the pathological 'third-window' hypothesis of superior canal dehiscence (SCD). The dehiscence, at the roof of the superior canal, allows sound energy to flow from the oval window, through the canal and out the dehiscence. The arrows depict the flow of sound energy through the vestibular canal, explaining the vestibular systems, and away from the inner ear accounting for the observed hearing loss.

canal, as well as SCD-induced changes in middle ear sound transmission, and reductions in sound-evoked cochlear potential in chinchillas. (A study by Sohmer *et al.* (2004) did not demonstrate a dehiscence evoked decrease in sensitivity to air-conducted sound in sand rats, but this failure may be attributed to their use of click stimuli and auditory brainstem response (ABR) measurements, both of which are relatively insensitive to changes in low-frequency hearing, whereas the clinical observations (Mikulec *et al.*, 2004) and the cochlear potential data of Songer and Rosowski (2005) demonstrate SCD has its largest effect on sound frequencies below 1000 Hz.) Also, anatomically constrained computational models of the dehiscence acting as a third window (Rosowski *et al.*, 2004; Songer & Rosowski, 2007b) show good qualitative and quantitative agreement between model predictions and the measured effect of dehiscence on hearing mechanics in animals and hearing thresholds in humans.

SCD has also been associated with increases in the sensitivity to bone-conducted sound of frequencies from 250 Hz to 2000 Hz (Minor, 2000; Mikulec *et al.*, 2004). Such increases have also been observed in chinchillas (Songer *et al.*, 2004) and sand rats (Sohmer *et al.*, 2004). In discussing bone conduction evoked by compression of the inner ear, Békésy (1960) suggested that the presence of any normal third window would contribute to the cochlea's response to bone conduction stimuli, by affecting the differences in the impedance of the sound pathways on either side of the cochlear partition and thereby affecting the sound–pressure difference across the partition evoked by bone conduction. In this light, a pathologically enlarged third window from the vestibule to the cranial cavity, might be expected to increase bone conduction sensitivity: it would 'short' the pressure on the vestibular side of the cochlear partition to near zero, and thereby increase the difference in pressure between the round window and the vestibule. The anatomically and physiologically constrained models of SCD that predicted the reduced sensitivity to airborne sound, have been successfully expanded to fit the observed increase in sensitivity to bone-conducted sound (Rosowski *et al.*, 2004; Songer, 2006).

There is a collection of other inner ear bone disorders that sometimes evoke decreases in the sensitivity to air-conducted sound as well as increases in the sensitivity to bone-conducted sound. These include: enlarged vestibular aqueduct syndrome, dehiscence of other semicircular canals, and Paget's disease (Merchant *et al.*, 2007; Merchant & Rosowski, 2008). The pathological third cochlear window model may also explain these other disorders. However, the effect on hearing of any pathological third window into the inner ear will depend on the location of the break in the inner ear bone. A pathological window on the vestibular side of the inner ear should shunt stapes-induced sound energy away from the cochlea and produce an air–bone gap. However, a window between the scala tympani and the brain or middle ear might actually increase the sensitivity to airborne sound by enhancing the pressure difference across the cochlear partition.

3.5.6 Understanding bone conduction

The advent of the bone-anchored hearing aid (BAHA) resulted in renewed interest in the mechanisms of bone conduction stimulation of the ear. This interest produced multiple studies of how best to stimulate the ear by a bone conduction actuator (Håkansson *et al.*, 1994, 1996; Carlsson *et al.*, 1995), including an extensive series of papers on the mechanism of bone conduction made in human temporal bones and cadaveric whole heads by Stenfelt and colleagues (Stenfelt *et al.*, 2000, 2002, 2003; Stenfelt & Goode, 2005a,b), and measurements in live humans (Aazh *et al.*, 2005). This data set represents the most extensive investigation of bone conduction mechanisms since the time of Tonndorf (1972). One of the main outcomes of this work is a better understanding of the role of the inertance of the cochlear fluids in bone conduction hearing.

Some authors, however, have questioned some of the Stenfelt group's interpretations of their data. One issue is the contribution of the compressive component of bone conduction (Tonndorf, 1972). Stenfelt and Goode (2005a) summarize their thoughts on this issue by arguing that bone conduction stimuli, over much of the important frequency range, set the entire head into motion, and that such bulk motions are inconsistent with a compressive stimulus. However, such bulk motions are not inconsistent with the simultaneous presence of a compressive stimulus component, and it is also difficult to explain the effect of SCD on bone conduction hearing without invoking compressive bone conduction (Rosowski *et al.*, 2004; Songer, 2006). Another issue is that Stenfelt and Goode (2005a) generally ignore a body of evidence suggesting that bone-conducted sound is at least partially transmitted to the inner ear by motions of fluid through the normal third windows. Sohmer and colleagues (e.g. Sohmer *et al.*, 2000) have demonstrated that a bone conduction vibrator placed on the surface of the brain of animals and humans is just as effective in evoking auditory responses. They have also performed animal experiments that clearly demonstrate the fluid coupling of auditory responses to bone conduction stimuli (Sohmer & Freeman, 2004). A complication in the distinction between 'bone 'or 'fluid' conduction of sound is that vibrations of the skull certainly produce vibrations of the fluids and tissues within it, just as vibrations of the tissues must produce vibrations of the skull bones that surround the tissues.

3.6 Areas of continuing research

3.6.1 Structure and function of the tympanic membrane

'How does the normal and pathological structure of the tympanic membrane affect its function?' and 'What is that function at high frequencies?' are continuing questions of research. We have discussed two opposing theories of how high-frequency motions of the tympanic membrane affect ossicular motion: The 'membrane breakup' theory of Tonndorf and Khanna (1976) and Shaw and Stinson (1983) suggests that the complicated patterns of tympanic membrane motion in response to sounds of frequencies above a few kHz are uncoupled from the ossicular chain at those frequencies. The 'discordant drum' theory of Fay and colleagues (2006) suggests that some complex summing of the near-chaotic motion of the tympanic membrane at high frequencies actually results in a smooth drive to the ossicular chain. We have also seen data that suggest the motion of the tympanic membrane at high frequencies is highly ordered, rather than chaotic (Rosowski et al., 2007). Additional measurements of tympanic membrane motion before and after controlled manipulations of the middle ear (e.g. Wada et al., 2002) will help answer these questions. For example, knowledge of whether the patterns of vibration on the tympanic membrane surface change when the ossicular or cochlear load on the tympanic membrane is altered, or how perforations of the tympanic membrane affect ossicular motion and the patterns of motion on the tympanic membrane, will help differentiate between membrane breakup and the summing of multiple membrane modes. Note that the high-frequency transmission found by Olson (1998) and Overstreet and Ruggero (2002) and demonstrated in Figure 3.15 argues against a dramatic decrease in transmission due to break up of the motion of the tympanic membrane at high frequencies.

3.6.2 Ossicular motion at high frequencies

'Is the sound-induced velocity of the ossicles limited as sound-frequency is increased above some limit?' and 'Do limitations in the motion of the ossicles at high frequencies contribute to the roll-off of hearing function?' are questions that require attention. Ruggero and Temchin (2002) argued that there is no essential limitation to ossicular motion as frequency increases and have also pointed out that the inner ear plays a large role in determining the high-frequency limits of hearing in many animals. This chapter has presented data from others (Ravicz et al., 2008) supported by other data (de La Rochefoucauld & Olson, 2007) suggesting that there is a marked decrease in stapes velocity in gerbils at sound frequencies above 40 kHz; indeed the high-frequency limit observed in those studies is similar to limit of hearing found in behavioral studies of gerbil hearing (Ryan, 1976).

While Ruggero and Temchin (2002) show data suggesting that the middle ear response of many vertebrates is of relatively broader band, middle ear gain data in human temporal bones (e.g. Puria et al., 1997; Aibara et al., 2001) show a clear high-frequency limit at frequencies above 10 kHz similar to the limits of human hearing (Puria et al., 1997). The work of Willi et al. (2002) suggests a mechanism for this difference in middle ear behavior between humans and other mammals. The animals with a demonstrated extended high-frequency middle ear response (cat, gerbil, chinchilla, and mouse) are known to have a fairly rigid connection between the malleus and the incus, while the human incudomalleal joint is loose (Willi et al., 2002; Nakajima et al., 2005a,b). As quantified by Willi et al. (2002), this loose connection between the incus and malleus leads to a decrease in incus and stapes motion (relative to malleus motion) as frequency increases above 1 kHz (Fig. 3.14B) and certainly contributes to the loss in middle ear output that matches the audiometric roll-off at high frequencies in humans (Puria et al., 1997).

3.6.3 Role of non-piston-like stapes motions

The contribution of non-piston-like motions to hearing sensitivity is a point of two ongoing studies. Decraemer et al. (2007) have described three-dimensional sound-induced motion of the stapes in gerbils, and have compared these motion components to subsequent measurements of middle ear pressure gain in the same ears. The results indicate that while the measured pressure gain shows little frequency dependence between 2 kHz and 40 kHz, the amplitude of the displacement of the three spatial components of footplate motion show multiple peaks and valleys, with the piston-like stapes displacement showing the smoothest response. There was no correlation between the occurrence of maxima and minima in non-piston-like motion components and in the vestibule sound pressure, and the piston-like translation component was most like the vestibule sound pressure in response shape. These data suggest that the piston-like component of stapes motion is the best indicator of middle ear output and the non-piston-like motions contribute little to inner ear stimulation.

Eiber and colleagues (Eiber *et al.*, 2007; Sequeira *et al.*, 2007) are using a different approach to the question of the importance of non-piston-like stapes motions. They have developed a set of mechanical actuators that allow them to produce controlled three-dimensional motions of the guinea pig stapes while recording physiological responses to these motions. The results so far indicate that the inner ear is most sensitive to piston-like translation, but that there is considerable sensitivity to pure rocking motions of the stapes. This group is continuing to refine their techniques and will address this issue again.

3.6.4 Improvements in middle ear diagnostic procedures

While oto-reflectance and laser-Doppler vibrometry have both been shown to reliably detect ossicular disorders, there are other issues to which these devices are insensitive. One area that needs to be investigated is the diagnosis of the causes of tympanoplasty failures. About 50% of tympanoplasty procedures yield less than optimal hearing results (Merchant *et al.*, 2003). The causes of these failures range from mechanical issues such as poor coupling of the new tympanic membrane to the replacement ossicles, poor aeration leading to fluid accumulation, fixation of the stapes (or its replacement) by fibrous tissue, etc. A technique to help distinguish these different forms of failure would be useful. For example, it would be very helpful to differentiate between a loose prosthesis or graft, and eustachian tube failure, as the former is relatively easy to repair. While some of these causes for failure are easily observed with a normal tympanic membrane, the thicker and more opaque replacement grafts interfere with such judgments.

Acknowledgments

I thank Lisa Olson, Mike Ravicz, and Saumil Merchant for their comments on earlier versions of this chapter as well as all of my other co-workers at the Eaton-Peabody Laboratory of the Massachusetts Eye and Ear Infirmary for their input to this work. I also thank the National Institute for Deafness and Other Communicative Disorders for the continuing support that allowed me to prepare this chapter.

References

Aazh H, Moore B, Peyvandi AA & Stenfelt S. (2005) Influence of ear canal occlusion and static pressure difference on bone conduction thresholds: implications for mechanisms of bone conduction. *Int J Audiol* **44**: 178–89.

Aibara R, Welsh JT, Puria S & Goode RL. (2001) Human middle-ear sound transfer function and cochlear input impedance. *Hear Res* **152**: 100–9.

Algazi VR, Avendano C & Duda RO. (2001) Elevation localization and head-related transfer function analysis at low frequencies. *J Acoust Soc Am* **109**: 1110–22.

Algazi VR, Duda RO, Duraiswami R, Gumerov NA & Tang Z. (2002) Approximating the head-related transfer function using simple geometric models of the head and torso. *J Acoust Soc Am* **112**: 2053–64.

Allen JB. (1986) Measurements of eardrum acoustic impedance. In: Allen JB, Hall JH, Hubbard A, Neely ST & Tubis A, eds. *Peripheral Auditory Mechanisms.* Springer-Verlag, New York, pp. 44–51.

Allen JB, Jeng PS & Levitt H. (2005) Evaluation of human middle ear function via an acoustic power assessment. *J Rehabil Res Dev.* **42**: 63–78.

Allin EF & Hopson JA. (1992) Evolution of the auditory system in synapsida ('mammal-like' reptiles and primitive mammals) as seen in the fossil record. In: Webster DB, Fay RR & Popper AN, eds. *The Evolutionary Biology of Hearing.* Springer-Verlag, New York, pp. 587–614.

Asai M, Huber AM & Goode RL. (1999) Analysis of the best site on the stapes footplate for ossicular chain reconstruction. *Acta Otolaryngol* **119**: 356–61.

Aytekin M, Grassi E, Sahota M & Moss CF. (2004) The bat head-related transfer function reveals binaural cues for sound localization in azimuth and elevation. *J Acoust Soc Am* **116**: 3594–605.

Bance M, Campos A, Wong L, Morris DP & van Wijhe, R. (2007a) How does prosthesis head size affect vibration transmission in ossiculoplasty?. *Otolaryngol Head Neck Surg* **137**: 70–3.

Bance M, Morris DP & Van Wijhe R. (2007b) Effects of ossicular prosthesis mass and section of the stapes tendon on middle ear transmission. *J Otolaryngol* **36**: 113–19.

Batteau DW. (1967) The role of the pinna in human localization. *Proc R Soc Lond B Biol Sci* **8168**: 158–80.

Békésy G von. (1947) The sound pressure difference between the round and the oval windows and the artificial window of labyrinthine fenestration. *Acta Otolaryngol* **35**: 301–15.

Békésy G von. (1960) *Experiments in Hearing.* McGraw-Hill, New York.

Bismarck G Von & Pfeiffer RR. (1967) On the sound pressure transformation from free field to eardrum of chinchilla. *J Acoust Soc Am* **42**: 1156.

Borg E. (1968) A quantitative study of the effect of the acoustic stapedius reflex on sound transmission through the middle ear of man. *Acta Otolaryngol* **66**: 461–72.

Borg E & Møller AR. (1968) The acoustic middle ear reflex in unanesthetized rabbits. *Acta Otolaryngol* **65**: 575–85.

Borg E & Zakrisson JE. (1975) The activity of the stapedius muscle in man during vocalization. *Acta otolaryngol* **79**: 325–33.

Brackmann DE, Sheehy JL & Luxford WM. (1984) TORPS and PORPS in tympanoplasty: A review of 1042 operations. *Otolaryngol Head Neck Surg* **92**: 32–7.

Browning GG & Granich MS. (1978) Surgical anatomy of the temporal bone in the chinchilla. *Ann Otol Rhinol Laryngol* **87**: 875–82.

Butler RA & Belendiuk K. (1977) Spectral cues utilized in the localization of sound in the median sagittal plane. *J Acoust Soc Am* **61**: 1264–9.

Carlsson P, Håkansson B & Ringdahl A. (1995) Force threshold for hearing by direct bone conduction. *J Acoust Soc Am* **97**: 1124–9.

Chan JCK & Geisler CD. (1990) Estimation of eardrum acoustic pressure and of ear canal length from remote points in the canal. *J Acoust Soc Am* **87**: 1237–47.

Cheng T, Dai C & Gan RZ. (2007) Viscoelastic properties of human tympanic membrane. *Ann Biomed Eng* **35**: 305–14.

Cherukupally SR, Merchant SN & Rosowski JJ. (1998) Correlations between stapes pathology and conductive hearing loss in otosclerosis. *Ann Otol Rhinol Laryngol* **107**: 319–26.

Chien W, Ravicz ME, Merchant SN & Rosowski JJ. (2006a) The effect of methodological differences in the measurement of stapes motion in live and cadaver ears. *Audiol Neurootol* **11**: 183–97.

Chien W, Rosowski JJ, Ravicz ME & Merchant SN. (2006b) Measurements of stapes velocity in live human ears. Abstracts of the Twenty-Ninth Meeting of the Association for Research in Otolaryngology, Baltimore, MD, USA, February 2006, p. 216.

Chien W, Ravicz ME, Rosowski JJ & Merchant SN. (2007) Measurements of human middle- and inner-ear mechanics with dehiscence of the superior semicircular canal. *Otol & Neurotol* **28**: 250–7.

Dahmann H. (1929) Zur Physiologie des Hörens; experimentelle Untersuchungen über die Mechanik der Gehörknöchelchenkette, sowie über deren Verhalten auf Ton und Luftdruck. *Z. Hals-Nasen-u Ohrenheilk* **24**: 462–97.

Dai C, Cheng T, Wood MW & RZ Gan. (2007) Fixation and detachment of superior and anterior malleolar ligaments in human middle ear: Experiment and modeling. *Hear Res* **230**: 23–33.

Dallos P. (1973) *The Auditory Periphery*. Academic Press, New York.

Dancer A & Franke R. (1980) Intracochlear sound pressure measurements in guinea pigs. *Hear Res* **2**: 191–205.

Décory L, Guilhaume A, Dancer A & Aran J-M. (1988) On the origin of interspecific differences in auditory susceptibility. In: Wilson JP, Kemp DT, eds. *Cochlear Mechanisms: Structure, Function and Models*. Plenum Press, New York, pp. 225–34.

Decraemer WF & Dirckx JJJ. (1998) Pressure regulation due to displacement of the pars flaccida and pars tensa of the tympanic membrane. *Otorhinolaryngol Nova* **8**: 277–81.

Decraemer WF & Khanna SM. (2004) Measurement, visualization and quantitative analysis of complete three-dimensional kinematical data sets of human and cat middle ear. In: Gyo K, Wada H, Hato N & Koike T, eds. *Middle Ear Mechanics in Research and Otology*. World Scientific, Singapore, pp. 3–10.

Decraemer WF, Khanna SM & Funnell WRJ. (1989) Interferometric measurement of the amplitude and phase of tympanic membrane vibrations in cat. *Hear Res* **38** (1/2): 1–18.

Decraemer WF, Khanna SM & Funnell WRJ. (1995) Bending of the manubrium in cat under normal sound stimulation. *Progress in Biomedical Optics* **2329**: 74–84.

Decraemer WF, Khanna SM & Funnell WRJ. (1999) Vibrations at a fine grid of points on the cat tympanic membrane measured with a heterodyne interferometer. Presented at the EOS/Spie International Symposia on Industrial Lasers and Inspection, Conference on Biomedical Laser and Metrology and Applications, Munich, August 1999.

Decraemer WF, Khanna SM & Funnell WRJ. (2000) Measurement and modeling of the three-dimensional vibrations of the stapes in cat. In: Wada H, Takasaka T, Ikeda K, Ohyama K & T Koike, eds. *Proceedings of the Symposium on Recent Developments in Auditory Mechanics*. World Scientific, Singapore, pp. 36–43.

Decraemer WF, Dirckx JJJ & Funnell WRJ. (2003) Three-dimensional modeling of the middle-ear ossicular chain using a commercial high-resolution X-ray CT scanner. *J Assoc Res Otolaryngol* **4**: 250–63.

Decraemer WF, de La Rochefoucauld O, Dong W, Khanna SM, Dirckx JJ & Olson ES. (2007) Scala vestibuli pressure and three-dimensional stapes velocity measured in direct succession in gerbil. *J Acoust Soc Am* **121**: 2774–91.

de La Rochefoucauld O & Olson E. (2007) Exploring sound transmission through the middle ear by tracing middle ear delay. Abstracts of the Thirtieth Meeting of the Association for Research in Otolaryngology, Denver, CO, USA, February 2007, p. 182.

Dirckx JJJ, Decraemer WF, Unge M von & Larsson C. (1998) Volume displacement of the gerbil eardrum pars flaccida as a function of middle ear pressure. *Hear Res* **118**: 35–46.

Doan DE, Erulkar JS & Saunders JC. (1996) Functional changes in the aging mouse middle ear. *Hear Res* **97**: 174–7.

Dong W & Olson ES. (2006) Middle ear forward and reverse transfer function. *J Neurophysiol* **95**: 2951–61.

Doyle WJ. (2000) Middle ear pressure regulation. In: Rosowski JJ & Merchant SN, eds. *The Function and Mechanics of Normal, Diseased and Reconstructed Middle Ears*. Kugler, The Hauge, pp. 3–21.

Eiber A, Breuninger C, Sequeira D, Huber A. (2007) Mechanical excitation of complex stapes motion in guinea pigs. In: Huber A, Eiber A, eds. *Middle Ear Mechanics in Research and Otology*. World Scientific, Singapore, pp. 123–129.

Fay JP, Puria S, Decraemer WF & Steele C. (2005) Three approaches for estimating the elastic modulus of the tympanic membrane. *J Biomech* **38**: 1807–15.

Fay JP, Puria S & Steele CR. (2006) The discordant eardrum. *Proc Natl Acad Sci U S A* **103**: 19743–8.

Feeney MP & Keefe DH. (1999) Acoustic reflex detection using wide-band acoustic reflectance, admittance, and power measurements. *J Speech Lang Hear Res* **42**: 1029–41.

Feeney MP & Sanford CA. (2004) Age effects in the human middle ear: Wideband acoustical measures. *J Acoust Soc Am* **116**: 3546–58.

Feeney MP, Grant IL & Marryott LP. (2003) Wideband energy reflectance in adults with middle-ear disorders. *J Speech Lang Hear Res* **46**: 901–11.

Firzlaff U & Schuller G. (2004) Directionality of hearing in two CF/FM bats, *Pteronotus parnellii* and *Rhinolophus rouxi*. *Hear Res* **197**: 74–86.

Fung YC. (1981) *Biomechanics: Mechanical Properties of Living Tissues*. Springer-Verlag, New York.

Funnell WRJ & Decraemer WF. (1996) On the incorporation of moiré shape measurements in finite-element models of the cat eardrum. *J Acoust Soc Am* **100**: 925–32.

Funnell WRJ & Laszlo CA. (1982) A critical review of experimental observations on ear-drum structure and function. *ORL J Otorhinolaryngol Relat Spec* **44**: 181–205.

Funnell WRJ, Decraemer WF & Khanna SM. (1987) On the damped frequency response of a finite-element model of the cat eardrum. *J Acoust Soc Am* **81**: 1851–9.

Funnell WRJ, Khanna SM & Decraemer WF. (1992) On the degree of rigidity of the manubrium in a finite-element model of the cat eardrum. *J Acoust Soc Am* **91**: 2082–90.

Funnell WRJ, Siah TH, McKee MD, Daniel SJ & Decraemer WF. (2005) On the coupling between the incus and the stapes in the cat. *J Assoc Res Otolaryngol* **6**: 9–18.

Furlong C & Pryputniewicz RJ. (1998) Hybrid computational and experimental approach for the study and optimization of mechanical components. *Opt Eng* **37**: 1448–55.

Furlong C & Pryputniewicz RJ. (2000) Absolute shape measurements using high-resolution optoelectronic holography methods. *Opt Eng* **39**: 216–23.

Gan RZ, Sun Q, Dyer RK jr, Chang KH & Dormer KJ. (2002) Three-dimensional modeling of middle-ear biomechanics and its applications. *Otol Neurotol* **23**: 271–80.

Gan RZ, Dai C & Wood MW. (2006a) Laser interferometry measurements of middle ear fluid and pressure effects on sound transmission. *J Acoust Soc Am* **120**: 3799–810.

Gan RZ, Sun Q, Feng B & Wood MW. (2006b) Acoustical-structural coupled finite element analysis for sound transmission in human ear-Pressure distributions. *Med Eng Phys* **28**: 395–404.

Goode RL & Nishihara S. (1994) Experimental models of ossiculoplasty. *Otolaryngol Clin North Am* **27**: 663–75.

Goode RL, Ball G & Nishihara S. (1993) Measurement of umbo vibration in human subjects- methods and possible clinical applications. *Am J Otol* **14**: 247–51.

Goode RL, Killion M, Nakamura K & Nishihara S. (1994) New knowledge about the function of the human middle ear: Development of an improved analog model. *Am J Otol* **15**: 145–54.

Goode RL, Ball G, Nishihara S & Nakamura K. (1996) Laser Doppler vibrometer (LDV) a new clinical tool for the otologist. *Am J Otol* **17**: 813–22.

Goodhill V. (1979) *Ear Diseases, Deafness and Dizziness*. Harper & Row, Hagerstown, MD, pp. 781.

Gotay-Rodriguez VM & Schuknecht HF. (1977) Experience with type IV tympanomastoidectomy. *Laryngoscope* **87**: 522–8.

Graves AJ. (2005) The effect of smooth muscle antagonists on the sound-induced motion of the tympanic membrane. Master's Thesis in Speech and Hearing Bioscience and Technology, MIT, Cambridge, MA.

Guinan JJ Jr & Peake WT. (1967) Middle-ear characteristics of anesthetized cats. *J Acoust Soc Am* **41**: 1237–61.

Gyo K, Goode RL & Miller C. (1986) Effect of middle ear modification on umbo vibration–human temporal bone experiments with a new vibration measuring system. *Arch Otolaryngol Head Neck Surg* **112**: 1262–8.

Gyo K, Aritomo H & Goode RL. (1987) Measurement of the ossicular vibration ratio in human temporal bones by use of a video measuring system. *Acta Otolaryngol* 103: 87–95.

Håkansson B, Brandt A & Carlsson P. (1994) Resonance frequencies of the human skull *in vivo. J Acoust Soc Am* 95: 1474–81.

Håkansson B, Carlsson P, Brandt A & Stenfelt S. (1996) Linearity of sound transmission through the human skull *in vivo. J Acoust Soc Am* 99: 2239–43.

Hammershøi D & Møller H. (1996) Sound transmission to and within the human ear canal. *J Acoust Soc Am* 100: 408–27.

Harrison WH, Shambaugh GE & Derlacki EL. (1964) Congenital absence of the round window: case report with surgical reconstruction by cochlear fenestration. *Laryngoscope* 74: 967–78.

Hato N, Stenfelt S & Goode RL. (2003) Three-dimensional stapes footplate motion in human temporal bones. *Audiol Neurootol* 8: 140–52.

Heiland KE, Goode RL, Asai M & Huber AM. (1999) A human temporal bone study of stapes footplate movement. *Am J Otol* 20: 81–6.

Hellstrom S & Stenfors L-E. (1983) The pressure equilibrating function of the pars flaccida in middle ear mechanics. *Acta Physiol Scand* 118: 337–41.

Helmholtz HL von. (1868) Die Mechanik der Gehörknöchelchen und des Trommelfells. *Pflugers Arch Gesamte Physiol* 1: 1–60.

Hemilä S, Nummela S & Reuter T. (1995) What middle ear parameters tell about impedance matching and high frequency hearing. *Hear Res* 85: 31–44.

Henson OW Jr. (1965) The activity and function of the middle-ear muscles in echo-locating bats. *J Physiol* 180: 871–87.

Henson OW Jr. (1974) Comparative anatomy of the middle ear. In: Kiedel WD & Neff WD, eds. *Handbook of Sensory Physiology: The Auditory System.* Springer-Verlag, New York, Vol 1, pp. 39–110.

Henson OW Jr & Henson MM. (2000) The tympanic membrane: Highly developed smooth muscle arrays in the annulus fibrosus of mustached bats. *J Assoc Res Otolaryngol* 1: 25–32.

Henson MM, Madden VJ, Rask-Andersen H & Henson OW Jr. (2005) Smooth muscle in the annulus fibrosus of the tympanic membrane in bats, rodents, insectivores and humans. *Hear Res* 200: 29–37.

Huang AY & May BJ. (1996) Spectral cues for sound localization in cats: effects of frequency domain on minimum audible angles in the median and horizontal planes. *J Acoust Soc Am* 100: 2341–8.

Huang GT, Rosowski JJ, Flandermeyer DT, Lynch TJ III & Peake WT. (1997) The middle ear of a lion: Comparison of structure and function to domestic cat. *J Acoust Soc Am* 101: 1532–49.

Huber AM, Linder T, Ferrazzini M, Schmid S, Dillier N, Stoeckli S & Fisch U. (2001a) Intraoperative assessment of stapes movement. *Ann Otol Rhinol Laryngol* 110: 31–5.

Huber AM, Schwab C, Linder T, Stoeckli SJ, Ferrazzinin M, Dillier N & Fisch U. (2001b) Evaluation of eardrum laser doppler interferometry as a diagnostic tool. *Laryngoscope* 111: 501–7.

Huber AM, Koike T, Wada H, Nandapalan V & Fisch U. (2003) Fixation of the anterior mallear ligament: diagnosis and consequences for hearing results in stapes surgery. *Ann Otol Rhinol Laryngol* 112: 348–55.

Hunt RM Jr. (1974) The auditory bulla in carnivora: An anatomical basis for reappraisal of carnivore evolution. *J Morphol* 143: 21–76.

Hunt RM Jr & Korth WW. (1980) The auditory region of *Dermoptera:* morphology and function relative to other living mammals. *J Morphol* 164: 167–211.

Hüttenbrink KB. (1988) The mechanics of the middle-ear at static air pressures. *Acta Otolaryngol Suppl* 451: 1–35.

Hyrtl J. (1844) *Vergleichend anatomische Untersuchungen über das innere Gehörgan des Menschen und der Säugertiere.* Prague.

Ingelstedt S & Jonson B. (1966) Mechanisms of gas exchange in the normal human middle ear. *Acta Otolaryngol Suppl* 224: 452–61.

Keefe DH, Bulen JC, Arehart KH & Burns EM. (1993) Ear-canal impedance and reflection coefficient in human infants and adults. *J Acoust Soc Am* 94: 2617–38.

Keefe DH, Bulen JC, Campbell SL & Burns EM. (1994) Pressure transfer function and absorption cross section from the diffuse field to the human infant ear canal. *J Acoust Soc Am* **95**: 355–71.

Keller CH, Hartung K & Takahashi TT. (1998) Head-related transfer functions of the barn-owl: measurements and neural response. *Hear Res* **118**: 13–34.

Khanna SM & Tonndorf J. (1972) Tympanic membrane vibrations in cats studied by time-averaged holography. *J Acoust Soc Am* **51**: 1904–20.

Kinsler LE, Frey AR, Coppens AB & Sanders JV. (1982) *Fundamentals of Acoustics*. Wiley & Sons, New York.

Kistler DJ & Wightman FL. (1992) A model of head-related transfer functions based on principal components analysis and minimum phase reconstruction. *J Acoust Soc Am* **91**: 1637–47.

Kobrak HG. (1959) *The Middle Ear*. University of Chicago Press, Chicago IL.

Kohllöffel LUE. (1984) Notes on the comparative mechanics of hearing. III. On Shrapnell's membrane. *Hear Res* **13**: 83–8.

Koike T, Wada H & Kobayashi T. (2002) Modeling of the human middle ear using the finite-element method. *J Acoust Soc Am* **111**: 1306–17.

Kringlebotn M. (1988) Network model for the human middle ear. *Scand Audiol* **17**: 75–85.

Kruger B & Tonndorf J. (1977) Middle ear transmission in cats with experimentally induced tympanic membrane perforations. *J Acoust Soc Am* **61**: 126–32.

Kruger B & Tonndorf J. (1978) Tympanic membrane perforation in cats: configuration of losses with and without ear canal extensions. *J Acoust Soc Am* **63**: 436–41.

Kuijpers W, Peters TA & Tonnaer ELGM. (1999) Nature of the tympanic membrane insertion into the tympanic bone of the rat. *Hear Res* **128**: 80–8.

Kulkarni A & Colburn HS. (1998) Role of spectral detail in sound-source localization. *Nature* **396**: 747–9.

Kulkarni A, Isabelle SK & Colburn HS. (1999) Sensitivity of human subjects to head-related transfer-function phase spectra. *J Acoust Soc Am* **105**: 2821–40.

Kuhn GF. (1977) Model for the interaural time differences in the azimuthal plane. *J Acoust Soc Am* **62**: 157–67.

Kurokawa H & Goode RL. (1995) Sound pressure gain produced by the human middle ear. *Am J Otol* **113**: 349–55.

Ladak J & Funnell WRJ. (1996) Finite-element modeling of the normal and surgically repaired cat middle ear. *J Acoust Soc Am* **100**: 933–44.

Langendijk EH & Bronkhorst AW. (2002) Contribution of spectral cues to human sound localization. *J Acoust Soc Am* **112**: 1583–96.

Lawton BW & Stinson MR. (1985) Standing wave patterns in the human ear canal used for estimation of acoustic energy reflectance at the eardrum. *J Acoust Soc Am* **79**: 1003–9.

Lee K & Schuknecht HF. (1971) Results of tympanoplasty and mastoidectomy at the Massachusetts Eye and Ear Infirmary. *Laryngoscope* **81**: 529–43.

Lim DJ. (1968a) Tympanic membrane. Part I. Pars tensa. *Acta Otolaryngol* **66**: 181–98.

Lim DJ. (1968b) Tympanic membrane. Part II. Pars flaccida. *Acta Otolaryngol* **66**: 515–32.

Lim DJ. (1970) Human tympanic membrane, an ultrastructural observation. *Acta Otolaryngol* **70**: 176–86.

Limb CJ, Carey JP, Srireddy S & Minor LB. (2006) Auditory function in patients with surgically treated superior semicircular canal dehiscence. *Otol Neurotol* **27**: 969–80.

Linder TE, Ma F & Huber A. (2003) Round window atresia and its effect on sound transmission. *Otol Neurotol* **24**: 259–63.

Lopez-Poveda EA & Meddis R. (1996) A physical model of sound diffraction and reflections in the human concha. *J Acoust Soc Am* **100**: 3248–59.

Luntz M & Sadé J. (1990) Daily fluctuations of middle ear pressure in atelectatic ears. *Ann Otol Rhinol Laryngol* **99**: 201–4.

Luntz M, Fuchs C & Sadé J. (1997) Correlations between retractions of the pars flaccida and the pars tensa. *J Laryngol Otol* 111: 322–4.

Lynch TJ III, Nedzelnitsky V & Peake WT. (1982) Input impedance of the cochlea in cat. *J Acoust Soc Am* 72: 108–30.

Lynch TJ III, Peake WT & Rosowski JJ. (1994) Measurements of the acoustic input-impedance of cat ears: 10Hz to 20kHz. *J Acoust Soc Am* 96: 2184–209.

Magnan P, Avan P, Dancer A, Smurzynski J & Probst R. (1997) Reverse middle-ear transfer function in the guinea pig measured with cubic difference tones. *Hear Res* 107: 41–5.

Maki K & Furukawa S. (2005) Acoustical cues for sound localization by the Mongolian gerbil *Meriones unguiculatus*. *J Acoust Soc Am* 118: 872–86.

Manley GA & Johnstone BM. (1974) Middle-ear function in the guinea pig. *J Acoust Soc Am* 56: 571–6.

Margolis RH, Saly GL & Keefe DH. (1999) Wideband reflectance tympanometry in normal adults. *J Acoust Soc Am* 106: 265–80.

Marquet J. (1981) The incudo-malleal joint. *J Laryngol Otol* 95: 542–65.

Mason MJ. (2001) Middle ear structures in fossorial mammals: A comparison with non-fossorial species. *J Zool (1987)* 255: 467–86.

Mehta RP, Ravicz ME, Rosowski JJ & Merchant SN. (2003) Middle-ear mechanics of type III tympanoplasty (stapes columella): I. Experimental studies. *Otol Neurotol* 24: 176–85.

Mehta RP, Rosowski JJ, Voss SE, O'Neil E & Merchant SN. (2006) Determinants of hearing loss in perforations of the tympanic membrane. *Otol Neurotol* 27: 136–43.

Merchant SN & Rosowski JJ. (2008) Conductive hearing loss caused by third-window lesions of the inner ear. *Otol Neurotol* 29: 282–9.

Merchant SN, Rosowski JJ, Ravicz ME. (1995) Mechanics of type IV and V tympanoplasty. II. Clinical analysis and surgical implications. *Am J Otol* 16: 565–75.

Merchant SN, Ravicz ME & Rosowski JJ. (1997) Mechanics of Type IV Tympanoplasty: experimental findings and surgical implications. *Ann Otol Rhinol Laryngol* 106: 49–60.

Merchant SN, Rosowski JJ & McKenna MJ. (2003) Tympanoplasty. *Operative Techniques in Otolaryngology-HNS.* 14: 224–36.

Merchant SN, Nakajima HH, Halpin C, Nadol JB Jr, Lee DJ, Innis WP, Curtin H & Rosowski JJ. (2007) Clinical investigation and mechanism of air-bone gaps in large vestibular aqueduct syndrome. *Ann Otol Rhinol Laryngol* 116: 532–41.

Middlebrooks JC. (1999) Individual differences in external-ear transfer functions reduced by scaling in frequency. *J Acoust Soc Am* 106: 1480–92.

Middlebrooks JC, Makous JC & Green DM. (1989) Directional sensitivity of sound-pressure levels in the human ear canal. *J Acoust Soc Am* 86: 89–108.

Mikulec AA, McKenna MJ, Ramsey MJ, Rosowski JJ, Herrmann BS, Rauch SD, Curtin HD & Merchant SN. (2004) Superior semicircular canal dehiscence presenting as conductive hearing loss without vertigo. *Otol Neurotol* 25: 121–9.

Mikulec AA, Poe DS & McKenna MJ. (2005) Operative management of superior semicircular canal dehiscence. *Laryngoscope* 115: 501–7.

Minor LB. (2000) Superior canal dehiscence syndrome. *Am J Otol* 21: 9–19.

Minor LB, Solomon D, Zinreich JS & Zee DS. (1998) Sound- and/or pressure-induces vertigo due to bone dehiscence of the superior semicircular canal. *Arch Otolaryngol* 124: 249–58.

Minor LB, Carey JP, Cremer PD, Lustig LR, Streubel SO & Ruckenstein MJ. (2003) Dehiscence of bone overlying the superior canal as a cause of apparent conductive hearing loss. *Otol Neurotol* 24: 270–8.

Møller AR. (1961) Network model of the middle ear. *J Acoust Soc Am* 33: 168–76.

Møller AR. (1964) Effect of tympanic muscle activity on movement of the eardrum, acoustic impedance and cochlear microphones. *Acta Otolaryngol* 58: 1–10.

Møller AR. (1965) Experimental study of the acoustic impedance of the middle ear and its transmission properties. *Acta Otolaryngol* **60**: 129–49.

Møller AR. (1974) The acoustic middle-ear muscle reflex. In: Keidel WD & Neff WD, eds. *Handbook of Sensory Physiology: Auditory System*. Springer-Verlag, New York, Vol. 1, pp. 519–48.

Møller AR. (1983) *Auditory Physiology*. Academic Press, New York.

Moore WJ. (1981) *The Mammalian Skull*. Cambridge University Press, Cambridge.

Morris DP, Wong L, van Wijhe RG & Bance ML. (2006) Effect of adhesion on the acoustic functioning of partial ossicular replacement prostheses in the cadaveric human ear. *J Otolaryngol* **35**: 22–5.

Nakajima HH, Ravicz ME, Merchant SN, Peake WT & Rosowski JJ. (2005a) Experimental ossicular fixations and the middle-ear's response to sound: Evidence for a flexible ossicular chain. *Hear Res* **204**: 60–77.

Nakajima HH, Ravicz ME, Rosowski JJ, Peake WT & Merchant SN. (2005b) Experimental and clinical studies of malleus fixation. *Laryngoscope* **115**: 147–54.

Nedzelnitsky V. (1980) Sound pressures in the basal turn of the cat cochlea. *J Acoust Soc Am* **68**: 1676–89.

Neely ST & Gorga MP. (1998) Comparison between intensity and pressure as measures of sound level in the ear canal. *J Acoust Soc Am* **104**: 2925–34.

Novacek MJ. (1977) Aspects of the problem of variation, origin and evolution of the eutherian auditory bulla. *Mammal Rev* **7**: 131–50.

Olson ES. (1998) Observing middle and inner ear mechanics with novel intracochlear pressure sensors. *J Acoust Soc Am* **103**: 3445–63.

Olson ES & Cooper N. (2000) Stapes motion and scala vestibuli pressure in gerbils. Abstracts of the Twenty-Third Meeting of the Association for Research in Otolaryngology, St Petersburg Beach, FL, USA, February 2000, p. 114.

Onchi Y. (1961) Mechanism of the middle ear. *J Acoust Soc Am* **33**: 794–805.

Overstreet EH III & Ruggero MA. (2002) Development of wide-band middle-ear transmission in the Mongolian gerbil. *J Acoust Soc Am* **111**: 261–70.

Pang XD & Peake WT. (1986) How do contractions of the stapedius muscle alter the acoustic properties of the middle ear? In: Allen JB, Hall JL, Hubbard A, Neely ST & Tubis A, eds. *Peripheral Auditory Mechanisms*. Springer-Verlag, New York, pp. 36–43.

Peake WT, Rosowski JJ & Lynch TJ III. (1992) Middle-ear transmission: Acoustic vs. ossicular coupling in cat and human. *Hear Res* **57**: 245–68.

Pearce M, Richter CP & Cheatham MA. (2001) A reconsideration of sound calibration in the mouse. *J Neurosci Methods* **106**: 57–67.

Pralong D. (1996) The role of individualized headphone calibration for the generation of high fidelity virtual auditory space. *J Acoust Soc Am* **100**: 3785–93.

Proctor B. (1964) Type 4 tympanoplasty: A critical review of 122 cases. *Arch Otolaryngol* **79**: 176–81.

Puria S. (2003) Measurements of human middle ear forward and reverse acoustics: Implications for otoacoustic emissions. *J Acoust Soc Am* **113**: 2773–89.

Puria S & Allen JB. (1991) A parametric study of cochlear input impedance. *J Acoust Soc Am* **89**: 287–309.

Puria S & Allen JB. (1998) Measurements and model of the cat middle ear: Evidence of tympanic membrane acoustic delay. *J Acoust Soc Am* **104**: 3463–81.

Puria S, Peake WT & Rosowski JJ. (1997) Sound-pressure measurements in the cochlear vestibule of human cadavers. *J Acoust Soc Am* **101**: 2745–70.

Puria S, Kunda LD, Roberson JB & Perkins RC. (2005) Malleus-to-footplate ossicular reconstruction prosthesis positioning: Cochleovestibular pressure optimization. *Otol Neurotol* **26**: 368–79.

Qi L, Liu H, Lutfy J, Funnell WRJ & Daniel SJ. (2006) A nonlinear finite-element model of the newborn ear canal. *J Acoust Soc Am* **120**: 3789–98.

Ranke OF. (1953) Physiologie des Gehörs. In: Ranke OF & Lullies H, eds. *Gehör-Stimme-Sprache*. Springer, Berlin, pp. 3–110.

Ravicz ME, Rosowski JJ & Voigt HF. (1992) Sound-power collection by the auditory periphery of the Mongolian gerbil *Meriones unguiculatus*: I. Middle-ear input impedance. *J Acoust Soc Am* **92**: 157–77.

Ravicz ME, Peake WT, Nakajima HH, Merchant SN, Rosowski JJ. (2004a) Modeling flexibility in the human ossicular chain: Comparison to ossicular fixation data. In: Gyo K, Wada H, Hato N, Koike T, eds. *The Proceedings of the Third International Symposium on Middle-Ear Mechanics in Research and Oto-Surgery*. World Scientific, Singapore, pp. 91–98.

Ravicz ME, Rosowski JJ & Merchant SN. (2004b) Mechanisms of hearing loss resulting from middle-ear fluid. *Hear Res* **195**: 105–30.

Ravicz ME, Olson ES & Rosowski JJ. (2007) Sound pressure distribution and energy flow within the gerbil ear canal from 100 Hz to 80 kHz. *J Acoust Soc Am* **122**: 2154–73.

Ravicz ME, Cooper N & Rosowski JJ. (2008) Gerbil middle-ear sound transmission from 100 Hz to 60 kHz. *J Acoust Soc Am* **124**: 363–80.

Rice JJ, May BJ, Spirou GA & Young ED. (1992) Pinna-based spectral cues for sound localization in cat. *Hear Res* **58**: 132–52.

Rodriguez Jorge J, Zenner H-P, Hemmert W, Burkhardt C & Gummer AW. (1997) Laservibrometrie: ein mittelohr- und Kochelaanalysator zur nicht-invasiven Untersuchung von Mittel-und Innenohrfunktionsstörungen. *HNO* **45**: 997–1007.

Rosowski JJ. (1991a) The effects of external- and middle-ear filtering on auditory threshold and noise-induced hearing loss. *J Acoust Soc Am* **90**: 124–35.

Rosowski JJ. (1991b) Erratum: The effects of external- and middle-ear filtering on auditory threshold and noise- induced hearing loss [*J Acoust Soc Am* 1991; 90: 124–35]. *J Acoust Soc Am* **90**: 3373.

Rosowski JJ. (1992) Hearing in transitional mammals: Predictions from the middle-ear anatomy and hearing capabilities of extant mammals. In: Webster DB, Popper AN & Fay RR, eds. *The Evolutionary Biology of Hearing*. Springer-Verlag, New York, pp. 615–31.

Rosowski JJ. (1994) Outer and middle ear. In: Popper AN & Fay RR, eds. *Springer Handbook of Auditory Research: Comparative Hearing: Mammals*. Vol. IV. Springer-Verlag, New York, pp. 172–247.

Rosowski JJ. (1996) Models of external and middle-ear function. In: Hawkins HL, McMullen TA, Popper AN & Fay RR, eds. *The Springer Handbook of Auditory Research Volume 6: Auditory Computation*. Springer-Verlag, New York, pp. 15–61.

Rosowski JJ & Lee C-Y. (2002) The effect of immobilizing the gerbil's pars flaccida on the middle-ear's response to static pressure. *Hear Res* **174**: 183–95.

Rosowski JJ, Carney LH, Lynch TJ III & Peake WT. (1986) The effectiveness of external and middle ears in coupling acoustic power into the cochlea. In: Allen JB, Hall JL, Hubbard A, Neely ST & Tubis A, eds. *Peripheral Auditory Mechanisms*. Springer-Verlag, New York, pp. 3–12.

Rosowski JJ, Davis PJ, Merchant SN, Donahue KM & Coltrera MD. (1990) Cadaver middle ears as models for living ears: Comparisons of middle-ear input immittance. *Ann Otol Rhinol Laryngol Suppl* **99**: 403–12.

Rosowski JJ, Teoh SW & Flandermeyer DT. (1997) The effect of the pars flaccida of the tympanic membrane on the ear's sensitivity to sound. In: Lewis ER, Long GR, Lyon RF, Narins PM, Steele CR & Hect-Poiner E, eds. *Diversity in Auditory Mechanics*. World Scientific, New Jersey, pp. 129–35.

Rosowski JJ, Mehta RP & Merchant SN. (2003a) Diagnostic utility of laser-Doppler vibrometry in conductive hearing loss with normal tympanic membrane. *Otol Neurotol* **24**: 165–75.

Rosowski JJ, Brinsko KM, Tempel BL & Kujawa SG. (2003b) The ageing of the middle ear in 129S6/SvEvTac and CBA/CaJ mice: Measurements of umbo velocity, hearing function and the incidence of pathology. *J Assoc Res Otolaryngol* **4**: 371–83.

Rosowski JJ, Songer JE, Nakajima HH, Brinsko KM & Merchant SN. (2004) Clinical, experimental, and theoretical investigations of the effect of superior canal dehiscence on hearing mechanisms. *Otol Neurotol* **25**: 323–32.

Rosowski JJ, Ravicz ME & Songer JE. (2006) Structures that contribute to middle-ear admittance in chinchilla. *J Comp Physiol A* **192**: 1287–311.

Rosowski JJ, Furlong C, Ravicz ME, Rodgers MT. (2007) Real-time opto-electronic holographic measurements of sound-induced tympanic membrane displacements. In: Huber A & Eiber A, eds. *Middle-Ear Mechanics in Research and Otology*. World Scientific, New Jersey, pp. 295–305.

Rosowski JJ, Nakajima HH & Merchant SN. (2008) Clinical utility of laser-Doppler vibrometer measurements in live normal and pathologic human ears. *Ear Hear* **29**: 3–19.

Ruggero MA & Temchin AN. (2002) The roles of the external, middle and inner ears in determining the bandwidth of hearing. *Proc Natl Acad Sci U S A* **99**: 13206–10.

Ryan A. (1976) Hearing sensitivity in the Mongolian gerbil. *J Acoust Soc Am* **59**: 1222–6.

Sadé J & Amos A. (1997) Middle ear and auditory tube: Middle ear clearance, gas exchange, and pressure regulation. *Arch Otolaryngol Head Neck Surg* **116**: 499–524.

Saunders JC & Summers RM. (1982) Auditory structure and function in the mouse middle ear: An evaluation by SEM and capacitive probe. *J Comp Physiol A.* **146**: 517–25.

Schuknecht HF. (1974) *Pathology of the Ear*. Harvard University Press, Cambridge.

Sequeira D, Breuninger C, Eiber A, Huber A. (2007) The effects of complex stapes motion on the response of the cochlea in guinea pigs. In: Huber A & Eiber A, eds. *Middle Ear Mechanics in Research and Otology*. World Scientific, Singapore, pp. 130–135.

Shaw EAG. (1974a) Transformation of sound pressure level from the free field to the eardrum in the horizontal plane. *J Acoust Soc Am* **56**: 1848–60.

Shaw EAG. (1974b) The external ear. In: Keidel WD & Neff WD, eds. *Handbook of Sensory Physiology: Vol V/1: Auditory System*. Springer-Verlag, New York, pp. 455–490.

Shaw EAG. (1982) 1979 Rayleigh Medal Lecture: The elusive connection. In: Gatehouse RW. *Localization of Sound: Theory and Applications*. Amphora Press, Groton, CT, pp. 13–29.

Shaw EAG & Stinson MR. (1983) The human external and middle ear: Models and concepts. In: deBoer E & Viergever MA, eds. *Mechanics of Hearing*. University Press, Delft, pp. 3–10.

Shaw EAG & Teranishi R. (1968) Sound pressure generated in an external-ear replica and real human ears by a nearby point source. *J Acoust Soc Am* **44**: 240–9.

Shera CA & Zweig G. (1992a) Middle-ear phenomenology: The view from the three windows. *J Acoust Soc Am* **92**: 1356–70.

Shera CA & Zweig G. (1992b) An empirical bound on the compressibility of the cochlea. *J Acoust Soc Am* **92**: 1382–8.

Shrapnell HJ. (1832) On the form and structure of the membrana tympani. *Lond Med Gazette* **10**: 120–4.

Siebert WM. (1973) Hearing and the ear. In: Brown JHU, ed. *Engineering Principles in Physiology Vol 1*. Academic Press, New York, pp. 139–84.

Silman S. (1984) *The Acoustic Reflex: Basic Principles and Clinical Applications*. Academic Press, New York.

Sim JH & Puria S. (2008) Soft tissue morphometry of the malleus-incus complex from micro-CT imaging. *J Assoc Res Otolaryngol* **9**: 5–21.

Sohmer H. (2006) Sound induced fluid pressure directly activates vestibular hair cells: Implications for activation of the cochlea. *Clin Neurophysiol* **117**: 933–4.

Sohmer H & Freeman S. (2004) Further evidence for a fluid pathway during bone conduction auditory stimulation. *Hear Res* **193**: 105–10.

Sohmer H, Freeman S, Geal-Dor M, Adelman C & Savion I. (2000) Bone conduction experiments in humans – a fluid pathway from bone to ear. *Hear Res* **146**: 81–8.

Sohmer H, Freeman S & Perez R. (2004) Semicircular canal fenestration – improvement of bone- but not air-conducted auditory thresholds. *Hear Res* **187**: 105–10.

Songer JE. (2006) Superior canal dehiscence: auditory mechanisms. Speech and Hearing Bioscience and Technology Division of Health Sciences and Technology, Cambridge, MA. PhD Thesis, p. 159.

Songer JE & Rosowski JJ. (2005) The effect of superior canal dehiscence on cochlear potential in response to air-conducted stimuli in chinchilla. *Hear Res* **210**: 53–62.

Songer JE & Rosowski JJ. (2006) The effect of superior-canal opening on middle-ear input admittance and air-conducted stapes velocity in chinchilla. *J Acoust Soc Am* **120**: 258–69.

Songer JE & Rosowski JJ. (2007a) Transmission matrix analysis of the chinchilla middle ear. *J Acoust Soc Am* **122**: 932–42.

Songer JE & Rosowski JJ. (2007b) A mechano-acoustic model of the effect of superior canal dehiscence on hearing in chinchilla. *J Acoust Soc Am* **122**: 943–50.

Songer JE, Brinsko KM & Rosowski JJ. (2004) Superior semicircular canal dehiscence and bone conduction in chinchilla. In: Gyo K, Wada H, Hato N & Koike T, eds. *Middle-ear Mechanics in Research and Otology*. World Scientific, Singapore, pp. 234–41.

Spezio ML, Keller CH, Marrocco RT & Takahashi TT. (2000) Head-related transfer functions of the Rhesus monkey. *Hear Res* **144**: 73–88.

Stenfelt S & Goode RL. (2005a) Bone-conducted sound: physiological and clinical aspects. *Otol Neurotol* **26**: 1245–61.

Stenfelt S & Goode RL. (2005b) Transmission properties of bone conducted sound: measurements in cadaver heads. *J Acoust Soc Am* **118**: 2373–91.

Stenfelt S, Håkansson B & Tjellström A. (2000) Vibration characteristics of bone conducted sound *in vitro*. *J Acoust Soc Am* **107**: 422–31.

Stenfelt S, Hato N & Goode RL. (2002) Factors contributing to bone conduction: the middle ear. *J Acoust Soc Am* **111**: 947–59.

Stenfelt S, Wild T, Hato N & Goode RL. (2003) Factors contributing to bone conduction: the outer ear. *J Acoust Soc Am* **113**: 902–13.

Stenfelt S, Hato N & Goode RL. (2004) Fluid volume displacement at the oval and round windows with air and bone conduction stimulation. *J Acoust Soc Am* **115**: 797–812.

Stenfors L-E, Salen B & Winblad B. (1979) The role of pars flaccida in the mechanics of the middle ear. *Acta Otolaryngol* **88**: 395–400.

Stinson MR. (1986) Spatial distribution of sound pressure in the ear canal. In: Allen JB, Hall JL, Hubbard A, Neely ST & Tubis A, eds. *Peripheral Auditory Mechanisms*. Springer-Verlag, New York, pp. 13–20.

Stinson MR & Khanna SM. (1989) Specification of the geometry of the human ear canal for the prediction of sound-pressure level distribution. *J Acoust Soc Am* **85**: 2492–503.

Stinson MR, Shaw EAG & Lawton BW. (1982) Estimation of acoustical energy reflectance at the eardrum from measurements of pressure distribution in the ear canal. *J Acoust Soc Am* **72**: 766–73.

Teoh SW, Flandermeyer DT & Rosowski JJ. (1997) Effects of pars flaccida on sound conduction in ears of Mongolian gerbil: acoustic and anatomical measurements. *Hear Res* **106**: 39–65.

Tonndorf J. (1972) Bone conduction. In: Tobias JV, ed. *Foundations of Auditory Theory Vol II*. Academic Press, New York, pp. 197–237.

Tonndorf J & Khanna SM. (1970) The role of the tympanic membrane in middle ear transmission. *Ann Otol Rhinol Laryngol* **79**: 743–53.

Tonndorf J & Khanna SM. (1972) Tympanic-membrane vibrations in human cadaver ears studied by time-averaged holography. *J Acoust Soc Am* **52**: 1221–33.

Tonndorf J & Khanna SM. (1976) Mechanics of the auditory system. In: Hinchcliffe R & Harrison D, eds. *Scientific Foundations of Otolaryngology*. William Heineman, London, pp. 237–52.

Tonndorf J & Tabor JR. (1962) Closure of the cochlear windows: its effects upon air and bone-conduction. *Ann Otol Rhinol Laryngol* **71**: 5–29.

Voss SE & Allen JB. (1994) Measurement of acoustic impedance and reflectance in the human ear canal. *J Acoust Soc Am* **95**: 372–84.

Voss SE, Rosowski JJ & Peake WT. (1996) Is the pressure difference between the oval and round windows the effective acoustic stimulus for the cochlea?. *J Acoust Soc Am* **100**: 1602–16.

Voss SE, Rosowski JJ, Merchant SN & Peake WT. (2000a) Acoustic response of the human middle ear. *Hear Res* **150**: 43–69.

Voss SE, Rosowski JJ, Shera CA & Peake WT. (2000b) Acoustic mechanisms that determine the ear-canal sound pressures generated by earphones. *J Acoust Soc Am* **107**: 1548–65.

Voss SE, Rosowski JJ, Merchant SN & Peake WT. (2001a) Middle-ear function with tympanic membrane perforations. I. Measurements and Mechanisms. *J Acoust Soc Am* **110**: 1432–44.

Voss SE, Rosowski JJ, Merchant SN & Peake WT. (2001b) Middle-ear function with tympanic membrane perforations. II. A simple model. *J Acoust Soc Am* **110**: 1445–52.

Voss SE, Rosowski JJ, Merchant SN & Peake WT. (2001c) How do tympanic-membrane perforations affect human middle-ear sound transmission?. *Acta Otolaryngol* **121**: 169–73.

Voss SE, Rosowski JJ, Merchant SN, Peake WT. (2007) Non-ossicular signal transmission in human middle ears: experimental assessment of the 'acoustic route' with perforated tympanic membranes. *J Acoust Soc Am* **122**: 2135–53.

Voss SE & Shera CA. (2004) Simultaneous measurement of middle-ear input impedance and forward/ reverse transmission in cat. *J Acoust Soc Am* **116**: 2187–98.

Vrettakos PA, Dear SP & Saunders JC. (1988) Middle-ear structure in the chinchilla: a quantitative study. *Am J Otolaryngol* **9**: 58–67.

Wada H, Ando M, Takeuchi A, Sugawara H, Koike T, Kobayashi T, Hozawa K, Gemma T & Nara M. (2002) Vibration measurement of the tympanic membrane of guinea pig temporal bones using time-averaged speckle pattern interferometry. *J Acoust Soc Am* **111**: 2189–99.

Wever EG & Lawrence M. (1950) The acoustic pathway to the cochlea. *J Acoust Soc Am* **22**: 460–7.

Wever EG & Lawrence M. (1954) *Physiological Acoustics*. Princeton University Press, Princeton, NJ.

Whittemore KR, Merchant SN & Rosowski JJ. (1998) Acoustic mechanisms: canal wall-up versus canal wall-down mastiodectomy. *Otolaryngol Head Neck Surg* **118**: 751–61.

Whittemore KR, Merchant SN, Poon BB & Rosowski JJ. (2004) A normative study of tympanic membrane motion in humans using a laser Doppler vibrometer (LDV). *Hear Res* **187**: 85–104.

Wiener FM & Ross DA. (1946) The pressure distribution in the auditory canal in a progressive sound field. *J Acoust Soc Am* **18**: 401–8.

Wiener FM, Pfeiffer RR & Backus ASN. (1966) On the sound pressure transformation by the head and auditory meatus of the cat. *Acta Otolaryngol* **61**: 255–69.

Wiggers HC. (1937) The functions of the intra-aural muscles. *Am J Physiol* **120**: 771–80.

Wightman FL & Kistler DJ. (1989) Headphone simulation of free-field listening. II: Psychophysical validation. *J Acoust Soc Am* **85**: 868–78.

Wightman FL & Kistler DJ. (1992) The dominant role of low-frequency interaural time differences in sound localization. *J Acoust Soc Am* **91**: 1648–61.

Willi UB, Ferrazzini MA & Huber AM. (2002) The incudo-malleolar joint and sound transmission loss. *Hear Res* **174**: 32–44.

Wüllstein H. (1956) The restoration of the function of the middle ear in chronic otitis media. *Ann Otol Rhinol Laryngol* **65**: 1020–41.

Xu L & Middlebrooks JC. (2000) Individual differences in external-ear transfer functions of cats. *J Acoust Soc Am* **107**: 1451–9.

Yang X & Henson OW Jr. (2002) Smooth muscle in the annulus fibrosus of the tympanic membrane: Physiological effects on sound transmission in the gerbil. *Hear Res* **164**: 105–14.

Young ED, Rice JJ & Tong SC. (1996) Effects of pinna position on head-related transfer functions in the cat. *J Acoust Soc Am* **99**: 3064–76.

Zwislocki J. (1950) Theory of the acoustical action of the cochlea. *J Acoust Soc Am* **22**: 778–84.

Zwislocki J. (1962) Analysis of the middle-ear function. Part I: Input impedance. *J Acoust Soc Am* **34**: 1514–23.

Zwislocki J. (1963) Analysis of the middle ear function. Part II. Guinea-pig ear. *J Acoust Soc Am* **35**: 1034–40.

Zwislocki J. (1965) Analysis of some auditory characteristics. In: Luce RD, Bush RR & Galanter E, eds. *Handbook of Mathematical Psychology*. John Wiley & Sons, New York, Vol. III, pp. 3–97.

Zwislocki JJ. (1980) An ear simulator for acoustic measurements: Rationale, principles and limitations. In: Studebaker GA & Hochberg I, eds. *Acoustical Factors Affecting Hearing Aid Performance*. University Park Press, Baltimore.

Chapter 4

Otoacoustic emissions and evoked potentials

David T Kemp

4.1 Introduction

Hearing is an energetic process generating acoustic and electrical signals that can be externally recorded and used for clinical and research purposes. The outer ear and ear drum capture sound energy from the air. The middle ear transfers this energy to the cochlea as vibration with great efficiency so as to maximize hearing sensitivity. Inside the cochlea the vibrational energy initiates a complex physical interaction between motions of the fluid filling the cochlea and displacements of the spiral elastic basilar membrane that partitions the cochlea in two longitudinally from base to apex (Fig. 4.1A). That interaction results in what is known as the cochlear travelling wave (see Fig. 4.2), a progressive wave of fluid and membrane vibration that carries stimulus energy along the cochlear spiral at a speed very much slower than that of sound. The physical construction of the cochlea causes the wave's energy to become concentrated onto a small region of the basilar membrane depending on its frequency of vibration, at which point stimulation at that frequency is most effectively transduced by the cochlea's sensory inner hair cells. However, as the wave progresses towards this point some of its energy is lost due to viscous damping as the cochlear fluid is forced to vibrate in confined spaces and adjacent to cochlear tissues. Remarkably, some of that lost stimulus energy is regained as a result of the synchronized physical response of special-ized sensory cells which form an array running along the outer portion of the basilar membrane spiral. The mechanism is known as the cochlear amplifier and it is the small fraction of this mechanism's energy leaking back to the ear drum that creates otoacoustic emissions (OAEs).

The two types of sensory cell in the cochlea, the inner and outer hair cells, reside in the organ of Corti, which sits on the basilar membrane. Outer hair cells are organized in three spiral arrays along the outer part of the cochlear spiral beside one inner row of quite different cells, the inner hair cells (Fig. 4.1B). Outer hair cells respond to stimulation by drawing electrical current through their stereocilia ('S' in Fig. 4.1C) from the endocochlear potential (EP) of the endolymph when the stereocilia are displaced outwards. The EP is a 90 mV potential that is maintained in the endol-ymph of the scala media by the stria vascularis. The apical surfaces of all the sensory cells together with their stereocilia are exposed to this potential whereas the remainder of their cell bodies are bathed in the surrounding perilymph at zero potential relative to the body. Outer hair cell trans-ducer currents are therefore synchronously modulated by stimulus-induced basilar membrane motion. The resulting modulation of each cell's receptor potential generates a motile response because of the piezoelectric-like properties of a protein prestin in their lateral cell membrane. The modulation of receptor current caused by stimulus vibration is therefore converted back into synchronized mechanical vibration, which is then communicated back to the basilar membrane. This mechanical-to-electrical-to-mechanical feedback loop brings the travelling wave under

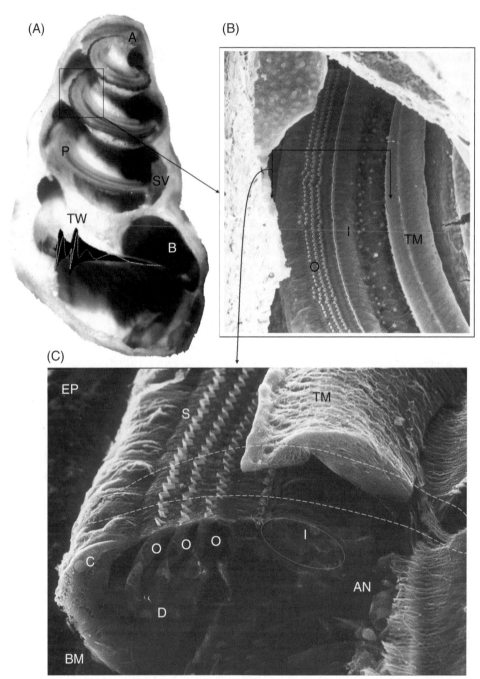

Fig. 4.1 The cochlea as a mechanism for sound processing, illustrated with a guinea pig ear. (A) The whole cochlea with bony encapsulation removed to show the spiral cochlear partition (P) incorporating the basilar membrane which makes three and a half turns from the basal end (B) to the apex (A). SV indicates the position of the stria vascularis that spirals around the outer wall. Superimposed on this photograph is a computer graphic showing two travelling waves (see text) of slightly differing high-frequency forming vibration peaks at two different places.

Fig. 4.1 *(Continued)* See also Figure 4.2. Note that these waves are grossly enlarged for illustration purposes. In fact the greatest vibration sound creates in the cochlea is of much less than cellular dimensions. (B) An enlargement under the electron microscope of the outlined section of cochlea in (A) shows the upper surface of the organ of Corti. The lines of stereocilia belonging to three outer (O) and one inner (I) row of hair cells are clearly visible. Distinct irregularities in the outer rows can be seen, and these could be the source of reflection-based otoacoustic emissions. The tectorial membrane (TM) is visible in this image but it is in the wrong location due to changes during tissue preparation. The higher magnification electron micrograph (C) of a section through the organ of Corti (C) shows the TM in more nearly the correct position but it is still distorted. The dashed white line shows the approximate *in vivo* location of the TM resting on the tops of the outer hair cell's stereocilia. This image also shows the bodies of the outer (O) and inner (I) hair cells. (The inner hair cell stereocilia have been disordered by the preparation method; they should be erect.) The outer hair cell bases rest on Dieter's cells (D) and the auditory nerve (AN) fibres synapse onto the base of the inner hair cell (not visible). The organ of Corti rests on the elastic basilar membrane (BM). The surfaces of all the structures above and on the surface of the organ of Corti are bathed in endolymph, which carries the endocochlear potential (EP) and fills the scala media. The inside of the organ of Corti and the hair cell bodies are bathed in the perilymph of the scale tympani, which is at body potential. The human cochlea differs from that of the guinea pig in that the spiral is wider at the base and has less height.

Figure 4.1A is a photograph by Ade Pye, used with permission; Figure 4.2B, C are electron microscope images by Andrew Forge, used with permission.

direct physiological control in a way that enhances the basilar membrane's physical responsiveness and greatly increases the sensitivity of hearing.

Of equal importance to the sensitivity of the cochlea is its capacity to analyse sounds into their component frequencies. The basilar membrane has uniquely tapered mechanical properties, being elastically stiff and narrow at the base and becoming wider and more flexible at the apex. As will be explained later this causes travelling waves of differing frequency to penetrate different distances along the spiral. Very low frequencies travel as far as the apex, about 3 cm distant, but very high frequencies reach only a millimetre or so from the base. As the stimulus-generated waves travel away from the base of the cochlea, their speed of progression reduces because of the basilar membrane tapering. This concentrates the incoming stimulus energy into a smaller and smaller space and so increases the amplitude of vibration. The amplitude of vibration continues to rise as the speed of progression slows and reaches a peak shortly before the place where the progression of that particular frequency wave would come to a physical stop. At the same time energy absorption accelerates and the vibration amplitude sinks very rapidly to zero. In this way stimulus components of different frequencies become spatially separated and focused onto different places along the basilar membrane (Fig. 4.2), paralleling the way a prism generates a coloured spectrum from white light. Each frequency in the range of hearing has its own 'frequency place' on the basilar membrane where maximum vibration to that frequency is found. This property is referred to as tonotopicity. It is the combination of this frequency-dispersive characteristic of wave transmission in the cochlea and the enhancement of that motion by the synchronous motility of outer hair cells which gives the mammalian cochlea its remarkably sensitive and frequency selective properties.

The fluid motion accompanying vibration of the basilar membrane and organ of Corti provides excitation to the inner hair cells. The crucial process of neurally encoding the stimulus begins only when fluid vibration surrounding the stereocilia of the inner hair cells reaches sufficient intensity. Like the outer hair cells, inner hair cells draw current from the EP and do so synchronously with

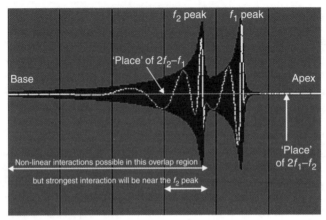

Fig. 4.2 A highly schematic representation of the travelling wave on the basilar membrane in response to two tones of frequency, f_1 and f_2. This was generated by a computer model of the cochlea written by David Brass (see Kemp, 2001). The undulating wave represents the greatly exaggerated displacement of the basilar membrane at a moment in time as the wave travels from left to right on the figure – from the base towards the apex in the cochlea. The dark filled area represents the envelope of the travelling wave. Note how the distance between wave peaks (the wavelength) reduces as the wave progresses from left to right. This is a consequence of a reduction in the speed of progression of the travelling wave due to anatomical tapering. Vibrations at frequency f_2 reach a peak first and stop, leaving the lower frequency f_1 to continue to form its own peak more apically (to the right on the figure). The position along the basilar membrane where a particular frequency peaks is called the 'frequency place'. The frequency places of f_1 and f_2 are marked. The long double-headed arrow shows the region of overlap of the two stimuli and the region of possible non-linear interactions between the two. There is no unique place where distortion is generated but the smaller double arrow marks the region where both waves have gained amplitude and where non-linear distortions are most likely to be generated. After generation, the distortion can travel, like a new stimulus, to its own frequency place. The frequency places of the two strongest distortion products are indicated. Note that the frequency place of the lower frequency distortion product $2f_1 - f_2$ is apical to the region stimulated by either f_1 or f_2.

the stimulus vibration. But inner hair cell transduction channels are more than 80% closed in the absence of stimulation so that the modulation of the receptor current by the stimulus is not simply a copy of the stimulus. It is very asymmetrical. Inner hair cell transduction channels open only to one phase of stimulation, the excitatory phase. In a process called rectification, sustained stimulation progressively depolarizes the cell. At some threshold level of depolarization, neurotransmitter is released causing the firing of one or more of the several afferent nerve fibres that synapse onto each inner hair cell. Firings can be synchronous with stimulus vibration for low frequencies.

The basilar membrane's frequency selective properties ensure that each place along the cochlear partition receives stimulation mainly from a restricted band of stimulus frequency components. We refer to this function as the 'auditory filter'. Each of the 3000 or so sensory inner hair cells arranged in a line around the cochlear spiral receives a frequency range around one-third of an octave wide, which is a 26% range of frequencies. The centre frequency of the auditory filter 'seen' at each inner hair cell location is different. However, adjacent inner hair cells' bands differs by only around 1/300 of an octave, or a 0.23% change in frequency, so there is a large degree of overlap. *Frequency resolution*, which is the separation of different simultaneously applied frequencies into different neural channels, is limited by the auditory filter to about one-third of an octave (a 26% frequency step). On the other hand, auditory frequency *discrimination*, which is the sensitivity to frequency changes, is limited by the ability of the cochlea to signal a change in the distribution of excitation along the basilar membrane. A musical semitone is about 1/11th of an octave or a 6.5% step in frequency and is readily detected even though the step is smaller than an auditory filter bandwidth. Musicians can detect much smaller differences in frequency than a semitone as they tune their instruments. The human potential for musical frequency discrimination is actually about hundred times finer than the cochlea's auditory filter bandwidth, and so it is important not to get the two terms confused. Frequency discrimination is enhanced by the precipitous termination of the travelling wave that is formed in response to a single frequency stimulus (see Fig. 4.2). This is because a minute change in the frequency of a pure tone can cause a great change in the excitation reaching the inner hair cells located near this termination. This mechanism does not assist the separation of simultaneously applied tones.

Since each inner hair cell receives a limited frequency band of the stimulation each of the afferent fibres synapsing on and excited by that cell (typically ten or more) appears to be 'tuned' or 'most sensitive to' that centre frequency. It is not of course the auditory nerve that is tuned but the 'place' where its inner hair cell resides. The nerve does not even need to carry nerve impulses at the correct stimulus frequency for the brain to work out what frequency is being received. That can be derived from its place of origin in the tonotopically organized cochlea. The crucial process of analysing and interpreting the cascade of sound-induced activity in the 30 000 or so primary auditory nerve fibres that emerge from the cochlea begins when they reach the cochlear nucleus. However, this chapter is concerned only with activity originating in the cochlea.

There is so much energetic activity occurring inside the cochlea that it is not surprising we can detect some of it from outside. We refer to a detectable electrical or mechanical signal arising from stimulus-related activity in the cochlea as an 'auditory response' to that stimulation. Externally detectable signals are not 'responses' in the sense of a functional reflex but just byproducts of cochlear function, that is, a leakage of energy which is of little consequence for hearing. Historically the discovery of each 'cochlear response' came as a surprise to auditory physiologists (e.g. cochlear microphonic: Wever & Bray, 1930; action potential: Galambos & Davis, 1948; Galambos, 1954; cochlear summating potential: Davis *et al.*, 1950; travelling waves: von Bekesy, 1950; otoacoustic emissions: Kemp, 1977). Each led to a reassessment of the contemporary understanding of cochlear function and each revealed something quite new and important about how the cochlea works. The 'revelationary' role of cochlear responses continues, with their evolving applications in auditory research, hearing screening, and clinical diagnosis.

4.2 **Cochlear responses**

The compact overview of cochlear function given above allows us to deduce what kind of responses might be measurable outside the cochlea. First, we would expect some externally detectable mechanical reaction to the development of the travelling wave and to its subsequent interaction with electromotile outer hair cells. Second, we would expect some external electrical signals to arise from the stimulus-driven currents flowing through both inner and outer hair cells. Third, we would expect to detect the gross action potential of the auditory nerve. This chapter seeks to introduce the nature, origin, and applications of externally observable correlates of normal cochlear function, namely:

- otoacoustic emissions (OAEs)
- cochlear input impedance (Zc)

- ◆ cochlear microphonic (CM)
- ◆ cochlear summating potential (SP)
- ◆ auditory compound action potential (CAP).

A distinctly biophysical approach will be taken to introduce each cochlear response. Most attention will be focused on the acoustic or rather 'otoacoustic' responses of the cochlea. This is partly because these responses tell us most specifically about the most vulnerable cochlear mechanism on which high sensitivity depends and which is most commonly found to be disabled in cases of hearing impairment, and partly because otoacoustic responses are the least well understood. This chapter does not consider signals emanating from the auditory brainstem, that is, the auditory brainstem response (ABR), of which the CAP forms just the initial component.

4.2.1 Auditory nerve response

The only truly functional 'response' of the cochlea is of course auditory nerve activity. With a stimulus of sufficient intensity and wide enough frequency range (e.g. loud 'pink noise') the 30 000 or so individual nerve fibres in the bundle emanating from the cochlea might each fire at a rate of many hundreds of spikes per second giving the whole bundle a staggering information capacity of may be 12 Mb/s. With today's data compression techniques this would be sufficient to carry a high-definition television channel. The cochlea uses data compression too, to achieve a remarkable working dynamic range of around 120 dB, that is, a 1 000 000:1 range of sound pressures.

Concentrations of neural activity within the brain result in small potential differences, of the order of microvolts or less, distributed over the scalp. But little of the electrical activity of the entire auditory nerve's continuous firing is detectable from surface electrodes. The bipolar nature of nerve spikes means that beyond a few millimetres away from the nerve the random positive and negative excursions of the individual action potentials tend to overlay and cancel each other out. The exception is when the stimulus changes rapidly. At the sudden onset of stimulation there are no 'negatives' from preceding spikes to balance the synchronized 'positives' due to the action potentials from newly excited neurones. Similarly, at the sudden termination of a sound there are no new 'positives' to cancel the negative excursions of the most recently excited neurones. As a result, at the sudden start and finish of a stimulus there is a remotely observable net electrical signal. The 'whole' nerve or 'compound' action potential from the auditory nerve resembles a single fibre action potential, with the terminal signal being the inverse of the onset signal (Fig. 4.3). The signal is less than 1 microvolt at the scalp and originates largely from the internal auditory meatus. This is where afferent fibres synapsing with the inner hair cells join the auditory and vestibular nerve bundles after passing through the spiral ganglion and become myelinated.

Of the infinite variety of stimuli that could be presented to the ear, single impulses (heard as 'clicks') are an ideal stimulus for observing the auditory nerve CAP. Their short duration physically embodies a wide spectrum of frequencies and so it can provide stimulation to all parts of the basilar membrane simultaneously. If its duration is less than the duration of a single action potential it ensures that all excited fibres are activated simultaneously (subject to delays in the stimulus propagating along the cochlea). This provides the maximum whole nerve remote response signal. Suitable click stimuli are generated by applying a 100 microsecond or shorter electrical impulse to a loudspeaker or earphone. CAP waveforms are independent of the stimulus polarity. This means that the response signal will be the same whether the click stimulus begins with sound compression or rarefaction (see Fig. 4.3). This is an important factor in the design of electrocochlear response capture and analysis systems.

To assess gross cochlear function, the potential difference between two scalp electrodes, one near the vertex and one near the ear (or sometimes in the ear canal), is recorded in response to repeated click presentations. These electrical signals are synchronously averaged (see later) to enhance the auditory response component relative to the higher background electroencephalographic (EEG), myogenic, and other electrical activity. If the peak sound level of the click is reduced in steps from say 80 dB SPL peak equivalent (pe) the CAP amplitude is seen to reduce systematically as fewer neurones fire synchronously with the stimulus. The response also becomes slightly more delayed as the adequacy of excitation becomes more dependent on the enhancement that the travelling wave provides over its peak. The delay is because the travelling wave peak takes time to develop. At some low stimulus level, the CAP not only becomes too small to distinguish against the noise floor (a problem which could be overcome by extending recording times), it eventually becomes non-existent. Below some absolute threshold stimulus level no neurone fires in response to the click. This level is known as the CAP click threshold. In practice time restraints preclude the determination of absolute threshold but the stimulus level at which CAP becomes practically undetectable is highly correlated with hearing threshold and is an excellent relative indicator of general cochlear condition.

The use of click stimuli to obtain CAP thresholds raises a number of issues of interpretation. A loud click will excite most auditory nerve fibres (as will loud noise). Lower level clicks will excite a smaller and smaller region of the cochlea centred on some frequency, which will depend on the frequency of maximum sensitivity of the individual ear and also on the frequency of maximum stimulus energy. The CAP click threshold is therefore the threshold of some undefined frequency place in the cochlea. What determines the place of maximum stimulation? A true acoustic impulse, that is, a very brief sound pressure excursion, say lasting around 50 microsecond, will deliver uniform stimulus energy in each equal frequency band up to above 10 kHz. But the tonotopic organization of the cochlea is not based on 'equal frequency bands'. The cochlea's filtering process tends to have equal *proportional* bandwidths across frequency. For example if the auditory filter centred on 1 kHz had a bandwidth of 250 Hz, then the bandwidth at 2 kHz would most likely be around double this at around 500 Hz wide, and at 4 kHz around 1000 Hz wide – thus maintaining a constant ratio of centre frequency to the range of frequencies transmitted (4:1 in this example). With a perfect click stimulus therefore the *energy* passing through the auditory filter and delivered to each sensory hair cell will increase by two times for each octave step up in frequency. Double the energy is equivalent to a 3 dB rise in stimulation so the cochlear frequency places for 2 kHz, 4 kHz, and 8 kHz will receive 3 dB, 6 dB, and 9 dB more stimulation, respectively, from a click compared with the 1 kHz place. In other words click stimuli are 'high-frequency biased' for auditory purposes. This in turn means that the CAP click threshold will most likely be the threshold of the most sensitive region in the higher frequency range of hearing, typically 3–6 kHz. Such a bias is quite convenient for clinical applications since it is high-frequency hearing that tends to be lost first, and it is high-frequency hearing that tends to be the most valuable in terms of speech discrimination. In practice, click stimuli are influenced by the click waveform and the sound delivery system and these therefore influence the place in the cochlea at which threshold is being measured.

The ratio of centre frequency over filter bandwidth is commonly referred to as 'Q', a term which has its historical roots in the 'quality' of electrical resonator filters. Larger Qs mean a proportionally narrower filter. It is should be noted that auditory bandwidth is normally measured across the frequency range within which transmission is within 32% (−10 dB) of the peak transmission and the Q derived in this way is properly referred to as $Q_{10\,dB}$. Engineers tend to use the half power or '−3 dB' bandwidth to calculate $Q_{3\,dB}$.

Returning to the topic of determining cochlear sensitivity through CAP threshold measurements, it is clear that a frequency-specific stimulus is necessary to determine threshold as a function of frequency. An intense single frequency tonal stimulus may excite all auditory nerves from the base up to its frequency place but as stimulus intensity is reduced the region of above-threshold excitation shrinks around the travelling wave peak at the frequency place. At near-threshold levels of stimulation this adequate stimulation extends over just a fraction of a millimetre length of the organ of Corti and involves fewer than 50 inner hair cells. By stepping the stimulus frequency through the hearing range, and measuring CAP threshold at each step, a complete cochlear sensitivity curve can be obtained. This might be thought of as the objective equivalent of the subjective hearing threshold audiogram. There are, however, some technical issues to consider. The first is that a stimulus of well-defined frequency has to have a long duration but a sustained stimulus does not evoke a practically measurable CAP. The major component of CAP will be a transient signal detectable only at the start and end of the tonal stimulus. But signal theory tells us that rapid changes to a signal, such as a sudden onset, greatly widen its frequency content and that undermines the concept of a frequency-specific stimulus. A practical compromise is to use a short burst of tonal stimulation known as a tone-pip, which starts and stops slowly enough for its centre frequency to be adequately defined but fast enough to generate a significant CAP response. A practical tone-pip could be one steadily increasing in amplitude for the first two cycles of the stimulus, then steady for one cycle and then falling smoothly for the last two cycles. At 8 kHz this stimulus would last 0.6 ms and evoke a good CAP response. At 1 kHz, however, such a stimulus would last 5 ms and produce an indistinct CAP response. Frequency-specific CAP threshold measurement therefore becomes increasing difficult at lower frequencies. Since the CAP response itself gives no indication of the frequency place originating the response, caution is needed in the interpretation of tone-pip thresholds in the case of irregular hearing loss with steep slopes. This is because the absence of a true frequency place response might be obscured by an off-frequency place response given sufficient stimulus level. Masking techniques can overcome this limitation (Schoonhoven, 2006). CAP threshold determination is a vital tool in the auditory physiology lab but it is not the response of choice clinically. In human subjects auditory evoked neural signals from the brainstem are more robust and easier to recognize because they conform to a consistent waveform. Brainstem responses have a greater tolerance to lack of synchrony in primary nerve fibres so that good responses can be obtained from tone-pips and frequency-specific thresholds can be defined more accurately. It is beyond the scope of this chapter to describe ABRs or their use but the literature is extensive (e.g. Buckard *et al.*, 2006).

4.2.2 The cochlear microphonic response

Action potentials are not the only physiological activity that generate far-field electrical signals. The sensory cells of the cochlea have receptor currents which are synchronous with the local vibration at each hair cell and these can summate to create externally measurable electrical signals. The voltage driving these receptor currents is the EP. It is maintained at around 90 mV by a spiral organ called the stria vascularis, which also tightly controls the ionic content of the endolymph of the scala media. Scala media is the wedge shaped spiral space between the apical surface of the organ of Corti and Reissner's membrane, and the stria vascularis forms the third surface. As the sensory cells draw current from the scala media, local potential will drop by Ohm's Law, that is, stimulus-driven receptor currents 'load' the EP. Local to the each hair cell therefore the electrical potential will be modulated by the stimulus vibration arriving at that place. This modulation of EP is the local CM signal and it tends to consist of an oscillatory modulation of the EP at a frequency reflecting the characteristic frequency of that place. The return current back to the stria vascularis forms an electrical circuit that creates small potential gradients throughout the head. Just as with individual nerve fibre signals, the far-fields from each hair cell circuit largely cancel each other because the stimulus vibration at each place has a different timing or phase. This is because the local stimulus vibration is derived from a travelling wave that progresses from base to apex. Each frequency component passes by each place at a different time, and with a different amplitude.

Figure 4.2 shows schematically the travelling wave to tonal stimuli. The distance between adjacent peaks and troughs in a travelling wave is called the wavelength. Within the peak amplitude region wavelength is short and this region contains simultaneously positive (current increasing) and negative (current decreasing) displacements closely packed together. Because of this the average modulation of the local EP across the excitation peak region of pure tone stimulus is small and the far-field signal will be negligible. Near to the base of the cochlea, however, travelling waves of any frequency have much larger wavelengths than at their frequency place (see Fig. 4.2). There is less opportunity here for complete cancellation of far-field potentials from the currents through these sensory cells. The majority of externally detectable CM signals therefore arise from hair cells near the base of the cochlea. Of course for any frequency the amplitude of vibration in the basal region is much smaller than at its frequency place so that the individual receptor currents will be smaller. Balancing this is the larger wavelength in the basal region, which means a much greater number of hair cells receive a similar phase of excitation and draw current synchronously than do so at the travelling wave peak. The net result is that the extracochlear microphonic signal is largely generated by the receptor currents of basal hair cells. It therefore reflects the stimulus as it *enters* the cochlea very much more than it reflects excitation reaching the travelling wave peak where the transduction is optimal. Because this signal reflects activity at the input of the cochlea its waveform closely follows the waveform of the incident sound – hence the term cochlear microphonic (see Fig. 4.3). An electrode placed near to the cochlea (on the promontory or the ear drum) will collect a signal which, when amplified and fed to a loudspeaker, clearly reproduces the sound being received by the ear.

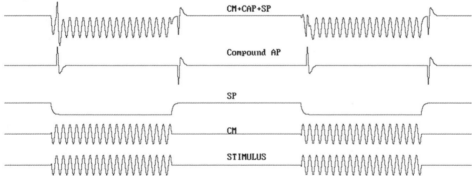

Fig. 4.3 Schematic representation of externally recordable electrical cochlear response waveforms and their relationships to each other. Time progresses from left to right. The stimulus (lower trace) consists of two 1 kHz tone bursts lasting about 18 ms. Note that the second tone burst is inverted in polarity with respect to the first. From the bottom up we see the stimulus and then the cochlear microphonic response (CM) exactly following both stimulus waveforms. Third up is the summating potential (SP), which is by definition non-oscillatory. It follows the envelope of the stimulus. Fourth up is the compound or whole nerve action potential (CAP), which consists of a spike at the start and end of each stimulation burst. The top trace shows the composite electrical signal as it would actually be recorded. The CM, SP, and CAP traces are simply added. The composite responses to the two stimuli look different only because of the polarity inversion of CM. Subtraction of the two composite waveforms from the two complementary stimuli would leave only the CM trace, whereas adding them together would eliminate CM and leave the sum of SP and CAP traces.

The characteristics of the CM contrasts in many important ways those of the CAP. CM is presynaptic, CAP is postsynaptic. Because CM follows the stimulus waveform its polarity will invert if the stimulus polarity inverts, whereas the CAP polarity is unchanged. The CM is sustained throughout continuous stimulation whereas the CAP is seen only at stimulus onset and termination. The CAP waveform is derived from and is similar to a single nerve action potential waveform and is largely independent of stimulus frequency and waveform. The nature of the evoking stimulus cannot be determined from the CAP it produces but it is fully manifest in the CM. With CM there is no overriding necessity to employ a frequency-specific stimulus to exploit CM to the full since an analysis of the frequency components present within the CM response to a click will provide essentially the same information as would be obtained by recording the CM in response to a series of frequency-specific stimuli. A frequency-specific stimulus must be used to obtain frequency-specific information with CAP.

The practical value of CM is limited compared to that of CAP. Since CM is presynaptic and comes largely from the base rather than the travelling wave peaks within the cochlea it cannot be used to provide a frequency-specific indication of cochlear sensitivity. Coming from the input of the cochlea and before the travelling wave has developed, it is not as sensitive to minor changes in cochlear status as is the CAP. CM does not show the increased latency with reducing stimulus level shown by CAP and it does not exhibit a true threshold. CM reduces proportionately as stimulus level is reduced and although it is eventually obscured by noise is never absolutely ceases to exist. CM is, however, a good indicator of general cochlear health and, in particular, of the environment and likely integrity of the outer sensory hair cells.

CM and CAP responses do not exist in isolation. A click stimulus will directly evoke a transient CM and the subsequent neural response will generate a transient CAP. These electrical responses overlap in time and, depending on the electrode configuration, can be of similar amplitude. The electrical response of the cochlea is always a mixture of these two quite different responses. Separation of the two can easily be achieved by exploiting their different polarity characteristics. Use of an alternating polarity click stimulus will leave the CAP waveform unaffected but the polarity of the CM will alternate. By recording cochlear responses to alternating polarity stimuli, some useful signal waveform 'arithmetic' can be performed. The positive click stimuli will evoke a composite response, $R_+ = +CAP + CM$. The response to the negative clicks will evoke $R_- = +CAP - CM$ (since CAP never inverts its waveform). From this we can derive separated CM and CAP responses, that is, $CM = (R_+ - R_-)/2$, $CAP = (R_+ + R_-)/2$. See also Figure 4.3.

4.2.3 The summating potential

For clarity in introducing the CM response an important consideration was omitted and this needs to be reintroduced to complete this survey of the cochlea's electrical responses. When the phase of a passing basilar membrane wave excites the sensory hair cells to draw greater current (the excitatory phase) then the local EP is reduced due the load and finite electrical source resistance. When the stimulus cycle causes the sensory cells to reduce their receptor current the local EP must rise. This is because the electrical 'load' on it is reduced. Provided there is symmetry between current reduction and current increase throughout each stimulus cycle, the mean local EP will remain unchanged. This is the case for the current drawn by outer hair cells in response to lower levels of stimulation. Receptor currents for small stimuli are proportional to basilar membrane displacement in both the 'up' and 'down' phases of vibration in these cells. For high stimulus levels the excitation will drive the ion channels between fully close and fully open rapidly through each cycle. This response is a *non-linear* situation – a term meaning that the effect is not proportionately related to the cause throughout each cycle. In the case of the cochlea it is a saturating non-linearity. The average current during saturating stimulation may not be the same as the unstimulated or resting current, depending on the cell's unstimulated operating point between the upper and lower saturated limits. There can therefore be a net change in average EP during stimulation (i.e. a 'DC shift'). Inner hair calls operate differently from outer hair cells in that they operate entirely in a non-linear mode. With no stimulation present they draw only a small fraction of the maximum possible current. Therefore stimulation can affect inner hair cell receptor currents much more during the excitatory half of each cycle. This extreme form of non-linearity gives rise to 'rectification'. It means that for inner hair cells the average current during stimulation is always higher than without stimulation. The net result of hair cell transducer non-linearity is that the mean current drawn from the EP is always greater during stimulation than in silence and therefore the local mean potential is always pulled lower over the region receiving stimulation. As this effect is unidirectional there is no 'cancellation' of the effect on one region by another. The summation of all the local stimulus-induced reductions in mean EP results in an externally measurable potential change which is sustained throughout stimulation. This is the 'summating potential' known as SP.

The terms 'DC' and 'AC' are used in a specific way in electrophysiology and need clarification. The far field CM potential is the residual from the summation of multiple stimulus-induced alternating currents (AC) throughout the cochlea and is therefore called an AC potential. The SP is due to the summation of small changes in the *average* unidirectional or 'direct current' over a stimulated region. It is the steady component of the potential changes caused by stimulation that creates the SP and so it is called a 'DC' potential. A similar logic is applied inside the cell where there are AC and DC receptor potentials.

The polarity of the SP does not change with stimulus polarity inversion as there is no difference in the mean current being drawn. In this respect the SP is like the CAP in that it is not removed from the composite averaged signal by stimulus polarity alternation as the CM is. But unlike the CAP the SP persists for the duration of the applied stimulus and this forms a basis for its identification (see Fig. 4.3).

4.2.4 Electrocochleography

Electrocochleography (often referred to as ECOG, and pronounced 'ee-cog' or 'ee-co-gee') is the term used to describe the clinical examination of the cochlea's three electrical responses – CM, SP, and CAP (Ferraro & Krishnan, 1997; Ferraro, 2000). Good clinical recordings of electrocochlear responses require the local electrode to be placed as close to the cochlea as possible. A sponge electrode in contact with the ear canal gives a good result but contacting the ear drum is better. Trans-tympanic recordings, in which a fine electrode punctures the drum and is settled into a bony hollow called the promontory, give the best signals, but this highly invasive technique would only be used under exceptional circumstances or for research. Figure 4.3 shows schematically the composite electrical signal arising from a short burst of tonal stimulus and the effects of polarity inversion. As already indicated, ABR analysis has totally replaced ECOG for the clinical purpose of screening and the derivation of an objective audiogram. ECOG remains valuable for research purposes and for clinical diagnostics.

Hearing loss can arise from a number of causes. Conductive loss due to middle ear infection is easily identified by air and bone conduction audiometry and is diagnosed by tympanometry but other forms of loss can be difficult to differentiate. With non-conductive peripheral hearing loss the CAP and ABR thresholds will be raised. The hearing loss could be due to a problem with neural transmission through the auditory nerve from the cochlea, caused, for example, by direct pressure from a tumour. However, this is extremely rare and non-conductive hearing loss is very much more likely to be caused by cochlear dysfunction than by auditory nerve pathology.

Hearing depends totally on the inner hair cell to transduce the stimulus and activate the auditory nerve. But the sensitivity of hearing depends strongly on *outer* hair cells, which ensure that enough of the right frequency reaches the appropriate inner hair cells during low level stimulation. Measurement of an elevated CAP or ABR threshold does not indicate the specific cause of the loss. But each of the three stages indicated above – the outer hair cell's *manipulation* of stimulation, the inner hair cell's *transduction* of stimulation, and the auditory pathway's *transmission* of stimulus information – contributes differently to the composite electrocochlear response and so a comparison of responses can help indicate the cause of a loss. It is the *relative* amplitudes of CM, SP, and CAP that can be important in diagnosis. The absolute levels are not important because the electrical pathway from cochlea to the electrodes is uncertain and cannot be calibrated. But this electrical path is similar for CM, SP, and CAP, and so relative difference remains significant. So, for example, a SP/CAP ratio above 0.5 is considered abnormal and indicative of Ménière's disease (Ferraro & Krishnan, 1997; Ferraro, 2000; Chung *et al.*, 2004).

4.2.5 Acoustic cochleography

'Acoustic cochleography' (Kemp *et al.*, 1986) is not a very widely used term and it is used here only to resonate with the term 'electrocochleography' and to emphasize that the cochlea's functional status can be examined though acoustic as well as electrical measurements. The introductory review made it clear that the cochlea does not simply 'absorb' sound energy. It reacts to it both physically and physiologically. The development of the travelling wave after the initial transfer of stimulus energy into the cochlea is physically and physiologically assisted by the outer hair cells and this is crucial to the efficient and frequency-specific delivery of stimulation to the inner sensory cells. Invasive cochlear studies show that the morphology of the travelling wave and, in particular, the sharpness of its peak, is critically dependent on the health of the sensory outer hair cells (e.g. Robles & Ruggero, 2001). These cells have electromotile properties that exert a physical influence on basilar membrane vibration. Excessive stimulation, anoxia, ischemia, endolymph contamination, infection, and ototoxic drugs, each quickly disable and can destroy outer hair cell function. Deprived of active support the travelling wave in response to a tone dies out before reaching a strong peak. This results in a serious loss of hearing sensitivity and frequency selectivity (i.e. resolution). Outer hair cell function is essential for the efficient transmission of stimulus along the basilar membrane. Degradation of this transmission results in elevation of the hearing threshold.

From a clinical perspective then, it would be highly desirable to directly observe the progression of stimulation inside the cochlea. Unfortunately no technique yet exists which is capable of non-invasively visualizing or directly recording the motion of the basilar membrane. This is due to the cochlea's anatomical inaccessibility and the extremely small motions involved in acoustic stimulation. Ear drum displacements in response to low to moderate sound levels are of atomic dimensions.

The possibility of 'acoustic cochleography', that is of examining the cochlea from outside with sound, is very attractive and arises from the very nature of the peripheral auditory apparatus. The middle ear mechanism has evolved to maximize the transfer of energy from airborne sound into the fluid-filled capsule that is the cochlea. This mechanism also works in reverse, ensuring that any audio frequency vibrations occurring at the base of the cochlea are efficiently coupled back to the ear drum. The middle ear is like a stethoscope permanently attached to the cochlea. By recording the sound pressure in sealed-up an ear canal during controlled sound stimulation it is possible to determine how well the cochlea absorbs sound and also how well the cochlea processes sound. The latter is only possible because the energetic action of the cochlea's outer hair cells, which create physical vibration. Some of their energy is not used to enhance hearing but instead escapes back to the middle ear. The sounds that these vibrations create when they reach the ear drum and vibrate the adjacent air in the ear canal are called *otoacoustic emissions,* and they complement the electrical responses of the auditory system. Absence of OAEs with normal middle ear function indicates abnormal cochlear function and hearing loss.

4.3 **The input to the cochlea and 'impedance'**

We will return to OAEs in detail but first it is useful to consider the action of the middle ear more closely. In physical terms the efficient transfer of stimulus energy from air to the cochlea requires 'impedance matching'. Air is very elastic and requires little force to compress or rarefy it. The ratio of pressure to movement is low. Air has low 'impedance'. In order for it to move easily in response to sound the ear drum needs to be of similar impedance to that of air. It needs to be light and flexible, that is, of low impedance. The thin tissue of the human drum achieves this quite well at the ear's most sensitive frequencies (2–3 kHz). Motion of the drum needs to be transmitted to the stapes and to the cochlear fluid before it can become a stimulus for hearing. Cochlear fluid is physically little different from water. It is often quoted as being 'incompressible'. Water is not in fact *in*compressible. It is actually 200 times *more* compressible than steel, but water is nevertheless almost a 100 000 times harder to compress than air. If the functional role of the middle ear was to transfer the stimulus energy collected by the drum into a sound wave inside the cochlear fluid, it would be an extremely inefficient mechanism. Fortunately the ear's sensory cells do not detect sound pressure waves but rather fluid motion. Fluid motion is much easier for the middle ear to create in the cochlea than a sound wave. Cochlear fluid can move backwards and forwards inside the cochlea without being compressed because the fluid has somewhere it can move to. This is the function of the round window. The round window of the cochlea opens onto the surface of the air-filled middle ear cavity. It is about the same size as the stapes footplate and is covered by an elastic membrane. Motion of the stapes is only possible without the compression of cochlear fluid because cochlea fluid can move the round window. What the middle ear mechanism has to achieve then is to match the low impedance of the ear drum to the only moderately higher impedance of the notional column of fluid that bridges the oval and round windows plus the impedance of the windows themselves. It is the motion of fluid between these two flexible windows, crucially intercepted by the basal basilar membrane, which initiates the cochlear travelling wave and ultimately hearing itself. How does the middle ear match ear drum impedance to that of the oval window? It does so because the area of the ear drum is much larger than that of the stapes footplate resting in the oval window, by more than 15 times. This area ratio ensures that the inertia of the cochlea fluid and the stiffness of the adjacent elastic components, *viz.* the stapedial ligament, basilar membrane and the round window membrane, do not exert an overriding influence on the motion of the ear drum as this would increase its impedance and reduce the efficiency of the drum for sound energy collection. Looked at another way the area reduction from ear drum to stapes transforms the small sound pressure at the ear drum into a higher pressure at the stapes which is better able to overcome fluid inertia and membrane stiffness at the input to the cochlea.

The cochlear input impedance does contribute to a small degree to the tympanic impedance and this is measurable by the acoustical analysis of ear canal sound. Standard clinical tympanometry primarily seeks to establish the flexibility or compliance of the ear drum and middle ear mechanism and this is most easily achieved with a low-frequency probe sound well below the ear drum's resonance of around 1 kHz. At these low frequencies (typically 220 Hz) the inertia of the middle ear bones is negligible and the input impedance to the cochlea is mainly due to the elastic stiffness of the oval and round windows. Above about 1 kHz, inertial factors become important. Rapid vibration of the ossicles and basal cochlear fluid increases the reactive component of the tympanic impedance. There is also a resistive or 'energy-absorbing' component of the impedance which originates in the cochlea and represents the absorption of energy into the cochlea, energy which goes to form the travelling wave. This cochlear absorption component is of course *the* most important thing for hearing. All other sound energy collected by the middle ear is either absorbed before reaching the cochlea or reflected back into the air and so is never heard.(Margolis & Shanks, 1985). The total energy absorbed by the ear can be clearly observed and measured with an advanced acoustic technique known as 'wideband reflectance' (Voss & Allen, 1994; Allen *et al.*, 2005). With this technique, a click or other wideband stimulus is applied via a highly calibrated ear canal probe for which the sound energy being delivered to an ear can be precisely calculated. The reflected sound energy is then computed from ear canal sound measurements as a function of frequency. Any energy missing from the reflected sound relative to the incidence sound must have been absorbed either usefully by the cochlea or functionlessly by the middle ear. Wideband reflectometry is gradually gaining popularity as means of analysing middle ear dysfunction with a detail not provided by standard tympanometry. It is particularly effective at detecting the presence of middle ear effusion (Keefe *et al.*, 2000, Allen *et al.* 2008) but reflectance also has the potential to detect abnormal cochlear status. An extension of the technique which encompasses non-linear reflectance, a phenomenon closely related to OAEs, registers the mechanical response of cellular activity (Keefe, 1997; see later).

4.4 **Otoacoustic emissions**

OAEs are sounds recorded with an acoustic 'probe' inserted into the ear canal as illustrated in Figure 4.4A. There are several sound sources in the head due to breathing, swallowing, chewing, blood flow, muscles, etc. These sounds all find their way to the ear canal through the skull and can

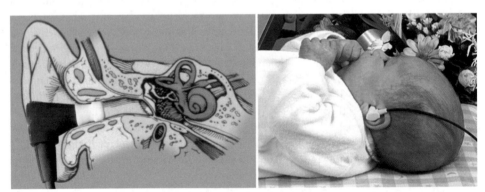

Fig. 4.4 The recording of otoacoustic emissions (OAEs). (A, left) Illustration of an otoacoustic emission probe inserted into the ear canal and communicating acoustically with the cochlea through the middle ear. There are no electrodes. The probe contains a miniature microphone to record sounds in the closed ear canal and one or two miniature loudspeakers, as used in hearing aids, to provide stimulation. (B, right) An infant fitted with an OAE probe for hearing screening. A tight and deep probe fit is valuable in gaining a good signal-to-noise ratio. OAEs are typically registered in 10–30 seconds in healthy newborns. Those not showing a strong OAE are retested since birth debris in the ear canal or fluid in the middle ear can block the response (Keefe, 2007). Babies who fail to show a good response are referred for audiological examination. Between one and two babies per 1000 are born with considerable hearing loss of cochlear origin and early provision of a hearing aid or implant greatly accelerates the normal development of speech and language.

be recorded via an ear canal microphone probe; but they are not OAEs! OAEs are the sounds found in the ear canal which are generated by ear drum vibrations originating in the cochlea and which are a direct byproduct of the hearing process (Kemp, 1978). In the following sections we consider how these vibrations arise in the cochlea, what causes their escape, what characteristics OAEs have, and how emissions can be validated, interpreted, and used clinically. See also Kemp (2001, 2007).

The emergence of an otoacoustic response from the auditory system is completely different from the emergence of an electrophysiological response. Except when constrained within a nerve by its myelin sheath, electrophysiological activity induces signals that can travel freely throughout the body because tissue conducts electricity. Vibration is physically different. Cellular tissue is a relatively poor conductor of audiofrequency sound vibration. Although bone is a better conductor, stimulus energy inside the cochlea does not escape through the bony surround. For the most part, the physical energy of stimulation does not reside in the cochlea as 'a sound' but as fluid and tissue vibration. There is also such a massive impedance mismatch between the slowly propagating transverse waves of the basilar membrane with its associated fluid motion and the bony periphery that little energy is transferred. In short there is no general 'far-field' vibration as a result of what happens physically deep inside in the cochlea. In the peripheral auditory system stimulus vibration travels along very specific pathways from ear drum to hair cell. In the production of OAEs, vibration travels in reverse, from hair cell to ear drum along the same pathways.

OAEs can arise in two ways: in response to applied external stimulation (i.e. evoked or stimulated OAEs) and as a result of internal self-stimulation and oscillation (spontaneous OAEs).

4.4.1 Spontaneous otoacoustic emissions

Spontaneous OAEs tend to consist of single or multiple pure tones continuously emitted by the ear. Figure 4.5 (upper panel) shows spontaneous emissions recorded from a baby's ear. Spontaneous OAEs are a result of a fortuitous feedback loop within the cochlea in which vibrations generated by outer hair cells are sent back to the middle ear and then reflected again back into the cochlea to restimulate the same hair cells. Self-sustained oscillation can develop in this way if the loop delivers a signal back to the originating region of the cochlea with just the right time delay to exactly synchronize with the existing oscillation. This means oscillations can only occur at very specific frequencies determined by the travelling wave speed and the reflecting cells' location. Furthermore the oscillations will only sustain themselves if the reflection arrives back with sufficient intensity to create an equally strong reflection the second time around. This means that all energy losses along the route have to be compensated for in some way. This demands amplification as the wave travels along the basilar membrane or as the internal reflection occurs – or during both. It is noteworthy that spontaneous OAEs are not rare. They occur in about one in three adult ears and even more frequently in infants ears (Bright, 2007) and in many animals. Spontaneous OAEs provided the first unambiguous evidence that a vibration-generating mechanism existed in the cochlea (Wilson, 1980a; Kemp, 1981) and they suggested that all cochleae have the capacity to amplify stimulus vibration (Kemp, 1979)

The clinical use of spontaneous OAEs is very limited because not all healthy ears have the right conditions to support them. In ears that do not have spontaneous OAEs it might be that the reflections that are present are not as strong as in ears that do, or that their cochlear amplifier might not be as strong. There is currently no way of interpreting the presence or absence of these oscillations in terms of cochlear health but measures of spontaneous activity are frequently included in research protocols. Spontaneous OAEs are believed by many to be a sign of overabundant outer hair cell activity but there are also indications that microscopic damage to the cochlea can trigger spontaneous emission in an otherwise 'quiet' cochlea (Clark et al., 1984). The author's

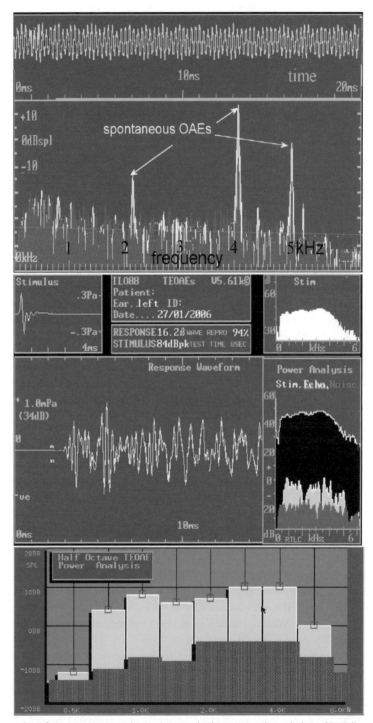

Fig. 4.5 Examples of spontaneous and transient evoked otoacoustic emissions (OAEs) and their analysis. Top panel: A spontaneous OAE from a neonate. Upper trace: The waveform of the emission sound in the ear canal showing the periodicity of the dominant component at 4.1 kHz.

Fig. 4.5 *(Continued)* The small modulation of intensity is due to the presence of other smaller spontaneous emissions. Lower trace: the frequency spectrum of this sound shows three clear spontaneous OAEs at 2.2 kHz, 4.1 kHz, and 5 kHz. The largest has an amplitude of 10 dB SPL. The darker shading is the noise contamination assessed by subtracting repeat recordings. Middle panel: A strong transient OAE recording from a different healthy human ear. Lower large section (left): A transient evoked OAE (TEOAE) response waveform showing ear canal oscillations lasting over 15 ms and peaking at 1 mPa, 34 dB SPL. The mean response level is 16.2 dB SPL. The trace is blanked (flattened) for the first 2.5 ms after the stimulus because the system is overloaded with stimulus oscillations during this period and cannot register the OAE. The initial portion of the waveform after 2.5 ms contains more high frequencies (4 waves/ms or more) than does the latter portion (about 1 wave/ms). Top left section shows the transient stimulus waveform on a much reduced amplitude scale. The main activity occurs in the first millisecond. This is the stimulus click modified by ear canal acoustics. Its peak sound level is 84 dB SPL, or approximately 300 times larger than the peak OAE response. Top right shows the stimulus spectrum which is wide and smooth. The measured stimulus intensity falls above 4 kHz partly due to antiphase reflections from the ear drum but the ear may still be stimulated and newborns typically produce an OAE at this frequency. Often clinically normal adult ears do not give detectable levels of high frequency OAE. Lower right: composite spectrum of the stimulus (line boundary for the dark area), OAE response (bright area) and noise estimate (shaded area). The noise estimate is obtained from the difference between repeat recordings. Two repeat recordings are actually superimposed on the response panel but overlap almost completely. The waveform reproducibility is 94% in this example (see text). Note that the response spectrum has a fine structure on a scale of approximately 100 Hz. If spontaneous emissions occurred in this ear they would be at frequencies close to TEOAE spectrum peaks. This TEOAE was recorded using 'non-linear clicks' (see text). Lower panel: A half octave spectrum analysis of the TEOAE shown in the centre panel. This is the most useful representation for clinical purposes. Light areas are validated TEOAE energy levels and the shaded area is the noise level. The decibel difference between OAE and noise is a good measure of measurement quality and reliability, that is the signal-to-noise ratio.

view is that there is an abundance of outer hair cell activity in healthy ears and that naturally occurring irregularities provide focal points for spontaneous OAEs to develop if their location and the wave travel time and middle ear properties all happen to be appropriate.

Spontaneous OAEs can often be heard by their owner when they are in a quiet environment. Occasionally this sensation gives rise to anxiety. A demonstration of the physical nature of this sensation (as in Fig. 4.5) can sometimes bring relief to those who are troubled by these specific sounds. However, this 'physiological' cause of tinnitus appears to be quite different from the sources of pathological tinnitus. The possible relationship of spontaneous OAEs to tinnitus initially aroused interest (Wilson & Sutton, 1981) but no systematic correlation with pathological tinnitus has been established. Spontaneous OAEs remain a remarkable phenomenon of considerable research interest.

4.4.2 **Stimulated otoacoustic emissions**

Most OAE observations are made in conjunction with acoustic stimulation. Almost any stimulus can be used to obtain an evoked or stimulated OAE, but it is most common to employ either a transient (a click) or tone pair stimulus. The resulting OAE is neither a copy of the evoking stimulus, as it is with CM, nor does it conform to a stimulus-independent template, unlike CAP and ABR. The correlation between an OAE and the evoking stimulus is very strong but so complex that it can be difficult to recognize in raw data. This contrast between stimulus and response often confuses the newcomer to OAE measurement. Another source of confusion is the practice of presenting OAE recordings in quite different formats depending on the nature of the applied stimulus and the type of signal processing used to extract the response. It is often wrongly concluded that these different modes of stimulation evoked different 'types' of OAE. More correctly the different methodologies used to record OAEs each extract different components of the total OAE from the cochlea. While OAEs are certainly driven by two different processes in the cochlea, *viz*. reflection and non-linearity (Shera & Guinan, 1999), both these emission-generation mechanisms are involved to some degree whatever the applied stimulus. The unifying factor is the common origin of all OAEs in the physical response of the mechanically active outer hair cells to the travelling wave.

4.4.3 Transient evoked otoacoustic emissions

OAEs can be evoked by click stimuli (see Fig. 4.4). The method is particularly effective with human ears and has been well established for infant hearing screening since 1983 (Johnsen & Elberling, 1983; Vohr & Kemp, 1991; Kemp & Ryan, 1993; Norton *et al.*, 2000; Bamford *et al.*, 2005; Hergils, 2007). It is the preferred method in some national universal newborn hearing screening programmes. Transient evoked OAEs (TEOAEs) also have important research applications (see later).

The results of a TEOAE recording are usually presented as a waveform representing the time course of ear drum motion for a period up to 20 ms after transient stimulation. Ear drum motion is not directly recorded although this would be possible to do using laser interferometry. What is actually measured and presented is the air pressure fluctuations in the closed ear canal created by the stimulus and later by ear drum vibrations driven by the cochlea.

Figure 4.5 (middle panel) shows a typical TEOAE recording (see also Kemp *et al.*, 1990). With a well-controlled click sound source and a well-fitted acoustic probe the stimulus waveform decays rapidly after about 1–2 ms. This early part of the ear canal waveform includes the acoustic response of the ear canal and ear drum to the briefer acoustic impulse delivered to the ear canal. Peak applied stimulus sound levels between 80 dB SPL and 90 dB SPL pe are usual. This level of click is not loud, due to its short duration, being 50–60 dB above click threshold. The response waveform is more than 100 times smaller than the stimulus waveform. It is typically long and complex, containing many different periodicities across time and contrasting with the much simpler and shorter stimulus waveform. Intersubject variance is high and mean sound levels during the response can range from 5 dB SPL to 35 dB SPL with clinically normal ears. Each ear's response waveform is unique but its detailed waveform tends to remain stable over years if not decades. An underlying waveform feature (not always visible) is for the higher frequencies (i.e. waves of smaller time periods) to be dominant in the earlier part of the response and for lower frequencies to dominate the later parts (Glattke & Robinette, 2007; see Fig. 4.6, lower half of lower panel).

Every component of the TEOAE response wave (Fig. 4.5 middle panel) is traceable back to the stimulus but the transformation is complex. What has happened is that the wide frequency range of 'virtual' oscillations that comprise the stimulus impulse have been separated out in time with the lowest frequency delayed of the longest. This effect is called frequency dispersion and is well known in physics when waves travel through a medium where the wave velocity is frequency dependent. The presence of frequency dispersion in TEOAEs is strong evidence that the sound has been into the cochlea because wave propagation in the cochlea is frequency dispersive (see later).

TEOAEs can be recorded using any short stimulus. The use of a tone burst stimulus illustrates the dispersion property of TEOAEs well. A short tone burst contains energy over a limited range of frequencies. TEOAEs can be obtained with such a stimulus but the response does not have the complex multi-frequency character of click evoked OAEs. Instead the response consists of oscillations similar to those in the stimulus (Fig. 4.6 upper panel). The delay of the peak of the packet

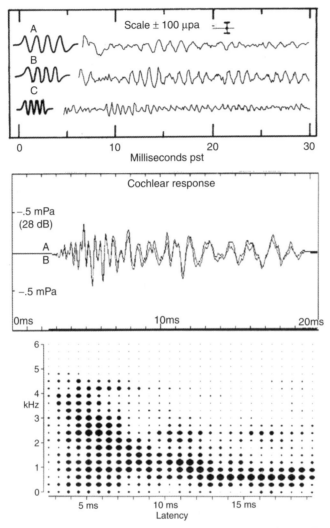

Fig. 4.6 Insights into the formation of otoacoustic emissions. Upper panel: Tone burst evoked otoacoustic emissions (OAEs) echo the period of the tone burst stimulus. The same ear is run with tone burst stimuli of three different frequencies, 800 Hz, 1100 Hz, and 1800 Hz, and this is indicated by the stimulus waveform on the right at greatly reduced size. In each case the response (left) is dominated by an oscillation of the same periodicity as the stimulus but lasting much longer. The response to the lower frequency (marked A) begins later than that to the higher frequency (marked C). This is evidence of frequency dispersion and was crucial in linking the new ear canal response to the cochlea in 1978. Lower two panels: An clear example of frequency dispersion in a transient evoked otoacoustic emission (OAE) response. Upper half shows the wavefom of a transient evoked OAE response clearly exhibiting a transition from a close wave (higher frequency) initial waveform to a more spaced (lower frequency) waveform out to 20 ms. Lower half shows a frequency time plot for this waveform revealing the downward glide of the dominant response frequency from around 4 kHz at 2.5 ms to about 700 Hz beyond 16 ms. This is a direct correlate of the frequency dispersion in the cochlear travelling wave.

Figure 4.6 data reprinted with permission from Kemp (1978) (© 1978; American Institute of Physics).

of oscillations depends on frequency – being longer the lower the frequency. Tone burst evoked OAEs are perhaps the simplest OAEs to appreciate. The response is visibly related to the stimulus and resembles an 'echo' of it. It demonstrates most clearly that the cochlear travelling wave is actually reflected and in fact the phenomenon was at first referred to as a cochlear 'echo' (Rutten, 1980; Wilson, 1980b).

The clinical value of TEOAEs rests on research findings that TEOAE generation is very closely associated with the cochlear hearing mechanism. The initial research findings indicated that TEOAEs were absent from ears with substantial hearing loss (Kemp, 1978) and this is been well substantiated (Robinette & Glattke, 2007). It was demonstrated that TEOAEs reduce in intensity as the hearing sensitivity of an ear reduces, for example following ototoxic drugs or noise exposure (Anderson & Kemp, 1979; Kemp, 1982). A similar reduction in OAE intensity takes place if reception of the click stimulus is masked by other more intense simultaneously presented sounds so that the click stimulus cant be heard (Kemp & Chum, 1980).

The individual frequency components comprising a TEOAE are of interest. TEOAE responses are 'frequency specific' in that, for example, a 1 kHz tone burst will generate a 1 kHz tone burst OAE response. It has this property in common with the CM. In addition there is good evidence from suppression tuning curve studies that TEOAEs are also frequency *place* specific, something that the CM is not. Frequency place specificity means that the emergence of a response to a particular stimulus frequency component involves hair cell activity predominantly at or near the appropriate frequency place for that stimulus in the cochlea. Consequently, if for that frequency there was a defective frequency place region on the organ of Corti it would lead to the response at that frequency being reduced or missing from the TEOAE. This is not a property shared by the CM because externally recorded CM originates mainly in the basal region whatever the stimulus frequency. The CAP is not intrinsically frequency place specific and only becomes so when near-threshold frequency-specific stimuli, for example tone bursts, are used. There is no way to obtain frequency-specific data from a click evoked CAP. However, TEOAEs retain their frequency place specificity even if wideband stimulation (e.g. clicks) is used. This makes the OAE a unique auditory response.

Evidence for the frequency-place specificity of all OAEs comes from experiments in which an additional tonal stimulus is applied to suppress the OAE response during a OAE recoding. The bandwidth of frequencies suppressed by a tone is restricted to a range comparable with the bandwidth of the auditory filter (Kemp & Chum, 1980). This is a characteristic that makes the frequency composition of a TEOAE of diagnostic interest.

The frequency spectrum of a click TEOAE response can be obtained by digital analysis and can be seen in Figure 4.5 (middle panel). There are two common ways to present these frequency data. A high-resolution spectral analysis (typically 50 Hz interval derived from a 20 ms poststimulus record as in the middle panel in Figure 4.5) reveals a detailed structure of peaks and dips. The sharp fine structure dips tend to be due to interference between different parallel pathways of OAE escape and the sharper peaks are related to the commencement of internal recirculation that can result in spontaneous OAEs. Neither feature is of great importance for hearing itself. They pose interesting research challenges but considerably complicate the clinical interpretation of OAEs. They also affect the audiogram because even when cochlear conditions are not sufficient for the creation of spontaneous emissions, the recirculation of stimulation inside the cochlea still enhances sensitivity at specific frequencies. This leads to a fine structure with frequency of hearing sensitivity due to standing wave resonances. High-resolution audiograms shown this fine structure phenomenon, as first reported, but not interpreted, by Elliot (1958). The same structure is also present in the spectrum of OAEs (Lutman & Deeks, 1999).

In practice, a lower resolution spectrum of TEOAEs is more useful clinically as it avoids the fine structure. Typically a clinical analysis consists of quarter, third, or half octave energy spectra showing the sound pressure level in each band (Fig. 4.5, lower panel). This type of presentation can be interpreted as representing outer hair cell activity at regular intervals along the basilar membrane. A strong TEOAE might have 10–15 dB SPL per half octave. A 0 dB SPL/half octave would be a low normal level. Less than −10 dB SPL/half octave would strongly indicate a problem.

Neonate screening is a major application of TEOAEs, which is assisted by the fact that newborn infants with clear ear canals usually have powerful emissions of up to 20 dB SPL/half octave from 2 kHz up to above 6 kHz (Hergils, 2007). The lower frequencies are more difficult to record in babies due to noise and the flaccid nature of their ear canals.

Frequency-specific TEOAE displays draw attention to the overall frequency balance of the emission across frequency and to any missing frequency regions. With ageing and with the onset of high frequency loss, the TEOAE spectrum is seen to slope down with increasing frequency. With increasing high-frequency loss, the response ultimately becomes confined to just the lower frequencies, that is, to 2 kHz and below, or the response becomes undetectable. Ears with serious high-frequency deafness can have near-normal low-frequency hearing and can continue to show a fairly normal looking TEOAE response waveform. However, this response will not include high-frequency components if the hearing loss is due to outer hair cell loss. It is therefore important to examine the frequency spectrum of TEOAEs and not just its waveform.

The long-term stability of individual TEOAE response waveforms has already been mentioned and demonstrates that both outer hair cell activity and whatever governs the leakage of electromotile energy back to the outer ear are both highly stable in the long term. But the mechanism does appear to be under some short-term physiological control. TEOAE responses to the same stimulus can vary in size by 1–2 dB (up to 20%) through the day and they do adapt to environmental factors. TEOAEs are readily depressed by a few decibels after listening to loud musical entertainment for an extended period, or after working in a noisy environment. These small changes in amplitude leave the waveform shape largely unchanged and the response amplitude typically returns to full size in an hour or less. There is clear evidence of some central control of cochlear sensitivity. Collet et al. (1990) discovered that a decrease of about 1–2 dB in the size of the TEOAE occurred if mild noise stimulation (about 60 dB SPL) was played into the opposite ear during OAE recording. This level of noise is too low to cause fatigue and also too low to pass through or round the head with enough intensity to influence the other ear directly. Collet proposed that the efferent neural pathway to the cochlea was being activated by the contralateral noise and that this was modifying the operating point of the outer hair cells on which efferent fibres synapse. His results have been widely confirmed and his hypothesis is well supported by laboratory studies in which electrical stimulation of the medial olivocochlear nerve produced similar reductions in cochlear activity (Kemp & Souter, 1988; Popelar et al., 2002). Collet's OAE measurement procedure is known as 'contralateral suppression' or the 'cochlear efferent' effect and the phenomenon itself has become known as the cochlear reflex (Guinan, 2006; Hood, 2007; Russell & Lukashkin, 2008). It demonstrates that cochlear function is at least to a small degree under central control. The functional importance of this effect is not yet well understood but could be far reaching.

TEOAEs increase in amplitude as stimulation level is increased, but not in direct proportion. TEOAEs are a non-linear phenomenon. This is wholly consistent with their physiological origin and quite uncharacteristic of a purely acoustic response such as the acoustic response of the ear canal to the stimulus or an acoustic echo. The type of non-linearity observed in TEOAEs is 'compressive', that is, it grows more slowly than the stimulus. It is found that the amplitude of the TEOAE increases roughly in proportion to the cube root of the stimulus increase (Kemp, 1978; Hauser et al., 1991). For example in decibel terms, a 6 dB increase in stimulus may only produce only a 2 dB increase in TEOAE level. Consequently, as stimulus level is increased TEOAEs constitute a smaller proportion of the total sound in the ear canal.

4.5 **Travelling waves, reflections, and otoacoustic emissions**

How are OAEs formed? Why for example is there a cascade of sound vibration in the ear canal for more than 1/50th second after a click stimulus? To answer these questions, it is necessary to consider the cochlear travelling wave in more detail. A click causes a mechanical impulse to be delivered to the oval window. This creates a sound impulse inside the cochlea, but this is very short lived and does not stimulate the sensory hair cells directly. What is important for hair cell stimulation and hearing is not sound pressure but fluid motion. A sound wave in water consists of a strong pressure wave but very little movement of fluid. Water has an acoustic impedance that is very high because it is very hard to compress. As explained above, the flexible membrane of the round window allows the stapes to create fluid motion within the closed capsule of the cochlea *without* high sound pressures. The basilar membrane, which lies between oval and round windows, stretches to allow this fluid motion to occur.

Displaced elastic membranes store energy, and the resulting tension causes them to spring back towards their rest positions when the applied force is removed. In the cochlea this restoration of position accelerates adjacent fluid in the opposite direction to the initial basal displacement. The force of this secondary (reactionary) local fluid motion reaches the stapes and influences the cochlear input impedance. More importantly it also reaches other more apical regions of the basilar membrane. This initiates a sequence of fluid and membrane interactions known as the cochlear travelling wave. The development of this travelling wave and its progression towards the apex of the cochlear spiral is governed by the elastic stiffness of the basilar membrane and by the inertial forces in the fluid that surrounds it. As mentioned in the introductory section there is a gradual increase in the width of the basilar membrane with distance into the cochlea and a corresponding reduction in its stiffness. Less stiffness and more inertia (as the wider membrane displaces more fluid) means slower apical progression of the travelling wave. As noted in the Introduction the slowdown in apical travel has the effect of concentrating the stimulus energy being carried into a smaller and smaller distance, which in turn increases the magnitude of the transverse excursions. The consequent magnification of stimulus vibration makes an important contribution to the sensitivity of hearing.

However, there is a more important physical effect that adds to cochlear sensitivity and also frequency selectivity. Basic physics tells us that once the displaced membrane's elastic restoring force has worked against the inertia of the surrounding fluid in order to get it back to its initial rest position, it remains in motion. This momentum then keeps the membrane in motion carrying the membrane beyond its rest position and creating a new and opposite displacement. The sequence then repeats in reverse. This seesaw behaviour is the fundamental physical 'recipe' for oscillation and resonance. Resonance occurs in an isolated system when the forces of inertia and elastic restoring force are of equal strength and opposite in direction so that they cancel each other. Crucial to the properties of the travelling wave is the fact that the force of inertia is intrinsically frequency dependent whereas the elastic restoring force is not. From Newton's second law the inertial force depends on the rate of change of velocity and so at any one place and for a given amplitude of vibration the inertial force increases with the applied frequency. Consequently for any frequency applied to the cochlea there will be one point along the basilar membrane where, for that frequency only, the forces of fluid inertia and of the elastic restoring force to basilar membrane displacement are equal and opposite. This results in minimum mechanical impedance to transverse oscillations at that place, and the vibration potentially reaches a maximum at that place for that frequency. The travelling wave amplitude builds up to maximum near to this point before its energy is rapidly absorbed and it ceases to propagate.

The above account describes the physics. To this must be added the electromotile contribution of the outer hair cells. So far as is known, the forces these cells generate work *with* the physical processes outlined above and serve to replace the energy lost by viscous drag which would otherwise absorb travelling wave energy before the wave could form a sharp peak at is the best frequency place. Most researchers believe that the outer hair cells do more that just replace lost energy. They believe that the energy injected more than compensates for viscous losses and that this amplifies the lowest levels of stimuli vibration by as much as 100-fold. Such an increase is seen in basilar membrane vibration (Robles & Ruggero, 2001). This process is known as 'cochlear amplification'. There remain some dissenting opinions about this concept (See Allen & Fahey, 1992; de Boer et al., 2005; Shera & Mountain, 2009), but without the capacity to amplify vibration it is impossible to explain the characteristics of spontaneous OAEs. See also Bialek and Wit (1984), van Dijk and Wit (1990), and Shera (2003).

Basilar membrane anatomy governs the progression of the travelling wave and the best frequency of each place. Its physical properties are tapered such that proportional steps in frequency (e.g. one octave step or a doubling in frequency) have their frequency places spaced at approximately equal distances along the cochlea. This characteristic is often referred to as octave or logarithmic 'scaling'. The spatial dimensions or sharpness of the travelling wave peak determines the range or bandwidth of frequencies that are delivered strongly to each place. This defines the bandwidth of the auditory filter and it tends to be a fixed fraction of the place frequency. For example a filter bandwidth equal to 25% its center frequency would have a one third octave bandwidth at all frequencies. The human cochlea is up to 3 cm long and hearing extends over ten octaves. Although each octave is not given an exactly equal share of the cochlear length – if it was then each octave would be served by just 3 mm of cochlea, and each human auditory filter band by less than 1 mm.

It takes time for the travelling wave to convey the stimulus and bring each frequency component to its own peak of maximum vibration. As already mentioned this time is frequency dependent, that is, there is frequency dispersion in the cochlea. The logarithmic scaling and semi-constant spatial width of the travelling wave peak mean that the Q of the cochlear filter changes only slowly with frequency. It also means that the number of stimulus periods between a stimulus entering the cochlea and it reaching its travelling wave peak is of the same order whatever the frequency. Evidence from OAEs suggest this number is between three and nine cycles in human ears in the middle frequency range. However, if the number of 'cycles' of delay were constant across frequency this would not mean that the *time* a stimulus took to reach its peak would be constant. The time is equal to the number of cycles N within the travelling wave envelope (see Fig. 4.2) multiplied by the time period of each cycle of the stimulus, which is $1/f$ where f is the frequency, so that travel time to peak would be N/f. For example in a cochlea with five stimulus cycles to its travelling wave peak – the latency of stimulation reaching the peak would be 5 ms at 1 kHz, 2.5 ms at 2 kHz, and 1.25 ms at 4 kHz. This is the origin of frequency dispersion in the cochlea and of the duration and frequency dispersion that is seen in TEOAE responses (see Figure 4.6, lower panel).

The physics and anatomy of the cochlea determine that however we stimulate the cochlea from outside a travelling wave will progress from base to apex (Schratzenstaller, 2000). How then does energy get back to the middle ear to form OAEs? The current theory of how TEOAEs arise is by reflection of the apically travelling wave. This model proposes that the positioning of the cells within the organ of Corti is not totally regular and/or that the level of activity of the outer hair cells are not all exactly equal.(see Fig. 4.1B). This does not have much effect until the wavelength of the travelling wave becomes very small and its intensity large, that is, at the travelling wave peak for any particular frequency. Small irregularities then become increasingly important and each one scatters or reflects a very small amount of the passing travelling wave energy back towards the base of the cochlea. Intuitively one would think that the summed effects of small, randomly spaced differences between the cellular components along the basilar membrane would cancel each other resulting in little or no net signal reaching the base to form an OAE. One possible explanation for the existence of a substantial level of reflection OAEs is to suppose that only a few discrete irregularities are responsible for most of the reflected signal. This turns out not to be able to explain the extensive frequency ranges which have fairly uniform OAE production. Notwithstanding the self-cancellation that undoubtedly occurs, Zweig and Shera (1995) have shown that coherent summation can also occur with densely but randomly distributed scattering points within the travelling wave's peak. The principle is that there will always be a subset of scattering points under the peak which happen to be distributed with just the right periodicity to form a Bragg reflector, which requires reflecting elements spaced at half wavelength intervals (Strube, 1989). Reflections from all other scattering points tend to cancel. Zweig and Shera (1995) demonstrated that what they call coherent reflection will be important if the travelling wave peak contains a sufficient number of wave periods of high amplitude. In their analysis, Zweig and Shera emphasize the passive and linear (i.e. proportional) nature of their proposed reflection mechanism. This is an important consideration as it suggests that the generator of OAEs (i.e. the mechanism returning energy to the middle ear) would not itself be a physiological process. Superficially this appears to contradict the evidence for an essentially physiological origin of TEOAEs. TEOAEs and other reflection-based OAEs always exhibit compressive non-linearity and vulnerability to acoustic physiological stress. But in the passive reflection model non-linearity and vulnerability stem from the linear reflection of a non-linearly amplified and therefore physiologically vulnerable travelling wave. However, if irregularities of outer hair cell motility rather than position were to be involved in the reflection process then non-linearity in the reflector mechanism itself might also play a part in OAE formation.

Accepting that coherent reflection creates a reverse travelling wave and that this wave accumulates the same number of cycles delay in travelling backwards as did the forward wave in reaching the reflection place then the waveform of the TEOAE response can be broadly understood. With our example of a five-cycle-to-peak travelling wave, the delay between stimulation and the reflected wave arriving back at the base of the cochlea would be 10 ms for 1 kHz, 5 ms for 2 kHz, and 2.5 ms for 4 kHz. This is very roughly right for human TEOAE response delays. After click (wideband) stimulation the higher-frequency components of the stimulus do emerge after the shortest time with medium- and low-frequency components following in sequence. This is clearly seen in Figure 4.6 (lower half of lower panel). The 'perfect' otoacoustic response to a click stimulus would consist of a downward gliding tone. In practice, irregularities in the amount of reflection with frequency and multiple reflections (see spontaneous OAEs above) usually obscure this feature.

The cochlear wave reflector acts on the travelling waves generated by any stimulus. Single tone stimulation evokes a single tone emission at the same frequency and this is known as stimulus frequency emission (SFOAE). The obvious difficulty of separating the SFOAE from the concurrent stimulus tone makes observations with a single tone much less practical than with the TEOAE technique but we know that the process of re-emission for a tone and for clicks is virtually the same. Stepping though the frequency range with a single frequency stimulus and recording the SFOAE level yield a frequency response closely matching the spectrum of a click TEOAE from the same ear (Brass & Kemp, 1991; Kalluri & Shera, 2007). Tracing the phase of the SFOAE relative to the stimulus phase reveals rapid changes with frequency. Rapid phase change with frequency is the continuous tone equivalent of delay and the two are simply related. If D is the delay in seconds (known as the group delay) then $D = \delta C/\delta F$ where δC is the number of additional stimulus cycles the SFOAE *lags* behind the input signal on increasing the stimulus frequency by δF Hz. For example in the case of an SFOAE whose phase (relative to the stimulus) changed by one complete cycle when the stimulus frequency was increased by 100 Hz, the delay in emission would be 10 ms.

4.6 **Non-linearity and otoacoustic emissions**

Non-linearity is an essential component of cochlear function and of OAEs. It has already been mentioned in relation to sensory cell transduction and to the compressive growth of TEOAEs with stimulus intensity. Non-linearity affects all aspects of hearing and all cochlear responses.

The effects of cochlear non-linearity can be demonstrated with two tones. When a pair of tones are simultaneously applied to the ear the stronger tone can mask perception of the weaker depending on the frequency separation. At the level of the travelling wave the lower frequency tone overlays and if strong enough can depress vibration in the higher tone's travelling wave making its peak smaller and less sharp. Tone pairs with a frequency ratio smaller than about 1.3 produce travelling waves whose peaks partially overlap so that even equal intensity tones will suppress each other's travelling waves. Consequently, any OAEs that derive from them will be reduced. This is called OAE two-tone suppression, and it should be noted that is a more general phenomenon than is defined as two-tone suppression in primary auditory nerve fibre recording.

The process of tone-on-tone OAE suppression can be understood as being due to 'competition' for the outer hair cells' limited electromotile energy resource between the two stimuli. When an outer hair cell is being driven at two different frequencies simultaneously, compressive (i.e. saturating) non-linearity means that the total energy in the hair cell's motile response will be less than the sum of the energies released in response to each of the two tones separately. The response to each tone is decreased when they are presented together. This is called direct suppression and it does more than affect the overall magnitude of the travelling waves. The response to each cycle of vibration of the combined vibration is distorted by the compressive non-linearity. The motile response of the outer hair cells to the composite stimulus is not an accurate summation of the two component stimulus frequencies but contains new frequency components called 'intermodulation distortions'.

It is possible to hear this non-linear process occurring when we listen to simple musical chords. Musicians may be familiar with the phenomenon. One can hear faint discordant tones not present in the original sound. These subjective 'intermodulation distortion products' (IMDs) are also known as combination tones. It is important to recognize that they are a physical and not a physiological phenomenon. They are the inevitable consequence of the distortion of complex waveforms and their production is not confined to the ear. When sounds are amplified electronically and reproduced via loudspeakers, intermodulation occurs if the amplifier or the loudspeaker system is minutely non-linear or if the size of the signal excursions approach the upper limit of the working range of any system component. The 'muddy', 'indistinct', and 'unsatisfactory' sound of poor quality sound amplification systems is due to intermodulation.

As intermodulation is a simple mechanical process its effects could be exactly predicted from the characteristics of the non-linearity. Even without knowledge of the specific non-linearity certain rules always apply concerning the possible new frequencies that can be added to the vibration. To gain an intuitive understanding of this consider two tones of differing frequencies f1 and f_2, with f_2 being higher than f_1. Their combined waveform has a modulated envelope due to the two signals periodically coming into and out of phase with each other (Fig. 4.7A). The periodicity of this modulation is that of the difference frequency given by $f_2 - f_1$. This modulation is not a non-linear phenomenon, but simply due to linear superposition. If we now pass this composite signal through a non-linear system, intermodulation occurs creating new periodic signals spaced at frequency intervals of precisely '$f_2 - f_1$' above and below the original signals, $viz.$ at $f_2 + (f_2 - f_1)$,

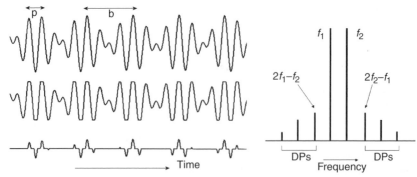

Fig. 4.7 Schematic illustration of intermodulation distortion production. (A) Top trace (left) shows the combined waveform of two tones of frequencies f_1 and f_2. The mean period of the oscillation is p. It is strongly modulated. The modulation is called 'beating' and occurs because the two tones slip in and out of step with each other. The period of the beats is 'b'. Beat period 'b' in this example is about four times 'p' but the principles apply to any ratio of f_2 and f_1. The beat frequency f_b is given by 1/b Hz where $f_b = f_2 - f_1$. The frequency f_b is called the 'difference frequency'. In the middle trace left the combined waveform has been exposed to a compressive non-linearity which has flattened (cut off) the positive and negative peaks of the largest excursions. The lower trace shows the difference between the original and distorted waveforms, which are concentrated at times of maximum overall stimulus size. This trace is the distortion. It consists of distortion products which combine to form pulses of oscillation with a period similar to f_1 and f_2 and synchronized to each beat (ie occurring at the difference frequency). (B, right) The frequency spectrum of such a distorted two-tone signal. The stimuli f_1 and f_2 are marked. In this representation the distortion products are seen as lines representing 'tones' either side of the primary tones f_1 and f_2, each separated by the difference frequency f_2-f_1. The degree of distortion on the right is actually much less severe in (B) than in the waveform example in (A), which has been exaggerated to make the distortion visible.

$f_2 + 2(f_2 - f_1)$ $f_2 + 3(f_2 - f_1)$, etc., and also $f_1 - (f_2 - f_1), f_1 - 2(f_2 - f_1), f_1 - 3(f_2 - f_1)$, etc. All these combinations are contained in the formula $f_{DP} = f_1 + N(f_2 - f_1)$ where N is a positive or negative whole number. Usually the intensity of these components decrease with increasing $|N|$. The characteristic pattern of intermodulation is shown in Figure 4.7B.

The most prominent subjective auditory distortion product is for $N = -1$ in the above formula for which $f_1 + N(f_2 - f_1)$ reduces to $2f_1 - f_2$. This is a frequency just below f_1. Kim *et al.* (1977) first indicated that during two-tone stimulation, vibration at $2f_1 - f_2$ is generated in the cochlea at the f_2 peak region where the f_1 and f_2 waves overlap and it then propagates as a travelling wave to its own frequency place apical to the f_1 place where it might be heard. Not all audible distortions belong to the same intermodulation family. We also perceive distortion at the primary modulation frequency $f_2 - f_1$, called the difference tone, but this component is not readily found as an OAE in human ears.

As our ears are so sensitive to any intermodulation in sound reproduction systems (which we invariably perceive as unpleasant) it is strange to find that our sensory mechanism generates such distortions itself. Until the discovery of OAEs in 1978 (Kemp, 1978, 1979) and of hair cell motility (Brownell *et al.*, 1985) the majority of workers considered aural distortion to be a purely neural phenomenon. The first suggestions that it could be a non-linear physical phenomenon were fiercely contended despite new evidence to the contrary (Kim, 1980). Non-linearity and distortion is certainly a prominent feature of *neural* signal transmission but auditory nerve signals are highly encoded and are not an analogue representation of the original sound. There is no necessity for non-linear distortion of neural signals to be perceived as sound. In contrast vibration on the basilar membrane *is* a direct stimulus analogue and any distortion in this peripheral location may be audible and will not be distinguished from a real stimulus. It must be heard as a sound.

How is it then that we can tolerate cochlear distortion and not tolerate distortion in a sound delivery system? The answer lies in the frequency selectivity of the cochlea. Intermodulation distortion occurs whenever two stimuli of different frequencies excite the same outer hair cells. But stimulus frequencies are spatially separated by the cochlea so that strong interactions between similar strength stimuli only occur between close frequencies. The distortion products from close frequencies are similar in frequency to the frequencies of the evoking stimuli and are always much lower in intensity and very often masked by the stimulus itself. In contrast, in a wideband electronic sound reproduction system, intermodulation distortion can occur between any and every frequency component, scattering inappropriate combination signals into frequency regions where they can be clearly heard. Hence, electronic distortion sounds 'bad', but cochlear distortion sounds 'normal'.

What function is performed by cochlea non-linearity? So far was we know there is no function associated with the production of distortion products, but great benefit is derived from the compressive non-linearity that causes them. Outer hair cell transduction channel non-linearity means that the mechanical forces generated by the cell's electromotility will not be proportional to the stimulus but compressed. With saturating wave amplification as provided by this motility the gain will be relatively high for small stimuli and progressively less for higher levels. This is very appropriate for cochlea function as very small stimuli actually require the most amplification to achieve vibration levels at the inner hair cell sufficient to cause the depolarization needed to excite neural firing. Higher levels of stimulation need progressively less help to stimulate the auditory nerve and the highest levels need no help at all. It is a question of dynamic range. Without the action of outer hair cells to increase threshold level travelling wave amplitude the inner hair cells would need sound about 60 dB above normal threshold levels to excite neural activity. A further 40–50 dB increase in stimulation would then begin to saturate the auditory nerves because the native dynamic range of the primary cochlear sensory system is only about 50 dB, an amplitude ratio of only 300:1. But *with* normal outer hair cell function this dynamics range expands to well over 100 dB (100 000:1). This is because the saturating amplification provided by the outer hair cells compresses the 100 000:1 dynamic range of useful stimulation *into* the 300:1 dynamic range that the sensorineural system can accommodate. This compression is clearly seen in the shape of the peak of the travelling wave in direct basilar membrane vibration measurements. Each 10 dB increase in stimulus level brings much less than a 10 dB increase in peak vibrational amplitude (Robles & Ruggero, 2001) paralleling what is seen externally in the TEOAE and SFOAE responses.

The value of compressive non-linearity in extending the ear's dynamic range is functionally immense, greatly outweighing any problems caused by distortion. However, because mechanical distortion is an inevitable byproduct of non-linearity the existence of distortion in OAEs is indirect evidence that outer hair cells are functioning normally and that they are achieving that vital stimulus compression. The detailed characteristic of that distortion has the potential to tell us in detail how well the outer hair cells are working.

4.7 Generation of distortion product otoacoustic emissions

Some of the distortion vibration generated by outer hair cell non-linearity finds its way back to the middle ear and creates distortion product OAEs (DPOAEs). This is of great research interest and clinical value in that it demonstrates that the outer hair cells are operating normally and presumably performing their primary function of supporting the travelling wave. However, the exact mode of DPOAE transmission back to the middle ear is complex, not fully understood, and is the subject of current debate (He *et al.*, 2008). An appreciation of these issues can be gained by considering their origin at the hair cell.

During two-tone stimulation each outer hair cell that is exposed to both stimuli generates a small amount of mechanical intermodulation distortion vibration. Some of this may be transmitted directly through the cochlear fluid as a pressure disturbance and drive the middle ear system in sympathetic vibration. However, it is generally assumed that most energy is transmitted to the basilar membrane, making each cell a potential source of a new travelling wave, that is a travelling wave at distortion product frequencies travelling apically and basally. In order for either the travelling wave or the direct route to cause sufficient vibration of the middle ear to generate DPOAEs – the small distortion vibrations from individual outer hair cells must arrive in step with each other and 'add up', that is, support and not cancel each other when they reach the middle ear. Close outer hair cells will receive almost identical stimulation and so will produce almost identical distortion waves in phase with each other. But cells further along the cochlear spiral will receive the stimuli a little later due to the finite velocity of the travelling waves. Furthermore, stimuli of two different frequencies are involved, f_1 and f_2, and these travel at different speeds as a result of frequency dispersion in the cochlea. In short, the timing or phase of distortion product vibrations generated along the length of the overlap of f_1 and f_2 will be 'scrambled' with apparently little chance of individual distortion components of the same frequency but from different places summating at the middle ear. This is just what occurs with the CM components generated by the same hair cells. It is the microphonic from the synchronously moving regions at the base of the cochlea that summate to create a substantial far-field CM. But there is a big difference between the transmission of vibration and of the conduction of CM. Electrical signals travel instantly to the scalp whereas distortion vibrations need time to travel. Distortion product vibrations appear to be able to propagate through the cochlea as a travelling wave as well as directly as a pressure wave (Ren *et al.*, 2006). However, delays in transmission provide a way for the 'scrambled' phases of individual hair cell distortions deep in the cochlea to reunite when they reach the middle ear.

Consider the distortion product generated by the interaction of two close tones, f_1 and f_2. The travelling wave due to the lower frequency stimulus f_1 penetrates further along the cochlea from the base than does the higher frequency f_2 wave as a consequence of the widening basilar membrane. The region of overlap between the two excitations, that is, the only region where distortion might be generated, extends from the base of the cochlea up to the f_2 frequency place (see Fig. 4.2). Close frequencies ensure substantial overlap of the travelling waves at nearly their peak amplitudes. Outer hair cell non-linearity is not itself frequency specific and so some distortion is generated throughout the overlap region but most is generated near to the f_2 peak where there is maximum f_2 stimulation and where the f_1 wave will have also grown substantially on its way to its own more apical peak. The above mentioned scrambling of distortion product phase with distance along the basilar membrane is systematically related to the phases of the two stimuli. If we imagine observing the waves at a point some way along the cochlea (but before the f_2 peak) then both f_1 and f_2 stimulus waves will arrive at that point with some time delay. That delay will increase the more apical a point we consider. The higher-frequency wave of f_2 will suffer more cycles of delay than that of f_1 at any point because its frequency place (its peak) is closer to the base. Another way to understand this is to note that in the cochlea the wavelength of f_1 is everywhere longer than that of the higher frequency f_2 wave. If frequencies f_1 and f_2 are very close their phases relative to that at the base will change almost identically with the distance of the observation point into the cochlea. In contrast, if f_1 and f_2 are dissimilar then the phase of f_2 will change more rapidly than that of f_1 with distance. The phase of, for example, the $2f_1 - f_2$ distortion product is given by the expression '$2\Phi_1 - \Phi_2$' where Φ_1 and Φ_2 are the local phases of f_1 and f_2, respectively, at the place considered. For close f_1 and f_2, Φ_1 and Φ_2 change almost identically and this expression indicates that the change in distortion product phase with distance along the basilar membrane will mirror the phase progression of the stimuli even though the frequency $(2f_1 - f_2)$ is different from and lower than that of the stimuli. Its spatial phase gradient will be in the same direction but steeper than the travelling wave of an externally applied stimulus at the distortion frequency. This situation is not conducive to the transmission of the distortion back to the middle ear nor to the summation of individual cell vibrations at the middle ear. It is an experimental fact that close stimulus frequencies do not generate the strongest DPOAEs even though the local conditions for distortion creation are near optimal. As the ratio of f_2/f_1 increases, the gradient of distortion phase with distance through the f_2 peak decreases and eventually reverses. This is possible because of the minus sign in $2\Phi_1 - \Phi_2$ and the fact that for greater f_2/f_1 the f_1 phase changes less than f_2 phase with distance through the f_2 place. There is a frequency ratio where the spatial distribution of distortion product vibrations along the basilar membrane becomes ideal for the propagation of distortion back to the middle ear and for the synchronous summation of each hair cell's contribution. At wider f_2/f_1 ratios the phase scrambling becomes severe again and the distortion-generating overlap occurs only in more basal regions were the f_1 stimulus is still small. Little distortion vibration arrives at the middle ear for frequency-wide ratios. For the distortion product $2f_1 - f_2$, it is found that an f_2/f_1 of about 1.2 elicits the maximum DPOAE output, that is, the 'optimum ratio' (Moulin, 2000). The optimum stimulus frequency ratio is used in nearly all DPOAE measurements. A more mathematical treatment of the process was given by Kemp and Tooman (2006). The interest in distortion phase is not confined to arguments about its escape route. DPOAE phase (or rather its phase gradient with stimulus frequency change) can be used to determine the travel time of stimulation within the cochlea (Mahoney & Kemp, 1995). Although no clinical use of this information has so far been found the technique has revealed that substantial functional differences exist between human and laboratory animal cochleae (e.g. Kemp & Brown, 1983).

There are further complexities in the emergence of DPOAEs. Maximum $2f_1 - f_2$ DPOAE level is found in the ear canal when f_2/f_1 is around 1.2. Distortion vibration appears to be strongly directed back to the base from its source at that ratio. But a second route is known to exist. As Kim demonstrated in 1977, some $2f_1 - f_2$ distortion product energy propagates from its source apically as a travelling wave and reaches the place in the cochlea tuned to that distortion frequency. Here it naturally reaches a peak of vibration and from there it can also be reflected back to the middle ear by the same mechanism that creates TEOAEs and SFOAEs (Gaskill & Brown, 1996). This second source of distortion product emission at $2f_1 - f_2$ contributes some energy to most DPOAEs. There are therefore commonly two components in DPOAE distinguishable by their different delays: one travelling directly from the source to the middle ear and one with greater delay having first travelled apically to its own frequency place. The proportion of each depends of the stimulus ratio. Small f_2/f_1 ratios produce mainly DPOAEs that have travelled apically and been reflected whereas at the optimum ratio (1.2) most DPOAEs usually come back directly from the site of generation (Shera & Guinan, 1999, 2008; Knight & Kemp, 2001). The 'direct' route back to the middle ear is not yet confirmed to be by the widely expected 'reverse' travelling wave. Recent evidence points to the possibility of a direct pressure wave route that is not fully understood (Ren *et al.*, 2006).

Important characteristics of DPOAEs can be predicted from an analysis of its origin in the overlap of the two stimulus travelling waves. At the optimum stimulus frequency ratio of 1.2, the f_2 and f_1 travelling wave peaks are separated by approximately one auditory filter bandwidth. The peak of the f_2 wave will be at a place where the f_1 wave is growing towards its peak but is not yet at its full size (see Fig. 4.2). As a physical process, non-linear intermodulation is optimal when both components are similar in amplitude. Referring to Figure 4.2 where the applied intensities L1 and L2 of stimuli f_1 and f_2, respectively, are equal, f_1 is much less intense than f_2 at the f_2 place. It is clear that an external increase in L1 would be needed for its travelling wave to reach internal equality with the f_2 travelling at the f_2 place. Raising the level of f_1 above that of f_2 should, and does, result in greater distortion production. Both the optimum intensity level ratio L1/L2 and the optimal f_2/f_1 ratio depend on the absolute f_2 stimulus intensity because the shape of the travelling wave envelope is dependent on the level. This is because of the compressive non-linearity of the electromotile forces that help sharpen travelling wave peak. The travelling wave receives relatively less amplification and less viscous loss compensation at higher stimulus levels so that envelope peaks become larger but broader. Higher stimulus levels therefore need more similar applied L1 and L2 levels to generate optimal DPOAE levels. At 70 dB SPL L2 = L1 is quite effective. Boege and Janssen (2002) have proposed a formula for estimating stimulus levels for optimum DPOAE production, *viz.* L1 = 0.4L2 + 39 (all quantities in dB SPL). This is an approximation only and individual differences are to be expected, but, in general, this formula assists in obtaining almost the maximum DPOAE output for a particular L2. The technique of reducing the intensity of stimulus f_1 more slowly than that of f_2 results in the cochlea exhibiting a clear L2 stimulus level threshold for DPOAE generation (see Fig. 4.9 below). This has been shown to have a greater intrinsic correlation with hearing threshold than 'threshold' assessments based on a fixed L2/L1 data.

We have focused so far on the distortion component '$2f_1 - f_2$', which has proved useful as an indicator of cochlear health. This component is always at a lower frequency than f_1 ($f_2 < f_1$). For example if $f_1 = 1000$ Hz and $f_2 = 1200$ Hz then the DPOAE '$2f_1 - f_2$' will be at 800 Hz. In contrast the distortion component '$2f_2 - f_1$' is of a higher frequency than either of the stimuli, that is, 1400 Hz, and so has its best frequency place more basal than that of either stimulus. The $2f_2 - f_1$ place will receive excitation before either stimulus has reached its own peak. Any distortion vibration that is generated at hair cell locations more apical than the $2f_2 - f_1$ frequency place cannot physically propagate in either direction as a travelling wave. This includes the $2f_2 - f_1$ distortion that will certainly be generated at the peak of the f_2 wave. In the region from the base up to the $2f_2 - f_1$ frequency place, this distortion can propagate provided its spatial phase distribution is appropriate. The possible distributions of $2f_2 - f_1$ phase are more limited than those for $2f_1 - f_2$. No value of f_2/f_1 favours direct transmission back to the middle ear. Its only route back to the middle ear is by reflection, probably from irregularities in the $2f_2 - f_1$ frequency place region. Experimental evidence supports this (Knight & Kemp, 2001). DPOAE $2f_2 - f_1$ shows greater normal inter-subject variability than does $2f_1 - f_2$ and is not used for clinical purposes. Whereas DPOAEs at $2f_1 - f_2$ logically provide information directly about sensory activity at the f_2 place, $2f_2 - f_1$ can only indicate indirectly the activity basal to this place.

Since outer hair cell non-linearity is the source of physical distortion in the cochlea it would be expected that distortions would also be found in the CM signal, since outer hair cells generate a major part of the CM. It is the case that the CM contains strong distortions at higher stimulus levels. Harmonic distortions (2f, 3f, 4f, etc.) are found in CM but these distortions are not found in OAEs. There is a clear reason for this. The externally recordable CM is largely generated by hair cells near to the base from where all components are readily conducted and summate. OAEs are mainly initiated near to travelling wave peaks. Vibrations at frequencies higher than the natural frequency of that place (and this includes all harmonics) cannot propagate away from that place. Harmonic distortions therefore cannot generate OAEs by a reverse travelling wave mechanism. Conversely, intermodulation distortions in the local CM in the regions where the travelling wave slows and peaks will consist of adjacent positive and negative phases which will tend to cancel remotely and not summate to create a CM 'DP'. Nevertheless intermodulation distortion products are found in the CM for moderate stimulation levels but Brown and Kemp (1985) have shown that these components are most likely due to basal hair cell CM responses to the DPOAE vibration arriving at the base.

4.7.1 Practical distortion product otoacoustic emission measurements

For practical purposes, DPOAEs are recorded via a probe which closes the ear canal to maximize emission sound pressure level and to exclude external noise. As for TEOAEs the microphone to record ear canal sound is either built into the ear piece or communicates with the ear canal via a fine tube passing through the canal closure. DPOAE observations require two-tonal stimuli and these generally need to be presented via two independent loudspeaker units to minimize inter-modulation within the transducers themselves, which would generate artefactual DPOAE. A typical clinical measurement might use levels of 65 dB SPL and 55 dB SPL for stimuli f_1 and f_2, respectively (often called the 'primaries'). This level of stimulation is sufficiently low to give a usefully sensitive test of normal cochlear function and high enough for good signal-to-noise ratios to be obtained in a reasonably short recording time. The frequency ratio f_2/f_1 would be fixed at around 1.2:1 to optimize $2f_1 - f_2$ intensity. During the measurement the stimulus pair would be shifted in frequency step by step over the range of interest in half, or one-third of an octave or even closer steps. At each frequency combination the instrument performs a high-resolution frequency analysis of the ear canal sound recorded by the probe's microphone. This would typically be per-formed on a one second or shorter sample of ear canal sound. Such an analysis would reveal the two stimuli and one or more intermodulation distortion products, the strongest of which would probably be $2f_1 - f_2$, as in Figure 4.8A. For clinical purposes results are normally presented as a

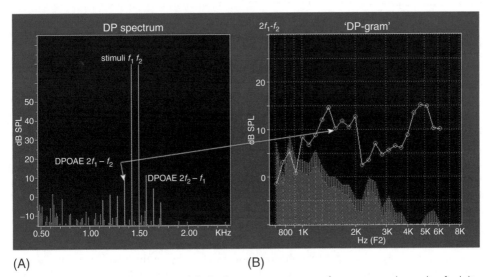

Fig. 4.8 Derivation of the 'DP-gram'. (A) The frequency spectrum of a one-second sample of adult ear canal sound during stimulation by two tones at 1425 Hz and 1500 Hz each at 70 dB SPL. The stimuli are seen in the spectrum as the two tallest lines. Either side are the distortion products. (B) The DP-gram is formed by taking the intensity of only the $2f_1 -f_1$ distortion from this spectrum and also from a series of other measurements at different f_1, f_2 frequencies, keeping f_2/f_1 constant. Eight frequencies per octave are plotted here. The shading on the right indicates the noise floor derived from the spectral level between distortion frequencies. The darkly shaded area is the level one standard deviation above the mean noise, and the lightly shaded area is two standard deviations above. This is a research recording with $f_2/f_1 = 1.05$. It was selected because it reveals the potential for multiple distortions. In clinical practice only one component $2f_1 - f_2$ is used. For a clinical DP-gram the f_2/f_1 ratio would be about 1.2, making the two stimuli further apart than on this spectrum (A). The distortion products for $f_2/f_1 = 1.2$ would also be more widely spaced. Fewer would be seen, perhaps only the $2f_1 - f_2$ and $2f_2 - f_1$ components. Stimulus levels for a screening test might be 65 dB and 55 dB SPL. Measurements would typically be made at two or three points per octave.

graph of DPOAE $2f_1 - f_2$ intensity in dB SPL as a function of the frequency of stimulus f_2 (see Fig. 4.8B). This graph is known as a 'DP-gram'. The DPOAE level is plotted against the f_2 frequency and not the DP or the f_1 frequency because evidence suggests that the $2f_1 - f_2$ DPOAE comes mostly from near the f_2 place. It certainly cannot be generated at the frequency places of f_1 or of DP since the f_2 travelling wave stops basal to those places and both stimuli are needed for intermodulation. Consequently the $2f_1 - f_2$ DPOAE level informs us about hair cell activity just prior to or at the f_2 place.

The normal DP-gram is approximately uniform across frequency but the inter- and intra-subject variance is quite high. An individual might show substantial variations in intensity across frequency with no obvious audiological correlate. A strong DPOAE from a young person might reach 25–30 dB SPL at some frequencies. A mature ear with clinically normal hearing might produce only 5–10 dB SPL across frequency. Levels below 0 dB SPL are usually an indication of clinically important hearing loss. Practical measurement systems are able to record DPOAEs well below −10 dB SPL. There are no internationally agreed norms for DPOAE measurement or interpretation. Levels of DPOAE obtained from an ear depend strongly on the relative intensity and relative frequency of the stimuli, as well as on their absolute levels. The literature provides useful guidance on the probability of, and probable utility of different DPOAE levels (e.g. Gorga et al., 1997, 2007), but if such guidance is adopted then it is essential that the stimulus parameters originally used to obtain the normative values are also adopted. The alternative is to develop local normative data with the specific protocol in use.

As the absolute level of stimulation is changed some systematic changes are seen in the DP-gram. At lower stimulus levels DPOAE intensity become less uniform across frequency. This is due in part to interference between the directly transmitted and reflected DPOAE emission sources. This creates a fine structure with frequency on a scale of 100–200 Hz which is not resolved by typical one-third or half octave interval measurements. Low stimulus level DPOAE measurements are more sensitive to milder hearing losses and the first effect of this is to reduce the degree of fine structure present. With high stimulus levels, for example L1 = L2 = 70 dB SPL or 75 dB SPL the normal DP-gram becomes more uniform across frequency. Sensitivity to mild hearing loss is lost but also the vagaries the emission process become less important. As a diagnostic measure of gross outer hair cell integrity (rather than as a hearing sensitivity screen) high levels are to be preferred and sometimes succeed in demonstrating residual outer hair cell function when 'screening' level DPOAEs are absent. (See below on recognizing artefactual responses.)

Counterintuitively for a non-linear phenomenon, in a healthy ear the intensity of DPOAE normally changes approximately proportionally to changes in stimulation level provided L2/L1 and F_2/F_1 are held constant. This represents a growth rate of 1 (i.e. 1 dB/dB). Ears with slight to moderate hearing loss often display steeper distortion product growth rates, with the distortion product being robust at high stimulus level but rapidly falling to the noise floor with smaller stimuli. With all ears, at some low stimulus level the DPOAE becomes undetectable in the noise floor. This is often referred to as 'DP threshold' but it is not a true physiological threshold, just a detection threshold (see Fig. 4.9A) Nevertheless the stimulus level at this crude DP threshold is found to correlate broadly with hearing threshold within a population. Some correlation is to be expected because both hearing threshold and DPOAEs depend on the efficient flow of energy through the cochlea and the activity of outer hair cells. As discussed earlier, Boege and Jannsen (2002) demonstrated a method of varying L2/L1 that optimizes DPOAE output when performing DPOAE input–output function measurements. This procedure manifests a true DPOAE threshold where distortion product levels reach zero sound pressure (see Fig. 4.9B). Although the method enhances the correlation between DPOAE threshold and hearing threshold in a population the accuracy in individual patients remains limited. This is understandable as hearing threshold is determined as

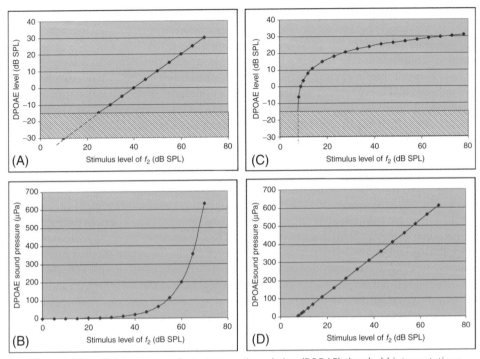

Fig. 4.9 Exposition of distortion product otoacoustic emission (DPOAE) threshold interpretations. DPOAEs are recorded with pure tone stimuli and this encourages comparison with measurements of audiometric threshold. However, the two are quite different measurements. DPOAE threshold requires careful definition, as illustrated here in schematic form based on an abstracted DPOAE $2f_1 - f_2$ growth function with stimulus level. (A, B) Illustration of DPOAE intensity level as a function of stimulus intensity for L2/L1 and f_2/f_1 fixed. (A) DPOAE level expressed as decibel sound pressure level (dB SPL). This typically exhibits steady decibel decrease in DPOAE per dB decrease in stimulation. The linear slope on this dB – dB plot is 1. The shaded area represent the noise floor of the instrument. The DPOAE becomes indistinguishable from the noise floor of −15 dB SPL at a stimulus level 'threshold' of about 23 dB SPL. This is the threshold for distortion product 'detection' and not a physiological threshold. This is clear in (B). Here the distortion product sound *pressure* is plotted in micro-pascals rather than decibels. It is clear that the absolute level of the distortion product is asymptoting to zero but that there is no specific threshold level where it actually reaches zero, that is, there is no physiological threshold. (C, D) In contrast, if L2/L2 is allowed to vary to achieve optimum DPOAE level at each L2 stimulus level then the level of the distortion product is maintained relatively constant over a wide range of L2 levels but the decibel level of DPOAE is found to drop abruptly at some low level of L2, as shown schematically to be at ~L2 = 8 dB SPL in this example (C). The absolute micro-pascal amplitude of distortion product for this condition is plotted in Fig. 4.9D. This shows there is now a true threshold. The DPOAE sound level linearly approaches zero at L2 = ~8 dB SPL. In this case the behaviour of the higher response levels predicts the eventual threshold level. The biophysical meaning of this threshold is uncertain because of the changing excitation patterns in the cochlea with level. It could represent the threshold of outer hair cell non-linearity. How this relates to the cochlear amplifier and hearing threshold is an open question. Better correlations are found with this method between this DPOAE threshold and hearing threshold, but this may be partly because of the methodological benefits of having a true intercept type threshold to measure.

much by the inner hair cells and their synaptic connections as by the outer hair cells which create OAEs. It must always be remembered that OAEs do not measure inner hair cell function. Also, as a consequence of stimulus compression by the action of outer hair cells a small decrease in the sensitivity of inner hair cells requires a large change in external stimulation to compensate, that is, inner hair cell threshold changes are 'expanded' when translated to audiometric threshold. This indicates that inner hair cell variance will play a disproportionate role in determining hearing threshold compared with factors influencing DPOAEs. It is unlikely that DPOAEs alone will ever provide sufficiently precise hearing threshold estimates but it is likely that the *difference* between the DPOAE threshold and the subjective threshold indicates an aspect of inner hair cell status.

Clinical DP-grams currently use only the '$2f_1 - f_2$' distortion component and it is important to remember that this is only one part of the total OAE generated in response to the stimuli. Little attention is currently paid to the other distortion products commonly present (e.g. $2f_2 - f_1$) although these have the potential to provide additional information. They can occasionally be present when $2f_1 - f_2$ is absent due to cancellation. The simultaneous production of SFOAEs at f_1 and f_2 during DPOAE measurement is totally ignored by the distortion product method as it requires a totally different extraction method (see later). SFOAEs together with TEOAEs provide additional information about cochlear amplification not present in DPOAEs. SFOAEs and TEOAEs are more directly related to the strength of the stimulating travelling wave can be more sensitive to minor abnormalities and changes in cochlear status than are distortion products OAEs.

4.8 Technical considerations with otoacoustic emissions

OAEs are a complex topic not only because of their complex origin but also because of the complex methods used in their stimulation, recording, and processing. In this section, attention is paid to calibration issues and to some technical factors that affect OAE recording quality.

4.8.1 Calibration

Calibration of OAE measurement systems involves independent consideration of both the systems stimulation and response measurement aspects. The importance of closing the ear canal and its effect on stimulation levels has already been mentioned. Concerning response measurement, OAEs are sound pressure fluctuations in the air of the ear canal caused by vibrations of the ear drum. The ear drum can only create measurable sound pressure changes if the air in the ear canal is impeded from moving backwards and forwards with the ear drum. In an open ear canal it is only at higher frequencies (>6 kHz) that the air in the ear canal has sufficient inertia on its own to oppose ear drum motion allowing sound pressure to be developed. Closing the ear canal with an OAE probe (Fig. 4.1) ensures drum vibration is converted to sound pressure at all frequencies and it also blocks external noise. A perfectly airtight seal in not essential at OAE frequencies but substantial leakage can result in the loss of low-frequency data and in resonance of the cavity, which can magnify oscillatory stimulus artefacts. The conversion of ear drum vibration to sound pressure is a function of the volume of the air in the ear canal and of the distance between the probe and the drum. The smaller the volume of air in the closed ear canal, the greater the sound pressure level developed, emphasizing the point that the absolute level of OAE is not in itself a primary physiological parameter.

Concerning stimulus calibration, stimulus levels must be calibrated *in situ* since the ear canal, and to some degree the ear drum, become components of the sound delivery system once the probe is inserted. Individual ear canal sizes vary considerable. Although the probe's microphone can be used to measure in-the-ear sound levels, accuracy is limited at higher frequencies by standing waves in the ear canal. These are due to reflections that cause the sound level to vary along the length of the ear canal so that the sound level measured by the probe may not equal the sound level present at the ear drum. The greater the distance 'x' between the probe tip and the drum the lower will be the frequency of the first 'closed ear canal' standing wave null. At this null frequency the stimulus reflected back from the drum arrives at the microphone in antiphase (i.e. ½ wave delayed) and falsifies the measurement of stimulus level at the probe. This makes accurate in-the-ear setting of the stimulus levels very difficult. Very approximately the null occurs at a frequency of $f_n = s/(4x)$ where 's' is the speed of sound. In the case of a well-fitted probe and an average ear, x might be 1.5 cm. Taking $s = 340$ m/s gives $f_n = 5.7$ kHz. Probe measurements may grossly underestimate the stimulus level being delivered to the drum around this frequency. The severity of this calibration problem varies from ear to ear. It is therefore preferable not to allow automatic in-the-ear stimulus calibration adjustments at null frequencies but to rely on prior probe calibrations (Siegel & Hirohata, 1994). The problem of knowing the exact stimulus level at the ear drum together with the sometimes critical dependence of DPOAE on the L2/L1 and f_2/f_1 ratios exacerbates calibration problems and make it difficult to obtain accurate and reliable OAE measurements above 5 kHz in adult ears and above may be 8 kHz in infants with commercial OAE instruments currently available. This is problematic if accuracy is needed say for long-term monitoring. Different fittings of the same probe can result in OAE level difference of a few decibels even with stimulus level calibration.

Transient OAE measurement methods also pose calibration difficulties. It is common to express the intensity of a click stimulus by its peak sound level or the peak positive to peak negative sound pressure difference, or 'peak-to-peak' level. The dB SPL level of a continuous tone with the same peak sound pressure values is used to express click level as dB SPL pe. This is useful where the stimulus drive waveform remains constant but it does not define the distribution of click stimulus energy across frequency and so it does not facilitate comparisons between instruments using different click waveforms.

Most OAE instruments do calibrate stimulus levels in the ear but they may adopt different procedures for doing so and this makes comparisons difficult. There are additional factors affecting calibration and accuracy. It is usual to cover the probe sound tubes by a sheath or disposable 'tip' for hygiene and comfort reasons. If this tip encloses or restricts the sound tubes or is badly fitted then errors of calibration can arise.

4.8.2 Otoacoustic emission identification, isolation, and validation

In all OAE measurements the response has to be identified and separated from the stimulus and validated as a true OAE. The following techniques for doing so exploit the inherent properties of OAEs:

◆ time windowing

◆ non-linear differences

◆ frequency analysis

◆ suppression

Different combinations of these techniques are used for DPOAEs, TEOAEs, and SFOAEs.

For DPOAEs measurement frequency analysis is the primary method of separating distortion from the stimuli. This very powerful since distortion product frequencies are precisely defined by the stimuli and not by the ear. It is then necessary to ensure that the measured level of distortion is well above the noise floor and other artefactual signals. Since electronic and electro-acoustic systems can produce distortion a control measurement needs to be made in a cavity modelled on the ear canal. A supposed DPOAE in an ear has to be shown to be well above the noise floor and any instrumental distortion. Since probes and equipment can deteriorate, frequent tests for arte-factual DPOAEs are recommended. Additional validation of a DPOAE can be achieved by dem-onstrating that it has a delay characteristic of the cochlea. As introduced in relation to SFOAEs, a change of distortion product phase with frequency indicates the inherent delay. In the simplest DPOAE delay procedure f_2 is incremented in frequency while f_1 is held constant. Group delay in seconds is given by $D = \delta C/\delta F$ where δC is the number of complete cycles of distortion product phase change (relative to a distortion product notionally generated from the stimuli in the ear canal) and δF is the f_2 frequency change in hertz. Typical values for human ears are 8 ms at 1 kHz, 5 ms at 3 kHz and 3 ms at 6 kHz (see Mahoney & Kemp, 1995). The key point for validation, however, is that the cochlear distortion product delay will exceed any likely delay in distortion generated in the instrumentation, which is typically less than 1 ms.

With TEOAEs, time delay is the primary method of separating the OAE from the stimulus. The transient stimulus excites an acoustic response from the ear canal and ear drum which usu-ally decays quickly, allowing the OAE to be seen after a time of about 2.5 ms. The technique of starting the recording after a time delay is called gating or windowing. However, this is not always sufficient for clinical purposes. In practice, in some ears with a well-fitted probe and in most ears with a badly fitted probe the initial acoustic response continues longer than 2.5 ms and so con-taminates the TEOAE recording. This is particularly problematic if the TEOAE is small or actually absent as then the acoustic artefact might be mistaken for evidence of cochlear activity. To mini-mize this risk the putative TEOAE response is routinely tested for compressive non-linearity – a defining feature of the cochlea. A special stimulus is used with clicks (or tone-pips) of two differ-ent intensities. In a common implementation every fourth stimulus is made three times larger. The responses to the three smaller clicks are added together and the response to the larger click is subtracted. This process would leave no response at all if its origin was purely acoustic and linear. But because true cochlear responses have compressive non-linearity the subtracted response can-cels little more than one of the three lower stimulus responses, leaving a validated artefact-free TEOAE response signal. This technique is referred to as the non-linear TEOAE method using a 'non-linear click' stimulus (see Kemp & Bray, 1986).

OAEs in response to single tone stimulation i.e. SFOAEs are included here for completeness but are not at present used clinically. SFOAEs arrive in the ear canal during stimulation. Their pres-ence can be recognized by applying a low level stimulus tone via a high impedance probe and sweeping its frequency through a range of say 1–2 kHz and observing the ear canal sound level. The ear canal sound level characteristically undulates by 1–3 dB with a period of 100–200 Hz. The undulation is due to interference between the stimulus and the delayed SFOAE. The magnitude of the undulations is greatest for near-threshold stimuli (e.g. 20 dB SPL) when it can be more than 6 dB peak to peak. Due to the compressive non-linearity of the cochlea, the effect is completely undetectable at high levels of stimulation (e.g. 80 dB SPL). SFOAEs can be isolated from the stimulus is several ways. The simplest way is proportionately scaling down the ear canal signal obtained at a high level of stimulation and then subtract it from the response obtained at low levels. This removes the stimulus and linear acoustic components leaving just the SFOAE (see Kemp & Chum, 1980; Brass & Kemp, 1993; Kalluri & Shera, 2007).

4.8.3 Noise, signal enhancement, and statistical response validity

All cochlear responses, that is, electrophysiological and otoacoustic, are inevitably contaminated by unwanted signals either temporally unconnected to the stimulus and collectively called 'noise' or signals related to the stimulus but not a response and collectively called 'artefacts'. For efficient recordings these contaminations have to be minimized at source as far as possible. The required signal then has to be enhanced relative to the noise and artefacts in order to make it detectable and measurable. Finally there needs to be a quantitative assessment of the quality or reliability of the response so obtained.

The CM, TEOAE, SFOAE responses have the problem that stimulus and response are very closely related. Minimizing electrical pickup from the transducers in the case of CM, and cancelling or otherwise minimizing stimulus contamination with OAEs is an essential process to avoid artefacts. Body noise can contaminate OAEs and because this is usually associated with muscle activity electrophysiological recordings are also affected by body movement. Keeping the subject comfortable, still, and quiet can control these noise sources. Environmental acoustic noise is especially problematic with OAEs as response levels are less than 30 dB SPL. Good probe fitting excludes noise well in adults but in not in infants. Firm deep probe fitting is key. Most OAE systems have noise rejection systems that temporarily halt the recording during sudden noise so that testing can continue usefully in between noisy events including occasional speech. But this technique is not helpful with continuous noise, such as air conditioning airflow noise. Such noise sources should be avoided completely. Conditions should be as quiet for OAE measurement as for audiometry. Environmental electrical noise for electrical apparatus is problematic for electrophysiological recording. It can be controlled by electrical screening and its effect is minimized by ensuring low electrode impedance and differential recording. However, such precautions are not needed at all for OAEs. Just as important as minimizing noise is maximizing response capture. Noise that is outside the frequency bandwidth of the response being measured can be rejected by filtering. Each physiological response has a different bandwidth with SP being the lowest frequency and smallest bandwidth (<100 Hz), CAP the next (<1000 Hz), and CM and OAE being potentially the widest being limited only by the frequency range of stimulation. With tonal stimulation such as is used for DPOAE, SFOAE, or tone-pip TEOAE or CM, strongly filtering the signal around the stimulation frequency is useful.

When everything possible has been done to reduce noise contamination to the minimum the response is still usually not detectable in the raw data stream. Signal enhancement is needed but this requires time and some knowledge of the specific characteristics of the response. With click evoked responses such as CM, TEOAE, and CAP the response is known to repeat exactly after each stimulus. Synchronous averaging of the responses to multiple stimulus repetitions reduces the noise contamination because the noise contributions in each sample are different and tend to partially cancel each other over time, whereas the identical response signals summate. With synchronous averaging the ratio of signal-to-noise amplitudes improves by a factor equal to square root of N, where N is the number of repeated responses that have been averaged. For example, a response drowned in noise ten times larger than the response would begin to emerge from the background after 100 responses were averaged.

The level of noise present is not precisely known in advance and neither is the expected level of the response so that the number of averages required for synchronous averaging to facilitate accurate measurement of the response cannot be predicted. What is needed is a measure of the balance of response to noise *during* the averaging process. One way to do this is to measure reproducibility. A response badly contaminated by noise will not produce repeatable values. Two independently collected averaged responses are needed – call them A and B. With a clear response and little noise signal contamination A should be almost identical to B. With waveform-based techniques it is useful to superimpose the waveforms of A and B as this makes it easy to see if the supposed response wave in A has been reproduced in B. For uncertain and emerging responses a more quantitative and objective method is desirable. A useful estimate of the noise present can be obtained by subtracting the two independently averaged recordings, that is, A – B. If we assume that the response is invariant and that the noise is random this subtraction leaves a residual signal, which contains only the noise present in the data. (Actually the noise present in A or B is 3 dB less than that obtained from the 'A − B' operation because the residual is a combination of the noise in both signals.)

The ratio of the total signal activity present, 'T' (i.e. the average of A and B) to the estimated non-repeated noise present (obtained by subtracting 3 dB from the level of the signal 'A − B') will be approximately unity while the response is much smaller than the noise 'n', but it will begin to rise above unity with continued averaging as the ratio of true signal to noise increases. This provides the simplest method to validate a response. A ratio of 'T' to 'n' greater than 2 (or + 6 dB) can be a useful minimum target condition for ensuring reliable measurement. If the total signal (response and noise) is twice the size of the noise estimate, it can be shown that the response energy is three times the noise energy, or 1.7 times its amplitude, and the true response should be detectable with a fair degree of reliability. This simple data ratio can be crudely converted into a true response signal-to-noise ratio estimate, *viz.* $(T − n)/n$. This relationship approximates to 's/n' where 's' is the repeatable or true response signal. With TEOAE recordings this estimate of signal-to-noise ratio is often refined by using the cross-power of the A and B recordings as a more accurate estimate of the response component, s. A signal-to-noise ratio of 2 times (or 6 dB) is commonly accepted as adequate for reliable detection of OAEs but accuracy in OAE level measurement benefits from longer averaging and higher signal-to-noise ratios.

A closely related data quality index known as 'reproducibility' is also in common usage with TEOAEs. Reproducibility is simply 100 times the Pearson's correlation coefficient computed from the two time series representing the two independently averaged response waveforms A and B. This closely approximates to $100 \times (I_{response}/I_{total})$, where '$I_{response}$' represents the intensity (rms amplitude squared) of the repeatable response and 'I_{total}' the total signal within the average. This index ranges from 0 for no repeatable response to 100% for a response with no noise. R = 50% would represent an equal balance of response and noise energy. Reproducibility is related to the signal-to-noise ratio (SNR) according to:

$$R=100(SNR^2/(1+SNR^2)$$

so that the criterion of a 2:1 signal to noise amplitude ratio corresponds to a reproducibility of 80%.

These calculations can all be conducted on specific frequency bands of the collected data. It is useful to do this on each octave or half octave frequency band of interest. A signal-to-noise ratio exceeding 2 (more than 6 dB) or a reproducibility exceeding 80% for each a half octave band is commonly accepted as adequate for confirmation of the presence of a response in that band for clinical purposes. Provided several (two to four) confirmed frequency bands are present in the required frequency range the ear is said to have passed an OAE screen. Such band analysis is highly beneficial in screening where speed is important. Some frequency bands are often fortuitously obscured by noise, especially the lower frequency bands, whereas others are not. As averaging progresses, the whole signal quality measures may remain poor long after there is sufficient band-specific evidence that the ear is normal. The method safely increases test specificity.

These methods based on signal processing work very well with TEOAE signals because they are rich in detailed information (i.e. a high number of degrees of freedom). They can be effective with cochlear evoked potentials too but auditory brain stem potentials have the least degrees of freedom, and a different philosophy of quality assessment has evolved based on the expectation of peaks in particular time windows. The method is to statistically assess whether specific waveform features are present. It is known as the FSP method (see Don *et al.*, 1984). Related statistical methods have also been used with TEOAEs and these have the advantage over signal-to-noise methods in that they provide a measure of the probability that the response obtained is not spurious. (Giebel, 2001).

In contrast with most other cochlear response measurements, DPOAE analysis is conducted entirely in the frequency domain. Recording duration is still the key to enhancing the response. Frequency analysis of longer ear canal sound samples allows for higher resolution frequency analysis and so excludes more noise from the measurement at the DPOAE frequency. It is equally effective to average data from many shorter samples, provided this is a vector average which accounts for the amplitude and phase of the data. To validate the distortion product response an assessment of the residual contamination by noise has to be undertaken. A good noise estimate is readily available from the signal levels of sounds at frequencies other than the DPOAE frequency, assuming that the noise is fairly uniformly distributed. Signal-to-noise ratio is the ratio of the signal at the DPOAE frequency to an appropriate measure of the signal at nearby frequencies. The way the neighbouring noise level is computed is important. Taking the mean level can be statistically unsafe. Taking the peak noise level is safer, as is taking one or two standard deviations above the mean noise level so as to give 84% or 95% confidence, respectively, that signals are not due to noise contamination at the DP frequency. Acceptable data quality is based on the DPOAE level being well above (e.g. 6 dB) the noise level measure.

It should be remembered that these measures of signal-to-noise ratio and reproducibility are only measures of data quality and are not physiological quantities in themselves. Reproducibility and signal-to-noise ratios compound cochlear and measurement-specific factors and should not be used to characterize an ear's response. For example a long averaging session might achieve a high signal-to-noise ratio and high reproducibility for an OAE response that was so small as to be well below the normal range and clinically abnormal. Conversely a short recording in noisy conditions could result in no evidence of a response even though a response was present. Because of this danger it is wrong to report an absent response when the noise present could have obscured a normal response. Noise contamination in the final result can be so high as to obscure even the most robust response. Assessment of an evoked response therefore needs to include an assessment of both the absolute levels of response and the noise present.

Clear pass criteria are particularly necessary for screening applications. The criteria need to include measures of both the adequacy and quality of the evidence collected. Most newborn screening programmes which use TEOAE or DPOAE have frequency-specific pass criteria requiring adequate signal-to-noise ratios (e.g. 6 dB) at a set minimum number of frequencies (e.g. in three half octave bands for TEOAE, or at three DPOAE frequencies made with half octave resolution. Such criteria are statistically safe only if minimum recording times are complied with. In addition, a minimum absolute signal level criterion should be set to avoid physiologically insignificant signals begin passed as normal.

The widespread use of frequency-specific criteria for infant screening with OAEs is a little strange when ABR is accepted as the gold standard for screening in its non-frequency specific mode, that is, with click stimulation. Frequency-specific criteria for TEOAEs were initially introduced as a means of overcoming the problem of patient and room noise because wideband measures of reproducibility and signal-to-noise suffered badly from such noise, causing low test specificity. As this noise tends to be irregular and low-frequency biased, the subdivision of the response by frequency greatly increases the chances of seeing a true response through the noise. The same logic applies to DPOAE screening. It has since become common for specific ranges of frequencies to be *required* as part of the OAE pass criteria. This extends the scope of hearing screening towards the diagnostic direction. Nevertheless the practical aim of infant screening remains the confirmation of 'adequate function' for the development of speech and language and not to demonstrate absolutely normal function at every audiometric frequency. The requirement for frequency specificity has not been applied to ABR screening perhaps because it would be impractical, or perhaps because this technique's inherent high-frequency bias is already ideal. ABR also has a special role with the at-risk baby population, in which OAE screening is insufficient due to the significant incidence of damage to auditory neural pathways.

4.9 Applications and interpretation of auditory responses

Of the cochlear responses reviewed here CAP, TEOAEs, and DPOAEs are each sensitive enough to be used as screening tests for normal cochlear function. It needs to be remembered that all OAE techniques rely on the middle ear for stimulus delivery and (unlike CM, CAP, and ABR) also for response collection. OAE measurements are therefore doubly sensitive to middle ear disorders. In the general population the absence or inadequacy of an OAE response is more likely to be due to middle ear problems than to the cochlea but this can readily be determined by tympanometry. CAP, TEOAE, and DPOAE each have the potential to give frequency-specific information about cochlear function but only CAP and ABR have the potential for accurate hearing threshold determination when used with frequency-specific stimuli. In all practical respects such as speed and ease of use, CAP is out-performed by ABR response methodology. TEOAE and DPOAE techniques rival and in some ways outperform ABR for speed, sensitivity, and easy of use. OAE and ABR tests should be seen as complementary. ABR provides a measure of total cochlear sensitivity including outer and inner hair cell contributions provided that the auditory pathway is normal. CAP comes even closer to being a purely cochlear assessment but is less practical. OAEs test only the transmission of stimulation inside the cochlea and the response of outer hair cells. They do not test transduction and so are highly focused on one stage of hearing albeit the most vulnerable. It is important to remember that OAE measurements are not 'hearing' tests. The limited extent of the hearing system tested by OAEs would severely limit their value was it not the case that it is the transmission function tested by OAEs that is most easily damaged and that is involved in the vast majority of sensory hearing losses. The majority of sensory hearing losses are in fact sensory transmissive losses. It was only because of the widespread adoption of OAEs as an infant 'hearing' screening test (Maxon et al., 1993; Vohr et al., 1998) that examples of other forms of sensory loss were identified. Cases where OAEs are strong and yet ABR and CAP were absent are defined as having 'auditory neuropathy' (Berlin et al., 2003). Previously known only in association with pathologies that disrupted the peripheral auditory pathway it became clear that this new class of cases had no recordable ABR because of either a malfunction of inner hair cell function (sensory transductive loss) or a disorder in the encoding of stimulation (neural dys-synchrony). In contrast to OAE and CAP, the CM and SP responses must be regarded as gross, whole cochlear status indictors of relatively low sensitivity to hearing loss. They are, however, important for establishing the health of inner hair cells.

Current techniques for otoacoustic and ECOG may be developed employing, for example more sensitive detectors, more informative stimulus paradigms, and better signal processing. The otoacoustic equivalent of the summating potential has not yet been clearly identified. This component is anticipated because outer hair cell motility is compressive and becomes asymmetric at higher levels. It is also likely that a functional part of outer hair cell motility consists of a DC component, a cell length change during stimulation. The former effect should give rise to a difference tone distortion product with two-tone stimulation, which has so far been seen only in laboratory preparations, for example Brown (1993). The latter should result in a 'summating mechanical response' producing a small inwards or outwards movement of the ear drum during stimulation (Lepage, 1987).

Ear canal acoustic reflectance measurements have the capacity to bridge middle ear and cochlear measurements. Although energy absorption in the middle ear can mask the crucial cochlear sound absorption, the use of multiple stimulus levels (as used with non-linear TEOAE and SFOAEs) allows non-linear reflectance to be measured, and this is a purely cochlear parameter. (Keefe, 1997). OAEs appear in ear drum reflectance measures as dense modulations in the ear drum frequency response (as with SFOAEs) and distortion products appear as a non-linear component of impedance.

A special clinical application of current OAE techniques is in the detection of acute changes in cochlear function and in long-term cochlear status monitoring. The normal stability of OAEs, their ease of use, and, with the right stimulation, their extreme sensitivity makes them ideal for this purpose. We have already mentioned the small suppression of OAEs observed with contralateral noise stimulation due to the activation of the cochlear reflex via the medial cochlear efferent system. Small oscillatory swings in OAE level occur as part of the cochlea's normal adaptation to moderately high stimulus levels (Kemp, 1986). These occur with a time period of approximately 200 seconds and do not appear to be centrally mediated (Kirk & Patuzzi, 1997). Observation of these swings and changes allow tracing of the dynamics of the cochlea's homeostatic system for the maintenance of sensitivity (Kemp & Brill, 2009). Abnormalities in this mechanism might be precursors of acquired hearing loss. Threshold elevation may only occur after the control system has lost its ability to maintain normal threshold. The ability of OAEs to indicate and track subtle cochlear changes will become important in the future clinical evaluation of oto-protective and oto-therapeutic drugs (e.g. McFadden & Pasanen, 1997).

Normally strong infant OAEs are sometimes found to be depressed just after birth and then recover over a 24-hour period. This reduces the specificity of newborn OAE screening. The most likely cause is retained fluid in the ear canal and middle ear – but there is a suspicion that it might also arise from birth-related stresses (Thornton *et al.*, 1993). Remarkably one study found a retrospective correlation between an unusual right–left asymmetry in newborn TEOAE levels and sudden infant death syndrome (Rubens *et al.*, 2008). There is also a definite gender effect on OAE intensity (Loehlin & McFadden, 2003; McFadden *et al.*, 2006) and in several studies a correlation has been found between atypical sexual partner preferences in females and unusually low levels of TEOAE (McFadden & Champlin, 2000) which has been speculatively attributed to adverse effects on the cochlea during hormone surges in gestation.

The cochlea has surprised us many times in the past as new 'responses' have been found that contradict contemporary models of its function. Doubts still persist about the precise role of outer hair cells. Is their motility simply to 'amplify' the travelling wave or do outer hair cells play a more complex role in bringing stimulation to the inner hair cells within the organ of Corti. (Drexl *et al.*, 2008). Do OAEs travel out as a reverse travelling wave? If so then why is there so far no direct evidence of this (see Wilson, 2008)? It could be that new understandings of the micromechanics of the organ of Corti and the role of outer hair cells are just around the corner. Effective pharmaceutical means of protecting and even restoring hearing may be developed soon, increasing the importance of our ability to objectively monitor changes in cochlear status through treatment via the recording of cochlear responses.

References

Allen JB & Fahey PF. (1992) Using acoustic distortion products to measure the cochlear amplifier gain on the basilar membrane. *J Acoust Soc Am* **92**: 178–88.

Allen JB, Jeng PS & Levitt H. (2008) Evaluation of human middle ear function via an acoustic power assessment. *J Rehabil Res Dev* **42** (**suppl 2**): 63–78.

Anderson SD & Kemp DT. (1979) The evoked cochlear mechanical response in laboratory primates. A preliminary report. *Arch Otorhinolaryngol* **224**: 47–54.

Bamford J, Uus K & Davis A. (2005) Screening for hearing loss in childhood: issues, evidence and current approaches in the UK. *J Med Screen* **12** (**suppl 3**): 119–24.

Berlin CI, Morlet T & Hood LJ. (2003) Auditory neuropathy/dyssynchrony: its diagnosis and management. *Pediatr Clin North Am* **50** (**suppl 2**): 331–40.

Bialek W & Wit HP. (1984) Quantum limits to oscillator stability: Theory and experiments on an acoustic emission from the human ear. *Phys Lett A* **104**: 173–8.

Boege P & Janssen TH. (2002) Pure tone threshold estimation from extrapolated distortion product otoacoustic emission I/O-functions in normal and cochlear hearing loss ears. *J Acoust Soc Am* **111**: 1810–18.

Brass D & Kemp DT. (1991) Time-domain observation of otoacoustic emissions during constant tone stimulation. *J Acoust Soc Am* **90**: 2415–27.

Brass D & Kemp DT. (1993). Suppression of stimulus frequency otoacoustic emissions. *J Acoust Soc Am* **93**: 920–39.

Bright KE. (2007) Spontaneous otoacoustic emissions in populations with normal hearing sensitivity. In: Robinette M & Glattke TJ, eds. *Otoacoustic Emissions: Clinical Applications*, 3rd edn. Theime, New York, pp. 69–86.

Brown AM. (1993) Distortion in the cochlea: acoustic $f_2 - f_1$ at low stimulus levels. *Hear Res* **70**: 160–6.

Brown AM & Kemp DT. (1985) Intermodulation distortion in the cochlea: could basal vibration be the major cause of round window CM distortion? *Hear Res* **19**: 191–8.

Brownell WE, Bader CR, Bertrand D & de Ribaupierre Y. (1985) Evoked mechanical responses of isolated cochlear hair cells. *Science* **227**: 194–6.

Buckard RF, Eggermont JJ & Don M. (2006) *Auditory Evoked Potentials: Basic Principles*. Lippincott Williams & Wilkins, Philadelphia.

Chung WH, Cho DY, Choi JY & Hong SH. (2004) Clinical usefulness of extratympanic electrocochleography in the diagnosis of Meniere's disease. *Otol Neurotol* **25**: 144–9.

Clark WW, Kim DO, Zurek PM & Bohne BA. (1984) Spontaneous otoacoustic emissions in chinchilla ear canals: correlation with histopathology and suppression by external tones. *Hear Res* **16**: 299–314.

Collet L, Kemp DT, Veuillet E, Duclaux R, Moulin A & Morgon A. (1990) Effect of contralateral auditory stimuli on active cochlear micro-mechanical properties in human subjects. *Hear Res* **43**: 251–61.

Davis H, Fernandez C & McAuliffe DR. (1950) The excitatory process in the cochlea. *Proc Natl Acad Sci* **36**: 580–7.

de Boer E, Nuttall AL, Hu N, Zou Y & Zheng J. (2005) The Allen-Fahey experiment extended. *J Acoust Soc Am* **117**: 1260–6.

Don M, Elberling C & Waring M. (1984) Objective detection of averaged auditory brainstem responses. *Scand Audiol* **13**: 219–28.

Drexl M, Lagarde MM, Zuo J, Lukashkin AN & Russell IJ. (2008) The role of prestin in the generation of electrically evoked otoacoustic emissions in mice. *J Neurophysiol* **99**: 1607–15.

Elliot E. (1958) A ripple effect on the audiogram. *Nature* **181**: 1076.

Ferraro JA. (2000) Electrocochleography. In: RJ Roeser, M Valente & Hosfort-Dunn H, eds. *Audiology Diagnosis*. Thieme, New York, pp. 425–50.

Ferraro JA & Kishnan G. (1997) Cochlear potentials in clinical audiology. *Audiol Neurootol* **2**: 241–56.

Galambos R. (1954) Neural mechanisms of audition. *Physiol Rev* **34**: 497–528.

Galambos R & Davis H. (1948) Action potentials from single auditory-nerve fibers? *Science* **108**: 513.

Gaskill SA, Brown AM. (1996) Suppression of human acoustic distortion product: dual origin of $2f_1 - f_2$. *J Acoust Soc Am* **100**: 3268–74.

Giebel A. (2001) Applying signal statistical analysis to TEOAE measurements. *Scand Audiol Suppl* **52**: 130–2.

Glattke TJ & Robinette M. (2007) Transient evoked otoacoustic emissions in populations with normal hearing. In: Robinette M & Glattke TJ, eds. *Otoacoustic Emissions: Clinical Applications*, 3rd edn. Theime, New York, pp. 87–106.

Gorga MP, Neely ST, Ohlrich B, Hoover B, Redner J & Peters J. (1997) From laboratory to clinic: a large scale study of distortion product otoacoustic emissions in ears with normal hearing and ears with hearing loss. *Ear Hear* **18**: 440–55.

Gorga MP, Neely ST, Johnson TA, Dierking DM & Garner CA. (2007) Distortion Product Otoacoustic emissions in relation to hearing loss. In: Robinette M & Glattke TJ, eds. *Otoacoustic Emissions: Clinical Applications*, 3rd edn. Theime, New York, pp. 197–225.

Guinan JJ Jr. (2006) Olivocochlear efferents: anatomy, physiology, function, and the measurement of efferent effects in humans. *Ear Hear* 27: 589–607.

Hauser R, Probst R & Löhle E. (1991) Click-and tone-burst-evoked otoacoustic emissions in normally hearing ears and in ears with high-frequency sensorineural hearing loss. *Eur Arch Otorhinolaryngol* 248: 345–52.

He W, Fridberger A, Porsov E, Grosh K & Ren T. (2008) Reverse wave propagation in the cochlea. *Proc Natl Acad Sci U S A* 105: 2729–33.

Hergils L. (2007) Analysis of measurements from the first Swedish universal neonatal hearing screening program. *Int J Audiol* 46: 680–5.

Hood LJ. (2007) Suppression of otoacoustic emissions in normal individuals and in patients with auditory disorders. In Robinette M & Glattke TJ, eds. *Otoacoustic Emissions: Clinical Applications*, 3rd edn. Theime, New York, pp. 97–320.

Johnsen NJ & Elberling C. (1983) Evoked acoustic emissions from the human ear. III. Findings in neonates. *Scand Audiol* 12: 17–24.

Kalluri R, Shera CA. (2007) Near equivalence of human click-evoked and stimulus-frequency otoacoustic emissions. *J Acoust Soc Am* 121: 2097–110.

Keefe DH. (1997) Otoreflectance of the cochlea and middle ear. *J Acoust Soc Am* 102: 2849–59.

Keefe DH. (2007) Influence of middle-ear function and pathology on otoacoustic emissions. In: Robinette M & Glattke TJ, eds. *Otoacoustic Emissions: Clinical Applications*, 3rd edn. Theime, New York, 163–96.

Keefe DH, Folsom RC, Gorga MP, Vohr BR, Bulen JC & Norton SJ. (2000) Identification of neonatal hearing impairment: ear-canal measurements of acoustic admittance and reflectance in neonates. *Ear Hear* 21: 443–61.

Kemp DT. (1978) Stimulated acoustic emissions from within the human auditory system. *J Acoust Soc Am* 64: 1386–91.

Kemp DT. (1979) The evoked cochlear mechanical response and the auditory microstructure – evidence for a new element in cochlear mechanics. *Scand Audiol Suppl* 9: 35–47.

Kemp DT. (1981) Physiologically active cochlear micromechanics-one source of tinnitus. In: Evered D & Lawrenson G, eds. *Tinnitus. Ciba Foundation Symposium.* Pitman Books, London, pp. 54-81.

Kemp DT. (1982) Cochlear echoes: Implications for noise-induced hearing loss. In: Hamernik RP, Henderson D & Salvi R, eds. *New Perspectives on Noise-Induced Hearing Loss.* Raven Press, New York, pp. 189–207.

Kemp DT. (1986) Otoacoustic emissions, travelling waves and cochlear mechanisms. *Hear Res* 22: 95–104.

Kemp DT. (2001) Exploring Cochlear Status with OAEs – the potential for new clinical applications. In: Robinette M & Glattke TJ, eds. *Otoacoustic Emissions: Clinical Applications*, 2nd edn. Theime, New York, pp. 1–47.

Kemp DT. (2007) Otoacoustic emissions: the basics, the science and the future potential. In: Robinette M & Glattke TJ, eds. *Otoacoustic Emissions: Clinical Applications*, 3rd edn. Theime, New York, pp. 87–106.

Kemp DT & Brill OJ. (2009) Slow oscillatory cochlear adaptation to brief over stimulation: cochlear homeostasis dynamics. In: Cooper N & Kemp DT, eds. *Concepts and Challenges in the Biophysics of Hearing. Proceedings of the 10th International Workshop on the Mechanics of Hearing.* World Scientific, New Jersey, pp. 168–74.

Kemp DT & Brown AM. (1983) A comparison of mechanical nonlinearities in the cochleae of man and gerbil from ear canal measurements. In: Klinke R & Hartmann R, eds. *Hearing – Physiological Bases and Psychophysics.* Springer-Verlag, Berlin, pp. 82–8.

Kemp DT & Chum R. (1980) Properties of the generator of stimulated acoustic emissions. *Hear Res* 2: 213–32.

Kemp DT & Ryan S (1993). The use of transient evoked otoacoustic emissions in neonatal hearing screening programs. *Semin Hear* 14: 30–45.

Kemp DT & Souter M. (1988) A new rapid component in the cochlear response to brief electrical efferent stimulation: CM and otoacoustic observations. *Hear Res* **34**: 49–62.

Kemp DT & Tooman PF. (2006) DPOAE micro and macrostructure – their origin and significance. In: Nuttall A, Gilespie RP, Grosh K, & de Boer E, eds. *Auditory Mechanisms: Processes and Models. Proceedings of the Ninth International Symposium, New Jersey*. World Scientific, New York, pp. 308–14.

Kemp DT, Bray P, Alexander L & Brown AM. (1986) Acoustic emission cochleography-practical aspects. *Scand Audiol Suppl* **25**: 71–95.

Kemp DT, Ryan S & Bray P. (1990) A guide to the effective use of otoacoustic emissions. *Ear Hear* **11**: 93–105.

Kim DO. (1980) Transcript of the mid-symposium discussion of the symposium on nonlinear and active mechanical processes in the cochlea. *(Chairman) Hear Res* **2**: 581–7.

Kim DO, Siegel LH & Molnar CE. (1977) Cochlear distortion product: Inconsistency with linear motion of the cochlear partition. *J Acoust Soc Am* **61**: S2 (A).

Kirk DL & Patuzzi RB. (1997) Transient changes in cochlear potentials and DPOAEs after low-frequency tones: the 'two minute bounce' revisited. *Hear Res* **112**: 49–68.

Knight RD & Kemp DT. (2001) Wave and Place fixed DPOAE maps of the human ear. *J Acoust Soc Am* **109**: 1513–25.

LePage EL. (1987) Frequency-dependent self-induced bias of the basilar membrane and its potential for controlling sensitivity and tuning in the mammalian cochlea. *J Acoust Soc Am* **82**: 139–54.

Loehlin JC & McFadden D. (2003) Otoacoustic emissions, auditory evoked potentials, and traits related to sex and sexual orientation. *Arch Sex Behav* **32**: 115–27.

Lutman ME & Deeks J. (1999) Correspondence amongst microstructure patterns observed in otoacoustic emissions and Békésy audiometry. *Audiology* **38**: 263–6.

Mahoney CF & Kemp DT. (1995) Distortion product otoacoustic emission delay measurement in human ears. *J Acoust Soc Am* **97**: 3721–35.

Margolis R & Shanks J. (1985) Tympanometry. In: Katz J, ed. *Handbook of Clinical Audiology*. Williams & Wilkins, Baltimore, pp. 438–75.

Maxon AB, White KR, Vohr BR & Behrens TR. (1993) Using transient evoked otoacoustic emissions for neonatal hearing screening. *Br J Audiol* **27**: 149–53.

McFadden D & Champlin CA. (2000) Comparison of auditory evoked potentials in heterosexual, homosexual, and bisexual males and females. *J Assoc Res Otolaryngol* **1**: 89–99.

McFadden D & Pasanen EG. (1997) Otoacoustic emissions and quinine sulfate. *J Acoust Soc Am* **102**: 2849–59.

McFadden D, Pasanen EG, Raper J, Lange HS & Wallen K. (2006) Sex differences in otoacoustic emissions measured in rhesus monkeys (*Macaca mulatta*). *Horm Behav* **50**: 274–84.

Moulin A. (2000) Influence of primary frequencies ratio on distortion product otoacoustic emissions amplitude. I. Intersubject variability and consequences on the DPOAE-gram. *J Acoust Soc Am* **107**: 1460–70.

Norton SJ, Gorga MP, Widen JE, Folsom RC, Sininger Y, Cone-Wesson B, Vohr BR, Mascher K & Fletcher K. (2000) Identification of neonatal hearing impairment: Evaluation of transient evoked otoacoustic emission, distortion product otoacoustic emission and auditory brain stem response test performance. *Ear Hear* **21**: 508–28.

Popelar J, Mazelová J & Syka J. (2002) Effects of electrical stimulation of the inferior colliculus on $2f_1 - f_2$ distortion product otoacoustic emissions in anesthetized guinea pigs. 1. *Hear Res* **170**: 116–26.

Ren T, He W, Scott M & Nuttall AL. (2006) Group delay of acoustic emissions in the ear. *J Neurophysiol* **96**: 2785–91.

Robinette M & Glattke TJ. (2007) Otoacoustic emissions in relation to hearing loss. In: M Robinette & TJ Glattke, eds. *Otoacoustic Emissions: Clinical Applications*, 3rd edn. Theime, New York, pp. 197–225.

Robles L & Ruggero MA. (2001) Mechanics of the mammalian cochlea. *Physiol Rev* **81**: 1305–52.

Rubens DD, Vohr BR, Tucker R, O'Neil CA & Chung W. (2008) Newborn oto-acoustic emission hearing screening tests. Preliminary evidence for a marker of susceptibility to SIDS. *Early Hum Dev* **84**: 225–9.

Russell IJ & Lukashkin AN. (2008) Cellular and molecular mechanisms in the efferent control of cochlear nonlinearities. In: Manley GA, Fay RR & Popper AN, eds. *Active Processes and Otoacoustic Emissions in Hearing*. Springer Science and Business Media, New York, pp. 343–79.

Rutten WL. (1980) Evoked acoustic emissions from within normal and abnormal human ears: comparison with audiometric and electrocochleographic findings. *Hear Res* 2: 263–71.

Schoonhoven R. (2006) Responses from the cochlea: Cochlear microphonic, summating potential and compound actions potential. In: Buckard RF, Eggermont JJ & Don M, eds. *Auditory Evoked Potentials*: Basic Principles. Lippincott Williams & Wilkins, Philadelphia, pp. 180–98.

Schratzenstaller B, Janssen T, Alexiou C & Arnold W. (2000) Confirmation of G. von Békésy's theory of paradoxical wave propagation along the cochlear partition by means of bone-conducted auditory brainstem responses. *ORL J Otorhinolaryngol Relat Spec* 62: 1–8.

Shera CA. (2003) Mammalian spontaneous otoacoustic emissions are amplitude-stabilized cochlear standing waves. *J Acoust Soc Am* 114: 244–62.

Shera CA & Guinan JJ. (1999) Evoked otoacoustic emissions arise by two fundamentally different mechanisms. *J Acoust Soc Am* 105: 782–98.

Shera CA & Guinan JJ. (2008) Mechanisms of mammalian otoacoustic emission. In: Manley GA, Fay RR & Popper AN, eds. *Active Processes and Otoacoustic Emissions in Hearing*. Springer Science and Business Media, New York, pp. 305–42.

Shera CA & Mountain DC. (2009) Transcript of the open discussion of the Mechanics of Hearing workshop. In: Cooper N & Kemp DT, eds. *Concepts and Challenges in the Biophysics of Hearing*. World Scientific, New Jersey, pp: 467–504.

Siegel JH, & Hirohata ET. (1994) Sound calibration and distortion product otoacoustic emissions at high frequencies. *Hear Res* 80: 146–52.

Strube HW. (1989) Evoked otoacoustic emissions as cochlear Bragg reflections. *Hear Res* 38: 35–45.

Thornton AR, Kimm L, Kennedy CR & Cafarelli-Dees D. (1993) External-and middle-ear factors affecting evoked otoacoustic emissions in neonates. *Br J Audiol* 27: 319–27.

Van Dijk P & Wit HP. (1990) Amplitude and frequency fluctuations of spontaneous otoacoustic emissions. *J Acoust Soc Am* 88: 1779–93.

Vohr BR & Kemp DT. (1991) Evoked otoacoustic emissions (EOAE) in the full term (FT) neonate. *Pediatr Res* 29: 270.

Vohr BR, Carty LM, Moore PE & Letourneau K. (1998) The Rhode Island Hearing Assessment Program: experience with statewide hearing screening (1993–1996). *J Pediatr* 133: 353–7.

von Bekesy G. (1950) DC potentials and energy balance of the cochlear partition. *J Acoust Soc Am* 22: 576–82.

Voss SE & Allen JB. (1994) Measurement of acoustic impedance and reflectance in the human ear canal. *J Acoust Soc Am* 95: 372–84.

Wever EG & Bray C. (1930) Action currents in the auditory nerve response to acoustic stimulation. *Proc Natl Acad Sci U S A* 16: 344–50.

Wilson JP. (1980a) Model for cochlear echoes and tinnitus based on an observed electrical correlate. *Hear Res* 2: 527–32.

Wilson JP. (1980b) Recording of the Kemp echo and tinnitus from the ear canal without averaging [proceedings]. *J Physiol* 298: 8P–9P.

Wilson JP, Sutton GJ. (1981) Acoustic correlates of tonal tinnitus. In: Evered D & Lawrenson G, eds. *Tinnitus. Ciba Foundation Symposium*. Pitman Books, London, 85: 82–107.

Wilson RM. (2008) Interferometry data challenges prevailing view of wave propagation in the cochlea. *Phys Today* 61: 26–7.

Zweig G & Shera CA. (1995) The origin of periodicity in the spectrum of evoked otoacoustic emissions. *J Acoust Soc Am* 98: 2018–47.

Chapter 5

Cochlear mechanics, tuning, non-linearities

Egbert de Boer and Alfred L Nuttall

5.1 Introduction

The cochlea is the place in the auditory pathway where the incoming signals are processed and analysed and where initiation of action potentials in primary auditory neurones occurs. Sounds come to the ear in the form of waves in air, impinge on the ear drum (tympanic membrane) and set the ossicles – the malleus (hammer), incus (anvil), and stapes (stirrup) – in motion. The stapes acts like a piston and moves the fluid with which the cochlea is filled. The reader is referred to Chapters 1 and 3 for reviews of anatomy and geometry of the cochlea and its immediate surroundings, in particular, the middle ear. In the present chapter we are concerned with the *signals* in the mammalian cochlea, mainly in the sense of physics, and the physiological processes that modify them.

The cochlea is, in the simplest possible sense, a system of fluid-filled channels, membranes, and cells in the temporal bone of the skull. Two channels play an important part, the scala vestibuli (of which the fluid is set into motion by the stapes) and the scala tympani (which contains the – flexible – round window to equalize the fluid flow). Between these channels lies the 'cochlear partition' with the organ of Corti containing, among others, the sensory cells. The entire structure has the shape of a helix; at the top the two main channels are connected by a tiny hole, the helicotrema. When the cochlea is stimulated by the stapes, a transversal wave develops that travels along the length of the cochlear partition. The way in which this wave originates, propagates, and dies out is a major subject of the discipline of 'cochlear mechanics'. The most remarkable thing about this cochlear wave is that, along its propagation path, the signal it carries is *analysed*. That is, the various signal components that it contains are deposited at different places along its path. Those components are actually sinusoidal components; we will specify signal analysis in more detail further on. On its way from the stapes to the helicotrema first the high-frequency components are removed from the signal and deposited at the corresponding location (thereby activating the associated nerve fibres), next the middle frequencies and lastly the low frequencies. The point of the present – necessarily somewhat vague – description is to make the reader aware that different locations in the cochlea handle different parts of the signal. The precise nature of this signal analysis in the cochlea will become clear in the further course of this chapter. Because different parts of the cochlea are, by way of afferent nerve fibres, connected to different parts of the first neural station, the cochlear nucleus, the tonotopic arrangement is preserved to within that station.

The present chapter is divided into nine parts. In this introductory section, we will describe a few concepts that are needed to follow the more detailed analysis in the remainder of this chapter. The next section 'Measurement of mechanics and physiology of the cochlea' describes the instrumentation necessary for mechanical research of the cochlea. The third section entitled 'Modern mechanical data – frequency selectivity and non-linearity' describes the experimental basis for modern cochlear mechanics. The next two sections, called 'Basic modelling of the cochlea' and 'The "active" cochlea', respectively, present the steps in the formulation and the solution of a model of the mechanics of the cochlea and illustrate the 'active' process (also known as the 'cochlear amplifier'). At the end of the procedure a model is created of which the response imitates most of the features and properties of the real cochlea. The sixth section describes 'Non-linear effects in the basilar membrane response' as a byproduct of cochlear amplification and the next section, dedicated to 'Organ of Corti micromechanics and the excitation of hair cells', elucidates many of the possible mechanisms behind cochlear amplification and discusses how the so-amplified motion is connected to inner hair cell (IHC) stereocilia. The eighth section treats 'Internal reflections and otoacoustic emissions' in some detail, and the chapter ends with 'Additional effects, puzzles, conclusions'. It should be noted at this point that many subjects in cochlear mechanics are complex, and have several different aspects, for example, otoacoustic emissions. Therefore, these subjects have been distributed over different sections in this chapter.

A number of tools and concepts are needed to understand the cochlea (to the degree that nowadays has been reached). We now describe the most important ones, starting with signal analysis. The waveform of a sound or of a signal inside the cochlea can be periodic or aperiodic. A very special type of signal that is periodic is a *sinusoidal* signal. In view of how it sounds it is often called a 'pure tone': it has a most neutral timbre (this has been one of the reasons why sinusoidal signals are used so much in auditory research – another reason will become clear below). Mathematically, all signals can be considered as *sums of sinusoidal signals*, which we refer to as 'analysis into sinusoidal components'. For a periodic signal such an analysis is fundamentally simple: if the frequency of the periodic signal is f_0, the constituent components have the frequencies f_0, $2f_0$, $3f_0$, $4f_0$, etc. In fact, sinusoidal oscillations with these frequencies can always be chosen (with proper amplitudes and phases) so that their sum equals the original periodic signal. This statement implies that signals can be *added*, and that idea constitutes the focus of signal analysis. When we put sinusoidal signals and the addition of signals at the centre of our attention we are in fact considering a system that is *linear*. Linear systems are extremely important, and not only in the cochlea. A linear system has the following fundamental property:

- When you put two signals at the input, the output signal will consist of the sum of the output signals that correspond to each of the two input signals separately.

It follows that:

- When you put in an input signal, and observe the output signal, the latter will be two times as large when the former is given with two times the amplitude. The number 'two' is arbitrary here.

The fundamental underlying property is: *the presence of one signal has no effect on the way a second signal is handled*, and this property is valid for all signals in a linear system. It can be shown mathematically that for a linear system a sinusoidal input signal always corresponds to a sinusoidal output signal. Actually, all a linear system can do to a sinusoidal signal is to alter its amplitude and phase, it cannot change the frequency. As a matter of fact, when the input signal is not sinusoidal, a linear system can modify amplitudes and phases of the component sinusoidal signals, and does this for every component independently of the others. For the sounds in our daily life the air carrying them to us is linear. One sound, in that case, can never be drowned out by another one. That we sometimes do not hear a sound in the presence of another, generally stronger, sound is not due to the properties of the air surrounding us but is a specific property of our ears.

Coming back to more general linear systems, many linear systems modify different frequencies differentially: they may cut off low frequencies, or high frequencies, or enhance a certain region of frequencies. In the latter case there often is a resonance at play. The curve of amplitude versus frequency is called the 'frequency response' although it would be better to include the phase with the amplitude. In general, the phase is not independent of the amplitude: certain phase patterns are characteristic for low-pass, high-pass, or band-pass systems. Owing to space constraints, we cannot explain these connections in detail here, but there are several textbooks and tutorial programmes dealing with this issue. One aspect of phase needs to be mentioned, however. Consider a signal with two components, with frequencies f_1 and f_2 very close together. The waveform of this signal has a slowly varying envelope and rapid oscillations with a frequency equal to the average of the frequencies f_1 and f_2. Assume this signal to pass through a linear system, where the components undergo a phase change. It can be shown that the time delay that the signal waveform (as well as the envelope waveform) undergoes is related to the derivative of the phase change with respect to frequency. That derivative is called the *group delay*. This concept plays an important part in present-day discussion about the cochlea as we will see later on.

Above we referred to the decomposition of an arbitrary periodic signal into sinusoidal components. This analysis is known as *Fourier analysis*. Actually, Fourier analysis of a periodic signal is but a special case. A signal may be non-periodic yet consist of the sum of a number of sinusoidal components. We already encountered such a signal: the one containing two components with nearly equal frequencies. Even a completely random signal (a noise signal) can be Fourier analysed, that is, considered as the sum of sinusoidal components. Since in this chapter we do not need this specific type of Fourier analysis, we will not define it. A linear system, when it handles a complex signal consisting of a number of sinusoidal components, can do nothing else but change amplitudes and phases of those components, for each component independently of all others. It can never create new frequency components.

The mechanics of the organ of Corti (which is dominated by the mechanics of the basilar membrane [BM]) can be considered as a linear system – we will encounter exceptions later. In that case the mechanics of the BM can be described by its 'mechanical impedance'. In the simplest form the BM impedance is defined as the quotient of the *pressure* difference across the BM and the *velocity* of the BM. However, a complication is due to possible phase differences between pressure difference and velocity. Let us consider the simple case of stiffness of a spring, for instance. In this case deflection and pressure are proportional. For a sinusoidal vibration – as we are considering here – velocity is proportional to deflection but there is a 90° phase difference between deflection and velocity (velocity is zero when deflection is maximal, and vice versa). The impedance (pressure divided by velocity) associated with the stiffness thus has to be marked in a special way to indicate that phase difference. The quotient of pressure and velocity is therefore given the mathematical form of a *complex number* – this is a number that has two parts, a real and an imaginary part, which are treated separately. The real part is concerned with variables that are in phase, and the imaginary part with variables that are 90° out of phase. In the case of stiffness, the impedance is *negative imaginary*, whereas a mass is represented by a *positive* imaginary value. Without going into more detail about mathematical concepts it is stated that stiffness and mass effects are lumped into one number, and together form the *imaginary* part of the impedance. The impedance component that has to do with friction and power loss forms the *real* part of the impedance. In the case of friction, the pressure or force is proportional to the velocity and the impedance, and thus the quotient is a real quantity. It is normally positive but – again – we will encounter exceptions later.

Processing of signals is different in a non-linear system (tacitly we will consider only stable, time-invariant non-linearities). Components are not processed independently any more, and new components can be generated. For a sinusoidal input signal with frequency f_0, the output signal is periodic but no longer sinusoidal in waveform. It may therefore contain not only the original frequency f_0 but also distortion products (DPs). These are called 'harmonics', and they are components with frequencies $2 f_0$, $3 f_0$, $4 f_0$ etc., none of them being present in the input signal. The situation is more interesting when a signal with two primary components, having frequencies f_1 and f_2 (where $f_2 > f_1$), is presented to a non-linear system. The output signal will then contain, apart from the harmonics of the two primary frequencies, other DPs, also known as combination tones (CTs), of which the frequencies are combinations of f_1 and f_2. In point of fact, the frequencies of these DPs are simple whole number combinations, such as $2 f_1 - f_2$, $3 f_1 - 2 f_2$, $2 f_2 - f_1$, $3 f_2 - 2 f_1$, and this range can be arbitrarily extended (even with plus signs instead of minus signs but these DPs are not important for our purpose). Assume now that the two frequencies f_1 and f_2 are close together. The first two of the DP frequencies can also be written as: $f_1 - (f_2 - f_1)$ and $f_1 - 2(f_2 - f_1)$, respectively, demonstrating that they are near (and below) f_1. Under certain conditions, when we listen to two simultaneous pure tones, the first of these DPs can even be heard! The second pair can, similarly, be seen to lie near (and above) f_2. The pair of signals with frequencies $f_2 - f_1$ and $f_2 + f_1$ is a member of a different class of DPs. In view of the theory of the cochlea these products are slightly less interesting (although the former one is sometimes audible), and we will further on concentrate on the DP components with frequencies $2 f_1 - f_2$, etc.

A completely different manifestation of non-linearity is found in the effect one tone has upon another. Take the case of the presentation of a tone with frequency f_0 to a non-linear system and observe the component with the same frequency in the output signal. Now, add another, generally stronger, tone (with a different frequency) to the input, then the component with frequency f_0 may well be changed. In the case of the cochlea it will generally be reduced in amplitude, and we speak of 'two-tone suppression'. When each tone is capable of suppressing the other one, we speak of 'mutual suppression'. In the case of suppression individual signal components are clearly not handled independently.

It should be noted at this point that 'suppression' is not the same as 'masking'. We consider suppression purely in the mechanical sense, as a phenomenon that can be measured directly. Masking belongs to the domain of psychophysics – one sound is made inaudible by the presence of another sound – and in this case 'perception' is involved. Actually, it has proven to be fairly difficult to detect evidence of suppression (formerly called inhibition) in the cochlea by way of a psychophysical measurement (Houtgast, 1972). A peripheral analogy to 'perceptual masking' is found in recording of responses of the auditory nerve. In this field of study, the relation between nerve-fibre masking (in this case rightly called inhibition) and suppression on the mechanical level is far from transparent (Schmiedt, 1982; Prijs, 1989; Ruggero *et al.*, 1992).

5.2 Measurement of mechanics and physiology of the cochlea

Cochlear mechanics is all about measurement (and mathematics). The structures of the inner ear, lying deep within the skull, are extremely delicate and vulnerable to damage, tiny in size, and miniscule in motion. They have only reluctantly given up some of their secrets and to this day retain several mysteries for auditory scientists to solve. Moreover, the cochlea as a system is not only mechanical, but its physiology is also tightly interwoven with electrical processes. In a very real sense the organ of Corti is an electromechanical machine specialized in real-time analysis of complex acoustic signals, that is, analysis of acoustic signals made up of many signal components each having differing intensity levels and varying with time such as in human speech or animal cries.

The motion of the structures in the cochlea can thus be measured using electrical as well as mechanical approaches. In the electrical domain, a voltage is recorded from one or more electrodes. The forms that the electrodes take vary from simple tiny wires to sharp glass pipettes with pointed tips sufficiently small to fit within single cells. A cleverly designed experiment and analysis of the voltage signals can reveal much information about the motion of cochlear structures and the mode of operation of cochlear cells.

The field of cochlear electrophysiology may be defined as having its start with the discovery of the Wever–Bray effect (Wever & Bray, 1930). This microvolt-level signal, now long known as the cochlear microphonic (CM), on its discovery was immediately shrouded in controversy over its origin – was it a neural response or not? It came to be understood much later (Dallos, 1973; Dallos & Cheatham, 1976) that the CM is mainly generated by outer hair cells (OHCs). By positioning electrodes in different turns of the cochlea one learns that the sensitivity to sound stimulation has a topographic arrangement. High-frequency tones give maximum signals at the base of the cochlea and low-frequency sounds at the apex. Finally, the tonotopic map of frequency distribution first described as a mechanical function by von Békésy (his collected works in von Békésy ([1960]) and explored by sharp electrode recording of action potentials in the population of afferent nerve fibres (Kiang et al., 1965), was confirmed by labelling of auditory nerve fibres (Liberman, 1982).

Direct measurement of mechanical motion has always been the main goal of specialists studying the vibration of the organ of Corti. The seminal work of Georg von Békésy (for which he received the Nobel Prize in Physiology in 1961) was accomplished in the human temporal bone using light microscopy with stroboscopic illumination (von Békésy, 1960). His approach was state of the art and very sensitive, having a resolution of displacement well below 1 μm. By observing the spiral-shaped BM in the apical region of the dissected human temporal bone he showed that different stimulus frequencies mapped to different places along the longitudinal direction. The lower the frequency the further from the stapes was the peak of BM motion. (We will discuss representative results of his work below.) This finding has stood the test of time but von Békésy's data also caused one of the biggest puzzles of cochlear physiology of the mid-twentieth century: the apparent subatomic size of the extrapolated threshold of BM motion (von Békésy, 1948). For a BM displacement of 1 μm, von Békésy had to use sound levels well over 100 dB SPL. The displacement was found to be linear with sound level and thus all one has to do is to extrapolate this linear function to that expected from a 0 dB level sound. The result is an astounding 10^{-11}m, 0.01 nm, or 0.1 Å (Ångström), much smaller than the diameter of the hydrogen atom (1.2 Å).

It took a wholly different technology to resolve the problem – it turned out to be not a problem at all – and to provide one of the great discoveries of twentieth-century cochlear mechanics (see Section 5.3). The new technology was the Mössbauer technique for measurement of velocity, and the discovery was the physiologically vulnerable mechanical non-linearity of the cochlea (Rhode, 1971). This technique uses a radioactive source placed on the BM and a tuned gamma-ray detector. Mechanical motion causes frequency modulation of the gamma radiation and this causes variations of the captured radiation by the detector. The method has a fundamentally non-linear response for velocity magnitude and thus requires care in calibration but the sensitivity is sufficient to measure BM velocity for sound levels as low as 10 dB SPL (e.g. Sellick et al., 1982). In addition to the intrinsic non-linearity of the method there are other shortcomings: the tiny gamma-ray source itself causes difficulties because of its mass and its radioactivity. At any rate, these experiments have resulted in a revolution in cochlear mechanics. More details about this pioneering work is given in Section 5.3.

A light-amplitude modulation method has been used to study BM motion induced by sound (Xue et al., 1993). Electrical stimulation of the cochlea (Xue et al., 1995) allowed the detection of a complex vibration across the width of the BM. Electrical stimulation was found to induce rocking at the outer pillar cell footplate (e.g. Nuttall et al., 1999). Optical methods with laser interferometry have advantages over all other methods and are in common use at this time. The sensitivity for either velocity (with laser-Doppler velocimetry) or for displacement (with homodyne interferometry) exceeds that needed to detect organ of Corti motion at the hearing threshold, especially when reflective objects, such as beads, are placed on the tissue surface. In the first implementation of laser interferometry for *in vivo* cochlear responses, Khanna and Leonard (1982) placed a reflective mirror on the BM in the high-frequency region of the cochlea in the cat. The apical low-frequency response of the guinea pig cochlea was examined in a unique *ex vivo* preparation that preserved the endocochlear potential (Ulfendahl *et al.*, 1989). Other custom-built instruments (Cooper, 2000) and adaptations of commercial laser-Doppler velocimeters (Nuttall *et al.*, 1991; Ruggero & Rich, 1991) have generated the large corpus of data on cochlear mechanics *in vivo* with preservation of normal or near-normal cochlear sensitivity, on which modern cochlear research relies. Two other implementations of laser interferometry warrant mention. The laser self-mixing method has allowed measurement of BM motion in the intact cochlea via a view through the round window membrane (Lukashkin *et al.*, 2005). The power of this approach is shown in studies of mice with mutations affecting the mechanics of the tectorial membrane (see Section 5.7). The other method is optical low-coherence interferometry (or tomography, OCT) where the illumination source is wide wavelength and not a coherent laser (Choudhury *et al.*, 2006; Hong and Freeman, 2006; Chen *et al.*, 2007). With OCT one has the ability to image and measure from the organ of Corti at the cellular level without reflective objects.

One should bear in mind that the choice of measurement method not only enables certain mechanical experiments, but also promotes creative preparations of the cochlea. Thus, with the use of fluorescent dyes and sound-synchronized laser confocal microscopy, Fridberger *et al.* (2004b) were able to show the three-dimensional motion of the apical organ of Corti. Whole mounts of cochlear turns (Mammano & Ashmore, 1993; Nowotny & Gummer, 2006), cochlear hemislices (Hu *et al.*, 1999; Richter *et al.*, 2000), or the organ of Corti in fluid-partitioned chambers (Chan & Hudspeth, 2005) have been studied. In some studies combinations were used of laser interferometry for optical axis motion with differential photodiodes for lateral motion. Results of all this work will be treated later.

In the field of instrumentation we should include the measurement of 'otoacoustic emissions'. These are weak sounds that are emitted by the ear, without and with specific stimulation. A tiny microphone is placed in the external ear canal, together with the miniature transducers ('loudspeakers') that are used to stimulate the ear. Chapter 4 is dedicated to otoacoustic emissions (its author Kemp discovered emissions in 1978). Some of these emissions are 'spontaneous', that is, they arise without a stimulus to the ear (e.g. Wilson, 1980; Zurek, 1981). All the others are evoked emissions, and they require an acoustical (or, in some cases, an electrical) stimulus signal. Otoacoustic emissions are important in the theoretical sense because they can tell us something about what is going on inside the cochlea, without having to anaesthetize the subject or surgically open the cochlea. These signals have also become increasingly important for the diagnostics of hearing loss, for example, in infants. The genesis of emissions will be treated at greater length in Section 5.8.

Let us now return to the very beginning of the era on measurements in cochlear mechanics. Using illumination with normal light and stroboscopy to measure vibration, Georg von Békésy (his work has been collected in von Békésy, 1960) set out to measure BM motion in human cochleae dissected from cadavers. We mentioned these measurements above but now we show an actual illustration. Figure 5.1A depicts response curves for a human cochlea. It shows these responses as functions of frequency, for six different locations along the length of the BM (von Békésy, 1949). A fairly wide range of frequencies was covered here. Each curve shows a maximum at a particular frequency, which is the 'best frequency' (BF) associated with the location of measurement. Figure 5.1B shows response curves of a human cochlea in a different way, namely, as functions of location, that is distance from the stapes, for a small number of low frequencies (von Békésy, 1947). To this figure the phase curves have been added. At the location of the peak

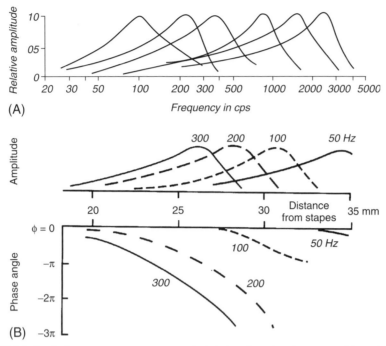

Fig. 5.1 (A) Mechanical response curves measured at six locations in a human cochlea, plotted as functions of frequency (*f*). All curves made to have the same maximum. (B) Mechanical response curves measured at four low frequencies in a human cochlea, plotted as functions of location (*x*). Upper panel: amplitude (all curves made to have the same maximum). Lower panel: phase, referred to the phase at the stapes.
Figure 5.1A reprinted with permission from Figure 7 of von Békésy (1949), © 1949, Acoustical Society of America. Figure 5.1B reprinted with permission from Figure 5 of von Békésy (1947), © 1947, Acoustical Society of America.

of the response the total phase shift accumulated is greater than one cycle, 2π radians. Because simple filters never accumulate a larger phase shift than π radians, these phase curves demonstrate that a wave is travelling along the length of the BM (of which the phase slope obviously depends on frequency and location). It is clear from Figure 5.1B that the location of maximum response is closer to the stapes for higher frequencies. From this result originates the fundamental principle: '*frequency*' is transformed into '*place*'. More precisely, it can be said that at each location the cochlea acts as a mechanical band-pass filter. We must add that von Békésy also provided the cue to this frequency-to-place transformation. He measured the stiffness of the BM and found it to decrease by a very large factor from the stapes to the helicotrema region (von Békésy, 1948, 1960). Later measurements in animal ears (Olson & Mountain, 1991, 1994; Naidu & Mountain, 1998; Emadi *et al.*, 2004) have substantiated the basic nature of these findings. We should add that the principle of spatial projection was predicted by von Helmholtz (1862, 1954).

Since the time of these measurements we know approximately how the cochlea projects frequency to space – and that knowledge has been extended to include many mammals. For a review and later refinements of this concept see two papers by Greenwood (1961, 1990), published 29(!) years apart. In Figure 5.2 we have schematically illustrated the two ways in which we can view the

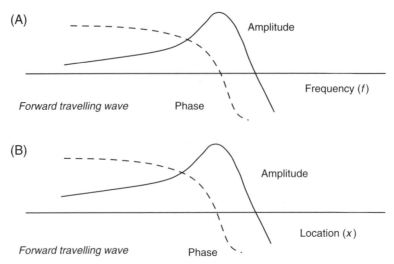

Fig. 5.2 The two ways of considering frequency-to-place transformation in the cochlea. (A) Frequency response, measured at one location, plotted as a function of frequency (*f*). (B) 'Cochlear pattern', or 'panoramic view', plotted as a function of location (*x*), for one frequency.

transformation from frequency to place and *vice versa*. Figure 5.2A shows the frequency response of the cochlea in stylized form (compare this with one of the curves of Fig. 5.1A). Stimulation is assumed to occur at the stapes, with constant velocity and zero phase. Amplitude and phase of the velocity of the BM for a sinusoidal stimulus at a *fixed location* are plotted as functions of frequency *f*, by a solid and a dashed curve, respectively. The frequency scale is logarithmic. The amplitude is assumed to be plotted on a decibel scale, and the form of the curve is based on more modern experiments and is therefore more detailed than Figure 5.1A. The frequency corresponding to the peak is the BF. The response phase (plotted linearly) has a monotonic course, starting at a value close to $+\pi/2$ (the sign depends on the polarity convention adopted), the phase lag is increasing with frequency – which indicates a delay. Consider next, in Figure 5.2B, the response for a *fixed frequency* plotted as a function of cochlear location *x*, that is the distance to the stapes measured along the length of the BM. We will call this a 'cochlear pattern', although some authors prefer the more illustrative term 'panoramic view'. Compare Figure 5.2B with one of the curves in Figure 5.1B. The abscissa scale (location) is linear rather than logarithmic. In this case the phase curve directly indicates a wave that is travelling to the right (towards the helicotrema). It is clear that the two representations resemble one another very much. When we move the observation location to the left, the BF is higher, and the frequency response as shown by Figure 5.2A moves to the right. Correspondingly, when we increase the frequency, the pattern of Figure 5.2B will shift to the left. Note that the two curves shift in opposite directions – it is good to be aware of this possible source of confusion. We emphasize once more that the cochlea not only transforms frequency into place, it also provides, at each location, a band-pass filter. This entails that at every location not a single frequency component but a certain band of frequencies acts as the stimulus signal. The term 'tuning of the cochlea' thus has a broader meaning. What has been said in Section 5.1 about signal analysis in the cochlea has to be interpreted in this sense.

5.3 **Modern mechanical data – frequency selectivity and non-linearity**

The study of cochlear mechanics is now nearly 75 years old but the era of greatest increase in knowledge started in the early 1970s. With the use of the Mössbauer technique to measure BM velocity, William S Rhode (1971, 1978) succeeded in demonstrating:

- high frequency *selectivity* of the cochlea for weak acoustical stimuli
- intrinsic *non-linearity* of cochlear responses for stronger stimuli.

Let us first concentrate on the former property, and use an illustration from a different labora-tory. To set the picture, in those days cochlear frequency selectivity was generally measured from responses of auditory nerve fibres. It was customary to determine at each frequency the *threshold* of response, that is to vary the tone intensity to the point where the fibre under study showed a discernible increase in average firing rate. Plotting the so-determined neural threshold as a func-tion of frequency resulted in what was called the 'frequency threshold curve' (FTC). In the case of mechanical responses of the BM, a threshold does not exist, and instead, the sound level required for *constant BM velocity* or *constant BM amplitude* was used as the criterion.

Figure 5.3, taken from Sellick *et al.* (1982), shows a characteristic picture for the basal turn of the guinea pig. In the amplitude versus frequency diagram the curves connect the points that obey the assumed condition. The figure shows as solid lines two mechanical responses, one the sound level required for constant BM velocity (0.04 mm/s) and the other one the level required for con-stant BM amplitude (3.5 Å). Both curves show a pronounced minimum around 18 kHz. This frequency is, apparently, the BF for the location at which the measurement was done. For com-parison the FTC is shown of an auditory nerve fibre that happens to have its BF (note: for audi-tory nerve fibres the term 'characteristic frequency', CF, is usually used) in the same range, and is

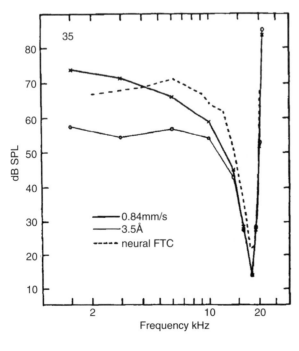

Fig. 5.3 Mechanical and neural equi-response curves. Solid curves: lines of constant velocity (thick line), and constant amplitude (thin line). Dashed line: neural frequency threshold curve (FTC). Reprinted with permission from Figure 10 of Sellick *et al.* (1982), © 1982, Acoustical Society of America.

presumably innervating the same region of the cochlea. It is evident that, as far as frequency selectivity in the region of maximal sensitivity is concerned, the neural and the mechanical responses show approximately the same bandwidth. Outside that region the neural curve is steeper (as found in later studies). Still further from the frequency region of maximal sensitivity, the neural equi-response curve (the FTC) differs markedly from either the constant-velocity or the constant-amplitude curve for the BM. The finding of comparable narrow band selectivities of nerve fibres and BM constituted the first major breakthrough in cochlear mechanics in those years. In one step it made obsolete various theories of 'sharpening' in the cochlea (reviewed by Evans, 1975).

The second basic finding involved non-linearity. To illustrate this aspect we return to the pioneering work of Rhode. Figure 5.4 has been borrowed from Rhode (1978), four sets of data are shown, taken in four chinchillas. In this animal, the BF of the region in which measurements were done is around 9.5 kHz, against 18 kHz for the guinea pig. The measured BM velocity is plotted against frequency for several levels of stimulation. Actually, each response is normalized, that is divided by the velocity of the malleus ossicle at the corresponding level. If the cochlea were linear, the response curves at different levels would coincide. Figure 5.4 shows that this is not so: the cochlea is fundamentally non-linear, particularly in the region of the peak. Weaker stimuli give rise to steeper curves; due to problems with data acquisition the curves at the lowest stimulation levels are not all complete. One very fundamental thing is clear: frequency selectivity is greatest for the weakest stimuli. When the stimulus level increases, the (relative) level of the maximum response as well as the frequency selectivity decreases.

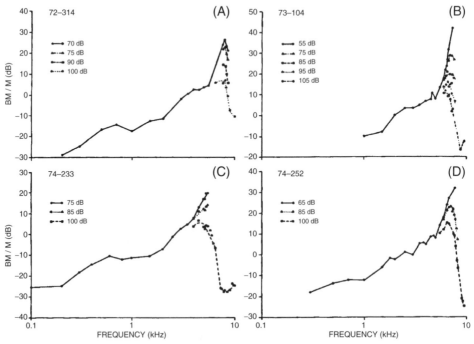

Fig. 5.4 Frequency responses measured in four chinchillas. The curves have been measured with different intensities of the stimulus tones (see the labels). The amplitudes are normalized with respect to the signal at the malleus. The data show that the cochlea is mechanically non-linear. Reprinted with permission from Figure 9 of Rhode (1978), © 1978, Acoustical Society of America.

The three data sets we have described (compiled by Rhode, 1971, 1978 and Sellick *et al.*, 1982) were seminal in setting up the theory of cochlear mechanics in the 1980s as we shall see in the next two sections. There is one aspect we must emphasize: vulnerability. The sharply peaked responses at low levels illustrated by Figures 5.3 and 5.4 can only be attained in a preparation that is in excellent physiological condition. The slightest damage to the cochlea causes a sensitivity loss that makes it impossible to measure reliable responses to low-level sounds. Accordingly, achieving minimal damage to the cochlea has been a major concern of experimentalists who have been performing these experiments, up to this very day.

The next acceleration of knowledge about cochlear mechanics research involved measurements with laser interferometers. Rhode's findings were confirmed and extended. In particular, Mario Ruggero and co-workers have gathered extensive data on mechanical responses from chinchillas, at first for pure tones only (Robles *et al.*, 1986) but later for other stimuli, for instance, clicks (Recio *et al.*, 1998). They also studied DPs (see Section 5.1) (Robles *et al.*, 1990, 1991, 1997), and two-tone suppression – one of the manifestations of non-linearity as described in Section 5.1 (Ruggero *et al.*, 1992). All of this work has been reviewed in Robles and Ruggero (2001). Quite recently Rhode (2007a) extended his work with the use of a displacement-sensitive interferometer and also investigated another form of cochlear non-linearity, mutual suppression (Rhode, 2007b). In a different study attention was given to peculiar oscillations in the response that occur in the frequency range above the BF (Rhode & Recio, 2000). A definite explanation of this puzzling effect has not yet been given. It also remains a mystery why these oscillations do not show up in the high-frequency branch of neural FTCs.

From Figure 5.4 we infer that strong sounds give rise to non-linear effects inside the cochlea. According to the duality shown by Figure 5.2 the degree of non-linearity will not be the same everywhere along the BM. Would it be possible to avoid this condition? With this question in mind, a different route to measure cochlear frequency selectivity and non-linearity was taken by de Boer and Nuttall (starting in 1997). The physiological technique was conventional (see Section 5.2), and a laser velocimeter was used to measure BM and stapes velocity, and the location studied was the basal turn of the guinea pig cochlea. Stimulation occurred not with sinusoidal signals but with *wide bands of noise*. Such a signal contains a multitude of closely spaced frequency components covering a large frequency range (ideally from 50 Hz to 50 kHz). The amplitudes of those components are equal, we express this by saying that the spectrum is flat. The phases of the components are random. The analytical background for this method was published by de Boer in 1997. Assume for a moment that the cochlea is linear. A noise stimulus with a flat spectrum will result in a noise signal with a peaked spectrum on the BM. This is because frequency components near the BF will be enhanced in amplitude. There exist various techniques to extract details of the frequency selectivity from the two signals, the stimulus noise signal and the recorded BM signal, as obtained with the cross-correlation function (Lee, 1969). That method is focused on the *similarity* in waveform of two signals and can be applied to signals of arbitrary bandwidth and waveform. Application of this method in a linear system is straightforward. In the aforementioned publication, de Boer (1997) showed in which way to interpret the findings in the presence of (weak and distributed) non-linearity as it exists in the cochlea.

Figure 5.5 shows representative results of this type of work, in the form of frequency responses for a number of stimulus levels. The functions are shown on a logarithmic frequency scale. All responses are normalized by the stimulus signal at the stapes. Figure 5.5A shows the amplitude. For the lowest levels the response curves almost coincide, and we can conclude that the BM response rises (nearly) linearly with the stimulus level and that there is little or no non-linearity. In that case, all components are processed independently (see Section 5.1), and each curve can be considered as the response to a sinusoidal signal presented at the stapes. Non-linearity is only

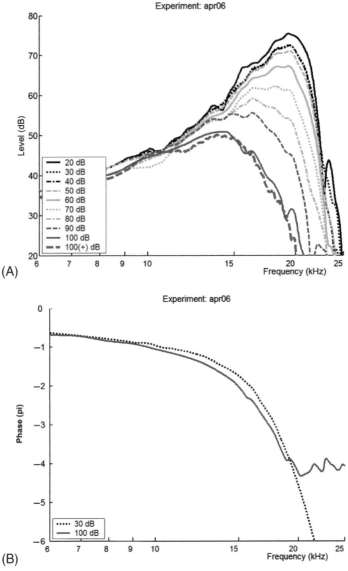

Fig. 5.5 (A) Response functions – amplitudes – derived from measurements performed in the basal turn of the guinea pig cochlea with wide-band noise signals as stimuli (unpublished data). The stimulus levels actually indicate the sound pressure level per octave of bandwidth. The measurement and analysis techniques have been published by de Boer and Nuttall (1997) and are summarized in the text. As in Figure 5.4, the curves measured at lower levels are sharper. Conversely, frequency selectivity decreases with increasing stimulus level. (B) Phase values corresponding to two of the curves of Figure 5.5A. See text for description.

involved at levels of 30 dB and above. In this case, each response should be considered as being obtained in the presence of other components that together produce approximately the same degree of non-linearity on all points of the BM. This results from the fact that the actual stimulus was a wide band of noise.

The response peak is highest and sharpest for the weakest stimuli, and is smaller for stronger stimuli (*cf.* Fig. 5.4 from Rhode). To the amplitude plot a fat red curve marked by a coarse dashed line has been added, labelled 100(+) dB, this is the response measured postmortem. It is curious that the 100– dB amplitude curve for the live animal is so close to the postmortem curve: apparently the mechanism that is responsible for the pronounced peak at low levels almost ceases to work at levels around 100 dB. When we remember the extreme vulnerability of the cochlea we can well understand why continuous sounds as loud as 100 dB can be damaging to the ear. In our present society damage to the ear due to loud sounds is a serious problem.

Figure 5.5B shows the associated phase. Because the phase does not vary much with level only two curves are shown, for a low (30 dB) and for a high level (100 dB). Two properties catch the eye. In the region where the amplitude rises towards the peak the phase curve is somewhat shallower for the lower level than for the higher level. Since the slope of the phase curve indicates group delay (see Section 5.1) this means that below the BF the group delay is smaller at low than at high levels. In the region around and above the BF this is inverted, at low levels the phase of the low-level phase curve is definitely steeper, and the group delay is larger at low than at high levels.

An important property that Figures 5.4 and 5.5A demonstrate is *compression* of strong stimuli. It is this property that partly solves the paradox that was mentioned in Section 5.2. In Figure 5.5A the ratio of the strongest to the weakest response is not 80 dB (i.e. the range in stimulus levels) but considerably smaller, of the order of 55 dB. Hence, von Békésy's high-level data cannot simply be extended downwards to a ridiculously low threshold level, we can guess that we would arrive at threshold values about 100 times larger than what has been stated above, that is, around 1 nm. This holds true for low frequencies. Still, the data in Figure 5.3, when extrapolated down to 0 dB yield a threshold value of 0.35 Å, that is 0.035 nm, a truly subatomic value. We should keep in mind the enormous difference in frequency, though.

The property of compression can be expressed in two ways: weak signals are enhanced; and strong signals are attenuated. Both interpretations are true as it has turned out. The former property has made it possible for us to hear extremely weak sounds. It is evident why such a property would be advantageous in evolution. The latter property is useful to adapt the large range of sound levels in nature to the limited range of signals that can be handled by neural circuits. There is an additional aspect of compression that merits discussion, and we might call it 'survival of filtering'. Recall what has been said in Section 5.1 about the way the cochlear wave, while propagating along the BM, gradually 'loses' signal components, starting with the highest frequencies. Figure 5.5 shows that at low to moderate levels the cochlea displays, despite its non-linearity, all the characteristics of filtering, and it acts as a band-pass filter. At the location of measurement, the BF is near 17 kHz, and signal components with frequencies in the 17 kHz range are amplified. If we now mentally apply the transformation of 'frequency response' into the 'cochlear pattern' illustrated in Figure 5.2, we can well imagine (observing the rapid cut-off towards the right in Fig. 5.2B) that these components will be absorbed as the cochlear wave moves further on. As it has been phrased in the introduction: first the high-frequency components are 'deposited' at the corresponding location, next the middle frequencies, and lastly the low frequencies. What is essential here is that our data in Figure 5.5 have been obtained with a wide-band stimulus, a stimulus signal that contains a multitude of frequency components, from very low to very high. The filtering action of the cochlea is manifest despite the intrinsic non-linearity of the cochlea, and this is true for any kind of sound stimulus and for weak to medium-loud sounds. It should be clear that this fundamental property can only be demonstrated via the use of a wide-band stimulus signal.

In comparison to the basal turn of the cochlea, the region of low frequencies and the apex of the cochlea have been studied only rarely, at least *in vivo*. A major reason is the inaccessibility of the apex – actually, it has been the 'upper' side of the organ, the tectorial membrane (TM), the reticular lamina (RL), or the Hensen cells from which measurements were performed rather than the BM (see various chapters in Ulfendahl *et al.*, 1989). Cooper and Rhode (1995, 1996) and Rhode and Cooper (1996) found moderate degrees of compressive non-linearity in the apical turns. In one case an expansive non-linearity was reported (Zinn *et al.*, 2000). In addition, there is uncertainty about the extent and significance of DC shifts in the apex (Rhode & Cooper, 1996).

5.4 **Basic modelling of the cochlea**

Several types of waves can exist in fluid. When we swim under water and hear a sound, that sound is carried to us by a 'compression' wave. A compression wave in water is like a sound wave in air; the medium is locally compressed and this disturbance propagates. Because fluid is 'stiff' and 'dense' compared with air, the speed of wave propagation is large (1500 m/s) in water, against 340 m/s in air. On the surface of the fluid there are 'surface waves', like the waves on a lake seemingly moved on by the wind. When the surface elevates, it exerts a force (pressure) on the underlying layers – the force of gravity. That force wants to lower the elevated fluid and to move adjacent fluid 'out of the way'. Because of the inevitable sluggishness caused by the fluid's mass any equilibration takes time and therefore a wave starts to propagate along the surface. This surface wave is considerably slower than the compression wave. In principle, surface waves on a lake can propagate in all directions. The waves in the cochlea are in many respects like surface waves but generally run in one direction, from the stapes towards the helicotrema – do not worry, we will encounter exceptions later. The BM, a rather stiff membrane, combined with the cells of the organ of Corti, acts more or less like the surface of a fluid. When you bend the BM, it exerts a force – just like the gravity force mentioned above. The fluid inside the cochlea acts like the mass, tending to slow down movements and thereby creating a wave. Hence, a wave will propagate along the length of the BM. Note that, just like the surface waves on the lake, the excursions of the cochlear wave are perpendicular to the surface of the BM. These cochlear waves are therefore known as 'transversal' waves. It goes without saying that these perpendicular movements are not limited to the BM, they will be present throughout the entire fluid – note that longitudinal fluid movements will also be involved. It is not only the mass of the fluid that plays a role in wave formation, the mass of the BM and the cells of the entire organ of Corti is also involved but to a smaller degree (Steele & Taber, 1979, 1981; de La Rochefoucauld & Olson, 2007).

The mechanical and dynamical behaviours of the fluid constitute the subject called 'hydrodynamics'. In mathematical physics we want to simplify all processes to their absolute minimum, and in cochlear mechanics it is the same. Therefore, fluid hydrodynamics is formulated for an ideal fluid (which is homogeneous, incompressible, and has no internal friction – zero viscosity). The relation between fluid pressure and fluid velocity can be expressed in mathematical form. The boundaries of the fluid as determined by the cochlea are simplified to be those of a rectangular box with solid walls, with holes in the walls for the oval and round windows, and a connection (helicotrema) at one end between the two main compartments. See Figure 5.6 for a stylized drawing of the geometry involved. The model contains two compartments, called channels. Restrictions on fluid movements due to the boundaries of the model must be taken into account in the mathematical equations.

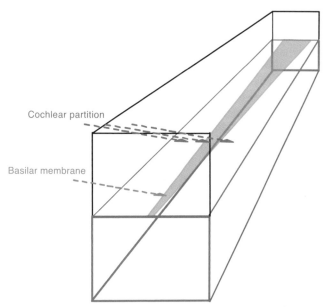

Cochlear partition

Basilar membrane

Fig. 5.6 Geometry of the *model* used to analyse the mechanics of the cochlea. The black part corresponds to the scala vestibuli, and the red part to the scala tympani. Geometrically, the model is simplified to the extreme. In the computations the model is taken as uniform in its dimensions and the taper of the BM is omitted. The cochlear windows and the helicotrema have been omitted in this drawing. The scala media and organ of Corti have been lumped into one membrane, the cochlear partition (magenta). The flexible part of the partition is the actual BM, and is shown in green. In most animals the BM is tapered as shown, but in the guinea pig its width is almost constant. The mechanics of the BM, actually those of the entire partition, are described by the BM impedance (see text).

The cochlear partition includes the BM plus the organ of Corti, and this combination will in what follows simply be called BM. To show that the movable part of the partition is narrower than the width of the channel, the BM in Figure 5.6 is narrower than the partition. Additionally, the mechanics of the BM, with all their complexity, are reduced to that of a membrane, or even simpler, to those of a set of adjacent independent springs. The dynamics of the BM are assumed to be linear and can therefore be represented by the BM impedance (see Section 5.1 for the introduction of the concept of impedance). Longitudinal coupling in the x-direction is neglected. Stiffness and mass of the BM are combined in the imaginary part of this impedance as has already been mentioned. Of course, friction has to be included; in the model the real part of the BM impedance is the only parameter that contributes damping to the mechanism of the cochlea. In the cochlea the movements of the fluid are tightly coupled with the movements of the BM and its associated structures, and this constitutes the 'coupling' between the mathematical descriptions of fluid and BM. Taking all those factors together leads to the conception of a *cochlear model*. It assumes the form of a set of equations that, in principle, can be solved (Allen, 1977; Steele & Taber, 1979, 1981; de Boer, 1981; Mammano & Nobili, 1993). A concise formulation can be found in de Boer *et al.* (2007). In this way the model yields a model response which can be compared to the actual response resulting from a physiological experiment. Waves computed from the model are inhomogeneous, near the stapes the wavelength is 'long' (that is, larger than the height or the width of the model), further on it rapidly becomes smaller. This variation of the wavelength corresponds to that found in experiments. In the interest of brevity we must omit a more detailed description of the properties of 'long' and 'short' waves generated by the model.

To achieve a realistic projection of frequency to place, the stiffness of the BM must decrease from stapes to helicotrema by a very large factor (von Békésy, 1960). In other words, it will be a strongly varying function of the longitudinal coordinate x (measured along the length of the BM). As a result of this property the BM will turn out to have its maximum vibration at a position that depends upon the frequency, just as is required by the results of experiments (Sections 5.2 and 5.3). Inversely, at every position there will be a frequency at which that location shows maximum response, the BF.

The friction (represented by the real part of the BM impedance) causes the response of this type of model to show a moderate peak, comparable with the postmortem response shown in Figure 5.5A. Assuming a smaller friction leads to a higher peak but that turns out to be far too narrow. In fact, researchers have always been relatively successful with the response of a dead cochlea (e.g. Zwislocki, 1948, 1950; Dallos, 1973). However, they consistently have encountered the obstacle that the response of a viable, alive cochlea could not be simulated by such a model. 'Something' seems to be missing in the model.

5.5 The 'active' cochlea

The experience that mathematical computations on a simple type of model of the viable cochlea never produce a realistic response has led to speculations (Kim et al., 1980), mathematical exercises (de Boer, 1983), and to more practical solutions (Zweig, 1991, for a one-dimensional model; de Boer, 1995a,b for a three-dimensional model) to resolve the dilemma. In straightforward terms, the problem posed was: when we have complete freedom to choose how the mechanical properties of the BM depend on the longitudinal coordinate x of the cochlea, how should we choose them to achieve a realistic response of the model? In mathematical terms, this is an example of an 'inverse problem': the cochlear response is given and the impedance of the BM to produce that response is to be determined. One introductory step is needed: the input (the cochlear response) must be given in the form of a cochlear pattern, that is as a function of x (the variable describing longitudinal position along the length of the BM) for a fixed frequency. Actual measurement results generally appear as functions of frequency f, for a fixed location. With the use of frequency-to-location scaling (Section 5.2) the measured response as a function of frequency f can easily be converted to a hypothetical response as a function of location x.

With modern-day computers the inverse solution is carried out readily. The inverse-solution technique is summarized in de Boer et al. (2007). The result of the inverse procedure is unexpected but conforms to de Boer's (1983) theoretical prediction. One typical result is shown in Figure 5.7 (modified from de Boer et al., 2007; data are taken from a different experiment, '20017'). In Figure 5.7A the given response (of a guinea pig ear, to a tone of 20 dB SPL) is shown, converted into a function of location x, for a frequency of 17 kHz. The curves show the response of a viable cochlea to that weak tone, the amplitude (solid curve) as well as the phase (dashed curve). A three-dimensional model is constructed along the scenario described above, and the 'inverse solution' is carried out to find the impedance of the BM. Real and imaginary parts of the BM impedance are individually shown in Figure 5.7B. In this panel the abscissa is again location x. Note that the ordinate scale is non-linear, it is linear around the centre and compressed towards both ends. Let us start with the imaginary part of the BM impedance, as said earlier, this represents the combination of (BM) stiffness and (BM) mass. The curve is shown as a dash-dot line. From $x = 0$, the location of the stapes, on it is negative, it starts at a large negative value and

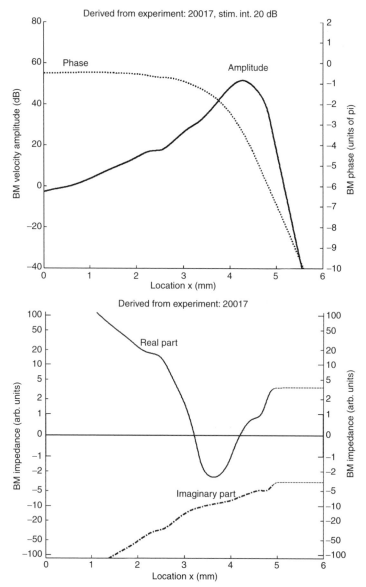

Fig. 5.7 (A) Input signal to inverse solution procedure. Result of one of our own guinea pig experiments (experiment code: '20017'; data not published). The BM response, measured as a function of frequency with a stimulus level of 20 dB, has been converted to a function of location x at 17 kHz and smoothed. Solid line: amplitude (in decibels with respect to stapes). Dotted curve: phase (in units of π radians, scale on the right side). (B) Result of the inverse procedure: real and imaginary parts of derived BM impedance. The three-dimensional model of Figure 5.6 was used. Ordinate scale is non-linear so as to show what happens around the zero point equally well as at larger distances. Around the zero point the scale is linear, at larger distances it is logarithmically compressed. Solid curve: real part, dash-dot curve: imaginary part of the BM impedance. Where the *real* part is negative, the BM–organ of Corti complex delivers acoustical power to the cochlear fluid.

decreases as a function of x. This tallies with what has been remarked before, on going along the length of the BM the stiffness should decrease rapidly.

If we had started with a post-mortem (dead) cochlea, the real part of the BM impedance should have remained positive – representing loss of power due to friction (damping). In a viable cochlea it is different: it is here where lies the surprise. In Figure 5.7B the real part of the impedance (solid curve) does not remain positive but is seen to bend down and to go through zero to become negative over some distance. Further on, it bends back and becomes positive again. A positive damping is easily understood: loss of power due to friction, and so we can understand positive resistance. But what about negative resistance? Negative resistance means that the BM is not absorbing power but is *creating* power. In more precise words, in the region of negative resistance the BM is delivering acoustical power to the fluid wave, and this is actually amplifying the wave – giving it a boost, so to speak. It is for this reason that we often speak of the *cochlear amplifier* (Davis, 1983; Neely, 1983). One reason to use this term has been that the amplification should almost certainly be effected by cellular structures in the organ of Corti. Amplification should then show all the characteristic signs of a cochlear physiological process – as will be confirmed presently. It is to be noted that the negative swing of the real part of the impedance occurs in the region before the wave reaches its peak (for $x < 4.3$ mm), this is where cochlear amplification occurs. Then the real part goes through zero at the peak of the response (at $x = 4.3$ mm). From that point on amplification is no longer needed and the response starts to decrease rapidly. It is generally agreed upon that the mechanism of the cochlear amplifier resides in the OHCs. It has proven to be very difficult to reliably measure the response properties of these cells (Dallos, 1985a,b) and we will come back to this topic later with more details.

It should come as no surprise that this peculiar behaviour of the real part is absent when the same analysis is applied to the response of a dead cochlea. It is the cochlear amplifier that forms the distinction between the 'active', viable, and living cochlea and its 'passive', dead counterpart. This cochlear amplifier, then, is characterized by a component of the BM impedance that is responsible for the amplification; we call this the 'active' impedance component, and it is completely dependent on the physiological state of the cochlea. This stands in direct relation to the extreme vulnerability that has been encountered in experimentation and the sensitivity of the cochlea to acoustical overstimulation (acoustical trauma). A physiological basis of cochlear amplification is also highly likely in view of the devastating influence of, for instance, furosemide on cochlear mechanics (Ruggero & Rich, 1991), or other chemicals. 'Activity' is not only evident in the real part of the BM impedance, there is a noticeable effect in the imaginary part, too. In a relative sense it is small; it is responsible, however, for the subtle but peculiar effects of stimulus intensity on the phase shown in Figure 5.5B.

The real and imaginary parts of the impedance shown in Figure 5.7B are derived by the 'inverse solution'. If, now, a hypothetical model is constructed on the basis of these impedance components, that model will have the response shown in Figure 5.7A. The inverse solution is, mathematically, not without pitfalls, and this reconstruction confirms the validity of the analysis. Therefore, this step is not superfluous.

In summary, with the use of a mathematical procedure, namely, the inverse solution, it has been possible to 'explain' the difference in response between the live and the dead cochlea. But what kind of explanation is this? At this stage it is not more than an abstract mathematical exercise. The impedance describes precisely the mechanical action that has to be associated with the cochlear partition (or the BM, for that matter). The impedance tells us what pressure (or force) must be developed in reaction to movements of the BM. How that pressure or force comes about is another matter, completely outside the domain of mathematics. We will come back to that topic in a later section. At this point it is appropriate to reveal that not all scientists working on the theory of cochlear mechanics agree that the cochlea should be 'locally active'. Indeed, it is correct to consider 'activity' as a hypothesis; it results from applying the inverse solution to a measured BM response function but it has proven to be extremely difficult to verify it experimentally (see Olson, 2000, 2001; Scherer & Gummer, 2004), or to falsify it. On the other hand, as has been stated above, it has proven impossible to explain the sharpness of the measured low-level BM response by way of a 'passive' model of the cochlea. In a paper by Allen and Neely (1992) the two possibilities, an extended 'passive' and an 'active' model, are set side by side. In order to achieve the same frequency selectivity at the level of the input to IHCs, both models had to include resonance of the tectorial membrane (we will come back to this subject in the concluding section of this chapter). In that way the 'passive' (Allen, 1980) and the 'active' (Neely, 1993) models are shown to be nearly equivalent. This holds, however, as far as the input to IHCs, and thus to the fibres of the auditory nerve, is concerned. With regard to the measured mechanical response of the BM (tuning as well as non-linearity) the 'active' model is definitely better (in the sense of 'more realistic').

The response and impedance functions shown in Figure 5.7 pertain to measurements of BM motion performed at a specific location along the BM in a guinea pig, approximately 4 mm from the stapes. That response location has a BF of approximately 17 kHz. It is easy to imagine that, were it possible to do similar measurements at other locations, the responses would show different BFs, and the impedance functions would appear as shifted in the x-direction.

As said earlier, it is generally assumed that the processes necessary to generate 'activity' are carried out by OHCs. The response shown and used as input in Figure 5.7 is a response measured at a very low sound level. At higher levels the measured response is, as said in Section 5.3 and demonstrated by Figures 5.4 and 5.5, compressed. A clear non-linear effect. Can we try to determine the BM impedance in the presence of this non-linearity? An orthodox theoretician would say 'stop' at this point: the concept of impedance is formally not allowed in a non-linear system. In the case of the cochlea, however, the degree of non-linearity is small and distributed over the length of the cochlea so that we can continue to use the concept of impedance. Remember that the use of a wide band of noise as stimulus causes an almost homogeneous degree of non-linearity over the entire length of the cochlea. A heuristic and a formal derivation to justify this procedure have been given by de Boer (1997). On carrying out the inverse solution on the compressed responses it was found that the negative 'swing' of the real part of the BM impedance is also compressed: it is smaller in size for louder stimuli (de Boer & Nuttall, 2000). This is a thought that harmonizes with the idea that the amplification process resides in OHCs and is of physiological origin. Any physiological mechanism is subject to overload by strong stimuli, whereby it decreases its quality of functioning. A further, logical, step is to find in the same feature the reason for other signs of cochlear non-linearity. After an excursion into the subject of compression we will return to this subject in the next section.

5.6 Non-linear effects in the basilar membrane response

We know that the cochlea is non-linear but what does this mean – apart from compression? It is good to reconsider at this point what is 'non-linearity' and what are its effects. The properties of linear systems have been defined in Section 5.1. A major property of linear systems is that they cannot create components with frequencies that do not exist in the input signal. This is different in a non-linear system. When a non-linear system is stimulated by two tones with frequencies f_1 and f_2, DPs with frequencies differing from those of the primary tones will be created. We mention DPs with frequencies $2f_1 - f_2$, $3f_1 - 2f_2$, $2f_2 - f_1$, and $3f_2 - 2f_1$ as being the most important ones for our purpose.

We now turn to another manifestation of non-linearity, distortion. Consider Figure 5.8, which shows a stylized form of the input-output characteristic (the transduction function) and typical input and output signals of an imaginary OHC. The form of the transduction function has been inspired by Hudspeth and Corey (1977). However, in our case the input is the deflection of the stereociliary bundle, and the output the local 'active' pressure that the cell produces. This figure demonstrates the linear as well as the non-linear aspects of OHC transduction. We have used an input signal that clearly illustrates the modification that the waveform undergoes; it is composed of two sinusoidal signals with closely spaced frequencies, together forming a beating signal. In Figure 5.8A the amplitude of the input signal is small, distortion is minimal and the output signal has almost the same waveform and amplitude as the input signal. In Figure 5.8B the input signal is large, and distortion is appreciable. To the picture of the heavily distorted output signal a fine green curve has been added. This curve shows the signal consisting of the main frequency components of the actual output signal. In other words, this is the signal whose waveform most closely resembles the input signal. On the transduction function in the centre of the figure a green dashed straight line is superimposed. This line depicts the average relation between the green output signal and the input signal. It clearly has a slope smaller than 1. Compare this with the similar green dashed line drawn in Figure 5.8A where it has a slope close to 1. In relating output (a pressure) and input (stereocilia deflection associated with BM velocity) of an OHC in this average way, and using the concept of impedance, we again invoke the technique of handling non-linear responses as it has been described and proven in de Boer (1997).

Two characteristics of the transduction curve in Figure 5.8 come to the fore. First, 'rectification', by this term we mean that negative excursions in this figure are handled completely differently from positive excursions. This effect tends to give rise to DPs with frequencies $f_2 - f_1$ and $f_2 + f_1$ that we mentioned in the foregoing and that we more or less dismissed as being of lesser importance to the study of the cochlea (at least if we limit ourselves to the high-frequency region of the cochlea). Second, the curve decreases in slope for large deflections of the stereociliary bundle. This effect causes large signals to be compressed in amplitude (see the green dashed line in panel B) and is also responsible for the creation of DPs with frequencies $2 f_1 - f_2$, etc. (as can be proven mathematically).

In view of the cross-correlation procedure mentioned in Section 5.3, we should compare input and output signals in terms of 'waveform similarity', and this is exactly what the green dashed lines in both parts of Figure 5.8 demonstrate. In this view, small signals will be transduced without distortion but large signals will, on the average, be transduced with a reduced amplitude. Large signals will thus give rise to less feedback. As a consequence, large signals will undergo less amplification by the mechanics of the cochlea than small signals. Here is where we find the origin of the compression that large stimuli undergo in the cochlea. In summary: large stimulus signals cause less-than-proportional output signals from OHCs, hence are amplified less. By the use of a typical non-linear transfer characteristic as the one in Figure 5.8 but brought into a stylized form it has even been possible to explain the compression of strong stimuli as measured in the cochlea in a *quantitative* way (de Boer & Nuttall, 2000). Every curve in Figure 5.5 can then be characterized by a single number that expresses the (average) factor with which OHC transduction is reduced.

The second effect of non-linearity of OHCs is that presenting tone pairs to the cochlea gives rise to the production of DPs on the BM. First, DPs are generated in the output signals of OHCs and second, these DP components generate *DP waves* along the BM having the same general properties as other waves. The DP waves on the BM can be measured in the same way as responses to tones or other signals. In Figure 5.9 we show a typical set of frequency components (amplitudes only) measured in the response of the BM to a tone pair (see the legend for details). The fat vertical lines denote the frequencies f_1 and f_2 of the two primary tones. The thinner lines show the DPs, several of these are marked with their respective frequencies. The over-all picture is that of the central set of pipes in the front of a church organ, in short, a 'church-organ front'. Distortion data of this nature have been published on the BM by, for example Robles *et al.* (1990, 1991, 1997), and on the intracochlear pressure by Dong and Olson (2005). The data shown in Figure 5.9 are from our own (unpublished) work. In this case, too, it has been possible to explain the amplitude distribution of these DPs in a quantitative way (de Boer *et al.*, 2002), starting from the same stylized rendition of the non-linear transfer characteristic of Figure 5.8 that was used to handle compression.

In order to present a coherent picture we have described the creation and solution of a cochlear model from a fairly narrow viewpoint, mainly because we wanted to justify the inverse solution. Other authors and groups have had entirely different aims. We will mention a few. General models with specific mechanisms for frequency-dependent 'activity' were published by, among others, Zweig (1991), Neely and Kim (1986), and Geisler (1993). Scientists including Shera, Talmadge, and Tubis have developed linear and non-linear cochlear models in great detail, and derived specific properties of them by ingenious means (Talmadge *et al.*, 1998a,b; Tubis *et al.*, 2000a,b; Shera, 2003; Shera *et al.*, 2005, 2007). Several of these models were specifically directed at otoacoustic emissions. More complicated models and more advanced computational techniques were used by

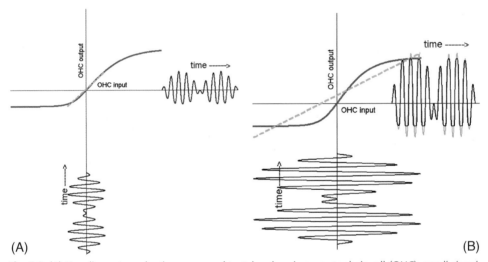

(A)   (B)

Fig. 5.8 (A) Non-linear transduction, assumed to take place in an outer hair cell (OHC), *small-signal case*. The input signal contains two frequency components, together forming a 'beating' signal. The OHC transduction function (blue) is curved, and on the left side it shows a more abrupt compression than on the right side. The input signal – plotted on a vertical time scale – is weak in this case, as a result the output signal – plotted on a horizontal time scale – has almost the same waveform; it is only slightly compressed. The green dashed line overlaying the transduction function shows the average relation between input and output waveforms. The slope of this line is very close to 1.0, actually equal to 0.90, denoting a small degree of compression. (B) Non-linear transduction, assumed to take place in an OHC, *large-signal case*. Layout as in Figure 5.8A. The input signal is four times larger than in Figure 5.8A. The output signal (black) is severely distorted in this case. The thin green waveform is the signal that has the closest resemblance to the input signal in the spectral sense. The green dashed line overlaying the transduction function shows the average relation between input and output waveforms (in the segment of the largest excursions). The slope of this line defines the average degree of compression and its value is 0.52, signifying a good deal of compression.

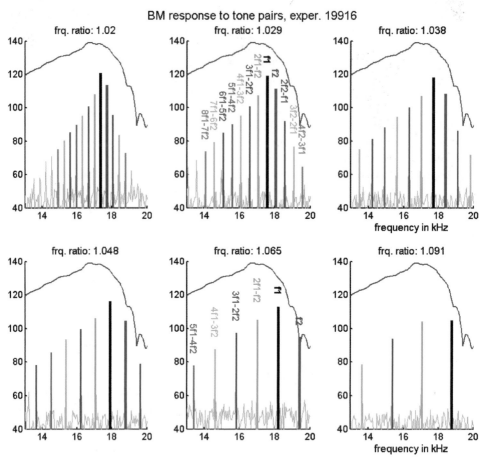

Fig. 5.9 Frequency spectrum of the response of the BM to a two-tone stimulus (the 'church-organ front' – look at the upper left panel). (Unpublished guinea pig data, experiment '19916'.) The two tones were presented at 70 dB SPL. The frequencies had the indicated ratio but the frequency $2f_1 - f_2$ of the principal DP always was equal to 17 kHz, approximately the BF of the location at which measurements were done. The blue curve illustrates the frequency response at that location, for the level of 70 dB, normalized to have its maximum at 140 dB. The primary tones (black and red) as well as a number of DPs are shown as vertical coloured bars, against an arbitrary but fixed reference. In two of the six panels the constituent frequencies, $2f_1 - f_2$, $3f_1 - 2f_2$, etc., are indicated. In each panel the thin green curve is the actual spectrum of the response.

Kolston and Ashmore (1996), Parthasarathi *et al.* (2000), and Ramamoorthy *et al.* (2007). Hubbard (1993), Chadwick *et al.* (1996), and Chadwick (1998) developed alternative multicompartment models (i.e. models with more than two channels) allowing for cochlear amplification, and Dimitriades and Chadwick (1999) published the inverse-solution method for the latter model. Models with 'feed-forward' will be introduced in the next section.

For the sake of completeness it should be revealed that in recent times an alternative theory of cochlear 'activity' and the genesis of cochlear oscillations has been put forward. It is based on the properties of a 'van der Pol oscillator', and the more extended concept is that all signal transformations and transitions in the cochlea can be described by what is known as a 'Hopf bifurcation' which is characteristic of such an oscillator. This theory is meant to unify the description of coch-lear processes and to derive *generic*, universal, properties that do not depend on a particular set of assumptions or parameters. A few seminal publications are by Camalet *et al.* (2000), Eguíluz *et al.* (2000), Jülicher *et al.* (2003), and Martin *et al.* (2000). This theory has deepened our insight into the fundamental boundaries between non-linearity, stability, and oscillation. In its most general form this theory is, however, at variance with the theory of non-linear cochlear mechanics as it has been unfolded in the foregoing (Zweig, 2006). The difference lies mainly in the transient and asymptotic behaviour of a van der Pol oscillator versus that of the frequency-selective, active and non-linear elements in a wave-supporting three-dimensional model of the cochlea.

5.7 Organ of Corti micromechanics and the excitation of hair cells

The operation of the organ of Corti is often described in terms of BM motion and micromechan-ics. Let us try to follow a logical chain of events but let us first have a short look at the end point. The end result of all micromechanical motion is stimulation of hair cells by the mechanical deflection of stereocilia, in particular, deflection of the stereocilia of IHCs, which results in excita-tion of afferent neurones via the release of neurotransmitter (see Chapter 9). The vibration of the BM couples to OHC stereocilia via a mechanical linkage that includes the TM. Figure 5.10 shows the classical idea that the different centres of rotation of the BM and the TM form a lever system that produces shear force between the motion of the TM and that of the reticular lamina (RL). The rigid triangle formed by the inner and outer pillar cells constitutes an essential link (in the figure extended to include the entire organ of Corti). This idea was published as early as 1900 (!) by ter Kuile (1900), and it is still adhered to. In the way depicted, stereocilia of OHCs are stimu-lated. The process that produces motion of the IHC stereocilia is more complex and still contro-versial. This is so because the IHC stereocilia are not connected to the TM but instead stand in the subtectorial space, that is, the narrow fluid-filled space between the RL and the bottom surface of the TM. Because of this lack of firm coupling to the TM, the IHC stereocilia are thought to feel a viscous force which is proportional to the local radial velocity of the fluid. Studies of hair cell receptor potentials confirmed that at least at low frequencies, IHCs are velocity coupled to BM motion (Sellick & Russell, 1980; Nuttall *et al.*, 1981; Russell & Sellick, 1983), whereas OHCs are displacement coupled (Dallos, 1986). At frequencies higher than a few hundred hertz the IHC stereocilia are thought to become displacement coupled by the thin fluid layer sandwiched between the RL and the TM (Ruggero & Rich 1987; Ruggero *et al.*, 2000).

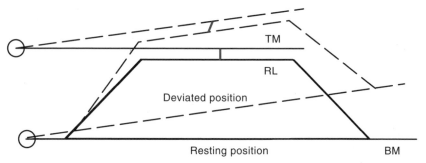

Fig. 5.10 Diagram of the transformation of transversal BM movements to radial displacements of stereocilia (red), according to ter Kuile (1900). The bending of the stereocilia (drawn red) is due to the differing rotation points of BM and TM (see text). Deviations from equilibrium positions are exaggerated in this figure.

As it has become clear in the foregoing, the cochlea harbours an amplification mechanism. In more precise terms: whenever the BM moves, the array of OHCs is excited, and these cells produce a pressure (actually, a pressure difference across the BM) which serves to amplify the wave on the BM. How OHCs can be excited by movements of the BM is illustrated by Figure 5.10. But what happens next? A highly remarkable property of OHCs has been discovered, called 'motility' or 'somatic motility' (Brownell *et al.*, 1985). Initially it was demonstrated on isolated OHCs, and later also in conglomerations of cells. Briefly, when an OHC is excited, it can change its length. Additionally, it can produce force (Hallworth, 1995). The force and length changes are correlated with a change of stiffness (He *et al.*, 2003). Either the length change or the force or the stiffness change could be the agent behind the 'active' mechanism as it has been described in Section 5.5. Let us assume this is true for the length change. Excised OHCs when stimulated by changing the electric potential difference across the cell membrane have length variations that can follow the electrical signal up to tens of kHz (Gale & Ashmore, 1997; Frank *et al.*, 1999). If we consider this type of transducer as involved in 'activity', that is, as the motor that powers the cochlear amplifier, we immediately hit upon a barrier. The internal voltage of a hair cell can only be varied by ionic current through the stereocilia. The resistance of the stereocilia and the capacitance of the cell membrane then form a low-pass filter (the resistance of the membrane should be thought of as in parallel with the resistance of the stereocilia). The cut-off frequency of that filter has been estimated to be of the order of 1 kHz (Santos-Sacchi, 1992). In this view OHC motility would not be able to function as required by the 'active' model at high frequencies. Various ideas have been proposed to counteract this effect of the membrane capacitance; one of these postulates a global influence on local potentials from OHCs further away (Dallos & Evans, 1995a,b). Recently, Fridberger *et al.* (2004a) have confirmed that this is a feasible idea. In point of fact, the protein that is responsible for OHC motility has been identified. It is called prestin (Zheng *et al.*, 2000) and resides in abundance in the lateral plasma membrane of OHCs (and not in IHCs). Since this discovery many publications have appeared on the distribution and properties of prestin; we mention Liberman *et al.* (2002) who proved that it is essential in the living and sensitive cochlea.

The force needed to counteract viscous energy loss need not come (only) from OHC somatic motility. There is considerable evidence that the stereocilia bundle can produce net energy from the binding of calcium (see Chan & Hudspeth, 2005, and LeMasurier & Gillespie, 2005, for reviews of this topic). This concept, stereocilia acting both as receivers of mechanical stimulation and sources of mechanical activity (reciprocal actions), forms an alternative hypothesis to implement 'activity'. Formally, a locally active model – as described in the two preceding sections – can operate with either OHC somatic motility or with stereociliary forces. The forces only have to have the correct amplitudes and phases and frequency dependence (as dictated by the 'active' component of the BM impedance). It should be added at this point that active movement of stereocilia is often detected in the presence of somatic motility, and cannot easily be separated from it (Jia & He, 2005; LeMasurier & Gillespie, 2005). Perhaps the two processes operate together.

From the work of Ricci *et al.* (2006) and Fettiplace (2006) it is clear that the OHC stereocilia of the rat show a calcium-dependent *adaptation* in the behaviour of the force-generation mechanism. Adaptation in mammalian OHCs is observed to have a submillisecond time constant, and is graded in a tonotopic fashion. At this time it is not at all clear in which way adaptation and force from stereociliary bundles will or can cooperate with somatic electromotility, but that these effects would work together is becoming an accepted idea (see the review by LeMasurier & Gillespie, 2005).

The property of somatic motility (as well as reciprocal excitability of stereocilia) makes it possible to stimulate the organ of Corti electrically and to expect mechanical effects specifically due to actions of OHCs that are measurable. In fact, several preparations of the cochlea have been developed whereby stimulation can be applied acoustically as well as electrically. These preparations were either *in vivo* or *in vitro*, and various optical methods were developed to measure the resulting motions in detail. It should be clear that the field of micromechanical studies has become very wide and multidimensional, and that we will only be able to describe a small subset of it. There is a fundamental difference between acoustical and electrical stimulation. With acoustical stimulation the entire organ of Corti is stimulated, or at less a large portion of the organ. In contrast, electrical stimulation produces forces (mainly) due to somatic motility inside the organ of Corti, in fact, two forces originating from apex and base of each OHC. In that case electrical stimulation produces a *deformation* of the organ of Corti.

The OHCs are not perpendicular to the BM, they are placed at an angle. Therefore, reactions to electrical stimulation have transversal as well as radial components of movement. In the base of the cochlea, Nilsen and Russell (1999, 2000) measured transversal movements of the BM due to acoustical stimuli at different radial positions without reflective objects. In the live animal they found characteristic differences in amplitude and phase over the width of the BM; in postmortem conditions most of these patterns had disappeared. The authors explain their finding as reflecting somatic motility. The phase pattern observed by Nilsen and Russell could not, however, be confirmed in other experiments also executed with acoustical stimulation and without reflective objects (Ren & Nuttall, 2001; Cooper, 2000). In contrast, a two- or multiple-mode vibration can definitely be seen when the organ is electrically stimulated (Nuttall *et al.*, 1999; Karavitaki & Mountain, 2007b). The explanation would be simple: this type of vibration could be due to the OHCs working against the arch formed by the inner and outer pillar cells. In later studies directed at details of radial movements, Fridberger *et al.* (2002, 2004b) also found lateral motions and expansions in the internal structure of the organ of Corti. In particular, individual OHCs in apical turns could be seen to bend during their motion. This (*in vitro*) work was accomplished using confocal microscopy and optical flow image analysis. It should be clear that simple models of OHC stimulation as shown in our Figure 5.10 and simple conceptions of the motions of OHCs have to be extended. The 'true' micromechanics of the organ of Corti is two-, perhaps three-dimensional, particularly in the upper turns.

The study of the organ of Corti has moved from the BM to the upper surface of the organ starting with the *in situ* and *in vivo* work of Khanna's laboratory (e.g. Ulfendahl *et al.*, 1989; Khanna & Hao, 1999). In other experiments the organ of Corti has completely been removed from the cochlea and electrically stimulated to evoke OHC motion. In this way Mammano and Ashmore (1993) found that the RL moves about 15 times more than the BM, an indication of the smaller stiffness of the RL. With the *in vitro* method and advanced optical techniques more complex modes of operation can be observed; the most recent work by Fridberger *et al.* (2004b) has just been mentioned. Chan and Hudspeth (2005) created a special multi-chamber preparation that allowed such measurements and also permitted the application of different ionic solutions to the upper and lower surfaces of the organ of Corti. They found that participation of stereocilia forces in micromechanics is different for acoustical and electrical stimulation. In the latter case there is clear evidence of hair-bundle and soma-based transduction. Nowotny and Gummer (2006) fastened isolated turns of the guinea-pig cochlea to a support in order to observe differential transverse movements of the RL and the TM. In the basal turn these structures were found to move in the same direction but in the second and third turns the movements were in counter-phase, this is valid near the corresponding BFs. The authors demonstrate by a physical-mathematical derivation that the counter-phase transverse movement would be capable of enhancing radial fluid movement. Of additional interest is that longitudinal fluid flow has been observed in the tunnel of Corti (Karavitaki & Mountain, 2007a).

As valuable as the *in vitro* preparation is, there is a critical need to obtain micromechanical vibration data from the intact *in vivo* organ of Corti. It appears now possible to move beyond the *in vitro* measurements by using novel imaging and interferometric methods. The low-coherence interferometry method mentioned in Section 5.2 is very promising in this respect. Furthermore, one must bear in mind that the organ of Corti is not only a mechanical but an *electro*-mechanical device. Various electrical and electro-mechanical cellular interactions can be distinguished. One component of a transmembrane voltage drive to OHCs can come from the cochlear microphonics generated by these cells farther away (Dallos & Evans, 1995a,b). This concept may be involved in the solution of the OHC membrane filter problem (see above). Intercellular coupling may modify passive mechanical properties of cells perhaps in the manner suggested by Zao and Santos-Sacchi (1999). Therefore, the effective stimulation of OHCs is possibly the sum of many different motions. This is even more true in the apical region of the cochlea, because the different structures have more empty fluid space between them and can move more freely.

Let us now consider the TM and its possible influence on cochlear tuning. Recent studies using targeted mutation of tectorin genes show that it is possible to modify the mechanical properties of the TM by molecular means. The mouse mutant with deletion of the alpha tectorin gene has a completely missing TM and a large (35 dB) loss of sensitivity, but it retains some mechanical tuning (Legan *et al.*, 2000, 2005). Russell *et al.* (2007) further found that the mutant which fails to produce the beta tectorin protein has an altered TM morphology and shows an unusual increase in sharpness of frequency tuning. Sensitivity is little changed but the altered nature of tuning suggests an influence on tuning from a possible resonance of the TM.

Each component of the organ of Corti has mechanical properties like stiffness and mass and may form a resonance at some frequency. The TM is particularly interesting from the resonance point of view because a TM resonance would greatly influence the stimulation of hair cell stereociliary bundles (for outer as well as IHCs). In a simple model the TM is a structure elastically hinged at one end and free at the other end. It has mass and stiffness (e.g. Masaki *et al.*, 2006) and these vary, as do its dimensions, along the longitudinal length of the cochlear partition (Richter *et al.*, 2007). The primary resonance of the TM would be in the *radial* direction (across the width of the organ). The radial type of TM resonance was proposed initially by Allen (1980) and Zwislocki and Kletsky (1979) to play a part in cochlear micromechanics. The same concept was used later to explain the 'tuning' of the cochlear amplification mechanism (Neely & Kim, 1986; Fukazawa, 1997; Fukazawa *et al.*, 1999). Indeed, resonance of the TM can serve a very important function in shifting the phase of stereocilia motion with respect to the phase of the BM motion. Such a phase shift is needed because in a simple system like that of Figure 5.10, bending of the stereocilia of OHCs is proportional to displacement of the BM. Thus maximum OHC force would occur when the stereocilia are maximally displaced, and this would coincide with minimum BM velocity. However, viscous drag is always in phase with velocity, and the maximum 'active' force (see Section 5.5) should be in opposite phase to viscous drag. A 90° phase shift is required to correct this problem and that can, in principle, be provided by TM resonance. TM resonance was confirmed experimentally by Gummer *et al.* (1996). Additional experimental evidence on possible involvement of TM resonance has recently been contributed by Lukashkin *et al.* (2007). A specific signal-analytical problem related to TM resonance will be discussed in the concluding section of this chapter.

Resonance in a structure depends on mass and stiffness, and its effect on other structures depends on relations to parameters of those other structures. The stiffness of the BM has been investigated since the time of von Békésy (1960). The stiffness of OHC stereocilia varies along the length of the organ (Billone & Raynor, 1973). The lateral and transverse stiffnesses of the TM have been determined *in vitro* and *in vivo* (Zwislocki & Cefaratti, 1989; Dallos, 2003; Freeman *et al.*,

2003a,b; Shoelson *et al.*, 2004; Richter *et al.*, 2007). All data indicate that it is reasonable to assume that the TM can influence deflection of OHC stereocilia, and that it may participate in resonance.

Evidence on multiple modes of vibration of the organ of Corti has been presented above. This subject has more aspects. As mentioned above, Karavitaki and Mountain (2007a) observed oscillatory fluid flow inside the tunnel of Corti, once more underlining the necessity to account for more complex vibrations in the organ of Corti. The first modelling steps to include fluid motion in the tunnel of Corti have been taken as early as 1993 by Hubbard (1993). A feature that has conspicuously been neglected in models of the organ of Corti is longitudinal stiffness of the tunnel of Corti. The tube-like form of it suggests some degree of torsional stiffness, yet it has not been fully taken into account. Experimental (Naidu & Mountain, 2000) and theoretical (Wickesberg & Geisler, 1986) approaches yielded the result that incorporation of longitudinal stiffness invariably broadens the response peak. Dimitriades and Chadwick (1999) express the need for including cell-to-cell interaction in modelling the organ of Corti. In the domain of fluid movements, the rocking action of the tunnel of Corti about its inner anchoring point might well provoke appreciable fluid flow in the inner spiral sulcus (ISS). Therefore, it might be necessary to take the mechanical action of that fluid into account (de Boer, 1993; Steele & Lim, 1999).

The unique morphology of the cochlea and the organ of Corti suggests further analysis of mechanical functions and interactions. For example, the curved shape of the cochlear duct in the apical turn has been modelled to show that centripetal force effects may enhance low-frequency signals by as much as 10 dB (Cai *et al.*, 2005). The 'V' or 'W' patterns and alignments of OHC stereocilia have intrigued auditory scientists but still remain somewhat a mystery. A basic thought is that they simply serve to increase stereociliary stiffness with respect to radial motion. Bell and Fletcher (2004) have suggested by model analysis that these arrangements could lead to local standing waves in the subtectorial fluid space.

Deiters' cells also are possible key structures in the mechanics of the organ. They not only connect the OHCs to the BM but each Deiters' cell sends a fine process (phalanx) from its body towards two or three OHCs located more apically. These phalangeal processes connect into the RL. Movements of OHCs at one location would be able to induce movements at more apical locations – a mechanism called *feed-forward*. The Deiters' cell–OHC phalanxes could be the cellular basis of such mechanical feed-forward. Steele *et al.* (1993), Geisler and Sang (1995), Lim and Steele (2003), and Wen and Boahen (2003) have modelled the organ of Corti to have feed-forward as a further refinement of locally active models. A combination of feed-forward and feed-backward (this is a mechanical coupling in the basal direction) was shown to have promising properties (de Boer & Nuttall, 2003). de Boer (2007, see also Section 5.9) has demonstrated that such 'non-classical' models have a special property, namely, asymmetrical amplification of cochlear waves. All these effects and problems have been studied more or less in isolation, and there is a need for more complex models of cochlear mechanics in the future.

5.8 Internal reflections and otoacoustic emissions

We continue with some general aspects of otoacoustic emissions (defined in Section 5.2). A stimulus is given and the sound pressure in the outer ear canal is measured (as a waveform, a function of time). One component of that sound pressure is the emission, it is generally much smaller than the primary sound pressure. There are many varieties of emissions and almost all of them are non-linear. Click evoked emissions (CEOAEs) were the first to be detected and analysed (Kemp, 1978). As the name implies, they are evoked by presenting a click-like sound to the cochlea and measuring the sound pressure in the external ear canal. The sound in the cochlea takes some time to travel (back and forth) so that detection of this type of emission is pretty straightforward: the emission signal is simply displaced in time (see e.g. Kalluri & Shera, 2007). Other types of OAEs are more difficult to detect. Stimulus frequency otoacoustic emissions (SFOAEs) arise with stimulation by a tone, are therefore simultaneous with that tone, and require specialized detection and analysis techniques because the frequency of the emission is the same as that of the stimulus. The main method used for this purpose is to present the tone two times, once with the target intensity and a second time with a larger intensity. In the second case cochlear non-linearity causes the stimulus evoked OEA level to be less than proportional to the sound pressure, whereas the basic sound pressure in the ear canal is proportional to it. Appropriate handling of the two responses yields the desired emission component (Brass & Kemp, 1993). Another method to isolate the SFOAE component is to employ suppression (Siegel *et al.*, 2005). Emissions can also be recorded for combination tones, or DPs as they have been called in the foregoing. These emissions are known as DPOAEs (distortion product otoacoustic emissions). In principle, detecting DPOAEs is easy because DPs have frequencies differing from the primary frequencies. A figure more or less similar to Figure 5.9 results for the DPOAEs, and the properties of each of the constituent DPs can be analysed fairly easily. Interpretation is, as we shall see, not that easy. After a digression into the subject of multiple spontaneous emissions we will return to the simpler types of emissions and more basic properties of them.

We now generally recognize that cochlear 'activity' arises from some sort of signal feedback in the cochlea and that many manifestations of cochlear non-linearity are intrinsically interwoven with it. Where activity gives rise to amplification this feedback is positive; this is true for a certain frequency range and in a certain domain of the BM. Therefore, it can be expected that in certain cases the positive feedback can lead to spontaneous oscillation. Such a spontaneous oscillation of the BM has indeed been observed (Nuttall *et al.*, 2004; de Boer & Nuttall, 2006b) but *spontaneous otoacoustic emissions* (SOAEs) have repeatedly been reported (Wilson, 1980; Zurek, 1981, just to mention two early reports) and analysed (e.g. Bialek & Wit, 1984; Talmadge *et al.*, 1991; Shera, 2003).

Often more than one emission frequency is found. Those multiple spontaneous otoacoustic emissions (multiple SOAEs) have the peculiar property that the spacing of their frequencies is more or less periodic, they are never close together. This property makes it unlikely that an SOAE is due to a *local* oscillation, and it is more likely due to a *global* series of events. In particular, it can be surmised that inside the cochlea a reflection occurs, and that the reflected wave travels back to the stapes region and is reflected there again. The doubly reflected wave can then interfere with the primary wave, thereby augmenting its amplitude, and this can occur for several, well-spaced frequencies. Deeper consideration has led to the formulation of the theory of *coherent reflection* (Zweig & Shera, 1995). The principle of coherent reflection can be explained as follows. A cochlea with parameters that are very smooth functions of x will not show reflection. Therefore, reflections will closely be connected with irregularities (of the anatomy or the physiology of the cells involved). Each irregularity sends off two waves, one of these travels in the backward direction and can be designated as 'reflected', the other one travels in the forward direction and can be labelled as 'scattered'. Where reflected waves coming from different locations add in a constructive way they can give rise to a sizeable reflected wave that travels with a non-negligible amplitude toward the stapes. Such a wave is then reflected at the stapes and travels forward again as described above. If this doubly reflected wave arrives with the correct phase and amplitude in the peak region, an oscillation may occur, leading to a spontaneous BM oscillation as well as an SOAE. In this way the entire process involves two reflections.

We will next consider the first reflection in more detail. Consider a single-frequency wave. As it travels along the length of the BM (BM), its propagation velocity decreases continually.

Its wavelength also decreases continually as we have seen. Consider for a moment the region where the wavelength is (on average) 2 mm. In that region two irregularities 1 mm apart could give rise to a reflected wave (both the incident and the reflected wave travel through that region and undergo a phase shift of π radians). At a location somewhat farther from the stapes the wavelength may have decreased to 1 mm, and in that region irregularities 0.5 mm apart may give rise to reflection, etc. Therefore, the average density of irregularities that might give rise to a noticeable reflected wave varies from location to location. For a sizable reflected wave to occur, the irregularities should have a more or less *random* distribution in the x-domain. This simplified reasoning explains why random irregularities are, in principle, capable of causing appreciable reflection in a non-homogeneous structure as the cochlea, for a limited number of frequency bands. The second point is that an oscillation can only occur when the original and the doubly reflected wave are in phase. It is this requirement that causes the frequencies of SOAEs to have a more or less constant spacing and can never be close together. The principle of coherent reflection has been evoked to explain the measured properties of the cochlea in which a spontaneous BM oscillation was detected (de Boer & Nuttall, 2006b). Actually, in this simulation the spacing of multiple response peaks was confirmed to correspond to steps of approximately π radians in the phase of the primary wave.

In a region where the primary wave is amplified, the reflected wave will be amplified, too. Therefore, as regards the ultimate amplitude of the wave reflected by coherent reflection and the stapes, this varies roughly as the *square* of the amplification factor. Therefore, coherent reflection can only occur in a region where there is appreciable amplification, and not in regions where there is no amplification. This description is necessarily somewhat vague. More quantitative details about the underlying mechanism are found in Zweig and Shera (1995), and examples of applications in Talmadge *et al.* (1998a), Shera (2003) and Shera *et al.* (2005). An illustrated recipe for actual computation of response peaks and their non-linearity as being generated by the coherent-reflection mechanism is found in de Boer and Nuttall (2006b).

Effects of coherent reflection are not only evident in spontaneous otoacoustic emissions. They may contribute to other types of emissions as well. As a result the interpretation of, for instance, measured group delays is not unequivocal. In general two classes of emissions can be distinguished (Shera & Guinan, 1999), called 'place-fixed' and 'wave-fixed', respectively. To the former class belong emissions that can be traced to local reflections. The group delay in this case is equal to the propagation delay of the original wave plus the (not yet properly understood – as we shall see) propagation delay of the returned wave. The second class of emissions arises directly from the active or the non-linear mechanism, the source of the returned wave is distributed around the peak of the response to the primary sound. Consider, for a moment, the case of a SFOAE, in which the primary sound is a single-frequency tone. When the frequency of that tone varies, the peak location moves with it and so does the origin of the returned wave. See Figure 5.1B and imagine the pattern to be moving back and forth. It was reported already in 1983 (Kemp & Brown, 1983) that theoretically the phase in this (moving) pattern is nearly invariant, and that therefore the intrinsic group delay is near zero. (It is tacitly assumed that phase delays between the transducers and the stapes are taken care of.) In the case of DPOAEs various definitions of group delay are possible. The first is the derivative $\delta\phi/\delta f_1$ with respect to the frequency f_1 whereby the frequency f_2 is kept constant. The second is the derivative $\delta\phi/\delta f_2$ with respect to the frequency f_2 whereby the frequency f_1 is kept constant. The third is defined as $(\delta\phi/\delta f_1)_{ratio}$ where both frequencies are varied but the frequency ratio is kept constant. In the literature it has been shown that there is a fixed relation between these three types of group delay (Prijs *et al.*, 2000; Shera, *et al.*, 2000). However, a full description of the intricacies involved in unravelling the phase of DPOAEs is beyond the scope of the present chapter.

In recent times, uncertainty has risen on the point of the cochlear waves that are associated with DPs. Detailed measurements of DPOAEs have shown that their group delays are remarkably short (Ruggero, 2004), and the same appears to be valid for SFOAEs (Siegel *et al.*, 2005). Theoretically, the propagation properties of forward and reverse travelling waves should be the same (de Boer *et al.*, 2007) but it should be remembered that the primary wave originates from one point, the stapes, whereas the returned wave always has a distributed origin. This basic symmetry property is true for a 'classical' model as described in Section 5.4. It is not true for a non-classical model, notably a model with feed-forward or feed-backward as described in Section 5.7 (de Boer, 2007). It has been found experimentally that forward-travelling DP waves on the BM are dominant (Ren *et al.*, 2006). In our own work we have confirmed that property experimentally: forward-propagating DP waves dominate over a larger stretch of the BM than can be accounted for by theory (de Boer *et al.*, 2008). It is clear that such effects constitute a challenge to theoreticians. Explanations have been posed and counteracted, even compression waves (see Section 5.4) have been called into action; smoke and the smell of powder are still hovering over this battlefield (de Boer & Nuttall, 2006a; Ren *et al.*, 2006; de Boer *et al.* 2008; He *et al.*, 2007; Shera *et al.*, 2007).

Otoacoustic emissions are frequently used to diagnose hearing disorders in humans (see Chapter 4). One frequently used method operates with CEOAEs (see above), another one with DPOAEs. Of course, the presence of SOAEs testifies to the viability of the cochlea. An important field of study is hearing estimation in infants. It is generally believed that from research in animals sufficient knowledge has been gathered about the human cochlea to make this approach fruitful. Recent studies have cast doubt on this idea. For once, there is evidence that the tuning in the cochlea of humans is finer, sharper than has been thought before (Shera *et al.*, 2002; Shera, 2007). The second body of knowledge concerns the travel time of the waves in the cochlea as it has been reviewed above. With respect to detailed diagnosis of hearing defects from measurements of otoacoustic emissions the field has evidently become somewhat more obscure.

5.9 **Additional effects, puzzles, conclusions**

The aforementioned problems are not the only remaining unsolved issues in the theory of the cochlea. In Section 5.7 we saw that many of the micromechanical processes that are involved are not understood at all. There exist alternative theories, for instance, one which takes into account the fact that the actual cochlea effectively contains three instead of two channels (e.g. Hubbard, 1993). More complications can arise because of multiple vibration modes, as reviewed in the foregoing sections.

On a final note, we should consider frequency selectivity. Cochlear 'activity' as it has been described above enhances frequency selectivity. It should be realized that at different locations along the BM the action of OHCs should be different. In other terms, a frequency- and location-dependent mechanism is involved that yields the correct frequency response at every location. Because the elements of this system are not (yet) accessible for experimentation it is mainly theory and hypothesis that have been brought in for better understanding.

A commonly considered mechanism – as mentioned and defended earlier, in Section 5.7 – is thought to reside in the TM. Its mass, in collaboration with the stiffness of the stereocilia and the stiffness of the TM's attachments, can give rise to resonance. Theoretically, with acceptable parameters, it is possible to construct a locally active cochlear model with a realistic type of response in which TM resonance ensures the proper feedback phase at all locations (Neely & Kim, 1986). However, objections to the concept of TM resonance have also been published: the presence of two resonances in the system (the resonance of the BM's stiffness with the total mass, and the TM resonance) would not tally with specific properties of the cochlea's impulse response (de Boer & Nuttall, 2000; Shera, 2001). However, in a recent study on a similar type of model the impulse-response problem did not turn up, for unknown reasons (Ramamoorthy *et al.*, 2007). Space does not permit a more complete description. This disagreement illustrates that we can describe, understand, and tie together many mechanical properties of the cochlea but that the end of this road is not yet in sight. In this connection the reader should be reminded that in this chapter cochlear mechanics has mainly been described for the high-frequency region, the basal turns of the cochlea. To this day the properties of regions of the cochlea tuned to lower frequencies have not been explored enough, and theoretical elaborations are scarce (e.g. Shera, 2007), to say the least. In this connection we might mention a singular fact: in the apical region of the cochlea DPs with frequencies $f_2 - f_1$ and $f_2 + f_1$ are dominant (Cooper, 2006), whereas in high-frequency regions they do not play an important part.

Acknowledgement

In this chapter a few figures show results from our own experiments. The authors want to acknowledge the invaluable and highly professional contributions of Dr Jiefu Zheng, in almost all aspects of these experiments and the ensuing discussions.

References

Allen JB. (1977) Two-dimensional cochlear fluid model: new results. *J Acoust Soc Am* **61**: 110–19.

Allen JB. (1980) Cochlear micromechanics – a physical model of transduction. *J Acoust Soc Am* **68**: 1660–70.

Allen JB & Neely ST. (1992) Micromechanical models of the cochlea. *Phys Today* **45**: 40–7.

Bell A & Fletcher NH. (2004) The cochlear amplifier as a standing wave: 'squirting' waves between rows of outer hair cells? *J Acoust Soc Am* **116**: 1016–24.

Bialek W & Wit HP. (1984) Quantum limits to oscillator stability: theory and experiments on acoustic emissions from the human ear. *Phys Lett A* **104**: 173–8.

Billone M & Raynor S. (1973) Transmission of radial shear forces to cochlear hair cells. *J Acoust Soc Am* **54**: 1143–56.

Brass D & Kemp DT. (1993) Suppression of stimulus frequency otoacoustic emissions. *J Acoust Soc Am* **93**: 920–1039.

Brownell WE, Bader CR, Bertrand D & de Ribaupierre Y. (1985) Evoked mechanical responses of isolated cochlear outer hair cells. *Science* **227**: 194–6.

Cai H, Manoussaki D & Chadwick R. (2005) Effects of coiling on the micromechanics of the mammalian cochlea. *J R Soc Interface* **2**: 341–8.

Camalet S, Duke T, Jülicher F & Probst J. (2000) Auditory sensitivity provided by self-tuned critical oscillations of hair cells. *Proc Natl Acad Sci U S A* **97**: 3183–8.

Chadwick RS. (1998) Compression, gain, and nonlinear distortion in an active cochlear model with subpartitions. *Proc Natl Acad Sci U S A* **95**: 14594–14599.

Chadwick RS, Dimitriades EK & Iwasa KH. (1996) Active control of waves in a cochlear model with subpartitions. *Proc Natl Acad Sci U S A* **93**: 2564–9.

Chan DK & Hudspeth AJ. (2005) Mechanical responses of the organ of Corti to acoustic and electrical stimulation in vitro. *Biophys J* **89**: 4382–95.

Chen F, Choudhury N, Zheng J, Matthews S, Nuttall AL & Jacques SL. (2007) In vivo imaging and low-coherence interferometry of organ of Corti vibration. *J Biomed Opt* **12**: 021006.

Choudhury H, Song G, Chen F, Matthews S, Tschinkel T, Zheng J, Jacques SL & Nuttall AL. (2006) Low coherence interferometry of the cochlear partition. *Hear Res* **220**: 1–9.

Cooper NP. (2000) Radial variation in the vibrations of the cochlear partition. In: Wada H, Takasaka T, Ikeda K, Ohyama K & Koike T, eds. *Recent developments in auditory mechanics*. World Scientific, Singapore, pp. 109–15.

Cooper NP. (2006) Mechanical preprocessing of amplitude-modulated sounds in the apex of the cochlea. *Orl Head Neck Surg* **68**: 353–8.

Cooper NP & Rhode WS. (1995) Nonlinear mechanics at the apex of the guinea-pig cochlea. *Hear Res* **82**: 225–43.

Cooper NP & Rhode WS. (1996) Fast traveling waves, slow traveling waves and their interactions in experimental studies of apical cochlear mechanics. *Audit Neurosci* **2**: 289–99.

Dallos P. (1973) *The Auditory Periphery. Biophysics and Physiology*. Academic Press, New York.

Dallos P. (1985a) Response characteristics of mammalian cochlear hair cells. *J Neurosci* **5**: 1591–608.

Dallos P. (1985b) Membrane potential and response changes in mammalian cochlear hair cells during intracellular recording. *J Neurosci* **5**: 1609–15.

Dallos P. (1986) Neurobiology of cochlear inner and outer hair cells: intracellular recordings. *Hear Res* **22**: 185–98.

Dallos P. (2003) Organ of Corti kinematics. *J Assoc Res Otolaryngol* **4**: 416–20.

Dallos P & Cheatham MA. (1976) Production of cochlear potentials by inner and outer hair cells. *J Acoust Soc Am* **60**: 510–12.

Dallos P & Evans BN. (1995a) High-frequency motility of outer hair cells and the cochlear amplifier. *Science* **267**: 2006–9.

Dallos P & Evans BN. (1995b) High-frequency outer hair cell motility: corrections and addendum. *Science* **268**: 1420–1.

Davis H. (1983) An active process in cochlear mechanics. *Hear Res* **9**: 79–90.

de Boer E. (1981) Short waves in three-dimensional cochlea models: Solution for a 'block' model. *Hear Res* **4**: 53–77.

de Boer E. (1983) No sharpening? A challenge for cochlear mechanics. *J Acoust Soc Am* **73**: 567–73.

de Boer E. (1993) The sulcus connection. On a mode of participation of outer hair cells in cochlear mechanics. *J Acoust Soc Am* **93**: 2845–59.

de Boer E. (1995a) The 'inverse problem' solved for a three-dimensional model of the cochlea. I Analysis. *J Acoust Soc Am* **98**: 896–903.

de Boer E. (1995b) The 'inverse problem' solved for a three-dimensional model of the cochlea. II Application to experimental data sets. *J Acoust Soc Am* **98**: 904–10.

de Boer E. (1997) Connecting frequency selectivity and nonlinearity for models of the cochlea. *Audit Neurosci* **3**: 377–88.

de Boer E. (2007) Forward and reverse waves in nonclassical models of the cochlea. *J Acoust Soc Am* **121**: 2819–21.

de Boer E & Nuttall AL. (1997) The mechanical waveform of the basilar membrane. I Frequency modulations ('glides') in impulse responses and cross-correlation functions. *J Acoust Soc Am* **101**: 3583–92.

de Boer E & Nuttall AL. (2000) The mechanical waveform of the basilar membrane. III Intensity effects. *J Acoust Soc Am* **107**: 1497–507.

de Boer E & Nuttall AL. (2003) Properties of amplifying elements in the cochlea. In: Gummer AW, Dalhoff E, Nowotny M & Scherer MP, eds. *Biophysics of the Cochlea: From Molecules to Models*. World Scientific, Singapore, pp. 331–342.

de Boer E & Nuttall AL. (2006a) Amplification via 'compression waves' in the cochlea – a parable. *Abstr. Midwinter Res. Meet. Assoc. Res. Otolaryngol.* **29**: 349.

de Boer E & Nuttall AL. (2006b) Spontaneous Basilar-Membrane Oscillation (SBMO) and Coherent Reflection. *J Assoc Res Otolaryngol* **7**: 26–37.

de Boer E, Nuttall AL & Zheng J. (2002) Towards explaining distortion products in basilar-membrane motion. *Abstr. Midwinter Res. Meet. Assoc. Res. Otolaryngol.* **25**: 192.

de Boer E, Nuttall AL & Shera CA. (2007) Wave propagation patterns in a 'classical' three-dimensional model of the cochlea. *J Acoust Soc Am* **121**: 352–62.

de Boer E, Zheng J, Porsov E & Nuttall AL. (2008) Inverted direction of wave propagation (IDWP) in the cochlea. *J Acoust Soc Am* **123**: 1513–21.

de La Rochefoucauld O & Olson ES. (2007) The role of organ of Corti mass in passive cochlear tuning. *Biophys J* **93**: 3434–50.

Dimitriades EK & Chadwick RS. (1999) Solution of the inverse problem for a linear cochlear model: A tonotopic cochlear amplifier. *J Acoust Soc Am* **106**: 1880–92.

Dong W & Olson ES. (2005) Two-tone distortion in intracochlear pressure. *J Acoust Soc Am* **117**: 2999–3015.

Eguíluz VM, Ospeck M, Choe Y, Hudspeth AJ & Magnasco M. (2000) Essential nonlinearities in hearing. *Phys Rev Lett* **84**: 5232–5.

Emadi G, Richter CP & Dallos P. (2004) Stiffness of the gerbil basilar membrane: radial and longitudinal variations. *J Neurophysiol* **91**: 474–88.

Evans EF. (1975) The sharpening of cochlear frequency selectivity in the normal and abnormal cochlea. *Am J Audiol* **14**: 419–42.

Fettiplace R. (2006) Active hair bundle movements in auditory hair cells. *Am J Physiol* **576**: 29–36.

Frank G, Hemmert W & Gummer AW. (1999) Limiting dynamics of high-frequency electromechanical transduction of outer hair cells. *Proc Natl Acad Sci U S A* **96**: 4420–5.

Freeman DM, Masaki. K, McAllister AR, Wei JL & Weiss TF. (2003a) Static material properties of the tectorial membrane: a summary. *Hear Res* **180**: 11–27.

Freeman DM, Abnet CC, Hemmert W, Tsai BS & Weiss TF. (2003b) Dynamic material properties of the tectorial membrane: a summary. *Hear Res* **180**: 1–10.

Fridberger A, Boutet de Monvel J & Ulfendahl M. (2002) Internal shearing within the hearing organ evoked by basilar membrane motion. *J Neurosci* **22**: 9850–7.

Fridberger A, Boutet de Monvel J, Zheng J, Hu N, Zou Y, Ren T & Nuttall AL. (2004a) Organ of Corti potentials and the motion of the basilar membrane. *J Neurosci* **24**: 10057–10062.

Fridberger A, Widengren J & Boutet de Monvel J. (2004b) Measuring hearing organ vibration patterns with confocal microscopy and optical flow. *Biophys J* **86**: 535–43.

Fukazawa T. (1997) A model of cochlear micromechanics. *Hear Res* **113**: 182–90.

Fukazawa T, Ishida K & Murai Y. (1999) A micromechanical model of the cochlea with radial movement of the tectorial membrane. *Hear Res* **137**: 59–67.

Gale JE & Ashmore JF. (1997) An intrinsic frequency limit to the cochlear amplifier. *Nature* **389**: 63–6.

Geisler CD. (1993) A realizable model of the effect of outer hair cell motility on cochlear vibrations. *Hear Res* **68**: 253–62.

Geisler CD & Sang C. (1995) A cochlear model using feed-forward outer-hair-cell forces. *Hear Res* **86**: 132–46.

Greenwood DD. (1961) Critical bandwidth and the frequency coordinates of the basilar membrane. *J Acoust Soc Am* **33**: 1344–56.

Greenwood DD. (1990) A cochlear frequency-position function for several species – 29 years later. *J Acoust Soc Am* **87**: 2592–605.

Gummer AW, Hemmert W & Zenner HP. (1996) Resonant tectorial membrane motion in the inner ear: its crucial role in frequency tuning. *Proc Natl Acad Sci U S A* **93**: 8727–32.

Hallworth R. (1995) Passive compliance and active force generation in the guinea pig outer hair cell. *J Neurophysiol* **74**: 2319–28.

He DZ, Jia S & Dallos P. (2003) Prestin and the dynamic stiffness of cochlear outer hair cells. *J Neurosci* **23**: 9089–96.

He W, Nuttall AL & Ren T. (2007) Two-tone distortion at different longitudinal locations on the basilar membrane. *Hear Res* **222**: 112–22.

Hong SS & Freeman DM. (2006) Doppler optical coherence microscopy for studies of cochlear mechanics. *J Biomed Opt* 11: 054014.

Houtgast T. (1972) Psychophysical evidence for lateral inhibition in hearing. *J Acoust Soc Am* 51: 1885–94.

Hu X, Evans BN & Dallos P. (1999) Direct visualization of organ of Corti kinematics in a hemicochlea. *Am J Physiol* 82: 2798–807.

Hubbard AE. (1993) A traveling wave-amplifier model of the cochlea. *Science* 259: 68–71.

Hudspeth AJ & Corey DP. (1977) Sensitivity, polarity, and conductance change in the response of vertebrate hair cells to controlled mechanical stimuli. *Proc Natl Acad Sci U S A* 74: 2407–11.

Jia S & He DZ. (2005) Motility-associated hair-bundle motion in mammalian outer hair cells. *Nat Neurosci* 8: 1028–34.

Jülicher F, Camalet S, Probst J & Duke TAJ. (2003) Active amplification by critical oscillations. In: Gummer AW, Dalhoff E, Nowotny M & Scherer MP, eds. *Biophysics of the Cochlea: from Molecules to Models.* World Scientific, Singapore, pp. 16–27.

Kalluri R & Shera CA. (2007) Near equivalence of human click-evoked and stimulus-frequency otoacoustic emissions. *J Acoust Soc Am* 121: 2097–110.

Karavitaki KD & Mountain DC. (2007a) Evidence for outer hair cell driven oscillatory fluid flow in the tunnel of corti. *Biophys J* 92: 3284–93.

Karavitaki KD & Mountain DC. (2007b) Imaging electrically evoked micromechanical motion within the organ of Corti of the excised gerbil cochlea. *Biophys J* 92: 3294–316.

Kemp DT. (1978) Stimulated acoustic emission from within the human auditory system. *J Acoust Soc Am* 64: 1386–91.

Kemp DT & Brown AM. (1983) An integrated view of cochlear mechanical nonlinearities observable from the ear canal. In: de Boer E & Viergever MA, eds. *Mechanics of Hearing.* Delft University Press, Delft, pp. 75–82.

Khanna SM & Hao LF. (1999) Reticular lamina vibrations in the apical turn of a living guinea pig cochlea. *Hear Res* 132: 15–33.

Khanna SM & Leonard DGB. (1982) Basilar membrane tuning in the cat cochlea. *Science* 215: 305–306.

Kiang NY-S, Watanabe T, Thomas EC & Clark LF. (1965) *Discharge patterns of single fibers in the cat's auditory nerve.* MIT Press, Cambridge, MA.

Kim DO, Neely ST, Molnar CE & Matthews JW. (1980) An active cochlear model with negative damping in the partition: Comparison with Rhode's ante-and post-mortem observations. In: Van Den Brink G & Bilsen FA, eds. *Psychophysical Physiological and Behavioural Studies in Hearing.* Delft University Press, Delft, pp. 7–14.

Kolston PJ & Ashmore JF. (1996) Finite element micromechanical modeling of the cochlea in three dimensions. *J Acoust Soc Am* 99: 455.

Lee YW. (1969) *Statistical Theory of Communication.* Wiley and Sons, New York.

Legan PK, Lukashkina VA, Goodyear RJ, Kössl M, Russell IJ & Richardson GP. (2000) A targeted deletion in α-tectorin reveals that the tectorial membrane is required for the gain and timing of cochlear feedback. *Neuron* 28: 273–85.

Legan PK, Lukashkina VA, Goodyear RJ, Lukashkin AN, Verhoeven K, Van Camp G, Russell IJ & Richardson GP. (2005) A deafness mutation isolates a second role for the tectorial membrane in hearing. *Nat Neurosci* 8: 1035–41.

LeMasurier M & Gillespie PG. (2005) Hair-cell mechanotransduction and cochlear amplification. *Neuron* 48: 403–15.

Liberman MC. (1982) The cochlear frequency map for the cat: labeling auditory-nerve fibers of known characteristic frequency. *J Acoust Soc Am* 72: 1441–9.

Liberman MC, Gao J, He DZ, Wu X & Zuo J. (2002) Prestin is required for electromotility of the outer hair cell and for the cochlear amplifier. *Nature* 419: 300–4.

Lim K-M & Steele CR. (2003) Response suppression and transient behavior in a nonlinear active cochlear model with feed-forward. *Int J Solids Struct* 40: 5097–107.

Lukashkin AN, Bashtanov ME & Russell IJ. (2005) A self-mixing laser-diode interferometer for measuring basilar membrane vibrations without opening the cochlea. *J Neurosci Methods* **148**: 122–9.

Lukashkin AN, Smith JK & Russell IJ. (2007) Properties of distortion product otoacoustic emissions and neural suppression tuning curves attributable to the tectorial membrane resonance. *J Acoust Soc Am* **121**: 337–43.

Mammano F & Ashmore JF. (1993) Reverse transduction measured in the isolated cochlea by laser Michelson interferometry. *Nature* **365**: 838–41.

Mammano F & Nobili R. (1993) Biophysics of the cochlea: Linear approximation. *J Acoust Soc Am* **93**: 3320–32.

Masaki K, Weiss TF & Freeman DM. (2006) Poroelastic bulk properties of the tectorial membrane measured with osmotic stress. *Biophys J* **9**: 2356–70.

Naidu RC & Mountain DC. (1998) Measurements of the stiffness map challenge a basic tenet of cochlear theories. *Hear Res* **124**: 124–31.

Naidu RC & Mountain DC. (2000) Longitudinal coupling within the basilar membrane and reticular lamina. In: Wada H, Takasaka T, Ikeda K, Ohyama K & Koike T, eds. *Recent developments in auditory mechanics*. World Scientific, Singapore, pp.123–129.

Neely ST. (1983) The cochlear amplifier. In: de Boer E & Viergever MA, eds. *Mechanics of hearing*. Delft University Press, Delft, pp. 111–118.

Neely ST. (1993) A model of cochlear mechanics with outer hair cell motility. *J Acoust Soc Am* **94**: 137–46.

Neely ST & Kim DO. (1986) A model for active elements in cochlear biomechanics. *J Acoust Soc Am* **79**: 1472–80.

Nilsen KE & Russell IJ. (1999) Timing of cochlear feedback: spatial and temporal representation of a tone across the basilar membrane. *Nat Neurosci* **2**: 642–8.

Nilsen KE & Russell IJ. (2000) The spatial and temporal representation of a tone on the guinea pig basilar membrane. *Proc Natl Acad Sci U S A* **97**: 11751–8.

Nowotny M & Gummer AW. (2006) Nanomechanics of the subtectorial space caused by electromechanics of cochlear outer hair cells. *Proc Natl Acad Sci U S A* **103**: 2120–5.

Nuttall AL, Brown MC, Masta RI & Lawrence M. (1981) Inner hair cell responses to the velocity of basilar membrane motion in the guinea pig. *Brain Res* **211**: 171–4.

Nuttall AL, Dolan DF & Avinash G. (1991) Laser Doppler velocimetry of basilar membrane vibration. *Hear Res* **51**: 203–14.

Nuttall AL, Guo M & Ren T. (1999) The radial pattern of basilar membrane motion evoked by electric stimulation of the cochlea. *Hear Res* **131**: 39–46.

Nuttall AL, Grosh K, Zheng J, de Boer E, Zou Y & Ren T. (2004) Spontaneous basilar membrane oscillation and otoacoustic emission at 15 kHz in a guinea pig. *J Assoc Res Otolaryngol* **5**: 337–49.

Olson ES. (2000) The use of intracochlear pressure to find the impedance of the organ of Corti. In: Wada H, Takasaka T, Ikeda K, Ohyama K & Koike T. *Recent Developments in Auditory Mechanics*. World Scientific, Singapore, pp. 144–150.

Olson ES. (2001) Intracochlear pressure measurements related to cochlear tuning. *J Acoust Soc Am* **110**: 349–67.

Olson ES & Mountain DC. (1991) In vivo measurement of basilar membrane stiffness. *J Acoust Soc Am* **89**: 1262–75.

Olson ES & Mountain DC. (1994) Mapping the cochlear partition's stiffness to its cellular architecture. *J Acoust Soc Am* **95**: 395–400.

Parthasarathi AA, Grosh K, & Nuttall AL. (2000) Three-dimensional numerical modeling for global cochlear dynamics. *J Acoust Soc Am* **107**: 474–85.

Prijs VF. (1989) Lower boundaries of two-tone suppression regions in the guinea pig. *Hear Res* **42**: 73–81.

Prijs VF, Schneider S & Schoonhoven R. (2000) Group delays of distortion product otoacoustic emissions: relating delays measured with f_1- and f_2-sweep paradigms. *J Acoust Soc Am* **107**: 3298–307.

Ramamoorthy S, Deo NV & Grosh K. (2007) A mechano-acoustical model for the cochlea: Response to acoustical stimuli. *J Acoust Soc Am* 121: 2758–73.

Recio A, Rich NC, Narayan S & Ruggero MA. (1998) Basilar-membrane responses to clicks at the base of the chinchilla cochlea. *J Acoust Soc Am* 103: 1972–89.

Ren T & Nuttall AL. (2001) Basilar membrane vibration in the basal turn of the sensitive gerbil cochlea. *Hear Res* 151: 48–60.

Ren T, He W, Matthews S & Nuttall AL. (2006) Group delay of acoustic emissions in the ear. *J Neurophysiol* 96: 2785–91.

Rhode WS. (1971) Observations of the vibration of the basilar membrane in squirrel monkeys using the Mössbauer technique. *J Acoust Soc Am* 49: 1218–1231.

Rhode WS. (1978) Some observations on cochlear mechanics. *J Acoust Soc Am* 64: 158–176.

Rhode WS. (2007a) Basilar membrane mechanics in the 6–9 kHz region of sensitive chinchilla cochleae. *J Acoust Soc Am* 121: 2792–804.

Rhode WS. (2007b) Mutual suppression in the 6 kHz region of sensitive chinchilla cochleae. *J Acoust Soc Am* 121: 2892–04.

Rhode WS & Cooper NP. (1996) Nonlinear mechanics in the apical turn of the chinchilla cochlea in vivo. *Audit Neurosci* 3: 101–21.

Rhode WS & Recio A. (2000) Study of mechanical motions in the basal region of the chinchilla cochlea. *J Acoust Soc Am* 107: 3317–32.

Ricci AJ, Kachar B, Gale J, & van Netten SM. (2006) Mechano-electrical transduction: new insights into old ideas. *J Membr Biol* 209: 71–88.

Richter CP, Edge R, He DZ & Dallos P. (2000) Development of the gerbil inner ear observed in the hemicochlea. *J Assoc Res Otolaryngol* 1: 195–210.

Richter CP, Emadi G, Getnick G, Quesnel A & Dallos P. (2007) Tectorial membrane stiffness gradients. *Biophys J* 2007 (published online).

Robles L & Ruggero MA. (2001) Mechanics of the mammalian ear. *Physiol Res* 81: 1305–52.

Robles L, Ruggero MA & Rich NC. (1986) Basilar membrane mechanics at the base of the chinchilla cochlea. I Input-output functions, tuning curves, and response phases. *J Acoust Soc Am* 80: 1364–74.

Robles L, Ruggero MA & Rich NC. (1990) Two-tone distortion products in the basilar membrane of the chinchilla cochlea. In: Dallos P, Matthews JW, Geisler CD, Ruggero MA & Steele CR, eds. *The Mechanics and Biophysics of Hearing*. Springer-Verlag, Berlin, pp. 304–311.

Robles L, Ruggero MA & Rich NC. (1991) Two-tone distortion in the basilar membrane of the chinchilla cochlea. *Nature* 349: 413–14.

Robles L, Ruggero MA & Rich NC. (1997) Two-tone distortion on the basilar membrane of the chinchilla cochlea. *J Neurophysiol* 77: 2385–99.

Ruggero MA. (2004) Comparison of group delay of $2 f_1 - f_2$ distortion product otoacoustic emissions and cochlear travel times. *Acoust Res Lett Online* 5: 143–7.

Ruggero MA & Rich NC. (1987) Timing of spike initiation in cochlear afferents: dependence on site of innervation. *J Neurophysiol* 58: 379–403.

Ruggero MA & Rich NC. (1991) Furosemide alters organ of Corti mechanics. *J Neurosci* 11: 1057–67.

Ruggero MA, Robles L & Rich NC. (1992) Two-tone suppression in the basilar membrane of the cochlea: mechanical basis of auditory-nerve rate suppression. *J Neurophysiol* 68: 1087–99.

Ruggero MA, Narayan SS, Temchin AN & Recio A. (2000) Mechanical bases of frequency tuning and neural excitation at the base of the cochlea: comparison of basilar-membrane vibrations and auditory-nerve-fiber responses in chinchilla. *Proc Natl Acad Sci U S A* 97: 11744–50.

Russell IJ & Sellick PM. (1983) Low-frequency characteristics of intracellularly recorded receptor potentials in guinea-pig cochlear hair cells. *Am J Physiol* 338: 179–206.

Russell IJ, Legan PK, Lukashkina VA, Lukashkin AN, Goodyear RJ & Richardson GP. (2007) Sharpened cochlear tuning in a mouse with a genetically modified tectorial membrane. *Nat Neurosci* 10: 215–23.

Santos-Sacchi J. (1992) On the frequency limit and phase of outer hair cell motility: effects of the membrane filter. *J Neurosci* **12**: 1906–16.

Scherer MP & Gummer AP. (2004) Impedance analysis of the organ of Corti with magnetically actuated probes. *Biophys J* **87**: 1378–91.

Schmiedt RA. (1982) Boundaries of two-tone rate suppression of cochlear-nerve activity. *Hear Res* **7**: 335–51.

Sellick PM & Russell IJ. (1980) The responses of inner hair cells to basilar membrane velocity during low frequency auditory stimulation in the guinea pig cochlea. *Hear Res* **2**: 439–45.

Sellick PM, Patuzzi R & Johnstone BM. (1982) Measurement of basilar membrane motion in the guinea pig using the Mössbauer technique. *J Acoust Soc Am* **72**: 131–141.

Shera CA. (2001) Intensity-invariance of fine time structures in basilar-membrane click responses: Implications for cochlear mechanics. *J Acoust Soc Am* **110**: 332–48.

Shera CA. (2003) Mammalian spontaneous otoacoustic emissions are amplitude-stabilized cochlear standing waves. *J Acoust Soc Am* **114**: 244–62.

Shera CA. (2007) Laser amplification with a twist: traveling-wave propagation and gain functions throughout the cochlea. *J Acoust Soc Am* **122**: 2738–58.

Shera CA & Guinan JJ. (1999) Evoked otoacoustic emissions arise by two fundamentally different mechanisms: A taxonomy for mammalian OAEs. *J Acoust Soc Am* **105**: 782–98.

Shera CA, Talmadge CL & Tubis A. (2000) Interrelations among distortion-product phase-gradient delays: their connection to scaling symmetry and its breaking. *J Acoust Soc Am* **108**: 2933–48.

Shera CA, Guinan JJ & Oxenham AJ. (2002) Revised estimates of human cochlear tuning from otoacoustic and behavioral measurements. *Proc Natl Acad Sci U S A* **99**: 3318–23.

Shera CA, Tubis A & Talmadge CL. (2005) Coherent reflection in a 2-dimensional cochlea: Short-wave versus long-wave scattering in the generation of reflection-source otoacoustic emissions. *J Acoust Soc Am* **118**: 287.

Shera CA, Tubis A, Talmadge CL, de Boer E, Fahey PA & Guinan JJ. (2007) Allen–Fahey and related experiments support the predominance of cochlear slow-wave otoacoustic emissions. *J Acoust Soc Am* **121**: 1564–75.

Shoelson B, Dimitriadis EK, Cai H, Kachar B & Chadwick RS. (2004) Evidence and implications of inhomogeneity in tectorial membrane elasticity. *Biophys J* **87**: 2768–77.

Siegel JH, Cerka AJ, Recio-Spinoso A, Temchin AN, van Dijk P & Ruggero MA. (2005) Delays of stimulus-frequency otoacoustic emissions and cochlear vibrations contradict the theory of coherent reflection filtering. *J Acoust Soc Am* **118**: 2434–43.

Steele CR & Lim K-M. (1999) Cochlear model with three-dimensional fluid, inner sulcus and feed-forward mechanism. *Audiol Neurootol* **4**: 197–203.

Steele CR & Taber LA. (1979) Comparison of WKB and finite difference calculations for a two-dimensional cochlear model. *J Acoust Soc Am* **65**: 1001–6.

Steele CR & Taber LA. (1981) Three-dimensional model calculations for guinea pig cochlea. *J Acoust Soc Am* **69**: 1107–11.

Steele CR, Baker G, Tolomeo J & Zetes D. (1993) Electro-mechanical models of the outer hair cell. In: Duifhuis H, Horst JW, van Dijk P & van Netten SM, eds. *Biophysics of Hair-Cell Sensory Systems.* World Scientific, Singapore, pp. 207–14.

Talmadge C, Tubis A, Long GR & Piskorski P. (1998a) Modeling otoacoustic emissions and hearing threshold fine structures. *J Acoust Soc Am* **104**: 1517–43.

Talmadge CL, Tubis A, Piskorski P & Long GR. (1998b) Modeling otoacoustic emission. In: Lewis ER, Long GR, Lyon RF, Narins PM, Steele CR & Poinar E, eds. *Diversity in Auditory Mechanisms.* World Scientific, Singapore, pp. 462–71.

Talmadge CL, Tubis A, Wit HP & Long GR. (1991) Are spontaneous otoacoustic emissions generated by self-sustained cochlear oscillators? *J Acoust Soc Am* **89**: 2391–9.

ter Kuile E. (1900) Die Übertragung der Energie von der Grundmembran auf die Haarzellen. *Pflügers Archiv* **79**: 146–57.

Tubis A, Talmadge CL & Tong C. (2000a) Modeling the temporal behavior of distortion product otoacoustic emissions. *J Acoust Soc Am* **107**: 2112–27.

Tubis A, Talmadge CL, Tong C & Dhar S. (2000b) On the relationships between the fixed- f_1, fixed- f_2, and fixed-ratio phase derivatives of the $2 f_1 - f_2$ distortion product otoacoustic emission. *J Acoust Soc Am* **108**: 1772–85.

Ulfendahl M, Flock Å & Khanna SM. (1989) Isolated cochlea preparation for the study of cellular vibrations and motility. *Acta Otolaryngol Suppl* **467**: 91–6 and other contributions.

von Békésy G. (1947) The variation of phase along the basilar membrane with sinusoidal vibrations. *J Acoust Soc Am* **19**: 452–60.

von Békésy G. (1948) On the elasticity of the cochlear partition. *J Acoust Soc Am* **20**: 227–41.

von Békésy G. (1949) On the resonance curve and the decay period at various points on the cochlear partition. *J Acoust Soc Am* **21**: 245–54.

von Békésy G. (1960) *Experiments in Hearing*. McGraw-Hill, New York.

von Helmholtz H. (1862) Original ed. *Die Lehre von den Tonempfindungen als physiologische Grundlage für die Theorie der Musik*. Vieweg, Braunschweig. 1st English ed (1954) *On the Sensations of Tone as a Physiological Basis For the Theory of Music* Paperback ed, Dover, New York.

Wen B & Boahen K. (2003) A linear cochlear model with active bi-directional coupling. *Conf Proc IEEE Eng Med Biol Soc.* **3**: 2013–16.

Wever EG & Bray C. (1930) Action currents in the auditory nerve in response to acoustic stimulation. *Proc Natl Acad Sci U S A* **16**: 344–50.

Wickesberg RE & Geisler CD. (1986) Longitudinal stiffness coupling in a 1-dimensional model of the peripheral ear. In: Allen JB, Hall JL, Hubbard A, Neely ST & Tubis A, eds. *Peripheral Auditory Mechanisms*. Springer-Verlag, Berlin, pp. 113–120.

Wilson JP. (1980) Evidence for a cochlear origin for acoustic re-emissions, threshold fine structure and tonal tinnitus. *Hear Res* **2**: 233–52.

Xue S, Mountain DC & Hubbard AE. (1993) Direct measurement of electrically-evoked basilar membrane motion. In: Duifhuis H, Horst JW, van Dijk P, & van Netten SM, eds. *Proceedings of the International Symposium on Biophysics of Hair Cell Sensory Systems*. World Scientific, New Jersey, pp. 361–69.

Xue S, Mountain DC & Hubbard AE. (1995) Electrically evoked basilar membrane motion. *J Acoust Soc Am* **97**: 3030–41.

Zao H-B & Santos-Sacchi J. (1999) Auditory collusion and a coupled couple of outer hair cells. *Nature* **399**: 359–62.

Zheng J, Shen W, He DZ, Long KB, Madison LD & Dallos P. (2000) Prestin is the motor protein of cochlear outer hair cells. *Nature* **405**: 149–55.

Zinn C, Maier H, Zenner HP & Gummer AW. (2000) Evidence for active, nonlinear, negative feedback in the vibration response of the apical region of the in vivo guinea-pig cochlea. *Hear Res* **142**: 159–83.

Zurek PM. (1981) Spontaneous narrowband acoustic signals emitted by human ears. *J Acoust Soc Am* **69**: 514–23.

Zweig G. (1991) Finding the impedance of the organ of Corti. *J Acoust Soc Am* **89**: 1229–54.

Zweig G. (2006) Cellular cooperation in cochlea mechanics. In: Gummer AW, Dalhoff E, Nowotny M & Scherer MP, eds. *Biophysics of the Cochlea: from Molecules to Models*. World Scientific, Singapore, pp. 315–322, discussion pp. 322–329.

Zweig G & Shera CA. (1995) The origin of periodicity in the spectrum of evoked otoacoustic emissions. *J Acoust Soc Am* **98**: 2018–47.

Zwislocki JJ. (1948) Theorie der Schneckenmechanik: Qualitative und quantitative Analyse. *Acta Otolaryngol Suppl* 72.

Zwislocki JJ. (1950) Theory of the acoustical action of the cochlea. *J Acoust Soc Am* **22**: 778–84.

Zwislocki JJ & Cefaratti LK. (1989) Tectorial membrane. II Stiffness measurement in vivo. *Hear Res* **42**: 211–28.

Zwislocki JJ & Kletsky EJ. (1979) Tectorial membrane: a possible effect on frequency analysis in the cochlea. *Science* **204**: 639–41.

Chapter 6

Electromotility of outer hair cells

Kuni H Iwasa

6.1 Introduction

Both inner and outer hair cells in the cochlea perform mechanoelectrical transduction in response to oscillation of the basilar membrane during acoustic stimulation. While inner hair cells (IHCs) directly send signals to the brain through fast myelinated fibers, outer hair cells (OHCs) are involved in enhancing the frequency selectivity and in increasing cochlear gain. Specifically, gain increase is limited to low intensity sounds. This non-linearity increases the dynamic range of the ear. Such a biological role of outer hair cells can be realized if these mechanoreceptor cells provide mechanical feedback to amplify the vibration of the basilar membrane that stimulates them. Indeed, OHCs have two reverse transduction mechanisms, one in their hair bundles (Chan & Hudspeth, 2005; Kennedy *et al.*, 2005) and another in the lateral wall of their cell body (Brownell *et al.*, 1985; Ashmore, 1987) to function as *cochlear amplifier*.

The reverse transduction mechanism in hair bundles is directly associated with the mechano-electric transducer (MET) channels. It is called fast adaptation because it closes the transducer channels at a fast rate, less than 1 ms as opposed to slow adaptation, which depends on myosin and has a time constant of ~10 ms. The reverse transduction mechanism in the cell body, which is referred to as electromotility, the voltage-dependent motility, or the somatic motility, is indirectly associated with the MET channels because this motile response of the lateral membrane of OHCs depends on the receptor potential that is generated by transducer currents through the MET channels. Because hair cells in non-mammalian ears do not have electromotility, electromotility is considered a mammalian innovation. Since non-mammalian ears must depend on hair bundle motility as a cochlear amplifier, it may not be too surprising if hair bundle motility functions as cochlear amplifier to some degree in the mammalian ear. A logical question is then, why the mammalian ear needs electromotility as well? One possibility is to encompass the higher frequency range of mammalian hearing.

Electromotility turned out to be unique in that it does not depend on chemical energy, which most, if not all, biological motilities use, but it uses electrical energy available at the plasma membrane in a manner similar to piezoelectricity. The idea that reverse transduction is required in the inner ear goes back to Thomas Gold's paper published in 1948. His reasoning was that viscous drag must be counteracted to achieve the sharp tuning of the ear. Amazingly, he predicted piezoelectricity as a likely mechanism for such an activity (Gold, 1948).

In this chapter, electromotility is described from a mechanistic viewpoint. Because of the limitation on the number of citations, an extensive list of references could not be provided. Some of the areas that this chapter does not cover can be found in reviews (Holley, 1996; Dallos *et al.*, 2006; Frolenkov, 2006; He *et al.*, 2006).

6.2 **Outer hair cells in the organ of Corti**

The apical surface of the OHC forms tight junctions with supporting cells and is a part of the reticular lamina, a stiff fiber-rich plate. The hair bundles of OHCs, which extend from the apical surface, are arranged in a V-shape, which points in the excitatory direction. The tallest stereocilia are embedded into the tectorial membrane. The apical surface of these cells is exposed to the endolymphatic fluid, which is high in potassium ion (~140 mM) and low in calcium ion (~10 μM), unusual for an extracellular fluid. This composition of the endolymphatic fluid helps OHCs to maintain the intracellular potassium ion concentration when hair cells are mechanically stimulated and MET channels open. In addition, this extracellular compartment has a positive potential of about + 80 mV, which is called the endocochlear potential, referenced to the perilymph. Combined with OHCs' resting membrane potential of about –70 mV, which is more negative than that of IHCs, this potential contributes to a ~150 mV voltage drop across the apical membrane of OHCs. This large voltage drop makes the MET channels in OHCs very effective in producing receptor currents (see Fig. 6.1A below).

The cell body of OHCs has a cylindrical shape. The basal part of OHCs has synaptic endings and up to the height of the nucleus it is wrapped around by Deiters' cup, which is connected to the basilar membrane. In addition to giving mechanical support to OHCs, Deiters' cup is thought to be important in recapturing K^+, which is released from OHCs, to pass on to other supporting cells for recycling. The lateral surface of the OHC does not have contacts with other cells and it is exposed to the perilymph, which is high in sodium ion and calcium ion, a typical extracellular fluid. These features are common in all three rows of OHCs in the cochlea.

6.3 **Structure of the outer hair cell**

6.3.1 **The length of the cell body and hair bundles**

As briefly described earlier, an OHC consists of a cylindrical cell body and a hair bundle on the apical surface. The radius of the cell body is about 10 μm. The length of the cell body varies from about 15 μm to about 100 μm, depending on its location. OHCs are long at the apical end and they are shorter toward the base. These cells are also longer in the outer row and shorter in the inner row. This row dependence is marked among the apical turn of the cochlea but is insignificant in the basal turn (Lim, 1980).

The length of the tallest stereocilia in hair bundles ranges from ~0.7 μm to 5.5 μm (in chinchilla). The height of stereocilia is well correlated with the length of the cell body. The tallest stereocilia are in OHCs in the outer row in the apex and the shortest ones are in the base, where the length is about the same in all three rows (Lim, 1980). These features are shared with most mammals.

6.3.2 **The apical end**

The apical part of OHCs is rich in actin filaments. Actin filaments also extend from the apical part of the cell body into the stereocilia, forming stiff backbones. Hair bundles have MET channels that are associated with tip links. The MET channels have non-zero open probability in the resting condition. Bending of hair bundles in the excitatory direction (toward the tallest hairs) pulls tip links and increases the open probability of those MET channels. Bending of hair bundles in the opposite direction decreases the open probability. The apical surface also has ATP-gated channels that can modulate mechanosensitivity of the cell (Housely et al., 1992). The plasma membrane Ca^{2+}-ATPase is also located in the apical surface, particularly of the hair bundles (Crouch &

Schulte, 1995). This ion pump is important for maintaining the cytosolic Ca^{2+} level because Ca^{2+}-influx occurs through the open MET channels.

6.3.3 The basal end

OHCs have their nuclei near the basal, synaptic pole. The plasma membrane of OHCs has nicotinic acetylcholine receptors. Their α subunits include $\alpha 9$ and $\alpha 10$, forming heteromers (Elgoyhen *et al.*, 2001). These receptors are involved in efferent inhibition of OHCs and attenuate the sensitivity of the ear. Calcium-activated potassium (SK_{Ca}) channels are also located in the basal end. Acetylcholine opens those acetylcholine receptors and induces the flux of extracellular Ca^{2+} into the cell. This in turn opens SK_{Ca} and hyperpolarizes the cell (see Chapter 10).

6.3.4 The lateral wall

The lateral wall of the OHCs above the nucleus includes the cortical lattice, and the submembranous cisternae that line the plasma membrane. Next to the submembranous cisternae are numerous mitochondria (Fig. 6.1B). The lateral plasma membrane has dense particles of about 10 nm in diameter (10 nm particles). The cortical cytoskeleton consists of actin filaments and bridges made of spectrin. The plasma membrane and the cortical cytoskeleton are linked by pillars (see Holley, 1996, for review). Unlike other elongated cellular structure such as axons, the bulk of OHC interior is devoid of the cytoskeleton. For this reason, OHCs collapse and flatten when they are exposed to hyperosmotic media.

At least three kinds of stretch-sensitive channels are located in the lateral membrane of the cell. One is a potassium channel with about 130 pS unitary conductance (Ding *et al.*, 1991; Iwasa *et al.*, 1991). Currents through these channels are observed not only in a sealed membrane patch but also in the whole cell on increased membrane tension (Iwasa *et al.*, 1991). The mean open time of this channel is about 2.7 ms. It is still not clear how effectively these channels can be stimulated by axial force applied to OHCs. The lateral membrane also has stretch-sensitive, non-selective cation channels with unitary conductance between 38 pS and 50 pS found in the on-cell membrane patch configuration (Ding *et al.*, 1991). The other kind is channels with much smaller unit conductance, which are non-selective and pass anions (Rybalchenko & Santos-Sacchi, 2003). Because of the low conductance, these channels are unlikely to affect the membrane potential directly. However, their effect could be important because electromotility depends on Cl^- concentration on the cytosolic side of the plasma membrane (see the section on anion dependence).

This expectation is confirmed by an *in vivo* experiment in which internal Cl^- is altered by perfusing low Cl^- media in the scala tympani, thereby reducing the amplitude of basilar membrane vibration (Santos-Sacchi *et al.*, 2006). In addition, this channel could function as a sensor for the membrane motor if it could be stimulated by axial force applied to the cells (and could respond at the auditory frequencies) (Rybalchenko & Santos-Sacchi, 2003). However, that does not appear to be the case under physiological conditions because the Cl^- ionophore tributyltin can counteract the effect of reduced Cl^- concentration in the external medium (Santos-Sacchi *et al.*, 2006).

The plasma membrane is rich in prestin (Zheng *et al.*, 2000), which is essential for motile activity, and GLUT5, a glucose transporter protein (Géléoc *et al.*, 1999). Both of these proteins are reported to be involved in glucose transport. Glucose uptake in these cells is important because they are metabolically active and these cells are not in the immediate vicinity of blood vessels, the supply route for glucose. Glucose is the energy source of ATP synthesis in the mitochondria and ATP is required by calcium ATPase to pump out calcium ions entering from the MET channels. Prestin's role on motile responses will be described in a later section.

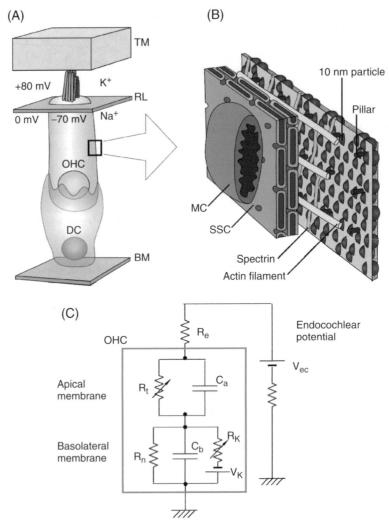

Fig. 6.1 An outer hair cell (OHC) and its equivalent circuit. (A) The environment of an OHC. The apical surface is exposed to the endolymph, which is high in K^+. The lateral surface is exposed to the perilymph. (B) Schematic representation of the lateral wall. The plasma membrane is packed with 10 nm particles. Under the plasma membrane, actin filaments run primarily in the circumferential direction and are bridged by spectrin. This cytoskeletal network is linked with the plasma membrane by structures called pillars. The subsurface cisternae (SSC) lie immediately inside of the lateral membrane. Numerous mitochondria (MC) are located next to the cisternae. (C) An equivalent circuit of an OHC (boxed). The apical membrane has the membrane capacitance C_a and resistance R_t, which is dominated by the MET channel. The basolateral membrane has the membrane capacitance C_b and membrane resistance R_b ($= R_n + R_K$). Receptor current through an external resistance R_e creates the cochlear microphonic. The time constant of the outer hair cell is $\sim R_b C_b$ because R_t is larger than R_b and C_b is larger than C_a. TM, tectorial membrane; RL, reticular lamina; DC, Deiters' cell; BM, basilar membrane.
Drawings in Figure 6.1A, B are credited to Janet Iwasa.

6.4 Electromotility: basic characterization

Here experimental and phenomenological observations are described that characterize electromotility. These descriptions will be re-examined in the section on modeling.

6.4.1 Length changes

With changes in membrane potential the cell body of OHCs undergoes graded changes in length called electromotility. Depolarization elicits shortening and hyperpolarization elongation (Fig. 6.2). The amplitude of length changes is up to 5% of the cell length in isolated cells without load. The membrane potential-dependence of the cell length L is well described by a two-state Boltzmann function (Ashmore, 1987),

$$L(V) = L_0 + \frac{\Delta L_{max}}{1 + \exp[\beta q^*(V - V_{1/2})]}$$

(6.1)

where V is the membrane potential, and $\beta = 1/k_B T$ with k_B Boltzmann's constant and T the temperature. ΔL_{max} and $V_{1/2}$ are constants representing the amplitude and the half-point potential, respectively. The quantity q^* represents phenomenological electric charge that determines the voltage sensitivity or 'voltage sensor', analogous to gating charge in voltage-gated ion channels. For this reason, it is sometimes called 'gating charge'.

The implication of Equation 6.1 is that motile responses of these cells are based on a motor with two conformational states, and that conformational changes between those states involve transfer of electric charge across the membrane. The phenomenological charge q^* has a value between 0.6 e and 1 e, which is rather variable. As shown later in modeling section, the quantity q^* is in most cases somewhat smaller than the real charge q, which is used to gain electrical energy that is converted into mechanical energy. This charge is perhaps more appropriately called 'unitary motor charge', because it is not associated with a control function as in 'gating' of ion channels. Equation (6.1) does not indicate whether the charge transferred is positive or negative because the effect of transferring a positive charge is energetically the same as transferring a negative charge in the opposite direction.

6.4.2 Charge transfer and non-linear capacitance

Length changes of OHCs are accompanied by transfer of charge across the plasma membrane (Ashmore, 1990) as expected from Equation (6.1), which can be analyzed in a manner similar to gating charge of voltage-gated ion channels. As with gating charge, this charge movement is elicited by changing the membrane potential. Thus, it can be observed as non-linear membrane capacitance (Santos-Sacchi, 1991). If changes in the cell length and charge transfer are tightly coupled, non-linear capacitance must have voltage dependence similar to dL/dV and thus we expect that the membrane capacitance C_m has two components,

$$C_m(V) = C_{lin} + 4C_{max} \frac{\exp[\beta q^*(V - V_{1/2})]}{1 + \exp[\beta q^*(V - V_{1/2})]^2}$$

(6.2)

where C_{lin} is the linear component due to the membrane structure and C_{max} is the peak of non-linear capacitance at $V_{1/2}$. Experimental data fit this relationship rather well (Santos-Sacchi, 1991).

The total charge Q of the motor transferred across the membrane is obtained by integrating non-linear capacitance over the voltage. Because Equation (6.2) assumes unitary charge transfer q^*, the number N^* of such motile units in the cell is phenomenologically obtained by $N^* = Q/q^*$.

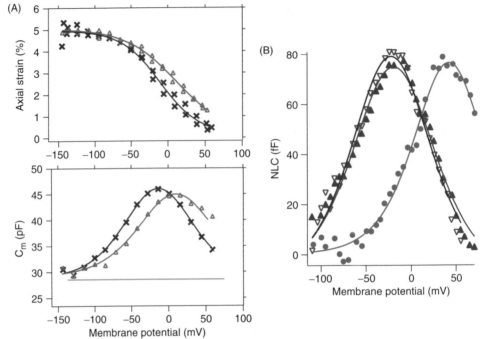

Fig. 6.2 Length changes and charge transfer of OHC elicited by voltage changes. (A) Length changes and (B) associated charge movement monitored as the membrane capacitance in response to changes in the membrane potential. When turgor pressure is increased by 0.4 kPa, the membrane potential dependence (×) shifts in the depolarizing direction by 27 mV (red). The charge parameter q^* slightly decreases from (0.81 ± 0.02) e to (0.75 ± 0.03) e. (B) In the experimental configuration of A and B, the pressure difference across the membrane depends not only on pipette pressure but on the membrane potential as well, bringing about negative cooperativity in voltage dependence and reducing q^* (see text in the model section). In the experimental configuration of C the pressure difference does not depend on the membrane potential. (C) Non-linear capacitance of a tight-sealed on cell patch formed at the lateral membrane. Zero pressure (control: Δ; recovery: ∇) and suction of 4 kPa at the pipette (red). The voltage shift is 60.3 mV. The charge parameter q^* is 1 e and it is unchanged. The data points are taken from Gale and Ashmore (1997b). Note that the value for the voltage sensitivity q is larger in Figure 6.2C than in Figure 6.2B. Figure 6.2A reproduced with permission from Adachi et al. (2000).

It has been noticed that the density of the motile units obtained with this method is $\sim 10^4/\mu m^2$, higher than the density of 10 nm particles by factor ~ 3 (Kalinec et al., 1992).

6.4.3 Axial stiffness and force production

For determining the axial stiffness and force production by OHCs, it is required to hold these cylindrical cells at two ends. One side needs to control or change the membrane potential, such as a patch pipette or suction pipette. The other side needs a force gauge such as a calibrated elastic probe made of glass fiber or an AFM tip (Fig. 6.3A). These force gauges either compress the cell at the cuticular place (Hallworth, 1995; Frank et al., 1999; He & Dallos, 1999) or pull the cell by the phalangeal process that connects with a neighboring OHC (Iwasa & Adachi, 1997).

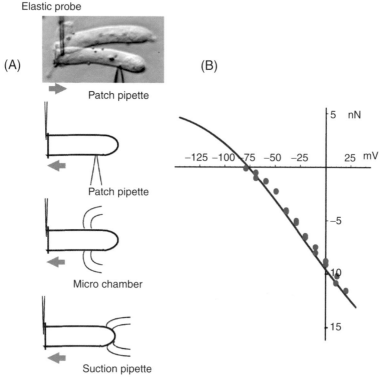

Fig. 6.3 Force produced by outer hair cells and methods for measurement. (A) Four recording configurations. From the top, the twin configuration in which the elastic probe is hooked to a remnant of the phalangeal process, the solo configuration, in which the cell is compressed by the probe at the apical surface, the microchamber configuration, and the suction pipette configuration. The arrows show the directions of force that the cell applies to the probe. (B) Isometric force production obtained by using the twin configuration. The slope is 0.1 nN/mV. Reproduced with permission from Iwasa and Adachi (1997).

The axial stiffness of OHCs reported is inversely proportional to the length as in ordinary elastic materials. In other words, the axial stiffness per unit length does not depend on cell length. The axial stiffness ranges between 40 nN and 750 nN per unit strain at about −70 mV (Hallworth, 1995; Iwasa & Adachi, 1997). These reported values depend on the laboratory where the experiments are performed, with some groups reporting a wider range of variability than others. It is likely that this variability is not an intrinsic property of these cells but it is due to some degree of damage inflicted on OHCs during the isolation process. Because it is hard to conceive that damage could lead to increased axial stiffness, it is likely that higher values for the stiffness reflect more intact conditions and therefore they are more physiological.

Isometric force production by OHCs can be obtained by using a probe much stiffer than the cell or by extrapolating to null displacement if the stiffness of the probe is comparable to that of the cell. In most cases, the reported values for isometric force are positively correlated with the values for the axial stiffness determined for the same preparation. The value for isometric force at peak slope is about 0.1 nN/mV (Fig. 6.3B) for those cells with the axial stiffness of about 500 nN per unit strain (Iwasa & Adachi, 1997).

6.4.4 Reciprocal effects

To examine the nature of the underlying mechanism of electromotility, it is important to determine whether or not imposed mechanical changes produce reciprocal changes in electrical properties. The effects of three types of mechanical conditions have been examined.

Axial displacement: reciprocal relationship

One such examination is to monitor membrane currents under voltage clamp while the length of the cell is changed. While the cell is being elongated by an external force applied in the axial direction, an inward current is observed. This current ceases when cell elongation ceases and reverses when the cell is being shortened. It is proportional to the speed of length changes. These properties are quite different from currents through mechanosensitive channels, which depend on the stress applied to the membrane. In addition, the current that is induced by length changes depends on the holding potential. It is maximal at the membrane potential where length change is most sensitive to voltage changes (Fig. 6.4A).

If the motile mechanism in the lateral wall of OHCs is based on mechanoelectric coupling analogous to piezoelectricity, a small increment ΔL in the cell length and a small increment ΔQ of motile charge can be related to a small increase ΔF of axial force and a small change ΔV of the membrane potential in the following manner,

$$\Delta L = c_{mm}\Delta F + c_{em}\Delta V, \tag{6.3}$$

$$\Delta Q = c_{me}\Delta F + c_{ee}\Delta V, \tag{6.4}$$

where c_{mm} is the axial compliance of the cell, c_{ee} is non-linear capacitance, and c_{me} and c_{em} are the coupling coefficients. Further, the coupling coefficients must satisfy Maxwell's reciprocal relationship $c_{me} = c_{em}$. This relationship leads to two testable expressions,

$$\left(\frac{\Delta Q}{\Delta F}\right)_V = \left(\frac{\Delta L}{\Delta V}\right)_V, \tag{6.5}$$

$$-\left(\frac{\Delta Q}{\Delta L}\right)_V = \left(\frac{\Delta F}{\Delta V}\right)_L. \tag{6.6}$$

To test the first equality, currents elicited by small axial force are measured under voltage clamp. The currents are then integrated over time to obtain charge transfer. This is to be compared the sensitivity of cell length to voltage changes in the load-free condition. The second equality is tested by measuring charge transfer induced by known length changes and isometric force production (Fig. 6.4B). The reciprocal relationship has been experimentally confirmed (Dong et al., 2002).

Pressure-induced membrane tension

Membrane tension can be increased by increasing the pressure difference across the plasma membrane. An increase in membrane tension induces a positive shift in the voltage dependence. Such shifts are observed in the whole-cell configuration by applying positive pressure through the recording pipette (Iwasa, 1993; Kakehata & Santos-Sacchi, 1995) as well as by applying negative pressure in a sealed patch configuration (Gale & Ashmore, 1997b). The tension sensitivity of the motor is determined as changes in the membrane area of the motor because the product of tension and membrane area is energy. It is analogous to the relationship between the membrane

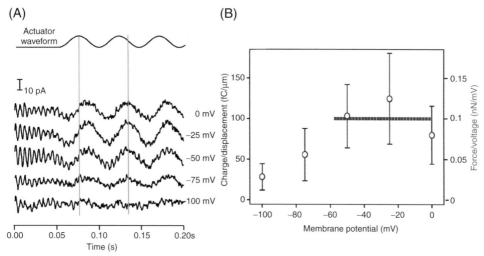

Fig. 6.4 The reciprocal relationship. (A) Currents elicited by stretching the cell. The cell was stretched with an elastic probe in the twin configuration (see Fig. 6.3) mounted in a piezoelectric actuator with a sinusoidal waveform (top). An upward deflection of the actuator waveform stretches the cell. The holding potential is indicated on the right. Downward deflections in the current trace correspond to inward currents. The phase of currents is advanced by about 90° from that of the stimulus (green lines). Ripples in the beginning show the resonance frequency of the system. (B) Charge transfer per length change (circles) and force produced per voltage changes (broken line) are plotted together to examine their equivalence.
Reproduced with permission from Dong *et al.* (2002).

potential and charge transfer. Tension sensitivity is therefore significant for modeling electromotility along with the voltage sensitivity. A more detailed account is given in Section 6.5.

Membrane area constraint

An OHC can be inflated into a sphere by applying positive pressure in the whole-cell recording configuration with a trypsin-containing patch pipette (see inset; Fig. 6.5). Using this configuration, it is possible to prevent the usual membrane area decrease by using a brief depolarization because the constriction at the tip of the recording pipette limits volume flow (Fig. 6.5B). Under this condition, if pressure applied from the pipette is above a certain threshold, the non-linear charge transfer evoked by a brief depolarization, which should reduce the membrane area, is suppressed (Fig. 6.5A,C). If the same depolarization is longer lasting, and fluid is allowed to pass the mouth of the pipette, a reduction of the radius, which corresponds to about 4% of the membrane area, is observed (Fig. 6.5F). These observations demonstrate that area changes and transfer of charge are tightly coupled (Adachi & Iwasa, 1999).

6.4.5 **Frequency response**

In order to test the frequency characteristics of electromotility, the voltage waveforms that drive the motile response must be delivered to the membrane without significant frequency-dependent attenuation. To achieve this bandwidth requirement, two experimental configurations are employed. One is the on-cell or detached patch mode of the patch clamping method. With this configuration, the membrane capacitance is monitored. Another is the microchamber configuration to monitor displacements of the cell.

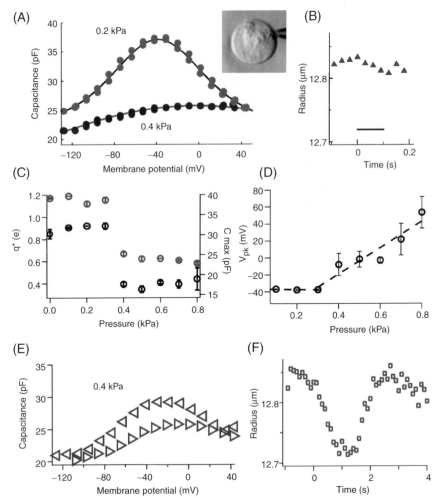

Fig. 6.5 A spherical cell with electromotility. An outer hair cell is inflated into a sphere with a patch pipette (inset). The waveform applied consists of a step from the holding potential of −75 mV to −130 mV, 10 mV steps to 50 mV, 10 mV steps back to −30 mV, and a step back to the holding potential. A–D are obtained when the waveform is run in 0.1 s (fast-run waveform), and E and F are obtained when it is run in 3.3 s (slow-run waveform). The fast-run waveform does not change the cell diameter (B) and non-linear capacitance becomes considerably flat when pressure exceeds 0.3 kPa (A, C). The voltage V_{pk} of flattened capacitance peak shifts with pressure above 0.3 kPa (D). The slow-run waveform decreases the diameter at depolarizing potentials and shows hysteresis in the membrane capacitance (E, F).
Reproduced with permission from Adachi and Iwasa (1999).

The microchamber configuration (see Fig. 6.3A) is formed by sucking the basal part of an OHC into a microchamber pipette. In this configuration, the lateral membrane is divided into two parts by the pipette wall and serves as capacitive voltage divider at high frequencies when waveforms are applied across the pipette. This allows application of high-frequency waveforms across the membrane without marked attenuation (Dallos & Evans, 1995a). In this configuration, load-free motion rolls off at between 10 kHz and 20 kHz (Fig. 6.6A). If a very stiff elastic probe is used to achieve near isometric condition, the frequency response is flat at least up to 50 kHz (Fig. 6.6B) (Frank *et al.*, 1999).

The membrane capacitance of sealed membrane patches formed on the lateral wall of OHCs rolls off at frequencies about 10 kHz (Fig. 6.6C) (Gale & Ashmore, 1997a; Dong *et al.*, 2000). Membrane noise, however, shows somewhat higher characteristic frequency of between 30 and 40 kHz (Fig. 6.6D). These experiments measure the speed of charge movement and not mechanical movement. However, these values should correspond to the frequency limit of membrane movement because charge movement is tightly coupled with mechanical movement. These results seem to imply that the intrinsic frequency limit of electromotility is hard to establish because of mechanoelectric coupling. Presumably, the frequency limits observed depend on the mode of vibration, indicating the importance of mechanical factors. This issue is discussed in the next section.

6.5 Modeling of electromotility

As the preceding section shows, various aspects of electromotility described phenomenologically on an *ad hoc* basis demonstrate that the underlying mechanism of electromotility is mechanoelectrical coupling. The objective of modeling is to describe these observations in a more unified manner for clearer understanding so that predictions for unexamined conditions can be made.

Several models have been proposed for electromotility. Those include models based on two-state membrane motor (Dallos *et al.*, 1993; Iwasa, 1993, 2001), piezoelectricity (Tolomeo & Steele, 1995), and membrane bending (Raphael *et al.*, 2000). Such models need to describe both the elastic property of OHCs and the voltage-sensitive motor. A model described in this section is a membrane model for OHCs combined with a two-state membrane motor model, which has the minimal number of adjustable parameters (Iwasa, 2001).

6.5.1 Cell geometry and membrane tension

Elastic displacements of OHCs can be described by a membrane model that assumes cylindrical geometry. Let the radius be R and the length L. If the pressure inside the cell is higher than outside by P, membrane tension T_1 in the axial direction is given by $\pi R^2 P / (2\pi R)$, and membrane tension T_2 in the circumferential direction is $2RLP/2L$. If the cell is held at both ends, it is possible to apply force F_{ex} in the axial direction, which results in tension $T_{ex} = F_{ex}/(2\pi R)$ in the axial direction. By choosing 1 for the suffix for the component in the axial direction and 2 in the circumferential direction, we obtain,

$$\begin{bmatrix} T_1 \\ T_2 \end{bmatrix} = \begin{bmatrix} \frac{1}{2}RP + T_{ex} \\ RP \end{bmatrix}$$

(6.7)

Membrane tension (T_1, T_2) must be balanced by elastic stress of the membrane. Here an elastic displacement $(\Delta x_1^e, \Delta x_2^e)$ is related to elastic strain $(\varepsilon_1^e, \varepsilon_2^e)$ by

$$\varepsilon_1^e = \Delta x_1^e / L,$$

(6.8)

$$\varepsilon_1^e = \Delta x_1^e / (2\pi R).$$

(6.9)

For a small elastic strain, the corresponding elastic stress is

$$\begin{bmatrix} g_{11} & g_{12} \\ g_{21} & g_{22} \end{bmatrix} \begin{bmatrix} \varepsilon_1^e \\ \varepsilon_2^e \end{bmatrix} = \begin{bmatrix} T_1 \\ T_2 \end{bmatrix}.$$

(6.10)

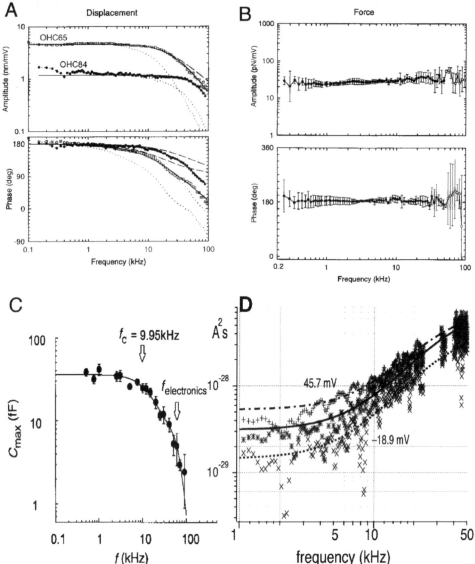

Fig. 6.6 The frequency dependence of electromotility. (A, B) Frequency dependence of axial movement. (C, D) Frequency of a tight-sealed membrane patch. (A) Load-free axial displacement. Amplitude (top) and phase (bottom) of two OHCs of different length. Recorded in the microchamber configuration. OHC65 is 83 μm long and has the corner frequencies of 9.5 kHz. OHC84 is 51 μm long and its corner frequency is 23.3 kHz. (B) Quasi-isometric force production. The cell is axially loaded by a stiff (6 N/m) AFM cantilever. Amplitude (top) and phase (bottom). The resonance above 50 kHz is instrumental, associated with the cantilever. (C) The voltage dependence of the membrane capacitance of sealed patches formed on the lateral membrane. Non-linear capacitance at high frequencies because the movement of motor charge cannot follow changes of the membrane potential. (D) The current noise spectra of a sealed patch. The traces are labeled with the pipette potential in on-cell configuration. The unlabeled middle traces are for 0 mV. Membrane noise is reduced at low frequencies by compensatory movement of motor charge. The effectiveness of this effect depends on the frequency response of the charge movement. The characteristic frequency is between 33 kHz and 40 kHz.
Figure 6.6A, B reproduced with permission from Frank *et al.* (1999), and Figure 6.6C reproduced with permission from Gale and Ashmore (1997b). Figure 6.6D reproduced with permission from Dong *et al.* (2000).

If the membrane is orthotropic, the elastic moduli satisfy $g_{12} = g_{21}$. If the membrane is isotropic, these moduli are expressed by an area modulus K and a shear modulus μ by $g_{11} = g_{22} = K + \mu$ and $g_{12} = g_{21} = K - \mu$.

If isotropy is assumed, the area and shear moduli can be determined by an experiment in which axial strain and circumferential strain is determined for a known pressure increase. During such an experiment, an increase in P results in an increase in the diameter and a reduction in length. The reason for this displacement is that the circumferential tension is twice as large as the axial tension due to the cylindrical geometry. The anisotropy in tension is combined with the property of the membrane that the area modulus K is larger than the shear modulus, that is, it needs less force to shear the membrane than changing its membrane area. If the stress–strain relationship in response to axial force is available in addition to the one for pressure, orthotropic assumptions for membrane elasticity can be used.

6.5.2 Models for membrane motor

Because a two-state Boltzmann function gives good fit to length changes and charge transfer across the membrane, it would be reasonable to assume that the membrane motor has two states analogous to open and closed states in ion channels. In the following, a simple two-state model and its predictions are described.

A two-state motor

In a two-state model, mechanoelectric coupling is realized by assuming that these two conformational states differ in charge as well as in membrane area. The free energy difference ΔG between the two states can be expressed by,

$$\Delta G = \Delta G_0 - qV - \mathbf{a} \cdot \mathbf{T}_m, \tag{6.11}$$

where the first term is a constant, the second term electrical energy due to unitary motor charge q, and the term mechanical energy associated with a difference in the membrane area $\mathbf{a}$ (Fig. 6.7).

Unitary motor charge q does not need to be an integer multiplied by the electronic charge e because this charge does not have to move from one surface of the membrane to the other. The mechanical part can be expressed by the sum of its axial and circumferential components as $a_1 T_1 + a_2 T_2$, where a_1 and a_2 are components of area change in the axial and the circumferential directions, respectively. Considering the two components in the area change is required because membrane tension $\mathbf{T}_m$ is anisotropic due to the cell's cylindrical geometry.

The probability P_e that the motor is in the extended conformation is then proportional to $\exp[-\beta \Delta G]$ with the Boltzmann factor $\beta = 1/k_B T$. With normalization this relationship is expressed,

$$P_e = \frac{1}{1 + \exp[\beta \Delta G]}. \tag{6.12}$$

This means that the surface area of the cell and the motor charge follows the Boltzmann distribution and that the non-linear capacitance is the voltage derivative of the Boltzmann function. Because the Boltzmann function has a sigmoidal voltage-dependence, its voltage derivative is bell-shaped, with a peak at $V_{1/2}$, the steepest slope of the Boltzmann function.

The total charge transfer, which is obtained by integrating the non-linear capacitance over the voltage, is given by Q_{max}. The number N of the motor is obtained by

$$N = Q_{max} / q. \tag{6.13}$$

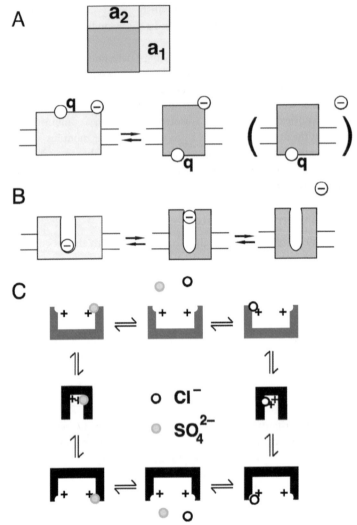

Fig. 6.7 Models for the membrane motor. (A) A two-state area motor model. The motor charge q can be positive or negative. The model does not assume the physical mechanism for the charge transfer. Ignoring the inactive state can be justified if transitions between the active and inactive states are slow. (B) An anion shuttle model proposed by Oliver et al. (2001) assumes three states for the motor, two of which bind an anion in different locations along the pore. (C) An anion counterporter model assumes six states for the motor. Cl$^-$ (unfilled circle) is transported from the cytosol to the extracellular space and SO$_4^{2-}$ (filled circle) is transported in the opposite direction. This model involves movement of ions as well as intrinsic charges of the motor protein. Reproduced with permission from Muallem and Ashmore (2006).

What is the effect of increasing membrane tension? An increase in membrane tension raises the energy of the state with smaller membrane area more than that of the state with larger membrane area. Thus such a change favors the extended state at a given voltage. The midpoint potential $V_{1/2}$ then shifts in the positive direction to enlarge the domain of the extended state, which dominates at negative membrane potentials.

What is the effect of a chemical that preferentially binds to one conformation of the motor? It does not change the motor charge but changes ΔG_0. This shifts the midpoint voltage $V_{1/2}$. If the motor charge q is affected by the binding of a chemical, the steepness of the voltage dependence is expected to change. Then the total charge transfer Q_{max} should also change to keep the number N of the motor constant.

Models with more than two states

Two-state models can provide a reasonable description of the experimental data. However, that does not exclude alternatives, such as three-state models and continuous models. One strong point of two-state models is that they are simpler than the alternative models. Another, more substantive, point is that numerous factors, such as changes in membrane tension, binding of chemicals, and mutation of molecules, tend to shift $V_{1/2}$, but not voltage sensitivity. In two-state models these interactions simply favor one state over another, resulting in shifts in the voltage dependence. There are, however, experimental data that cannot be explained by two-state models. This includes the effect of salicylate and the effect of reducing the cytosolic Cl^- concentration. Salicylate reduces voltage sensitivity. In two-state models, such a change would require a reduction of unitary charge transferred during conformational changes.

The replacement of Cl^- with pentanesulfonate results in reducing the total charge transfer Q_{max} without changing the motor charge q. To be able to explain this Cl^- concentration dependence, it is necessary to introduce at least one additional conformational state of the motor, which does not undergo conformational transitions in response to voltage changes. These issues are discussed in more detail in Section 6.7.1.

It is possible that a multiple state model is approximated in many situations by a simpler two-state model, given the success of two-state models. Such reduction can take place if those models have a small number of rate-limiting steps. In this regard, it would be of interest to determine whether or not such simplification is possible with an anion exchanger model, which has six conformational states (Muallem & Ashmore, 2006).

6.5.3 Incorporating the motor into the cell

The simplest way the membrane motor is incorporated into the cell model is to assume that the cell's displacement is the sum of elastic displacement (Δx_1, Δx_2) and motor displacement. By introducing the cell's strain ($\Delta x_1^e, \Delta x_2^e$),

$$\varepsilon_1 = \Delta x_1 / L, \tag{6.14}$$

$$\varepsilon_1 = \Delta x_2 / (2\pi R). \tag{6.15}$$

the assumption is expressed by,

$$\varepsilon_j = \varepsilon_j^e + nP_e a_j, \tag{6.16}$$

where n is the density of the motor molecule and the suffix j runs from 1 to 2, that is, the axial and the circumferential components. This equation also requires a *homogenization* approximation that the boundary effect between the motor and the rest of the membrane can be ignored. It also requires a simplifying assumption that the elastic moduli of the motor are the same as the rest of the membrane.

The response of the cell to electric and mechanical stimuli can be described by combining Equations 6.7, 6.10, 6.11, 6.12, and 6.16. In the following, the cell's response in a number of conditions will be examined.

Response to pressure changes

Here we consider an increase in the pressure across the plasma membrane either by hypo-osmotic perfusion or fluid injection through a patch pipette in the whole-cell recoding configuration. In both cases, cell volume increases. Cell displacement stops when the force due to the pressure difference is balanced by tension.

An increase in the pressure across the membrane increases membrane tension and lowers the free energy of the conformation with larger membrane area. This effect is in the opposite direction of the elastic response, which shortens the cell. Because the elastic response is dominant, the contribution of the motor is not distinctly observed in the displacements of the cell. The response of the motor to pressure is, however, clearly observed as voltage shifts in the non-linear capacitance. Let a voltage shift ΔV_p takes place due to a pressure increase ΔP. In the absence of externally applied axial force, the voltage shift is expressed by,

$$q\Delta V_p = \tfrac{1}{2}(a_1 + 2a_2)R\Delta P,$$ (6.17)

because the voltage shift ΔV_p and pressure increase ΔP have the same effect on the free energy ΔG, expressed by Equation 6.11, which determines P_e. This condition can be used to determine area changes from the unitary motor charge.

To determine the area change a $(=a_1+a_2)$ of the motor, membrane tension must be isotropic. This can be achieved by making the cell membrane spherical. One such configuration is a tight-sealed membrane patch formed on the lateral membrane of OHCs. The corresponding relationship between pressure increase and voltage shift for spherical geometry is

$$q\Delta V_p = \tfrac{1}{2}a_1 R_s \Delta P,$$ (6.18)

where R_s is the radius of the sphere. The main technical difficulty of determining the area difference a lies in measuring the radius R_s of the sealed membrane patch. An alternative experimental configuration is the whole-cell recording from a cell inflated into a sphere with trypsin-containing patch pipette. The radius R_s of curvature is readily available with this preparation (see Fig. 6.5). Using the spherical cell preparation affords alternative methods of determining the area change a, including a more direct one by measuring diameter changes during voltage waveforms imposed on the membrane while keeping a steady pressure difference across the membrane (Adachi & Iwasa, 1999).

Response to rapid voltage changes

During rapid voltage changes that last a fraction of a second, volume flow is usually negligible. For this reason, the response of the cell can be adequately described by the combined equations given above with a constant volume constraint. Under this condition, the phenomenological unitary motor charge q^* determined from non-linear capacitance is smaller than the real charge q.

Suppose the cell with cylindrical geometry has initial turgor pressure. A positive-going change in membrane potential V favors the compact conformation of the motor because of the electric term in the free energy difference ΔG. The resulting reduction in the membrane area would increase pressure, resulting in increased membrane tension. Increased membrane tension would favor the extended state owing to the mechanical term in the free energy difference ΔG. The opposite effect is expected for the response to a negative-going pulse. In both cases this negative feedback reduces conformational changes of the motor for a given change of the membrane potential. This reduced sensitivity to voltage changes leads to an apparent motor charge q^* that is smaller than the real value q.

The significance of negative cooperativity mediated by pressure can be experimentally tested by deflating and collapsing the cell with negative pressure applied to the recording patch pipette. Under this condition negative cooperativity between motor molecules is not expected because conformational changes of the motors can change the surface area without changing the pressure across the membrane. Experiments show that collapsing cells increases the apparent motor charge q^* by about 10%. Increased voltage sensitivity is accompanied by a negative shift in the voltage dependence due to nullified membrane tension that favors the compact conformation at a given membrane potential. This analysis indicates that the value for the phenomenological number N^* of motile units obtained from non-linear capacitance experiments is an overestimate of only 10% and does not markedly affect the comparison with the number of 10 nm particles. Thus the number of motile units is close to the number of 10 nm particles.

Another test of the model is to increase initial turgor pressure (see Fig. 6.2A). The model predicts positive shifts in the voltage dependence without changes in the steepness of voltage dependence. The pressure in the cell during application of a voltage waveform is the sum of the initial pressure and the component that depends only on the membrane potential provided that the cell is initially not collapsed. Thus a voltage shift obtained from experiments in which cell volume is held constant is determined by the difference in the initial pressure. The voltage sensitivity is less than that of collapsed cells due to voltage-dependent pressure changes. This means that Equations (6.17) and (6.18) can be used for determining the motor displacement a from experimental conditions under which cell volume does not change. However, using an apparent charge q^* that is determined by the slope of voltage dependence under such an experimental condition instead of q would lead to an error.

Experiments show that the voltage shifts indeed depend on applied pressure as predicted by the model (see Fig. 6.2A). However, experimental data often show reduced steepness, particularly when the pressure applied is large and the cell becomes barrel-shaped as the result. The departure from the prediction is attributed to the deformation of the cell in those cases. Since an inhomogeneity in the diameter leads to inhomogeneity of membrane tension, non-linear capacitance of the cell as a whole is expected to turn into a broader bell-shaped voltage dependence. This interpretation is supported by the observation that the capacitance of sealed patches formed on the lateral membrane shows voltage shifts (see Fig. 6.2B) without reducing the steepness of voltage dependence (Gale & Ashmore, 1997b).

In the following, an outline of a more mathematical analysis is presented. By using the constant volume condition $\varepsilon_1 + 2\varepsilon_2 = const$, the axial strain ε_1 can be expressed by

$$\varepsilon_1 = F_{ex} + b_1 P_e + b_0, \tag{6.19}$$

where b_1 and b_2 are constants. The initial volume of the cell, which is determined by turgor pressure is represented in b_0. The factor b_1, defined by,

$$b_1 = 2g[a_1(2d_1 - c) + a_2(2c - d_2)] \tag{6.20}$$

with

$$g = \frac{1}{4d_1 - 4c + d_2} \tag{6.21}$$

depends on the displacements of a motor molecule during its conformational changes and the elastic moduli of the cell. Here d_1, d_2, and c are the elastic moduli and a_1 and a_2 are the two components of motor's area changes. This is the efficiency with which axial external force F_{ex} affects the axial displacement of the cell. Here the factor g is the quantity that determines the axial compliance, as we will see later.

The free energy difference ΔG that determines the probability P_e of the extended state can be expressed as

$$\Delta G = -qV - b_1 F_{ex} + b_2 k_B T P_e + b_3 \qquad (6.22)$$

where a constant b_2, which is

$$b_2 = \beta gn(d_1 d_2 - c^2)(a_1 + 2a_2) \qquad (6.23)$$

introduces negative cooperativity between motor molecules. The constant b_3 depends on the initial volume of the cell, reflecting turgor pressure. The set of equations that describe the cell can be reduced to (Iwasa, 2001),

$$\beta(qV + b_1 F_{ex}) = b_2 P_e - \ln\left(\frac{1}{P_e} - 1\right) + b_3 \qquad (6.24)$$

This equation is somewhat complicated to solve if we attempt to obtain P_e for a given set of V and F_{ex}. However, it is simpler to solve in the opposite direction. If we fix the external force F_{ex} applied to the cell and give a value of the probability P_e to the extended state, the membrane potential V can be determined by the equation. Because the motor molecules have negative cooperativity, the membrane potential V is a monovalent function of the probability P_e. Once the value for V is determined for a given set of vales for F_{ex} and P_e, all variables including the cell displacements can be calculated.

Although the description presented above is for voltage changes, the result obtained, that is, Equation 6.24, is symmetrical with respect to the membrane potential V and axial force F_{ex}. This symmetry implies that the effect of axial force can be described in a manner similar to voltage dependence.

6.5.4 Piezoelectric description

The result of the model can be presented in a form more familiar to descriptions of piezoelectricity by examining the responses to small changes in the membrane potential V and axial force F_{ex}. An increment ΔQ in charge and an increment ΔL in the cell length can be expressed by

$$\Delta Q = Nq\Delta P_e + C_{lin}\Delta V, \qquad (6.25)$$

$$\Delta L = b_1 nL\Delta P_e + b_4\Delta F, \qquad (6.26)$$

where N is the total number of the motor molecules, C_{lin} is the linear, or regular, membrane capacitance of the cell due to its structure (somewhat less than $1\ \mu F/cm^2$), and b_4 is the axial compliance of the cell due to the material property, which is expressed by

$$b_4 = 2g\frac{L}{\pi R}, \qquad (6.27)$$

where g is defined by Equation (6.21).

By using Equation 6.24, we can obtain

$$\Delta Q = c_{ee}\Delta V + c_{em}\Delta F_{ex}, \qquad (6.28)$$

$$\Delta L = c_{me}\Delta V + c_{mm}\Delta F_{ex}, \qquad (6.29)$$

where the coefficients are now expressed with the model parameters,

$$c_{ee} = a\beta Nq^2 P_e(1 - P_e) + C_{lin},$$

(6.30)

$$c_{mm} = a\beta nb_1^2 \frac{L}{2\pi R} P_e(1 - P_e) + b_4,$$

(6.31)

$$c_{em} = c_{me} = a\beta nLqb_1 P_e(1 - P_e).$$

(6.32)

where the factor α ($= 1/[1 + b_2 P_e]$) represents the negative cooperativity factor.

Here c_{ee} is the membrane capacitance and c_{mm} is the axial compliance. They are symmetrical in having two components. One is based on the material property of the cell and the other is based on conformational changes of the motor molecules. Non-linear capacitance is the component of the membrane capacitance associated with conformational changes of the motor. The counterpart in the axial compliance is an analog of 'gating compliance' observed during hair bundle displacements.

The quantity c_{em}, which is the same as c_{me}, is the piezoelectric coefficient. The value for this coefficient is ~25 μC/N for OHCs 50 μm long at the optimal voltage at which $P_e = 0.5$. This value is much larger than 2.5 nC/N for the best man-made piezoelectric material, respectively (Iwasa, 2001). The values for quartz and Rochelle salt are between 2 and 4 pC/N and ~0.5 nC/N.

Another characteristic coefficient for piezoelectric materials is the coupling coefficient k, defined by

$$k^2 = \frac{c_{em}c_{me}}{c_{ee}c_{mm}}.$$

(6.33)

This quantity represents the fraction of energy converted from one form to another. The coupling coefficient k for OHCs is ~0.3. The coupling coefficients for quartz and Rochelle salt are 0.1 and 0.76, respectively.

Comparison with piezoelectric materials

OHCs have mechanoelectric coupling similar to piezoelectricity, but with two distinctive features:

◆ First, the mechanoelectric coupling mechanism in OHCs is non-linear instead of linear. One way of explaining this is that the motor in OHCs has only two states instead of the continuum of states in ordinary piezoelectric materials. However, that does not exclude other explanations and indeed alternative explanations for the non-linearity are also possible.

◆ Second, the piezoelectric coefficient of OHCs at the optimal operating point is orders of magnitude higher than the best man-made piezoelectric materials. However, this property is due to the cell's much higher compliance compared with those piezoelectric materials, which are solids. For this reason the coupling coefficient of OHCs is not particularly high.

Voltage dependence of the axial stiffness

The axial compliance depends on the material properties of the lateral membrane, which we assume are independent of the membrane potential or applied axial force. The axial compliance has another component that depends on conformational changes of the motor. Because an increase in the (extensive) axial force makes the extended state energetically more favorable to the compact state, it induces conformational changes that result in an additional elongation, which contributes to the compliance. This term is analogous to non-linear capacitance and maximizes

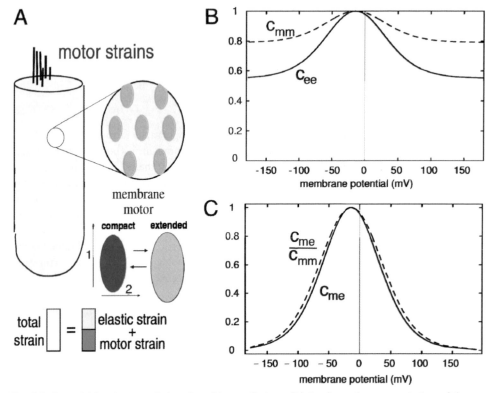

Fig. 6.8 A model for the outer hair cell and its predictions. (A) A schematic representation of the model. The cell is approximated by a cylinder with length L and radius R at the reference state. The total strains are the sum of elastic strains and motor strains. The motor strains are due to conformational changes of the motor, which involve transfer of charge and changes of its membrane area. The elastic strains are balanced with membrane tension due to pressure difference. (B) The membrane capacitance c_{ee} and the axial compliance c_{mm}, predicted by the model. (C) The piezoelectric coefficient c_{me} ($=c_{em}$), which corresponds to the load-free amplitude, and the ratio c_{me}/c_{mm}, which corresponds to isometric force production. The parameter values for the model are: for elastic moduli, $d_1 = c = 0.046$ N/m, and $d_2 = 0.068$ N/m. For the motor, $q = 0.9 e$, $a_1 = 4.5$ nm^2, and $a_2 = -0.75$ nm^2. The density n of the motor is 9×10^3 μm^{-2}. This set of values gives $c_{ee}-C_{lin} = 17$ pF, $c_{me} = 2 \times 10^{-5}$ m/V or C/N, and c_{mm}(max) $= 118$ m/N. See Iwasa (2001) for details. Figure 6.6B, C reproduced with permission from Iwasa (2001).

where the ratio of the two states is 1:1. Therefore it has a bell-shaped dependence on membrane potential (Fig. 6.8).

Experimental data on apical hair cells show a monotonic increase of compliance on depolarization. The predicted compliance reaches the maximum, which is about 20% higher than at –75 mV, at the membrane potential of about –20 mV that also maximizes the membrane capacitance. However, the experimental observation at the voltage is about 50% higher at this membrane potential and increases further with more depolarized potential (He & Dallos, 1999). This observation is in contrast to experimental data on more basal cells reported by another group. Those data do not show such large monotonic voltage-dependent changes in the axial compliance but are rather flat, allowing about 20% uncertainty (Hallworth, 2007). This result is compatible with the prediction of a 20% increase in the axial compliance even though it does not show an analog of gating compliance.

Is there any way of explaining these two starkly contrasting experimental observations? Suppose the two conformational states of the motor have different compliance as well as different membrane area. If the material compliance of the motor is important in determining the compliance of the lateral wall, the axial compliance would depend on the conformational state of the motor. That may not be unreasonable because the membrane motor occupies a substantial part of the plasma membrane (see next section on the role of cytoskeleton).

From the view point of protein structure, such an expectation could be reasonable to some extent. The compact conformation, which has more degrees of freedom toward extension, may be more compliant than the extended conformation. However, such a difference in stiffness may be valid only for a small stress. If it is also valid for a large stress, the compact state would have to become larger than the extended state! Such a reversal in size would be unphysical. According to a rough estimate, the critical stress for such a reversal corresponds to about 0.1 kPa turgor pressure (Iwasa, 2006). This could explain the variability of the data on the axial compliance. The experimental condition that shows monotonic voltage dependence would require turgor pressure below 0.1 kPa. If turgor pressure exceeds this threshold, two conformational states of the motor should have the same material compliance. Indeed, the difference in the motor's membrane area is determined in a pressure range much larger than 0.1 kPa.

Role of the cytoskeleton

The model presented is constructed in such a way that its parameters can be determined by experiments. This may leave some questions as to how physical the model is. In other words, how far is such a model useful in deducing molecular properties?

A specific issue is that the model does not include a factor that maintains the cylindrical shape of the cell. The characteristic cylindrical shape of the cell must be maintained by the cytoskeleton. Indeed, OHCs that are internally digested with trypsin cannot maintain their characteristic shape. The model simply assumes the cylindrical geometry of the cell. Another observation that could be related is that the elastic moduli of the membrane are smaller than the values expected from lipid bilayers. A possible explanation of these problems could be that the cortical cytoskeleton that underlies the plasma membrane itself contributes significantly to the mechanical properties of the lateral wall of OHCs. If the membrane motor is sensitive only to tension applied to the plasma membrane, which is a fraction of the total, the area changes of the motor during conformational changes must be much larger than the value obtained using the model described.

This issue can be experimentally examined by using OHCs that are internally treated with trypsin. Such a preparation can be created by injecting trypsin into the cell from the patch pipette in the whole-cell configuration. With this preparation, the absence of the cortical cytoskeleton is confirmed from their response to pressure. Positive pressure inflates those cells, transforming them into a spherical shape (see Fig. 6.5). Unlike untreated cells, those treated cells do not revert to the cylindrical shape but remain round even when suction is applied. The area modulus of the plasma membrane determined by measuring the diameter of the sphere for given values of pressure is (0.13 ± 0.02) N/m, somewhat larger than for the lateral wall of untreated cells. This value is within the range between 0.1 N/m to 0.2 N/m obtained for lipid bilayers (Evans & Rawicz, 1990). This observation indicates that the plasma membrane is an important factor in determining the area modulus of the intact lateral wall of OHCs.

The effects of internal digestion by trypsin suggest that the cortical cytoskeleton is indeed important for maintaining the cylindrical shape of these cells. However, it also suggests that a major part of the stress applied to the cell is applied to the motor through the plasma membrane.

For this reason, the estimate of area changes of the motor should be not grossly in error. Nonetheless it is clear that the functional significance of the highly organized structure of the lateral wall is largely unexplored. This structure includes the subsurface cisternae, the cortical cytoskeleton that involves actin and spectrin, the plasma membrane, of which a substantial part is made of 10 nm particles, and the pillars that bridge the cortical cytoskeleton to the plasma membrane (Fig. 6.1B). Among those factors, the predominantly circumferential orientation of actin filaments may be reflected in the anisotropy of the elastic moduli.

6.5.5 Non-elastic elements

Can the passive (non-motile) properties of OHCs be simply elastic? Polymeric and biological materials tend to have viscoelasticity. If that is the case for OHCs, such a property could have a marked effect on electromotility.

An experimental observation relevant to this is that non-linear capacitance shows hysteresis (Santos-Sacchi *et al.*, 1998). Holding the cell at a hyperpolarized potential has the effect of shifting the peak of non-linear capacitance in the depolarizing direction. The opposite is true for depolarization. This effect does not depend on turgor pressure and is explained as viscoelastic relaxation of the lateral membrane. The characteristic relaxation times are 1.3 s and 70 ms, even the slower being shorter than the cytoskeletal relaxation time of about 20 s (Ehrenstein & Iwasa, 1996). The shift in the voltage dependence is about 15 mV for a 160 mV difference in the holding potential. This observation is likely due to viscoelastic relaxation around motor molecules. However, these relaxation times are much longer than the periods of acoustic stimulation. The voltage differences that manifest this effect are much larger than those occurring physiologically. For these reasons, viscoelastic effects are unlikely to affect electromotility. Indeed, force measurements do not show clear frequency dependence (Frank *et al.*, 1999).

6.5.6 Frequency response

Because electromotility is based on mechanoelectric coupling, the frequency response can be determined by mechanical factors in a manner similar to piezoelectric materials. Absence of resonance in experimental data of isolated OHCs indicate that a kinetic term can be ignored in such experimental conditions. Then the equation of motion can be described in the form

$$\eta \frac{dx}{dt} = -kx + F(t)$$

(6.34)

where η is the drag coefficient, k the stiffness, and F the force generated by electromotility. The frequency response of such a system is determined by the ratio k/η. If the amplitude of the motion is constrained by an elastic load k_c, the frequency response is determined by $(k+k_c)/\eta$ unless the elastic load is accompanied by substantial drag. This explains why the frequency response is higher (> 50 kHz) at isometric condition than in load free condition (~ 20 kHz).

In addition, this explanation seems to be consistent with the observed frequency dependence. For example, the membrane capacitance of sealed membrane patches rolls off at a lower frequency (~ 10 kHz) than does the motile response of axial elongation and contraction (10–20 kHz). This may reflect a different stiffness/friction ratio in the two different modes of motion. The differing frequency dependence of membrane capacitance (~ 10 kHz), which is associated with collective motion of a tight-sealed membrane patch, and membrane noise (~ 30 kHz), which reflects movement of individual unitary motor charge, are other examples. These observations suggest that different modes of motion have different stiffness/drag ratios, leading to different frequency dependence (Dong *et al.*, 2000).

6.6 Effects of electromotility

The effects of electromotility have been examined by various means, *in vitro* as well as *in vivo*. These studies use pharmacological, molecular genetic, and electrophysiological means as well as the combination of any of the three. Here, this issue is discussed from a mechanistic viewpoint.

6.6.1 Displacement of the organ of Corti by electromotility

Perhaps the most direct approach of examining the effect of electromotility would be the application of an AC electric field applied across the cochlear partition *in vivo* as well and *in vitro* (Xue *et al.*, 1995). Those experiments show that such stimulation induces displacement of the organ of Corti as well as that of the basilar membrane. These effects are eliminated by inhibitors of electromotility such as salicylate. These experiments show that electromotility has a significant effect in the ear if the membrane potential across the cell body of OHC is large enough. The question is whether or not electromotility is important under physiological conditions.

6.6.2 RC time constant problem

Electromotile output is sufficiently fast to encompass auditory frequencies under isometric conditions (Frank *et al.*, 1999). However, it is driven by the receptor potential, which is highly attenuated at the OHC's operating frequencies due to the inherent electric circuit properties. Changing the membrane potential of the cell requires charging and discharging the capacitor formed by the plasma membrane (see Fig. 6.1B). Because capacitive conductance increases with the frequency whereas the ohmic conductance does not, the resulting electric characteristic of the circuit is low pass with the time constant determined by the resistor-capacitor (RC) circuit. Under *in vitro* conditions, the membrane resistance of OHCs in the third turn is about 50 MΩ and the membrane capacitance is about 20 pF. The roll-off frequency of the resulting low-pass filter is then 160 Hz, which is about one-tenth of the characteristic frequency of the location. Thus this factor would attenuate the amplitude by a factor 10. This is known as the 'RC time constant problem.'

Counteracting viscous damping

In examining the RC time constant problem, it is important to set a scale with which to assess the importance of the attenuation. Instead of seeking a sufficient condition for the cochlear amplifier, it would be much simpler to examine necessary conditions. One such condition is that the force must be sufficient for counteracting viscous damping. Since the shear motion between the tectorial membrane and the reticular lamina must be the major source of viscous drag (Allen, 1980), it would be reasonable to compare the magnitude of the force generated by electromotility with this viscous force to address this issue.

Viscous drag in the gap between the tectorial membrane and the reticular lamina can be estimated by assuming that the gap at a given location is the same as the length of the tallest stereocilia of OHCs, which is embedded in the tectorial membrane. Because the thickness of the boundary layer is larger than the gap, the formula for laminar flow should provide good estimates. The drag due to the stereocilia does not contribute if the fluid in the gap is driven by the shear motion between the two plates. However, certain assumptions regarding cochlear mechanics need to be made. These assumptions include that the ratio of basilar membrane motion and shear at the gap (we assume the ratio is 1:1) and that the phase of electromotility is optimal in counteracting drag. With these assumptions, it can be shown that electromotility counteracts viscous drag up to about 10 kHz (Ospeck *et al.*, 2003), which is appreciable but still does not reach the higher end of the auditory range. Thus a mechanism that counteracts capacitive currents and extends the frequency limit is required. One such mechanism can be fast potassium currents because such currents have, similar to an inductance, the opposite phase of capacitive currents, and can counteract capacitive current.

Indeed, in the guinea pig cochlea, fast K^+ currents are found in the basal turn, which is mapped to frequency higher than about 7 kHz. Such fast currents are not found in more apical turns. This may indicate that these fast K^+ currents help counteract capacitive currents and reduce the attenuation of the receptor potential by the RC filter. Thus, this finding supports this line of argument. However, the effectiveness of this current in counteracting capacitive currents still needs to be determined.

Role of the cochlear microphonic

Recall that a high-frequency electric potential can be applied effectively across the plasma membrane in the microchamber configuration (see Fig. 6.3A). The *in vivo* condition is somewhat similar to this experimental configuration because tight junctions that link OHCs with supporting cells at the cuticular plate divide the OHC membrane into two parts, apical and basolateral in a manner similar to the glass wall of the microchamber pipette.

If an AC electric field is applied across the reticular lamina, the apical and the basolateral membranes of OHCs work as a voltage divider. The voltage drop is determined by the ratio of the admittance between their apical and basolateral membranes. At low frequencies the potential is primarily determined by the ratio of ionic conductance and at high frequencies their potential is determined primarily by the ratio of membrane capacitance. If the capacitance and resistance ratios are similar, the membrane potential has a frequency dependence similar to that of the external field.

The cochlear microphonic is an AC electric field with a relatively small frequency dependence. This potential is produced primarily by transducer currents of OHCs flowing through extracellular space. This induces an AC potential across the lateral membrane of OHCs, including those not performing mechanoelectric transduction. The frequency dependence of this AC membrane potential is similar to that of the cochlear microphonic and is not subjected to the RC filter of the cell (Dallos & Evans, 1995b). However, OHCs that are performing mechanoelectric transduction and generating the cochlear microphonic have a receptor potential which is subject to the RC filter. That is because adding an extracellular resistance does not increase the receptor potential (see Fig. 6.1C). Thus, somewhat paradoxically, a non-performing cell can have a 'parasitic' receptor potential larger than the genuine receptor potential of performing cells at high frequencies. The reason for this 'paradox' is in the phase. The effect of the cochlear microphonic on the receptor potential of performing cells is canceled by their own transducer currents because of the phase difference at those high frequencies.

This effect is of little importance among OHCs in the same lateral location in the cochlea. However, it could be important as interaction between OHCs at different locations near the characteristic frequency where the wavelength of the traveling wave is short. That is, the cochlear microphonic generated by transducer current at the characteristic location of the stimulation frequency could drive OHCs which are located slightly more basally by generating a parasitic receptor potential. Those cells are indeed in the location logical for amplifying the traveling wave. Despite its possible importance, quantitative analysis of this effect has not been reported beyond measuring the cochlear microphonic.

6.7 Molecular mechanism and regulation

6.7.1 Significance of anions

Earlier studies of electromotility were performed in the whole-cell recording configuration of the patch clamp method using intracellular media that contain Cl^- at relatively high concentrations, and the dependence on Cl⁻ concentration was not noticed. To observe a clear effect of reduced Cl⁻, the concentration has to be reduced below 5 mM. When Cl⁻ is replaced by pentanesulfonate, electromotility is reversibly eliminated (Fig. 6.9A). At 150 mM concentration, charge transfer due to electromotility is in the order $I^- \approx Br^- > NO^- > Cl^- > HCO^- > F^-$ for monovalent anions (Oliver et al., 2001), consistent with the Hofmeister series (Cacace et al., 1997). Despite the difference in the peak capacitance, their voltage dependence is similar. The capacitance-voltage plots superpose well if their peaks are normalized.

The charge transfer due to electromotility also decreases with increasing alkyl chain length when carboxylic acids are used. However, in this case, the motor charge q decreases together with the total charge transfer with increasing chain length (Oliver et al., 2001). The important role of anions is further demonstrated by the observation that salicylate, which is an amphipathic anion and also an inhibitor of electromotility, competes with Cl⁻ for the anion-binding site of the motor molecule. That is, the inhibitive action of salicylate is to exclude Cl⁻ from the anion-binding site of the motor molecule (Oliver et al., 2001).

The effect of salicylate, however, does not fit the pattern of other anions. Salicylate reduces the voltage sensitivity, indicating that the unitary motor charge is reduced. However, the total charge transfer Q_{max}, which is obtained by integrating non-linear capacitance over the voltage, does not appear to be markedly affected (Fig. 6.9B). Thus the apparent number N^* of the motile units must increase.

Motor charge

A model proposed to explain the dependence on anions is that the movement of anions, Cl⁻ under physiological conditions, within the motor molecule is coupled with conformational transitions

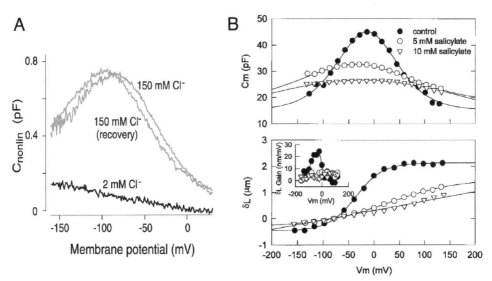

Fig. 6.9 Effect of anions. (A) Effect of cytosolic Cl⁻ concentration on the non-linear capacitance of a prestin-transfected CHO cell. Cl⁻ is replaced by pentanesulfonate. (B) Effects of salicylate on the membrane capacitance (top) and load-free displacement (bottom). Notice that salicylate reduces the peak height of non-linear capacitance but it elevates the capacitance at both ends of the membrane potential. The inset in the bottom figure shows the voltage sensitivity.

Figure 6.9A reproduced with permission from Oliver et al. (2001). Figure 6.9B reproduced with permission from Kakehata and Santos-Sacchi (1996).

of the motor (Oliver *et al.*, 2001). This model has certain attractiveness because anions with longer chain lengths would travel shorter distances in the cavity within the motor molecule in the direction of the electric field. Shorter distance of travel means smaller unitary charge q (Fig. 6.7B). This interpretation is reinforced by the observation that point mutations of charged residues of prestin only shift the voltage dependence (Oliver *et al.*, 2001). Namely, movements of an extrinsic anion may not be affected seriously by those mutations.

However, these observations do not rule out alternative explanations. For example, these observations also can be interpreted by extending two-state models. Anion dependence implies that anion binding is required for the motor molecules to be in the voltage-sensitive states. For simple ions such as Br⁻, Cl⁻, or HCO⁻, conformational transitions between active motor states are accompanied by transfer of the same unitary charge (Oliver *et al.*, 2001) across the membrane. Motor molecules that are not bound to an anion are in a third state that is voltage insensitive. This condition is realized if the transitions between active states and the inactive state are slower (Fig. 6.7A). Shifts in the voltage dependence associated with anion concentration can be explained by difference in the binding energy. The change in the unitary charge q by a class of anions can be explained by the extended two-state model, whereby the binding of those anions affects the charge of one or both of the motor states. Although this adjustment may appear rather *ad hoc* at first sight, such a systematic shift due to the interaction with those anions is not unreasonable.

The assumption of intrinsic charge movement is not limited to those phenomenological models but is also the case in more physical models. For example, anion antiporter models (Muallem & Ashmore, 2006) assume movement not only of anions but also of intrinsic charges (see Fig. 6.7C). Attempts to interpret the effect of salicylate forces some changes in these models because the apparent number of the motile units must increase with salicylate as explained earlier. Such a change would require more states and with smaller unitary charge transfer during conformational changes. If salicylate functions as the motor charge, as proposed by Oliver *et al.* (2001), its movement across the membrane is broken down into multiple steps and each step across the membrane must be short. Such effects of salicylate can be understood as the loss of cooperativity.

6.7.2 Lipid and cytoskeleton

The membrane motor of OHCs is similar to mechanosensitive channels in that it depends on membrane tension. Because cell membranes are usually supported by the underlying cytoskeleton, it is important to know how these membrane proteins interact with lipid bilayer and the cytoskeleton, directly or indirectly. Here experimental approaches to this problem are described.

Lipid environment

Because the motor responsible for electromotility must be in the plasma membrane to make use of electrical energy, and the density of pillars (see Fig. 6.1A) is much less than that of the motor, the motor must exert force through the lipid bilayer. If the cytoskeleton is connected in parallel and bears a substantial part of the stress, the two-state model that was described earlier must be regarded as phenomenological. Furthermore, the magnitude of area changes of the motor could be an underestimate of the physical membrane motor. However, this is not a serious problem because internal digestion by trypsin does not have a remarkable effect on the area modulus as discussed earlier. Injection of trypsin-containing medium dissolves the cytoskeleton. The area modulus under this configuration does not show a significant difference from that of the intact cell (Adachi & Iwasa, 1999).

Another issue is whether membrane bending is the physical mechanism for electromotility, which can be called the 'curvature motor' model (Raphael *et al.*, 2000). This model assumes that the lipid bilayer of the lateral plasma membrane has a natural curvature, which is supported by the cytoskeleton. This curvature change is enhanced by the presence of membrane proteins such as prestin, which behaves like dipole moments by twisting the lipid bilayer. This model can be tested by examining the effects of chemicals that bend lipid bilayers. Those chemicals that are incorporated into the inner leaf (cup-formers of red blood cells) such as chlorpromazine and procaine reduce the cell length up to about 5% (Fang & Iwasa, 2007) and positively shift the voltage dependence of electromotility up to 20 mV (Morimoto *et al.*, 2002). According to the curvature motor model, crenators of erythrocytes, such as trinitrophenol and dipyridamole, which are preferentially incorporated into the outer leaf, should have different, if not opposite, effect from cup-formers. However, trinitrophenol and dipyridamole have effects similar to cup-formers.

Although salicylate, a crenator anion, considerably reduces the slope of voltage sensitivity, it is an exception and not the rule. Because the effects of cup-formers and crenators are not associated with an elevation of turgor pressure, these experiments show that membrane bending in either direction has the same effect on electromotility, which is hard to explain by the curvature motor model. These results also show that the lipid bilayer bears a significant part of the stress applied to the cell.

Another experiment that shows the significance of lipid includes the use of methyl-β-cyclodextrins, water soluble molecules that binds to cholesterol in their hydrophobic cores and transports cholesterol between lipid bilayers and aqueous phases. Large voltage shifts of as much as 80 mV in the voltage-dependent capacitance of prestin (Sturm *et al.*, 2007) are induced by changing cholesterol content, which is essential for membrane rafts, in the plasma membrane.

Effect of the cytoskeleton

Spectrin is a structural protein that is thought to bridge actin filaments, which primarily run in the circumferential direction of the cylindrical cell. Thus it is likely that spectrin is oriented primarily in the axial direction and contributes to the axial elastic modulus d_1. Diamide is a reagent that affects spectrin by modifying its disulfide bonds. Indeed diamide treatment reduces the axial stiffness of OHCs up to threefold in a dose-dependent manner. A reduction of the axial stiffness is accompanied by an equally marked reduction in the force production by the cell. In contrast, the treatment also leads to some increases in the load-free motility (Adachi & Iwasa, 1997).

These observations can be reproduced by decreasing the axial elastic modulus d_1 in the model (Adachi & Iwasa, 1997). A reduction in the axial stiffness accompanies a reduction in force production and some increase in load-free amplitude. Although it is reasonable that spectrin reduces the axial modulus d_1, its effect on the cross modulus c is unclear. These results show the importance of the cytoskeleton in the axial stiffness and force production of OHCs. In the model presented earlier, the axial stiffness is determined by the factor $1/g$ in Equation (6.21), which is $4d_1 - 4c + d_2$. This indicates that the axial stiffness is determined by a delicate balance between the elastic moduli, in which a relatively small change in the cytoskeleton can be important.

This is illustrated by assuming mechanical isotropy of the membrane, replacing d_1 and d_2 with $K + \mu$, and c with $K - \mu$. Here K is the area modulus and μ the shear modulus. The axial stiffness is then proportional to $K + 9\mu$, which shows the importance of the shear modulus μ, and which can be attributed to the cytoskeleton because the shear modulus of lipid bilayers is small. The effect of diamide illustrates that load-free amplitude and isometric force generation may not always be related. Thus, it is important to measure not only load-free amplitude but also isometric force production to determine the significance of electromotility (see following discussion on the effects of the efferent neurotransmitter, acetylcholine).

6.7.3 Efferent stimulation

The interaction of efferent synaptic input with OHC electromotility is, at present, one of the least understood aspects of the cochlear amplifier. Efferent inhibition *in vivo* reduces the sensitivity of the ear, presumably by reducing the effect of the cochlear amplifier. Since the medial olivococh-lear efferents synapse directly with, and inhibit the OHCs, this interaction strongly supports the role of OHCs in cochlear amplification.

Efferent innervation of OHCs is mediated by nicotinic acetylcholine receptors. Application of acetylcholine to OHCs in whole-cell voltage-clamp at the physiological range of the holding potential, typically −70 mV, elicits a small, brief inward current followed by a pronounced out-ward potassium current (Housley & Ashmore, 1991). The small initial inward current is carried by Ca^{2+} influx through the acetylcholine receptor which is itself a ligand-gated cation channel (Fuchs & Murrow, 1992). The resulting increase in the cytosolic Ca^{2+} concentration activates Ca^{2+}-activated K^+ channels, leading to hyperpolarization (Housley & Ashmore, 1991; Blanchet et al., 1996). This hyperpolarization brings the operating point of electromotility to a less steep slope, reducing force production by OHCs. This could also lead to reduced displacements of OHCs under the load-free condition. However, with cholinergic stimulation, an increase of the load-free amplitude of electromotility accompanied with a reduction of the axial stiffness has been reported (Dallos et al., 1997).

Increased amplitude of electromotility has been considered paradoxical because efferent stimu-lation raises the hearing threshold, indicative of reduced gain of the cochlear amplifier. Efferent stimulation should reduce electromotility, which is responsible for cochlear amplifier. Why should an increase in the amplitude of electromotility result in reduced gain? This observation indicates that force production, and not load-free amplitude, is relevant to the cochlear amplifier. In this regard, it is important that applied acetylcholine also reduced axial stiffness, suggesting that force production may indeed be reduced. This would be equivalent to the dual effect of diamide on stiffness and load-free motility (Adachi & Iwasa, 1997).

What then is the mechanism by which acetylcholine reduces the axial stiffness? It is likely that a second messenger, Ca^{2+} for example, is involved and the target must be either the plasma mem-brane, the cytoskeleton, or both. A recent finding that the $\alpha 10$ subunit has undergone selective development in mammals together with prestin (Franchini & Elgoyhen, 2006) could be sugges-tive of a unique mechanism. Studying this issue has considerable technical hurdles because meas-urement of cellular force and patch clamp must be combined with chemical manipulations. Another factor that could be potentially important is the phase of the receptor potential that drives electromotility. This factor could be influenced by ionic conductance.

6.8 Molecular biology of prestin

6.8.1 Prestin

Prestin (SLC26A5) is an essential protein for electromotility (Zheng et al., 2000). It is a member of the solute carrier family 26, many members of which are anion exchangers. Orthologs of pres-tin are found not only in mammals but in other vertebrates, including opossum, chicken, xeno-pus, pufferfish, and zebrafish. Evolutionary analysis reveals that the sequence of prestin in mammals has amino acid polymorphism of significantly divergent from other animals and that it is highly conserved within mammals compared with other members of the SLC26 family, such as pendrin (Franchini & Elgoyhen, 2006). Parallel specialization is found in the $\alpha 10$ subunit of nico-tinic acetylcholine receptor, which is essential for efferent stimulation of OHCs (Franchini & Elgoyhen, 2006). These observations suggest that prestin (and $\alpha 10$) has undergone positive evo-lutionary selection to play a critical role in mammalian hearing.

Non-mammalian orthologs of prestin are not associated with motile function but they func-tion as electrogenic divalent-chloride anion exchangers (Schaechinger & Oliver, 2007). However, the zebrafish prestin does show non-linear capacitance with bell-shaped voltage dependence similar to that of mammalian prestin (Albert *et al.*, 2007). The main similarity is that the voltage dependence of the zebrafish prestin can be also described as a two-state Boltzmann function. Notable differences from the mammalian prestin are that the unitary charge q that is transferred across the membrane is smaller and that the response time of charge transfer is longer (~0.2 ms).

The existence of non-linear capacitance in ion carriers can be expected from the high-pass characteristics (Kolb & Läuger, 1978) of their membrane noise spectra (Iwasa, 1997). This indicates the importance of charge transfer between conformational states in those membrane proteins relative to ionic conductance. In this regard, the identity of the electric charge that contributes to the non-linear capacitance and function of prestin is still not resolved. However, the existence of mechanoelectric coupling is the essential property of prestin and so mammalian-specific amino acid substitutions (Franchini & Elgoyhen, 2006) may be a key to this issue.

6.8.2 Dimerization

Dimerization of prestin has been shown by SDS electrophoresis (Zheng *et al.*, 2006) and FRET (Navaratnam *et al.*, 2005). It has been further reported that prestin self-assembles into particles with diameter of about 10 nm in the plasma membrane of prestin transfected cells (Murakoshi *et al.*, 2006). Is dimerization important for the function of prestin? A related issue is the composition and functional importance of 10 nm particles in the plasma membrane. Are 10 nm particles homologous oligomers, perhaps tetramers, of prestin or heterologous oligomers that include GLUT5 or possibly other molecules? Is oligomerization required for motor function or is it necessary for some regulatory function?

A recent report indicates that dimerization of prestin increases with increased cholesterol and vice versa. The effect of cholesterol is associated only with shifts in the voltage dependence of non-linear capacitance, without changing unitary motor charge or the total charge transferred (Sturm *et al.*, 2007). This observation suggests that dimerization is not essential to charge transfer. Rather, it is consistent with the assumption that the motile unit is a monomer. Furthermore, the observed voltage shift does not appear to be associated with dimerization. If dimerization changes the voltage dependence, then the sharpness of voltage dependence of the entire cell must be reduced in the transition range where monomers and dimers coexist. However, that is not the case. Therefore, the observed voltage shifts are most likely the result of interactions between prestin and cholesterol and not due to dimerization.

Even if dimerization does not affect the electrical characteristics of prestin; dimerization, oligomerization, or the formation of 10 nm particles, could still be important functionally. In particular, the characteristics of a molecule or an assembly of molecules as a motor cannot be determined by charge transfer alone but also depends on the mechanoelectric coupling. This emphasizes that measurements of tension sensitivity are indispensable to studies of prestin and OHCs.

6.8.3 Molecular mutants

Some mutations of a membrane protein are important for function and some other mutations affect its transport to the plasma membrane. Here a description is given for only some of the mutations which are important in addressing the structure–function relationship.

One focus of creating and examining mutant prestin is to identify the motor charge. Specifically, one would like to know whether the motor charge is intrinsic, as in voltage-gated channels or extrinsic and due to ions in the protein. If the motor charge is intrinsic, it could be expected that point mutations of charged residues could change the unitary motor charge, which is observed as the sensitivity to voltage changes. However, point mutations of charged residues resulted only in shifting $V_{1/2}$ (Fig. 6.10) (Oliver *et al.*, 2001).

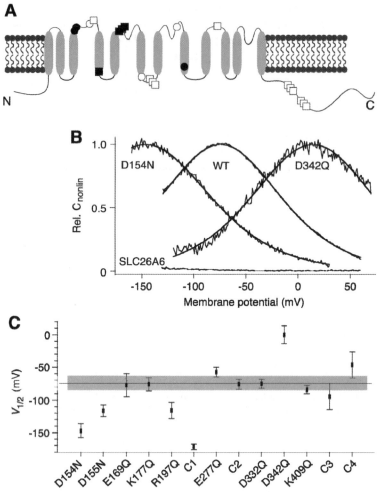

Fig. 6.10 Prestin and prestin mutants expressed in Chinese hamster ovary (CHO) cells. (A) A predicted membrane topology of prestin. Both N-terminus and C-terminus are in the cytosol. Circles: negatively charged amino acids; squares: positively charged amino acids. Filled ones show residues whose mutation lead to significant shifts in the voltage dependence. (B) Normalized non-linear capacitance. The wild-type (WT) is compared with two mutants in which aspartic acid at location 154 and 342 is replaced by asparagine. The capacitance peak shifts with mutations but the slope does not change. Another member, SLC26A6, of the same family SLC26A, does not show non-linear capacitance. (C) The peak potential $V_{1/2}$ of non-linear capacitance in mutants. C1–C4 are four clusters of charged amino acids from the N-terminus to the C-terminus (see A). Reproduced with permission from Oliver *et al.* (2001).

Prestin knock-out mice

To identify the role of prestin and electromotility based on it, prestin-deleted mice have been examined (Liberman *et al.*, 2002). OHCs in those mutant animals did not show electromotility and those animals have significantly higher hearing threshold. Thus this experiment proved that prestin is required for electromotility. However, these animals lose basal OHCs during development and the remaining OHCs are much shorter than those in wild-type mice. For this reason, the experiment cannot rule out the possibility that deformation in the organ of Corti is a factor in elevating the hearing threshold. To address this issue, new transgenic models with functionally altered forms of prestin will be constructed.

6.9 Summary

Electromotility is motility in the lateral membrane of OHCs based on electromechanical coupling similar to piezoelectricity. It is specific to the mammalian ear and uses electrical energy associated with the receptor potential, which is generated by the mechanotransducer channels in the hair bundles. It serves as one of the two molecular mechanisms for reciprocal transduction essential for cochlear amplifier, which is responsible for the sensitivity, frequency selectivity, and the dynamic range of the mammalian ear.

A current challenge in elucidating the mechanism of electromotility is to provide molecular or physical models. Our current understanding remains still more or less phenomenological. Unclarified issues include not only molecular details of conformational changes in prestin but also problems as basic as the functional unit of the membrane motor. Perhaps the most difficult scientific question would be how this motility contributes to this biological function as cochlear amplifier. Although many experiments do confirm the relationship between electromotility and cochlear amplifier, it is not clear, for example, how the RC time constant problem is going to be resolved. And how does efferent stimulation affect cochlear amplifier. Recent developments of molecular-based approaches should provide new tools for addressing these higher order problems.

Recently Dallos *et al.*, (2008) reported that mice with mutant prestin with operating voltage range positively shifted by 80 mV have normal organ of Corti morphology, unlike prestin knock-out mice. However, these animals have significantly elevated hearing threshold, similar to the knock-out animals. Therefore this report significantly strengthens the case for prestin's role in ear function.

Regarding the RC time constant problem, two papers were recently published: Iwasa & Sul (2008) and Mistrik *et al.*, (2009). These reports showed that the effect of the cochlear microphonic alone, as proposed by Dallos & Evans (1995b), is insufficient for resolving the RC time constant problem.

Acknowledgments

The author expresses his thanks to Drs Tom Friedman, Konrad Noben-Trauth, and Paul Fuchs for critical reading of the manuscript. This research was supported by the Intramural Research Program of the National Institute of Deafness and Other Communication Disorders, National Institutes of Health, USA.

References

Adachi M & Iwasa KH. (1997) Effect of diamide on force production and axial stiffness of the cochlear outer hair cell. *Biophys J* 73: 2809–18.

Adachi M & Iwasa KH. (1999) Electrically driven motor in the outer hair cell: Effect of a mechanical constraint. *Proc Natl Acad Sci U S A* 96: 7244–9.

Adachi M, Sugawara M & Iwasa KH. (2000) Effect of turgor pressure on outer hair cell motility. *J Acoust Soc Am* 108: 2299–306.

Albert JT, Winter H, Schaechinger TJ, Weber T, Wang X, He DZZ, Hendrich O, Geisler HS, Zimmermann U, Oelmann K, Knipper M, Gopfert MC & Oliver D. (2007) Voltage sensitive prestin orthologue expressed in zebrafish hair cells. *J Physiol* 580: 451–61.

Allen J. (1980) Cochlear micromechanics – a physical model of transduction. *J Acoust Soc Am* 68: 1660–70.

Ashmore JF. (1987) A fast motile response in guinea-pig outer hair cells: the molecular basis of the cochlear amplifier. *J Physiol* **388**: 323–47.

Ashmore JF. (1990) Forward and reverse transduction in guinea-pig outer hair cells: the cellular basis of the cochlear amplifier. *Neurosci Res Suppl* **12**: S39–50.

Blanchet C, Eróstegui C, Sugasawa M & Dulon D. (1996) Acetylcholine-induced potassium current of guinea pig outer hair cells: its dependence on a calcium influx through nicotinic-like receptors. *J Neurosci* **16**: 2574–84.

Brownell W, Bader C, Bertrand D & Ribaupierre Y. (1985) Evoked mechanical responses of isolated outer hair cells. *Science* **227**: 194–6.

Cacace MG, Landau EM & Ramsden JJ. (1997) The Hofmeister series: salt and solvent effects on interfacial phenomena. *Q Rev Biophys* **30**: 241–77.

Chan DK & Hudspeth AJ. (2005) Ca^{2+} current-driven nonlinear amplification by the mammalian cochlea *in vitro*. *Nat Neurosci* **8**: 149–55.

Crouch JJ & Schulte BA. (1995) Expression of plasma membrane Ca-ATPase in the adult and developing gerbil cochlea. *Hear Res* **92**: 112–19.

Dallos P & Evans B. (1995a) High-frequency motility of outer hair cells and the cochlear amplifier. *Science* **267**: 2006–9.

Dallos P & Evans BN. (1995b) High-frequency outer hair cell motility: corrections and addendum. *Science* **268**: 1420–1.

Dallos P, Hallworth R & Evans BN. (1993) Theory of electrically driven shape changes of cochlear outer hair cells. *J Neurophysiol* **70**: 299–323.

Dallos P, He DZ, Lin X, Sziklai I, Mehta S & Evans BN. (1997) Acetylcholine, outer hair cell electromotility, and the cochlear amplifier. *J Neurosci* **17**: 2212–26.

Dallos P, Wu X, Cheatham MA, Gao J, Zheng J, Anderson CT, Jia S, Wang X, Cheng WH, Sengupta S, He DZ, Zuo J. (2008) Prestin-based outer hair cell motility is necessary for mammalian cochlear amplification. *Neuron* **58**: 333–9.

Dallos P, Zheng J & Cheatham MA. (2006) Prestin and the cochlear amplifier. *J Physiol* **576**: 37–42.

Ding JP, Salvi RJ & Sachs F. (1991) Stretch-activated ion channels in guinea pig outer hair cells. *Hearing Res* **56**: 19–28.

Dong XX, Ehrenstein D & Iwasa KH. (2000) Fluctuation of motor charge in the lateral membrane of the cochlear outer hair cell. *Biophys J* **79**: 1876–82.

Dong XX, Ospeck M & Iwasa KH. (2002) Piezoelectric reciprocal relationship of the membrane motor in the cochlear outer hair cell. *Biophys J* **82**: 1254–9.

Ehrenstein D & Iwasa KH. (1996) Viscoelastic relaxation in the membrane of the auditory outer hair cell. *Biophys J* **71**: 1087–94.

Elgoyhen AB, Vetter DE, Katz E, Rothlin CV, Heinemann SF & Boulter J. (2001) α10: a determinant of nicotinic cholinergic receptor function in mammalian vestibular and cochlear mechanosensory hair cells. *Proc Natl Acad Sci U S A* **98**: 3501–6.

Evans & Rawicz. (1990) Entropy-driven tension and bending elasticity in condensed-uid membranes. *Phys Rev Lett* **64**: 2094–7.

Fang J & Iwasa KH. (2007) Effects of chlorpromazine and trinitrophenol on the membrane motor of outer hair cells. *Biophys J* **93**: 1809–17.

Franchini LF & Elgoyhen AB. (2006) Adaptive evolution in mammalian proteins involved in cochlear outer hair cell electromotility. *Mol Phylogenet Evol* **41**: 622–35.

Frank G, Hemmert W & Gummer AW. (1999) Limiting dynamics of high-frequency electromechanical transduction of outer hair cells. *Proc Natl Acad Sci U S A* **96**: 4420–5.

Frolenkov GI. (2006) Regulation of electromotility in the cochlear outer hair cell. *J Physiol* **576**: 43–8.

Fuchs PA & Murrow BW. (1992) Cholinergic inhibition of short (outer) hair cells of the chick's cochlea. *J Neurosci* **12**: 800–9.

Gale JE & Ashmore JF. (1997a) An intrinsic frequency limit to the cochlear amplifier. *Nature* **389**: 63–6.

Gale JE & Ashmore JF. (1997b) The outer hair cell motor in membrane patches. *Pflugers Arch* **434**: 267–71.

Géléoc GS, Casalotti SO, Forge A & Ashmore JF. (1999) A sugar transporter as a candidate for the outer hair cell motor. *Nat Neurosci* **2**: 713–19.

Gold T. (1948) Hearing. II. The physical basis of the action of the cochlea. *Proc R Soc Lond B Biol Sci* **135**: 492–8.

Hallworth R. (1995) Passive compliance and active force generation in the guinea pig outer hair cell. *J Neurophysiol* **74**: 2319–28.

Hallworth R. (2007) Absence of voltage-dependent compliance in high-frequency cochlear outer hair cells. *J Assoc Res Otolaryngol* **8**: 464–73.

He DZZ & Dallos P. (1999) Somatic stiffness of cochlear outer hair cells is voltage-dependent. *Proc Natl Acad Sci U S A* **96**: 8223–8.

He DZZ, Zheng J, Kalinec F, Kakehata S & Santos-Sacchi J. (2006) Tuning in to the amazing outer hair cell: membrane wizardry with a twist and shout. *J Membr Biol* **209**: 119–34.

Holley MC. (1996) Outer hair cell motility. In: Dallos P, Popper AN & Fay RR, eds. *The Cochlea*. Springer, New York, pp. 386–434.

Housley GD & Ashmore JF. (1991) Direct measurement of the action of acetylcholine on isolated outer hair cells of the guinea pig cochlea. *Proc Biol Sci* **244**: 161–7.

Housley GD, Greenwood D & Ashmore JF. (1992) Localization of cholinergic and purinergic receptors on outer hair cells isolated from the guinea-pig cochlea. *Proc Biol Sci* **249**: 265–73.

Iwasa KH. (1993) Effect of stress on the membrane capacitance of the auditory outer hair cell. *Biophys J* **65**: 492–8.

Iwasa KH. (1997) Current noise spectrum and capacitance due to the membrane motor of the outer hair cell: theory. *Biophys J* **73**: 2965–71.

Iwasa KH. (2001) A two-state piezoelectric model for outer hair cell motility. *Biophys J* **81**: 2495–506.

Iwasa KH. (2006) 'Area change paradox' in the membrane motor of outer hair cells. In: Nuttall A, ed. *Auditory Mechanisms: Processes and Models*. World Scientific, Singapore, pp. 155–61.

Iwasa KH & Sul B. (2008) Effect of the cochlear microphonic on the limiting frequency of the mammalian ear. *J Acoust Soc Am* **124**: 1607–12.

Iwasa KH & Adachi M. (1997) Force generation in the outer hair cell of the cochlea. *Biophys J* **73**: 546–55.

Iwasa KH, Li M, Jia M & Kachar B. (1991) Stretch sensitivity of the lateral wall of the auditory outer hair cell. *Neurosci Lett* **133**: 171–4.

Kakehata S & Santos-Sacchi J. (1995) Membrane tension directly shifts voltage dependence of outer hair cell motility and associated gating charge. *Biophys J* **68**: 2190–7.

Kakehata S & Santos-Sacchi J. (1996) Effects of salicylate and lanthanides on outer hair cell motility and associated gating charge. *J Neurosci* **16**: 4881–9.

Kalinec F, Holley M, Iwasa KH, Lim DJ & Kachar B. (1992) A membrane-based force generation mechanism in auditory sensory cells. *Proc Natl Acad Sci U S A* **89**: 8671–5.

Kennedy HJ, Crawford AC & Fettiplace R. (2005) Force generation by mammalian hair bundles supports a role in cochlear amplification. *Nature* **433**: 880–3.

Kolb HA & Läuger P. (1978) Spectral analysis of current noise generated by carrier mediated ion transport. *J Membr Biol* **41**: 167–87.

Liberman MC, Gao J, He DZ, Wu X, Jia S & Zuo J. (2002) Prestin is required for electromotility of the outer hair cell and for the cochlear amplifier. *Nature* **419**: 300–4.

Lim DJ. (1980) Cochlear anatomy related to cochlear micromechanics: a review. *J Acoust Soc Am* **67**: 1686–95.

Mistrik P, Mullaley C, Mammano F & Ashmore J. (2009) Three-dimensional current flow in a large-scale model of the cochlea and the mechanism of amplification of sound. *J Roy Soc Interface* **6**: 279–91.

Morimoto N, Raphael RM, Nygren A & Brownell WE. (2002) Excess plasma membrane and effects of ionic amphipaths on mechanics of outer hair cell lateral wall. *Am J Physiol Cell Physiol* **282**: C1076–86.

Muallem D & Ashmore JF. (2006) An anion antiporter model of prestin, the outer hair cell motor protein. *Biophys J* **90**: 4035–45.

Murakoshi M, Gomi T, Iida K, Kumano S, Tsumoto K, Kumagai I, Ikeda K, Kobayashi T & Wada H. (2006) Imaging by atomic force microscopy of the plasma membrane of prestin-transfected Chinese hamster ovary cells. *J Assoc Res Otolaryngol* **7**: 267–78.

Navaratnam D, Bai JP, Samaranayake H & Santos-Sacchi J. (2005) N-terminal-mediated homomultimerization of prestin, the outer hair cell motor protein. *Biophys J* **89**: 3345–52.

Oliver D, He DZ, Klocker N, Ludwig J, Schulte U, Waldegger S, Ruppersberg JP, Dallos P & Fakler B. (2001) Intracellular anions as the voltage sensor of prestin, the outer hair cell motor protein. *Science* **292**: 2340–3.

Ospeck M, Dong XX & Iwasa KH. (2003) Limiting frequency of the cochlear amplifier based on electromotility of outer hair cells. *Biophys J* **84**: 739–49.

Raphael RM, Popel AS & Brownell WE. (2000) A membrane bending model of outer hair cell electromotility. *Biophys J* **78**: 2844–62.

Rybalchenko V & Santos-Sacchi J. (2003) Cl⁻ flux through a non-selective, stretchsensitive conductance influences the outer hair cell motor of the guinea-pig. *J Physiol* **547**: 873–91.

Santos-Sacchi J. (1991) Reversible inhibition of voltage-dependent outer hair cell motility and capacitance. *J Neurophysiol* **11**: 3096–110.

Santos-Sacchi J, Kakehata S & Takahashi S. (1998) Effects of membrane potential on the voltage dependence of motility-related charge in outer hair cells of the guinea-pig. *J Physiol* **510**: 225–35.

Santos-Sacchi J, Song L, Zheng J & Nuttall AL. (2006) Control of mammalian cochlear amplification by chloride anions. *J Neurosci* **26**: 3992–8.

Schaechinger TJ & Oliver D. (2007) Non-mammalian orthologs of prestin (SLC26A5) are electrogenic divalent/chloride anion exchangers. *Proc Natl Acad Sci U S A* **104**: 7693–8.

Sturm AK, Rajagopalan L, Yoo D, Brownell WE & Pereira FA. (2007) Functional expression and microdomain localization of prestin in cultured cells. *Otolaryngol Head Neck Surg* **136**: 434–9.

Tolomeo JA & Steele CR. (1995) Orthotropic piezoelectric properties of the cochlear outer hair cell wall. *J Acoust Soc Am* **97**: 3006–11.

Xue S, Mountain DC & Hubbard AE. (1995) Electrically evoked basilar membrane motion. *J Acoust Soc Am* **97**: 3030–41.

Zheng J, Shen W, He DZZ, Long KB, Madison LD & Dallos P. (2000) Prestin is the motor protein of cochlear outer hair cells. *Nature* **405**: 149–55.

Zheng J, Du GG, Anderson CT, Keller JP, Orem A, Dallos P & Cheatham M. (2006) Analysis of the oligomeric structure of the motor protein prestin. *J Biol Chem* **281**: 19916–19924.

Chapter 7

Inner ear fluid homeostasis

Daniel C Marcus and Philine Wangemann

7.1 Introduction

The inner ear consists of an array of interconnected fluid compartments that include the cochlea, utricle, saccule, three ampullae and semicircular canals, the endolymphatic duct, and the endolymphatic sac (Fig. 7.1). Although the cochlear and vestibular organs serve different physiological functions, there is considerable conservation of mechanism at the cellular level between these organs. In addition to the similarities between cochlear and vestibular hair cells, there are functional homologies between strial marginal cells and vestibular dark cells, between cochlear outer sulcus cells and vestibular transitional cells, and between Reissner's membrane epithelium and semicircular canal duct cells. The mechanisms that these cells use to maintain the endolymphatic composition and volume necessary to sustain hearing and balance by secretion of K^+, Cl^-, Ca^{2+}, and HCO_3^- and absorption of K^+, Na^+, and Ca^{2+} will be described in this chapter.

The composition of the luminal fluid, endolymph, differs between different parts of the inner ear and from the surrounding fluid, the perilymph, and from cerebrospinal fluid and plasma (Table 7.1). The endolymph bathing the sensory cells in the cochlea and the vestibular labyrinth is a remarkable fluid in that it has a high concentration of K^+ concentration and low concentrations of Na^+ and Ca^{2+}. The high K^+ concentration makes K^+ the major charge carrier of sensory transduction. K^+ as charge carrier has several advantages compared with other ions. An influx of K^+ into the cytosol of the sensory hair cells causes minimal changes in the relative cellular ion composition since K^+ is the most abundant ion in the cytosol. In addition, both influx of K^+ via the sensory transduction channels in the apical membrane and efflux of K^+ across K^+ channels in the basolateral membrane occur down electrochemical gradients that do not require energy expenditure by the sensory cell. Consequently, the energetic requirements of the sensory hair cells are limited and sensory function does not require close approximation of blood vessels, which could provide a source of mechanical noise.

7.2 Epithelial cells and vectorial transport

Epithelial cells separate two defined extracellular spaces, one space being the nutritional source bathing the basolateral epithelial cell membrane and the other space comprising the lumen or other specialized compartment that is bordered by the apical cell membrane (Fig. 7.2A). The apical and basolateral membrane domains are separated by tight junctions, which perform both 'gate' and 'fence' functions. The gate function permits and limits the passage of solutes between the two extracellular fluid compartments. The fence function forms a barrier that prevents membrane proteins intrinsic to the outer leaflet of the plasma membrane lipid bilayer from diffusing between the apical and basolateral domains. Membrane proteins trafficked to either the apical or

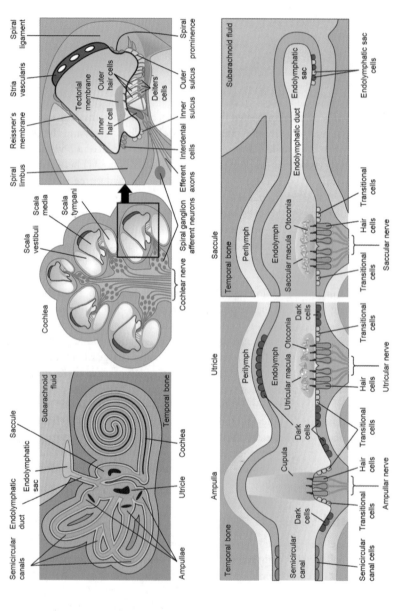

Fig. 7.1 Diagrammatic illustration of the inner ear and associated nomenclature. Top left panel: cochlea and vestibular labyrinth; top middle panel: cross-section of the cochlea; top right panel: expanded view of one cochlear turn; bottom left panel: utricle and semicircular canal with ampulla; bottom right panel: saccule and endolymphatic sac.

Parts of Figure 7.1 have been taken from Marcus and Wangemann (2009) with permission of the authors, editors, and publisher.

Table 7.1 Fluid composition of perilymph, cochlear and vestibular endolymph, and endolymph of the endolymphatic sac ('sac'), cerebrospinal fluid, and plasma*

	Cochlear perilymph	Cochlear endolymph	Utricular endolymph	Sac endolymph	Cerebrospinal fluid	Plasma
Na$^+$ (mM)	148	1.3	9	129	149	145
K$^+$ (mM)	4.2	157	149	8–13	3.1	5.0
Cl$^-$ (mM)	119	132	–	124	129	106
HCO$_3^-$ (mM)	21	31	–	–	19	18
Ca^{2+} (mM)	1.3	0.023	0.25	–	–	2.6
Protein (mg/dL)	178	38	–	–	24	4238
pH	7.3	7.5	7.5	6.7–7.1	7.3	7.3

*Values are taken from recent reviews (Wangemann & Schacht, 1996; Wangemann, 2006) and amended by additional data (Mori et al., 1987; Ikeda & Morizono, 1989a,b, 1991; Tsujikawa et al., 1992; Couloigner et al., 2000; Wangemann et al., 2007).

basolateral membrane will remain in place either by virtue of the junctional fence or by tethering to the cytoskeleton (Cereijido & Anderson, 2001).

The placement of different transport proteins in the apical or basolateral membrane leads to vectorial transepithelial transport. Movement from the basolateral to the apical fluid compartment results in *secretion*, while apical to basolateral movement results in *absorption* of solutes. Net absorption or secretion results in an accompanying osmotic movement of water (see below). Transport proteins fall into three broad categories: primary active 'pumps', transporters, and channels. The pumps catalytically transform metabolic energy (ATP) into the potential energy of ion concentration gradients across membranes, while transporters and channels selectively permit the movement of solutes down those gradients. The rate of transepithelial transport is under the control of a variety of hormonal and intracellular signaling pathways. In the face of changing transport rates, epithelial cells transport solutes at their own peril of disturbing their cytosolic homeostasis. An imbalance of transport rates across the apical and basolateral membranes would obviously result in an accumulation or deficit of the transported solute in the cytoplasm. Regulation of transepithelial transport rates for the control of luminal fluid composition therefore requires coordination of apical and basolateral cell membrane transport rates.

7.3 K$^+$ cycling

K$^+$ is the main charge carrier of sensory transduction in the cochlea and the vestibular labyrinth. Sensory transduction depends on a mechanically gated ion channel that is located in the hair bundles of the hair cells (Fig. 7.1). Opening of the transduction channel supports an influx of K$^+$ from endolymph into the hair cells, which depolarizes the basolateral membrane of these cells. This depolarization has different consequences depending on the type of hair cell. Depolarization of cochlear outer hair cells causes contraction of the motor protein prestin (SLC26A5), which shortens the outer hair cell and leads to an amplification of the mechanical stimulus. Depolarization of the cochlear inner hair cells or of vestibular hair cells leads to Ca^{2+} influx, vesicular neurotransmitter release and activation of the sensory neurons. Influx of K$^+$ from endolymph into the hair cells is balanced by an efflux of K^+ via basolateral K^+ channels into interstitial spaces that are continuous with perilymph.

Although the molecular identity of the mechanically gated ion channel in the apical membrane of hair cells has not yet been identified (Corey, 2006), the molecular identities of the major K^+ channels that mediate K^+ efflux from hair cells have been established. Most prominently, these include the voltage-gated K^+ channel KCNQ4 and the Ca^{2+}-activated K^+ channel KCNMA1 (Kros & Crawford, 1990; Housley & Ashmore, 1992; Mammano et al., 1996; Chambard & Ashmore, 2003; Thurm et al., 2005). Several splice variants of KCNQ4 are expressed in the inner ear of which one variant, KCNQ4v3, is preferentially expressed at the base of the cochlea (Beisel et al., 2005; Liang et al., 2005; Liang et al., 2006). The K^+ channel KCNQ4 associates with the beta-subunit KCNE1 and possibly with other KCNE subunits that are expressed in hair cells (Strutz-Seebohm et al., 2006). K^+ released from the sensory hair cells is recycled by uptake into spiral ligament fibrocytes, transferred into stria vascularis and secreted into endolymph (Figs 7.1 and 7.3). Several parallel pathways have been proposed for the path from the sensory cells toward the spiral ligament (Spicer & Schulte, 1996). The pathway through the open perilymph space of the scala tympani is supported by current measurements (Zidanic & Brownell, 1990). An additional pathway may involve uptake of K^+ into Deiters' cells, dispersion among cells via gap junctions and release of K^+ from root cells into the interstitial space of the spiral ligament (Kikuchi et al., 2000). Uptake of K^+ from the interstitial space of the spiral ligament that is continuous with perilymph occurs via specialized fibrocytes. Fibrocytes types II, IV, and V express Na^+/K^+-ATPase and the $Na^+/2Cl^-/K^+$ co-transporter SLC12A2 (NKCC1) and the Cl^- channels CLCNKA and CLCNKB (Schulte & Adams, 1989; Crouch et al., 1997; Mizuta et al., 1997; Maehara et al., 2003; Qu et al., 2006). Although functional data from fibrocytes are lacking, the resemblance of this array of transporters to the basolateral membrane of strial marginal cells and vestibular dark cells (see below) suggests that fibrocytes take up K^+ from perilymph. The K^+ taken up is thought to diffuse among types II, IV, and V fibrocytes and into the basal cells through gap junctions, in particular GJB2 (Cx26) and GJB6 (Cx30), and then via other gap junctions into the intermediate cells of the stria vascularis (see below).

7.4 K^+ buffering

Efflux of K^+ from sensory hair cells has been shown to lead to measurable increases in the extracellular K^+ concentration in the surrounding perilymph (Johnstone et al., 1989; Valli et al., 1990). K^+ buffering mechanisms may limit the magnitude of these increases in order to avoid depolarization of hair cells and adjacent neurons. Current measurements in scala tympani perilymph support the concept that the perilymph serves as an open fluid space into which K^+ can dissipate by diffusion (Zidanic & Brownell, 1990). Additional K^+ buffering may be provided by Deiters' cells and other supporting cells surrounding the hair cells (see Fig. 7.1). Deiters' cells have a membrane potential near the K^+ equilibrium potential (Oesterle & Dallos, 1990) and express the inward-rectifying K^+ channel KCNJ10 (Kir4.1), which is particularly abundant in the membrane area facing the outer hair cell, from which K^+ efflux occurs through KCNQ4 channels (Hibino et al., 1997; Ruttiger et al., 2004). Efflux of K^+ from the hair cells could lead to a local increase in the extracellular K^+ concentration, which would set the local K^+ equilibrium potential below the membrane potential and would promote K^+ influx into Deiters' cells. The ensuing elevation of the cytosolic K^+ concentration would promote K^+ efflux preferentially through inward-rectifying K^+ channels, outward-rectifying K^+ channels, or K/Cl co-transporters located away from the hair cell membrane (Boettger et al., 2002, 2003). A similar mechanism has been described in Müller glia of the retina (Reichenbach et al., 1992; Kofuji et al., 2002).

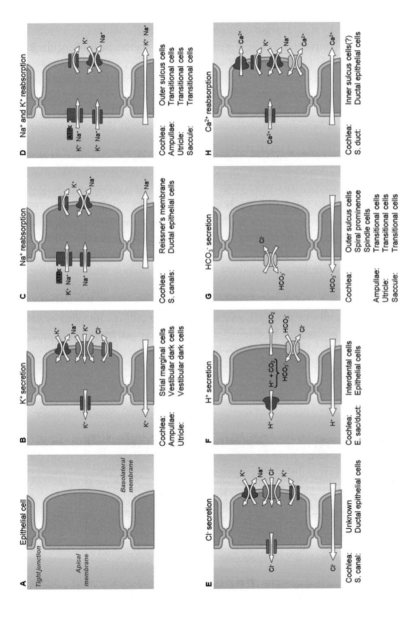

Fig. 7.2 A–H Ion transport models of cochlear and vestibular epithelial cells. ATP-ase ion 'pumps', carriers, and ion channels are shown. The arrow at the bottom of each diagram depicts the net absorption or net secretion resulting from apical and basolateral transport activity. See text for details about the specific genes that lead to the depicted transport function and the known regulatory pathways.

7.5 Strial marginal cells and vestibular dark cells

7.5.1 K⁺ secretion

K⁺ taken up by fibrocytes of the spiral ligament is dispersed via gap junctions among fibrocytes, basal and intermediate cells of stria vascularis (see Fig. 7.3). Intermediate cells release K⁺ into the intrastrial space via the K⁺ channel KCNJ10 that generates the endocochlear potential. From the intrastrial space, K⁺ is taken up by strial marginal cells and secreted into endolymph. Vestibular dark cells take up K⁺ from perilymph and secrete it into endolymph via mechanisms equivalent to strial marginal cells (Fig. 7.2B) (Wangemann *et al.*, 1995b). Both epithelial cells take up K⁺ across the basolateral membrane via the Na⁺/2Cl⁻/K⁺ co-transporter SLC12A2 and the Na⁺/K⁺-ATPase ATPA1/ATPB1 (Marcus & Marcus, 1987; Wangemann *et al.*, 1995a). The Na⁺/K⁺-ATPase takes up K⁺ and establishes a Na⁺ gradient that energizes further uptake of K⁺ via SLC12A2. The marginal cells of the stria vascularis, unlike vestibular dark cells, appear to express a K⁺/H⁺-ATPase in addition to Na⁺/K⁺-ATPase (Shibata *et al.*, 2006). The functional significance of this K⁺/H⁺-ATPase is currently unclear. K⁺ taken up across the basolateral membrane is secreted across the apical membrane via the K⁺ channel KCNQ1/KCNE1 (Marcus & Shen, 1994; Wangemann *et al.*, 1995a). The KCNQ1/KCNE1 K⁺ channel consists of an assembly of the pore-forming α-subunit KCNQ1 with the β-subunit KCNE1 (Barhanin *et al.*, 1996; Sanguinetti *et al.*, 1996). Na⁺ and Cl⁻ taken up via the Na⁺/2Cl⁻/K⁺ co-transporter are recycled in the basolateral membrane via the Na⁺/K⁺-ATPase and Cl⁻ channels (Wangemann & Marcus, 1992; Wangemann, 1995). Cl⁻ channels consist of the subunits CLCNKA/BSND (ClC-Ka/barttin) and CLCNKB/BSND (ClC-Kb/barttin) (Marcus *et al.*, 1993; Takeuchi & Irimajiri, 1994; Takeuchi *et al.*, 1995; Ando & Takeuchi, 2000; Estevez *et al.*, 2001; Sage & Marcus, 2001; Maehara *et al.*, 2003; Qu *et al.*, 2006).

The rate of K⁺ secretion in vestibular dark cells and strial marginal cells is controlled by ionic and osmotic stimuli as well as by receptors. K⁺ channel secretion is increased by lowering the apical or increasing the basolateral K⁺ concentration or by lowering the osmolarity on the basolateral

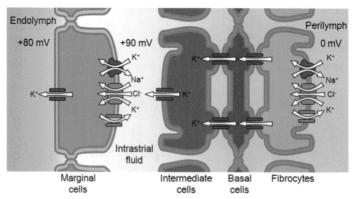

Fig. 7.3 Multicellular model of K⁺ transport and generation of the endocochlear potential by the stria vascularis. Fibrocytes of the spiral ligament act together with the basal, intermediate and marginal cells of the stria vascularis to secrete K⁺ into cochlear endolymph and to produce the endocochlear potential, both of which drive auditory transduction.

Parts of Figure 7.3 have been taken from Marcus and Wangemann (2009) with permission of the authors, editors, and publisher.

side (Marcus *et al.*, 1994; Wangemann *et al.*, 1995a,c, 1996). Further, the rate of K^+ secretion is increased by β_1-adrenergic receptors via cAMP (Sunose *et al.*, 1997a,b; Wangemann *et al.*, 1999b, 2000) and decreased by muscarinic and purinergic receptors (Wangemann *et al.*, 2001; Lee & Marcus, 2008).

7.6 Generation of the endocochlear potential

Sensory transduction in the cochlea depends on the endocochlear potential, which contributes significantly to the driving force of the transduction current. The endocochlear potential is a transepithelial potential that is generated by the stria vascularis (von Békésy, 1950; Tasaki & Spyropoulos, 1959; Wangemann & Schacht, 1996). The stria vascularis (see Figs 7.1 and 7.3) is a layered epithelium consisting of marginal, intermediate, and basal cells, as well as a network of embedded capillaries. The marginal and basal cells are each linked among themselves by tight junctions to form two epithelial barriers. The marginal cells form the barrier between endolymph and the intrastrial fluid space whereas the basal cells form the barrier between the intrastrial space and the interstitial fluid of the spiral ligament, which is continuous with the perilymph. The endocochlear potential is generated across the basal cell barrier (Salt *et al.*, 1987). The basal cell barrier is penetrated by tight capillaries that form a network within the intrastrial space (Jahnke, 1975). Tight junctions between basal cells differ from marginal cell tight junctions in that they contain only CLDN11 (claudin 11) whereas marginal cell tight junctions contain a multitude of different claudins (Florian *et al.*, 2003; Kitajiri *et al.*, 2004b). The inner membrane of the basal cell barrier, which faces the intrastrial fluid space, is connected via gap junctions to strial intermediate cells (Kikuchi *et al.*, 1994; Takeuchi S & Ando, 1998a). Gap junctions ensure that intermediate cells are electrically a part of the basal cell barrier. The molecular identity of these gap junctions has not yet been established. The outer membrane of the basal cell barrier is connected via gap junctions to type I fibrocytes of the spiral ligament. These gap junctions are mainly comprised of GJB2 (CX26) and GJB3 (CX30) (Kikuchi *et al.*, 1995; Lautermann *et al.*, 1998; Xia *et al.*, 2001; Ahmad *et al.*, 2003; Forge *et al.*, 2003).

The endocochlear potential is essentially a K^+ equilibrium potential that is generated by the K^+ channel KCNJ10 (Kir4.1) in the intermediate cells of the stria vascularis in conjunction with a low extracellular K^+ concentration in the intrastrial fluid space and a high cytosolic K^+ concentration in intermediate cells (Takeuchi *et al.*, 2000; Marcus *et al.*, 2002). The marginal cells of the stria vascularis and the fibrocytes of the spiral ligament support the generation of the endocochlear potential by maintaining, respectively, a low K^+ concentration in the intrastrial fluid space and by ensuring a high cytosolic K^+ concentration in the cytosol of strial intermediate cells (Marcus *et al.*, 1985; Wangemann *et al.*, 1995a; Takeuchi *et al.*, 2000). A detailed analytical model of K^+ secretion and endocochlear potential generation by the stria vascularis has been developed by Quraishi and Raphael (2007, 2008). The endolymphatic potential of the utricle and the ampullae is near zero due to the absence of intermediate and basal cells.

Numerous clinical and experimental conditions are associated with a loss of the endocochlear potential, which results in hearing loss or deafness. First, loop diuretics such as furosemide or bumetanide reduce the endocochlear potential by inhibiting K^+ uptake into the strial marginal cells, which increases the K^+ concentration in the intrastrial fluid space and thereby abolishes the steep K^+ gradient at the intermediate cells necessary for the generation of the endocochlear potential (Kusakari *et al.*, 1978a,b; Marcus *et al.*, 1985). Similarly, increases in the K^+ concentration in the intrastrial fluid space via vascular perfusion of elevated K^+ concentrations or via perfusion of other inhibitors of K^+ uptake by marginal cells cause a rapid inhibition of the endocochlear potential (Konishi & Mendelsohn, 1970; Kuijpers & Bonting, 1970; Kusakari *et al.*, 1978a,b;

Marcus *et al.*, 1985). Second, a mouse model that lacks the K^+ channel KCNJ10 fails to generate the endocochlear potential (Marcus *et al.*, 2002). Third, pharmacological inhibition of the K^+ channel KCNJ10 inhibits the endocochlear potential (Marcus *et al.*, 1985; Takeuchi *et al.*, 1996; Takeuchi & Ando, 1998b; Marcus *et al.*, 2002). Fourth, the anticancer drug difluoromethyl-ornithine (DMFO) inhibits the endocochlear potential by reducing inward-rectification of the KCNJ10 K^+ channels via inhibition of polyamine synthesis (Lourdel *et al.*, 2002; Nie *et al.*, 2005). Removal of inward-rectification may increase the efflux of K^+ into the intrastrial space, which abolishes the steep K^+ gradient necessary for the generation of the endocochlear potential. Fifth, loss of functional SLC26A4 in a mouse model of Pendred's syndrome leads to a loss of KCNJ10 channel expression and a loss of the endocochlear potential (Wangemann *et al.*, 2004, 2007; Singh & Wangemann, 2008). Sixth, loss of GJB6 (Cx30) in a clinical model of connexin-mediated deafness renders capillaries of the stria vascularis leaky to the intrastrial space, which provides an electrical short circuit for the endocochlear potential and a complete loss of the endocochlear potential (Cohen-Salmon *et al.*, 2007). Seventh, loss of tight junction integrity among basal cells due to a loss of CLDN11 (claudin 11) renders the basal cell barrier leaky and leads to a loss of the endocochlear potential (Gow *et al.*, 2004; Kitajiri *et al.*, 2004a). Taken together, these data underscore that the endocochlear potential depends critically on functional KCNJ10 K^+ channels, a large K^+ concentration gradient across this channel and on tight epithelial and endothelial barriers.

7.7 Reissner's membrane and semicircular canal duct

Both Reissner's membrane and semicircular canal duct epithelial cells absorb Na^+ from the endolymph (Lee & Marcus, 2003; Kim *et al.*, 2009; Pondugula *et al.*, 2004, 2006). Remarkably, the semicircular canal ducts also support the independent vectorial transport of Ca^{2+} and Cl^- and each is under the control of different hormone systems: glucocorticoids and vitamin D regulate Na^+ and Ca^{2+} absorption, respectively, through genomic control of regulatory genes whereas adrenergic agonists acutely control Cl^- secretion (Milhaud *et al.*, 2002; Pondugula *et al.*, 2004, 2006).

7.7.1 Na^+ absorption

Na^+ is absorbed from endolymph via entry into the cell across the apical membrane of Reissner's membrane and semicircular canal duct through an epithelial Na^+ channel, ENaC, that is a heteromultimer consisting of α, β and, γ subunits (Couloigner *et al.*, 2001; Pondugula *et al.*, 2006) (Figs 7.1 and 7.2C). Basolateral Na^+/K^+-ATPase transports the cytosolic Na^+ to the perilymph. K^+ entering the epithelial cells from perilymph on the Na^+/K^+-ATPase subsequently diffuses back into perilymph through basolateral K^+ channels. These K^+ channels also are expected to contribute to a cell-negative basolateral membrane voltage that pulls the positively charged Na^+ from endolymph into the cytosol. In Reissner's membrane, this electrical 'pull' on Na^+ is assisted by the 'push' from the positive endolymphatic potential.

Genes for subunits of each of these transporters in semicircular canal duct are upregulated by the synthetic glucocorticoid dexamethasone (e.g. α-ENaC, Kir7.1, β3-Na^+,K^+-ATPase), consistent with the markedly increased Na^+ transport in response to glucocorticoids (Pondugula *et al.*, 2004, 2006). Known regulatory genes are also found to be expressed and regulated by dexamethasone, including α-glucocorticoid receptor, 11β-HSD1, SGK1, and Nedd4-2. Additional support for the mediation of Na^+ absorption by ENaC was obtained from measurements of transepithelial Na^+ current. The Na^+ current was reduced when canal cells were transfected with siRNA against α-ENaC but not with a control nonsense siRNA (Marcus *et al.*, 2006).

Reissner's membrane has an additional Na^+ entry pathway in the apical membrane (Fig. 7.2C) that is also permeable to K^+ and is gated by extracellular ATP (Thorne *et al.*, 2004). This ionotropic

$P2X_2$ purinoceptor becomes active when ATP in endolymph increases, as during acoustic stimulation. This cation-selective channel is thought to provide a protective parasensory shunt during intense stimulation (reviewed in Lee & Marcus, 2008).

7.7.2 Ca^{2+} absorption

Homeostasis of the endolymphatic Ca^{2+} level is essential for inner ear function. The transduction of sound and acceleration into nerve impulses is known to be highly dependent on the homeostasis of endolymphatic calcium for multiple cellular processes (Ricci & Fettiplace, 1998). The calcium concentration of endolymph is very much lower than that of perilymph in both the cochlea and the vestibule (see Table 7.1). Although vestibular endolymphatic Ca^{2+} concentration is below electrochemical equilibrium, cochlear endolymphatic Ca^{2+} concentration is actually higher than equilibrium due to the positive endocochlear potential. Nonetheless, it is likely that there are both secretory and absorptive processes for Ca^{2+} within the cochlear duct. The non-selective cation channels found in outer sulcus cells and vestibular transitional cells (see below) are probably permeable to Ca^{2+} in addition to monovalent cations, but the relatively small extent of this epithelial domain makes it likely that there are other Ca^{2+} absorbing mechanisms employed by the inner ear to maintain endolymphatic Ca^{2+} levels. Indeed, a novel Ca^{2+} absorptive process has been identified in the vestibular labyrinth and there is evidence suggesting its occurrence in the cochlea as well.

Semicircular canal duct epithelial cells absorb Ca^{2+} from endolymph by the scheme modeled in Figure 7.2H. Entry of Ca^{2+} from the endolymph into the cell is through epithelial Ca^{2+} channels (TRPV5; also called CaT2, ECaC1; and TRPV6; also called CaT1, ECaC2) where the Ca^{2+} becomes buffered by the cytosolic Ca^{2+}-binding proteins calbindin-D9k and/or calbindin-D28k. The bound Ca^{2+} diffuses across the cell, where it is released and extruded by a plasma membrane ATPase (PMCA) and a Na^+-Ca^{2+} exchanger (NCX). Ca^{2+} absorption is stimulated by the active form of vitamin D (1,25-dihydroxyvitamin D_3) via activation of the vitamin D receptor. This model is supported by the expression of transcripts for all components of this Ca^{2+} absorptive pathway, including the vitamin D receptor, in primary cultures of canal duct epithelial cells (Yamauchi et al., 2005). Further, TRPV5 mRNA expression is strongly upregulated by incubation with 1,25-dihydroxyvitamin D_3 (Yamauchi et al., 2005). Importantly, functional studies showed that: tracer fluxes of Ca^{2+} were greater from the apical surface into the cells than from the basolateral side; this absorptive flux was increased by incubation with 1,25-dihydroxyvitamin D_3; and the absorptive flux was inhibited by known blockers of TRPV5/6 Ca^{2+} channels and by extracellular apical acidification (Nakaya et al., 2007). These findings point to a powerful system for maintenance of endolymphatic Ca^{2+} levels in the vestibular system. This transport pathway was previously demonstrated in the kidney and intestine (Hoenderop et al., 2002; Nijenhuis et al., 2003; Peng et al., 2003; van Abel et al., 2003). The TRPV5/TRPV6 entry channel is strongly inhibited by lowered extracellular pH (Yeh et al., 2006). This pH sensitivity is thought to play an important role in both the cochlea and the vestibular system, for example when there is a mutation of the bicarbonate transporter pendrin (Nakaya et al., 2007; Wangemann et al., 2007). One result of pendrin mutation is the concomitant decrease in pH and elevation of Ca^{2+} concentration in the endolymph (see below). The fact that this occurs in the cochlea as well as in the vestibular system and that immunoreactivity is seen for TRPV5 and TRPV6 in cochlear epithelial cells points to the likely importance of this Ca^{2+} absorptive system in the cochlea.

It is of clinical importance that bilateral sensorineural hearing loss (BSNHL) has been reported to occur in conjunction with low serum vitamin D (Brookes, 1983; Ikeda et al., 1989). Importantly, the patients with BSNHL and low serum vitamin D had normal serum Ca^{2+}, consistent with a local effect of vitamin D deficiency in the auditory and vestibular periphery. Vitamin D deficiency in rats also led to impairment of hearing, however the perilymphatic $[Ca^{2+}]$ level was reduced (Ikeda *et al.*, 1987), making the interpretation less clear. Interestingly, the locus of *DFNB13* autosomal recessive non-syndromic deafness encompasses the gene locations of TRPV5 and TRPV6, leading to the speculation that mutations in those Ca^{2+} channel genes may disrupt Ca^{2+} absorption and thereby lead to deafness (Yamauchi *et al.*, 2005).

7.7.3 Cl⁻ secretion

The largest cochlear cation flux is that of K^+ (Konishi *et al.*, 1978; Sterkers *et al.*, 1982), which is under control of basolateral β-adrenergic agonists, such as norepinephrine (see above) (Wangemann *et al.*, 1999a, 2000). Given that the cochlear and vestibular epithelia support very large ionic concentration differences between the endolymph and perilymph, the junctions between the epithelial cells are probably very tight. This would potentially pose a problem for transport of the anion(s) required to maintain bulk electroneutrality. Most commonly, epithelia transport one ion actively through a transcellular route and the accompanying counter ion moves passively through the paracellular route. The inner ear apparently solves this problem by employing another cell type, the semicircular canal duct epithelium in the vestibule, to carry the anion and puts it under the control of the same hormones. This regulated Cl⁻ secretory function in the canal probably has a counterpart in the cochlea, but has not yet been identified (Lee & Marcus, 2003; Kim *et al.*, 2009).

Indeed, Cl⁻ is secreted by semicircular canal duct cells under adrenergic control as modeled in Figure 7.2E. Cl⁻ is taken up from the perilymph via the $Na^+/K^+/2Cl^-$ co-transporter (NKCC1) in the basolateral membrane. This secondary-active transport is driven by the Na^+ gradient created by the basolateral Na^+/K^+-ATPase. K^+ taken up by both of these transport proteins is recycled through basolateral K^+ channels. Cytosolic Cl⁻ is then secreted into endolymph through apical Cl⁻ channels. One type of Cl⁻ channel identified by pharmacological action, CFTR, is known to be activated by cAMP stimulation via protein kinase A (PKA). Cl⁻ secretion by SCCD is indeed stimulated by elevation of intracellular cAMP (either directly or via activation of $β_2$-adrenergic receptors (Milhaud *et al.*, 2002)).

7.8 Outer sulcus and vestibular transitional cells

7.8.1 pH regulation

The outer sulcus, spiral prominence, strial spindle, and vestibular transitional epithelial cells all secrete HCO_3^- into endolymph via the Cl^-/HCO_3^- exchanger pendrin, SLC26A4 (Fig. 7.2G). Spindle cells are morphologically dissimilar to marginal cells but are surface epithelial cells that occur in the first row inside the strial border with spiral prominence and the border with Reissner's membrane. Pendrin protein is expressed in the apical membranes of these cells (Wangemann *et al.*, 2004) and the pH of both the cochlear and vestibular endolymph is more acidic (less basic) in transgenic mice lacking expression of functional pendrin (Nakaya *et al.*, 2007; Wangemann *et al.*, 2007). Further, spiral prominence cells were found to transport base equivalents out of their cytosol by a process that was inhibited by DIDS (4,4′-diisothiocyanatostilbene-2,2′-disulfonic acid) and stimulated by formate, a signature for pendrin activity (Wangemann *et al.*, 2004). These findings, taken together, are consistent with significant secretion of HCO_3^- into the endolymph by pendrin. All of the ramifications are not yet clear, but the lowered endolymphatic pH due to disruption of pendrin function in mice is now known to lead to greatly increased endolymphatic Ca^{2+} concentration (Nakaya *et al.*, 2007; Wangemann *et al.*, 2007) and probably to increased K^+ secretion (Wangemann *et al.*, 1995d; Singh & Wangemann, 2008). Increased K^+ secretion, in turn, leads to oxidative stress in the stria vascularis (Singh & Wangemann, 2008) and consequent loss of KCNJ10 K$^+$ channel expression (Singh & Wangemann, 2008) and loss of the endocochlear potential (Wangemann et al., 2004).

A late consequence is the invasion of the stria vascularis by macrophages in adult mice (Jabba et al., 2006). Endolymphatic pH is also known to affect the size/shape of the tectorial membrane and therefore probably impacts hearing (Weiss & Freeman, 1997). Additional pH regulation has been proposed via H$^+$-ATPase mediated acid secretion by interdental and/or marginal cells in the cochlea and by epithelial cells of the endolymphatic sac (Fig. 7.2F) (Lang et al., 2007).

7.8.2 Cation absorption

As discussed above, the inner ear has transepithelial pathways for absorption of K$^+$ and Na$^+$. Parasensory K$^+$ and Na$^+$ absorption has been found to occur in the cochlear outer sulcus and the vestibular transitional cell epithelia (Fig. 7.2D) (Marcus & Chiba, 1999; Chiba & Marcus, 2000, 2001). Outer sulcus epithelial cells take up Na$^+$ and K$^+$ via apical non-selective cation channels, BK K$^+$ channels, small-conductance K$^+$ channels and P2X2 receptor-gated non-selective cation channels. They release Na$^+$ and K$^+$ across the basolateral membrane via a Na$^+$/K$^+$-ATPase and K$^+$ channels, respectively (Marcus & Chiba, 1999; Chiba & Marcus, 2000, 2001; Lee et al., 2001). Similar transport mechanisms were found in the vestibular transitional cells (Lee et al., 2001). The P2X2 purinergic receptor ion channel is known to also be permeable to Ca^{2+} (Evans et al., 1996). The outer sulcus and transitional cells may therefore also absorb Ca^{2+} under stimulated conditions if there are Ca^{2+} transporters on the basolateral membrane to remove Ca^{2+} on the perilymphatic side of these epithelial cells.

7.9 Endolymph volume

Several genetic diseases and syndromes that result in deafness and/or vertigo are associated with an unusually distended (referred to as 'hydrops') or collapsed lumen of the inner ear. Hydrops in the cochlea was earlier thought to be a causative factor leading to deafness but is more recently thought to be an epiphenomenon (Merchant et al., 2005). Nonetheless, extreme distention of Reissner's membrane to its limits, as sometimes observed, is likely to cause deafness. Endolymphatic hydrops has been observed in Ménière's and Pendred syndromes. Shrinkage of the endolymphatic space has been observed in Scheibe's deformity (Anderson et al., 1968; Ryugo et al., 2003) and Jervell and Lange–Nielsen syndrome (Casimiro et al., 2001).

Hydrops can result from uncompensated overstimulation of ion secretion and/or reduction of absorption in the cochlea or vestibular labyrinth. Alternatively, interruption of fluid flow from the cochlea and vestibule to the endolymphatic sac (longitudinal flow) would be expected to have the same result (Kimura, 1967; Kimura et al., 1980), although longitudinal flow has been found to be slower than earlier thought (Salt et al., 1986). Altered net ion transport across inner ear epithelia will be accompanied by bulk volume changes in endolymph due to osmotically driven movement of water to accompany the solutes. Rapid water movements in the ear (Sterkers et al., 1982) are likely carried by aquaporins in the cell membranes (Huang et al., 2002; Verkman, 2002), since cell membranes are otherwise relatively water impermeable.

7.10 Summary

In summary, the establishment and maintenance of the specialized fluid composition and voltages in the inner ear rely on complex interactions between ion channels, pumps, transporters, barrier proteins, and regulatory signal pathways. The reviewed homology between epithelial cells of the cochlea and vestibular system emphasizes the conservation of sensory and homeostatic mechanisms.

Throughout this chapter we have provided examples of inner ear diseases that arise from dysfunction of constituent molecules. One of the great challenges facing otolaryngology is to understand inner ear homeostasis on the level of the genome, the proteome, and the physiome.

Acknowledgments

This work was supported by National Institutes of Health grants R01-DC000212 (DCM), R01-DC001098 (APW), and R01-DC04280 (APW).

References

Ahmad S, Chen S, Sun J & Lin X. (2003) Connexins 26 and 30 are co-assembled to form gap junctions in the cochlea of mice. *Biochem Biophys Res Commun* **307**: 362–8.

Anderson H, Henricson B, Lundquist PG, Wedenberg E & Wersall J. (1968) Genetic hearing impairment in the Dalmatian dog. An audiometric, genetic and morphologic study in 53 dogs. *Acta Otolaryngol* Suppl 3–4.

Ando M & Takeuchi S. (2000) mRNA encoding ClC-K1, a kidney Cl$^-$ channel is expressed in marginal cells of the stria vascularis of rat cochlea: its possible contribution to Cl$^-$ currents. *Neurosci Lett* **284**: 171–4.

Barhanin J, Lesage F, Guillemare E, Fink M, Lazdunski M & Romey G. (1996) KVLQT1 and IsK (minK) proteins associate to form the IKs cardiac potassium current. *Nature* **384**: 78–80.

Beisel KW, Rocha-Sanchez SM, Morris KA, Nie L, Feng F, Kachar B, Yamoah EN & Fritzsch B. (2005) Differential expression of KCNQ4 in inner hair cells and sensory neurons is the basis of progressive high-frequency hearing loss. *J Neurosci* **25**: 9285–93.

Boettger T, Hubner CA, Maier H, Rust MB, Beck FX & Jentsch TJ. (2002) Deafness and renal tubular acidosis in mice lacking the K-Cl co-transporter Kcc4. *Nature* **416**: 874–8.

Boettger T, Rust MB, Maier H, Seidenbecher T, Schweizer M, Keating DJ, Faulhaber J, Ehmke H, Pfeffer C, Scheel O, Lemcke B, Horst J, Leuwer R, Pape HC, Volkl H, Hubner CA & Jentsch TJ. (2003) Loss of K-Cl co-transporter KCC3 causes deafness, neurodegeneration and reduced seizure threshold. *EMBO J* **22**: 5422–34.

Brookes GB. (1983) Vitamin D deficiency – a new cause of cochlear deafness. *J Laryngol Otol* **97**: 405–20.

Casimiro MC, Knollmann BC, Ebert SN, Vary JC Jr, Greene AE, Franz MR, Grinberg A, Huang SP & Pfeifer K. (2001) Targeted disruption of the Kcnq1 gene produces a mouse model of Jervell and Lange-Nielsen Syndrome. *Proc Natl Acad Sci U S A* **98**: 2526–31.

Cereijido M & Anderson JM. (2001) Tight Junctions. In: Gonzalez-Mariscal L, Avila A & Betanzos A, eds. *The Relationship Between Structure and Function of Tight Junctions*, 2nd edn. Boca Raton, FL: CRC Press, pp. 89–119.

Chambard JM & Ashmore JF. (2003) Sugar transport by mammalian members of the SLC26 superfamily of anion-bicarbonate exchangers. *J Physiol* **550**: 667–77.

Chiba T & Marcus DC. (2000) Nonselective cation and BK channels in apical membrane of outer sulcus epithelial cells. *J Membr Biol* **174**: 167–79.

Chiba T & Marcus DC. (2001) Basolateral K$^+$ conductance establishes driving force for cation absorption by outer sulcus epithelial cells. *J Membr Biol* **184**: 101–12.

Cohen-Salmon M, Regnault B, Cayet N, Caille D, Demuth K, Hardelin JP, Janel N, Meda P & Petit C. (2007) Connexin30 deficiency causes instrastrial fluid-blood barrier disruption within the cochlear stria vascularis. *Proc Natl Acad Sci U S A* **104**: 6229–34.

Corey DP. (2006) What is the hair cell transduction channel? *J Physiol* **576**: 23–8.

Couloigner V, Fay M, Djelidi S, Farman N, Escoubet B, Runembert I, Sterkers O, Friedlander G & Ferrary E. (2001) Location and function of the epithelial Na channel in the cochlea. *Am J Physiol Renal Physiol* **280**: F214-F222.

Couloigner V, Teixeira M, Hulin P, Sterkers O, Bichara M, Escoubet B, Planelles G & Ferrary E. (2000) Effect of locally applied drugs on the pH of luminal fluid in the endolymphatic sac of guinea pig. *Am J Physiol Regul Integr Comp Physiol* **279**: R1695–700.

Crouch JJ, Sakaguchi N, Lytle C & Schulte BA. (1997) Immunohistochemical localization of the Na-K-Cl co-transporter (NKCC1) in the gerbil inner ear. *J Histochem Cytochem* **45**: 773–8.

Estevez R, Boettger T, Stein V, Birkenhager R, Otto E, Hildebrandt F & Jentsch TJ. (2001) Barttin is a Cl⁻ channel beta-subunit crucial for renal Cl⁻ reabsorption and inner ear K⁺ secretion. *Nature* **414**: 558–61.

Evans RJ, Lewis C, Virginio C, Lundstrom K, Buell G, Surprenant A & North RA. (1996) Ionic permeability of, and divalent cation effects on, two ATP-gated cation channels (P2X receptors) expressed in mammalian cells. *J Physiol* **497**: 413–22.

Florian P, Amasheh S, Lessidrensky M, Todt I, Bloedow A, Ernst A, Fromm M & Gitter AH. (2003) Claudins in the tight junctions of stria vascularis marginal cells. *Biochem Biophys Res Commun* **304**: 5–10.

Forge A, Becker D, Casalotti S, Edwards J, Marziano N & Nevill G. (2003) Gap junctions in the inner ear: comparison of distribution patterns in different vertebrates and assessment of connexin composition in mammals. *J Comp Neurol* **467**: 207–31.

Gow A, Davies C, Southwood CM, Frolenkov G, Chrustowski M, Ng L, Yamauchi D, Marcus DC & Kachar B. (2004) Deafness in Claudin 11-null mice reveals the critical contribution of basal cell tight junctions to stria vascularis function. *J Neurosci* **24**: 7051–62.

Hibino H, Horio Y, Inanobe A, Doi K, Ito M, Yamada M, Gotow T, Uchiyama Y, Kawamura M, Kubo T & Kurachi Y. (1997) An ATP-dependent inwardly rectifying potassium channel KAB-2 (Kir4.1), in cochlear stria vascularis of inner ear: Its specific subcellular localization and correlation with the formation of endocochlear potential. *J Neurosci* **17**: 4711–21.

Hoenderop JG, Dardenne O, van Abel M, Van der Kemp AW, Van Os CH, Arnaud R & Bindels RJ. (2002) Modulation of renal Ca²⁺ transport protein genes by dietary Ca²⁺ and 1,25-dihydroxyvitamin D3 in 25-hydroxyvitamin D₃–1alpha-hydroxylase knockout mice. *FASEB J* **16**: 1398–406.

Housley GD & Ashmore JF. (1992) Ionic currents of outer hair cells isolated from the guinea-pig cochlea. *J Physiol* **448**: 73–98.

Huang D, Chen P, Chen S, Nagura M, Lim DJ & Lin X. (2002) Expression patterns of aquaporins in the inner ear: evidence for concerted actions of multiple types of aquaporins to facilitate water transport in the cochlea. *Hear Res* **165**: 85–95.

Ikeda K, Kobayashi T, Itoh Z, Kusakari J & Takasaka T. (1989) Evaluation of vitamin D metabolism in patients with bilateral sensorineural hearing loss. *Am J Otol* **10**: 11–13.

Ikeda K, Kusakari J, Kobayashi T & Saito Y. (1987) The effect of vitamin D deficiency on the cochlear potentials and the perilymphatic ionized calcium concentration of rats. *Acta Otolaryngol Suppl* **435**: 64–72.

Ikeda K & Morizono T. (1989a) Effects of carbon dioxide in the middle ear cavity upon the cochlear potentials and cochlear pH. *Acta Otolaryngol* **108**: 88–93.

Ikeda K & Morizono T. (1989b) The preparation of acetic acid for use in otic drops and its effect on endocochlear potential and pH in inner ear fluid. *Am J Otolaryngol* **10**: 382–5.

Ikeda K & Morizono T. (1991) The ionic and electric environment in the endolymphatic sac of the chinchilla: relevance to the longitudinal flow. *Hear Res* **54**: 118–22.

Jabba SV, Oelke A, Singh R, Maganti RJ, Fleming SD, Wall SM, Green ED & Wangemann P. (2006) Macrophage invasion contributes to degeneration of stria vascularis in Pendred syndrome mouse model. *BMC Med* **4**: 37.

Jahnke K. (1975) The fine structure of freeze-fractured intercellular junctions in the guinea pig inner ear. *Acta Otolaryngol Suppl* **336**: 1–40.

Johnstone BM, Patuzzi R, Syka J & Sykova E. (1989) Stimulus-related potassium changes in the organ of Corti of guinea-pig. *J Physiol* **408**: 77–92.

Kikuchi T, Adams JC, Paul DL & Kimura RS. (1994) Gap junction systems in the rat vestibular labyrinth: Immunohistochemical and ultrastructural analysis. *Acta Otolaryngol* **114**: 520–8.

Kikuchi T, Kimura RS, Paul DL & Adams JC. (1995) Gap junctions in the rat cochlea: immunohistochemical and ultrastructural analysis. *Anat Embryol (Berl)* 191: 101–18.

Kikuchi T, Kimura RS, Paul DL, Takasaka T & Adams JC. (2000) Gap junction systems in the mammalian cochlea. *Brain Res Brain Res Rev* 32: 163–6.

Kim SH, Kim KX, Raveendran NN, Wu T, Pondugula SR, & Marcus DC. (2009) Regulation of ENaC-mediated sodium transport by glucocorticoids in Reissner's membrane epithelium. *Am.J.Physiol Cell Physiol* 296: C544–C557.

Kimura RS. (1967) Experimental blockage of the endolymphatic duct and sac and its effects on the inner ear of the guinea pig. A study on endolymphatic hydrops. *Ann Otol Rhinol Laryngol* 76: 664–87.

Kimura RS, Schuknecht HF, Ota CY & Jones DD. (1980) Obliteration of the ductus reuniens. *Acta Otolaryngol* 89: 295–309.

Kitajiri S, Miyamoto T, Mineharu A, Sonoda N, Furuse K, Hata M, Sasaki H, Mori Y, Kubota T, Ito J, Furuse M & Tsukita S. (2004a) Compartmentalization established by claudin-11-based tight junctions in stria vascularis is required for hearing through generation of endocochlear potential. *J Cell Sci* 117: 5087–96.

Kitajiri SI, Furuse M, Morita K, Saishin-Kiuchi Y, Kido H, Ito J & Tsukita S. (2004b) Expression patterns of claudins, tight junction adhesion molecules, in the inner ear. *Hear Res* 187: 25–34.

Kofuji P, Biedermann B, Siddharthan V, Raap M, Iandiev I, Milenkovic I, Thomzig A, Veh RW, Bringmann A & Reichenbach A. (2002) Kir potassium channel subunit expression in retinal glial cells: implications for spatial potassium buffering. *Glia* 39: 292–303.

Konishi T, Hamrick PE & Walsh PJ. (1978) Ion transport in guinea pig cochlea. I. Potassium and sodium transport. *Acta Otolaryngol* 86: 22–34.

Konishi T & Mendelsohn M. (1970) Effect of ouabain on cochlear potentials and endolymph composition in guinea pigs. *Acta Otolaryngol* 69: 192–9.

Kros CJ & Crawford AC. (1990) Potassium currents in inner hair cells isolated from the guinea-pig cochlea. *J Physiol* 421: 263–91.

Kuijpers W & Bonting SL. (1970) The cochlear potentials. I. The effect of ouabain on the cochlear potentials of the guinea pig. *Pflugers Arch* 320: 348–58.

Kusakari J, Ise I, Comegys TH, Thalmann I & Thalmann R. (1978a) Effect of ethacrynic acid, furosemide, and ouabain upon the endolymphatic potential and upon high energy phosphates of the stria vascularis. *Laryngoscope* 88: 12–37.

Kusakari J, Kambayashi J, Ise I & Kawamoto K. (1978b) Reduction of the endocochlear potential by the new 'loop' diuretic, bumetanide. *Acta Otolaryngol* 86: 336–41.

Lang F, Vallon V, Knipper M & Wangemann P. (2007) Functional significance of channels and transporters expressed in the inner ear and kidney. *Am J Physiol Cell Physiol* 293: C1187–208.

Lautermann J, ten Cate WJ, Altenhoff P, Grummer R, Traub O, Frank H, Jahnke K & Winterhager E. (1998) Expression of the gap-junction connexins 26 and 30 in the rat cochlea. *Cell Tissue Res* 294: 415–20.

Lee JH, Chiba T & Marcus DC. (2001) P2X2 receptor mediates stimulation of parasensory cation absorption by cochlear outer sulcus cells and vestibular transitional cells. *J Neurosci* 21: 9168–74.

Lee JH & Marcus DC. (2003) Endolymphatic sodium homeostasis by Reissner's membrane. *Neuroscience* 119: 3–8.

Lee JH & Marcus DC. (2008) Purinergic signaling in the inner ear. *Hear Res* 235: 1–7.

Liang G, Moore EJ, Ulfendahl M, Rydqvist B & Jarlebark L. (2005) An M-like potassium current in the guinea pig cochlea. *ORL J Otorhinolaryngol Relat Spec* 67: 75–82.

Liang GH, Jin Z, Ulfendahl M & Jarlebark L. (2006) Molecular analyses of KCNQ1–5 potassium channel mRNAs in rat and guinea pig inner ears: expression, cloning, and alternative splicing. *Acta Otolaryngol* 126: 346–52.

Lourdel S, Paulais M, Cluzeaud F, Bens M, Tanemoto M, Kurachi Y, Vandewalle A & Teulon J. (2002) An inward rectifier K^{+} channel at the basolateral membrane of the mouse distal convoluted tubule: similarities with Kir4-Kir5.1 heteromeric channels. *J Physiol* 538: 391–404.

Maehara H, Okamura HO, Kobayashi K, Uchida S, Sasaki S & Kitamura K. (2003) Expression of CLC-KB gene promoter in the mouse cochlea. *Neuroreport* 14: 1571–3.

Mammano F, Goodfellow SJ & Fountain E. (1996) Electrophysiological properties of Hensen's cells investigated in situ. *Neuroreport* 7: 537–42.

Marcus DC & Chiba T. (1999) K^+ and Na^+ absorption by outer sulcus epithelial cells. *Hear Res* 134: 48–56.

Marcus DC, Liu J & Wangemann P. (1994) Transepithelial voltage and resistance of vestibular dark cell epithelium from the gerbil ampulla. *Hear Res* 73: 101–8.

Marcus DC, Pondugula SR, Lee JH, Chiba T, Yamauchi D, Sanneman JD, Harbidge DG, Kampalli SB, Wu T & Wangemann P. (2006) Meniere's disease and inner ear homeostasis disorders. *Proceedings of the Fifth International Symposium. Ion Transport Pathways in the Cochlea and Vestibular Labyrinth.* Los Angeles, CA, pp. 31–35.

Marcus DC, Rokugo M & Thalmann R. (1985) Effects of barium and ion substitutions in artificial blood on endocochlear potential. *Hear Res* 17: 79–86.

Marcus DC & Shen Z. (1994) Slowly activating, voltage-dependent K^+ conductance is apical pathway for K^+ secretion in vestibular dark cells. *Am J Physiol* 267: C857-C864.

Marcus DC, Takeuchi S & Wangemann P. (1993) Two types of chloride channel in the basolateral membrane of vestibular dark cell epithelium. *Hear Res* 69: 124–32.

Marcus DC & Wangemann P. (2009) Cochlear and Vestibular Function and Dysfunction. In: Alvarez-Leefmans FJ & Delpire E, eds. *Physiology and Pathology of Chloride Transporters and Channels in the Nervous System – From Molecules to Diseases.* Academic Press, Elsevier, pp. 421–33.

Marcus DC, Wu T, Wangemann P & Kofuji P. (2002) KCNJ10 (Kir4.1) potassium channel knockout abolishes endocochlear potential. *Am J Physiol Cell Physiol* 282: C403-C407.

Marcus NY & Marcus DC. (1987) Potassium secretion by nonsensory region of gerbil utricle in vitro. *Am J Physiol* 253: F613–21.

Merchant SM, Adams JC & Nadol JB. (2005) Meniere's syndrome: are symptoms caused by endolymphatic hydrops? *The Registry* 12: 1–7.

Milhaud PG, Pondugula SR, Lee JH, Herzog M, Lehouelleur J, Wangemann P, Sans A & Marcus DC. (2002) Chloride secretion by semicircular canal duct epithelium is stimulated via β2-adrenergic receptors. *Am J Physiol Cell Physiol* 283: C1752–60.

Mizuta K, Adachi M & Iwasa KH. (1997) Ultrastructural localization of the Na-K-Cl⁻cotransporter in the lateral wall of the rabbit cochlear duct. *Hear Res* 106: 154–62.

Mori N, Ninoyu O & Morgenstern C. (1987) Cation transport in the ampulla of the semicircular canal and in the endolymphatic sac. *Arch Otorhinolaryngol* 244: 61–55.

Nakaya K, Harbidge DG, Wangemann P, Schultz BD, Green E, Wall SM & Marcus DC. (2007) Lack of pendrin HCO(3-) transport elevates vestibular endolymphatic $[Ca^{2+}]$ by inhibition of acid-sensitive TRPV5 and TRPV6. *Am J Physiol Renal Physiol* 292: 1314–21.

Nie L, Feng W, Diaz R, Gratton MA, Doyle KJ & Yamoah EN. (2005) Functional consequences of polyamine synthesis inhibition by L-alpha-difluoromethylornithine (DFMO): cellular mechanisms for DFMO-mediated ototoxicity. *J Biol Chem* 280: 15097–102.

Nijenhuis T, Hoenderop JG, Nilius B & Bindels RJ. (2003) (Patho)physiological implications of the novel epithelial Ca^{2+} channels TRPV5 and TRPV6. *Pflugers Arch* 446: 401–9.

Oesterle EC & Dallos P. (1990) Intracellular recordings from supporting cells in the guinea pig cochlea: DC potentials. *J Neurophysiol* 64: 617–36.

Peng JB, Brown EM & Hediger MA. (2003) Apical entry channels in calcium-transporting epithelia. *News Physiol Sci* 18: 158–63.

Pondugula SR, Raveendran NN, Ergonul Z, Deng Y, Chen J, Sanneman JD, Palmer LG & Marcus DC. (2006) Glucocorticoid regulation of genes in the amiloride-sensitive sodium transport pathway by semicircular canal duct epithelium of neonatal rat. *Physiol Genomics* 24: 114–23.

Pondugula SR, Sanneman JD, Wangemann P, Milhaud PG & Marcus DC. (2004) Glucocorticoids stimulate cation absorption by semicircular canal duct epithelium via epithelial sodium channel. *Am J Physiol Renal Physiol* **286**: F1127–35.

Qu C, Liang F, Hu W, Shen Z, Spicer SS & Schulte BA. (2006) Expression of CLC-K chloride channels in the rat cochlea. *Hear Res* **213**: 79–87.

Quraishi IH & Raphael RM. (2007) Computational model of vectorial potassium transport by cochlear marginal cells and vestibular dark cells. *Am J Physiol Cell Physiol* **292**: C591–C602.

Quraishi IH & Raphael RM. (2008) Generation of the endocochlear potential: a biophysical model. *Biophys J* **94**: L64-L66.

Reichenbach A, Henke A, Eberhardt W, Reichelt W & Dettmer D. (1992) K$^+$ ion regulation in retina. *Can J Physiol Pharmacol* **70** (**Suppl**): S239–47.

Ricci AJ & Fettiplace R. (1998) Calcium permeation of the turtle hair cell mechanotransducer channel and its relation to the composition of endolymph. *J Physiol* **506**: 159–73.

Ruttiger L, Sausbier M, Zimmermann U, Winter H, Braig C, Engel J, Knirsch M, Arntz C, Langer P, Hirt B, Muller M, Kopschall I, Pfister M, Munkner S, Rohbock K, Pfaff I, Rusch A, Ruth P & Knipper M. (2004) Deletion of the Ca^{2+}-activated potassium (BK) alpha-subunit but not the BKbeta1-subunit leads to progressive hearing loss. *Proc Natl Acad Sci U S A* **101**: 12922–12927.

Ryugo DK, Cahill HB, Rose LS, Rosenbaum BT, Schroeder ME & Wright AL. (2003) Separate forms of pathology in the cochlea of congenitally deaf white cats. *Hear Res* **181**: 73–84.

Sage CL & Marcus DC. (2001) Immunolocalization of ClC-K chloride channel in strial marginal cells and vestibular dark cells. *Hear Res* **160**: 1–9.

Salt AN, Melichar I & Thalmann R. (1987) Mechanisms of endocochlear potential generation by stria vascularis. *Laryngoscope* **97**: 984–91.

Salt AN, Thalmann R, Marcus DC & Bohne BA. (1986) Direct measurement of longitudinal endolymph flow rate in the guinea pig cochlea. *Hear Res* **23**: 141–51.

Sanguinetti MC, Curran ME, Zou A, Shen J, Spector PS, Atkinson DL & Keating MT. (1996) Coassembly of KVLQT1 and minK (IsK) proteins to form cardiac IKs potassium channel. *Nature* **384**: 80–3.

Schulte BA & Adams JC. (1989) Distribution of immunoreactive Na$^+$,K$^+$-ATPase in gerbil cochlea. *J Histochem Cytochem* **37**: 127–34.

Shibata T, Hibino H, Doi K, Suzuki T, Hisa Y & Kurachi Y. (2006) Gastric type H$^+$,K$^+$-ATPase in the cochlear lateral wall is critically involved in formation of the endocochlear potential. *Am J Physiol Cell Physiol* **291**: C1038–48.

Singh R & Wangemann P. (2008) Free radical stress mediated loss of Kcnj10 protein expression in stria vascularis contributes to deafness in Pendred syndrome mouse model. *Am J Physiol Renal Physiol* **294**: F139–48.

Spicer SS & Schulte BA. (1996) The fine structure of spiral ligament cells relates to ion return to the stria and varies with place-frequency. *Hear Res* **100**: 80–100.

Sterkers O, Saumon G, Tran Ba Huy P & Amiel C. (1982) K, Cl, and H$_2$O entry in endolymph, perilymph, and cerebrospinal fluid of the rat. *Am J Physiol* **243**: F173–80.

Strutz-Seebohm N, Seebohm G, Fedorenko O, Baltaev R, Engel J, Knirsch M & Lang F. (2006) Functional coassembly of KCNQ4 with KCNE-beta- subunits in Xenopus oocytes. *Cell Physiol Biochem* **18**: 57–66.

Sunose H, Liu J & Marcus DC. (1997a) cAMP increases K$^+$ secretion via activation of apical IsK/ KvLQT1 channels in strial marginal cells. *Hear Res* **114**: 107–16.

Sunose H, Liu J, Shen Z & Marcus DC. (1997b) cAMP increases apical IsK channel current and K$^+$ secretion in vestibular dark cells. *J Membr Biol* **156**: 25–35.

Takeuchi S & Ando M. (1998a) Dye-coupling of melanocytes with endothelial cells and pericytes in the cochlea of gerbils. *Cell Tissue Res* **293**: 271–5.

Takeuchi S & Ando M. (1998b) Inwardly rectifying K$^+$ currents in intermediate cells in the cochlea of gerbils: a possible contribution to the endocochlear potential. *Neurosci Lett* **247**: 175–8.

Takeuchi S, Ando M & Kakigi A. (2000) Mechanism generating endocochlear potential: role played by intermediate cells in stria vascularis. *Biophys J* **79**: 2572–82.

Takeuchi S, Ando M, Kozakura K, Saito H & Irimajiri A. (1995) Ion channels in basolateral membrane of marginal cells dissociated from gerbil stria vascularis. *Hear Res* **83**: 89–100.

Takeuchi S & Irimajiri A. (1994) Cl- and nonselective cation channels in the basolateral membrane of strial marginal cells. *Jpn J Physiol* **44**: s317–19.

Takeuchi S, Kakigi A, Takeda T, Saito H & Irimajiri A. (1996) Intravascularly applied K+-channel blockers suppress differently the positive endocochlear potential maintained by vascular perfusion. *Hear Res* **101**: 181–5.

Tasaki I & Spyropoulos CS. (1959) Stria vascularis as source of endocochlear potential. *J Neurophysiol* **22**: 149–55.

Thorne PR, Munoz DJ & Housley GD. (2004) Purinergic modulation of cochlear partition resistance and its effect on the endocochlear potential in the Guinea pig. *J Assoc Res Otolaryngol* **5**: 58–65.

Thurm H, Fakler B & Oliver D. (2005) Ca^{2+}-independent activation of BKCa channels at negative potentials in mammalian inner hair cells. *J Physiol* **569**: 137–51.

Tsujikawa S, Yamashita T, Amano H, Kumazawa T & Vosteen KH. (1992) Acidity in the endolymphatic sac fluid of guinea pigs. *ORL J Otorhinolaryngol Relat Spec* **54**: 198–200.

Valli P, Zucca G & Botta L. (1990) Perilymphatic potassium changes and potassium homeostasis in isolated semicircular canals of the frog. *J Physiol* **430**: 585–94.

van Abel M, Hoenderop JG, Van der Kemp AW, van Leeuwen JP & Bindels RJ. (2003) Regulation of the epithelial Ca^{2+} channels in small intestine as studied by quantitative mRNA detection. *Am J Physiol Gastrointest Liver Physiol* **285**: G78–85.

Verkman AS. (2002) Aquaporin water channels and endothelial cell function. *J Anat* **200**: 617–27.

von Békésy G. (1950) DC potentials and energy balance of the cochlear partition. *J Acoust Soc Am* **22**: 576–82.

Wangemann P. (1995) Comparison of ion transport mechanisms between vestibular dark cells and strial marginal cells. *Hear Res* **90**: 149–57.

Wangemann P. (2006) Supporting sensory transduction: cochlear fluid homeostasis and the endocochlear potential. *J Physiol* **576**: 11–21.

Wangemann P & Marcus DC. (1992) The membrane potential of vestibular dark cells is controlled by a large Cl- conductance. *Hear Res* **62**: 149–56.

Wangemann P & Schacht J. (1996) Homeostasic mechanisms in the cochlea. In: Dallos P, Popper AN & Fay R, eds. Springer Handbook of Auditory Research: The Cochlea. Springer, pp. 130–185.

Wangemann P, Liu J & Marcus DC. (1995a) Ion transport mechanisms responsible for K+ secretion and the transepithelial voltage across marginal cells of stria vascularis in vitro. *Hear Res* **84**: 19–29.

Wangemann P, Liu J, Shen Z & Marcus DC. (1995b) Similarity of ion transport properties between vestibular dark cells and strial marginal cells. *Proc Sendai Symp* **5**: 145–50.

Wangemann P, Liu J, Shen Z, Shipley A & Marcus DC. (1995c) Hypo-osmotic challenge stimulates transepithelial K+ secretion and activates apical IsK channel in vestibular dark cells. *J Membr Biol* **147**: 263–73.

Wangemann P, Liu J & Shiga N. (1995d) The pH-sensitivity of transepithelial K+ transport in vestibular dark cells. *J Membr Biol* **147**: 255–62.

Wangemann P, Shen Z & Liu J. (1996) K+-induced stimulation of K+ secretion involves activation of the IsK channel in vestibular dark cells. *Hear Res* **100**: 201–10.

Wangemann P, Liu J, Shimozono M & Scofield MA. (1999a) β1-adrenergic receptors but not β2-adrenergic or vasopressin receptors regulate K+ secretion in vestibular dark cells of the inner ear. *J Membr Biol* **170**: 67–77.

Wangemann P, Liu J, Shimozono M & Scofield MA. (1999b) β1-adrenergic receptors but not β2-adrenergic or vasopressin receptors regulate K+ secretion in vestibular dark cells of the inner ear. *J Membr Biol* **170**: 67–77.

Wangemann P, Liu J, Shimozono M, Schimanski S & Scofield MA. (2000) K^+ secretion in strial marginal cells is stimulated via β1-adrenergic receptors but not via β2-adrenergic or vasopressin receptors. *J Membr Biol* 175: 191–202.

Wangemann P, Liu J, Scherer EQ, Herzog M, Shimozono M & Scofield MA. (2001) Muscarinic receptors control K^+ secretion in inner ear strial marginal cells. *J Membr Biol* 182: 172–81.

Wangemann P, Itza EM, Albrecht B, Wu T, Jabba SV, Maganti RJ, Lee JH, Everett LA, Wall SM, Royaux IE, Green ED & Marcus DC. (2004) Loss of KCNJ10 protein expression abolishes endocochlear potential and causes deafness in Pendred syndrome mouse model. *BMC Med* 2: 30.

Wangemann P, Nakaya K, Wu T, Maganti R, Itza EM, Sanneman J, Harbidge D, Billings S & Marcus DC. (2007) Loss of cochlear HCO(3-) secretion causes deafness via endolymphatic acidification and inhibition of Ca(2+) reabsorption in a Pendred syndrome mouse model. *Am J Physiol Renal Physiol* 292: 1345–53.

Weiss TF & Freeman DM. (1997) Equilibrium behavior of an isotropic polyelectrolyte gel model of the tectorial membrane: effect of pH. *Hear Res* 111: 55–64.

Xia A, Katori Y, Oshima T, Watanabe K, Kikuchi T & Ikeda K. (2001) Expression of connexin 30 in the developing mouse cochlea. *Brain Res* 898: 364–7.

Yamauchi D, Raveendran NN, Pondugula SR, Kampalli SB, Sanneman JD, Harbidge DG & Marcus DC. (2005) Vitamin D upregulates expression of ECaC1 mRNA in semicircular canal. *Biochem Biophys Res Commun* 331: 1353–7.

Yeh BI, Yoon J & Huang CL. (2006) On the role of pore helix in regulation of TRPV5 by extracellular protons. *J Membr Biol* 212: 191–8.

Zidanic M & Brownell WE. (1990) Fine structure of the intracochlear potential field. I. The silent current. *Biophys J* 57: 1253–68.

Chapter 8

Hair bundle structure and mechanotransduction

Carole M Hackney and David N Furness

8.1 **Introduction**

The past three decades have seen substantial progress toward defining the structural and functional attributes of hair cell mechanotransduction. These insights into fundamental mechanisms have arisen from studies in various hair cell organs from all vertebrate classes. More recent research in human genetics and molecular biology has begun to identify some of the cellular and molecular mechanisms underlying hair cell mechanotransduction. This chapter will focus particularly on the information currently available on the structure, function and composition of the transduction apparatus of mammalian cochlear hair cells.

Hair cells are the sensory receptors of the vertebrate acousticolateralis system. These mechanosensors are characterized by an apical bundle of tiny hairs that are modified microvilli, the stereocilia (Fig. 8.1A–C). The stereocilia form rows increasing stepwise in height in a staircase pattern across the bundle. The stereocilia are interconnected by a variety of extracellular filaments, and mechanical displacement of the bundle unit produces gating of mechanoelectrical transduction (MET) channels (see reviews by Furness & Hackney, 2006, Phillips *et al.*, 2008).

Due to the mechanical tuning of basilar membrane motion (see Chapter 5), hair cells at the cochlear apex are subject to low-frequency vibration, whereas those at the cochlear base (nearest to the oval window) respond to high-frequency sounds, exceeding 100 kHz in some mammals, such as bats (Brown & Pye, 1975). Thus hair cell mechanotransduction must result from the fastest known ion channel kinetics (see reviews by Fettiplace, 2006; Vollrath *et al.*, 2007). The range of frequencies that can be detected is based on a number of structural modifications along the length of the cochlea including the size and shape of the stereociliary bundles as well as functional variation of the MET channels themselves (Ricci *et al.*, 2003).

In the cochlea, the hair cells and surrounding supporting cells form a multilayered epithelial sheet known as the organ of Corti that rests on the basilar membrane (Fig. 8.2). There are two types of hair cell, a single row of inner hair cells (IHCs), which are contacted by the majority of the type I afferents in the cochlear nerve, and three rows of outer hair cells (OHCs), which are innervated by medial efferent neurones originating in the superior olivary complex of the brain stem. In addition, type II afferents make extensively branched contacts with numerous OHCs, and a population of lateral efferents innervate type I afferents beneath IHCs. As their innervation pattern suggests, the IHCs provide most of the acoustic information to the brain (Chapter 9). OHCs, on the other hand, are electromotile and amplify cochlear vibrations in a manner that increases cochlear sensitivity (Chapter 6). Efferent neurones inhibit OHCs to modulate cochlear sensitivity (Chapter 10). Overlying the organ of Corti is an acellular matrix of collagen and glycoprotein, the tectorial membrane, which projects from the inner sulcus. The tallest stereocilia of the OHCs are embedded in this membrane, whereas the tips of IHC stereocilia approach, but

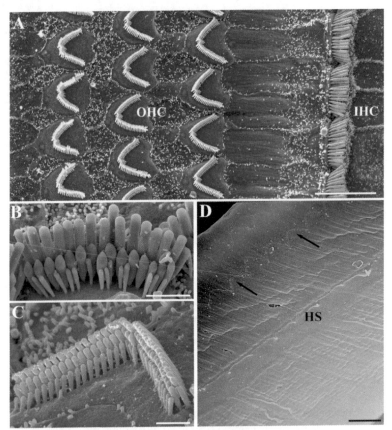

Fig. 8.1 Scanning electron micrographs of guinea-pig organ of Corti. (A) The tectorial membrane has been removed from this cochlear segment to reveal the upper surface (the reticular lamina) of the organ of Corti. One row of inner hair cell (IHC) stereociliary bundles and three rows of outer hair cell (OHC) stereociliary bundles can be seen protruding from the apices of the hair cells. In between are the apices of the surrounding supporting cells which are attached to the hair cells by tight junctions. Scale bar: 10 μm. (B, C) Higher magnification images showing (B) an IHC and (C) an OHC bundle taken from the apical and basal turn of the cochlea respectively. Note that although in both cases, the stereocilia are arranged in serried rows, there are differences in the shape and relative heights of the stereocilia in the bundle on the two types of hair cell. Scale bars: 2 μm (B) and 1 μm (C). (D) The under surface of the tectorial membrane, that is, the surface that normally lies over the tips of the stereocilia. Indentations (arrows) can be seen in the position that would normally correspond with the tips of that tallest row of OHC stereocilia and are thought to be where they insert into this membrane. A ridge, Hensen's stripe (HS), can also be seen in a position that corresponds to the tips of the tallest row of IHC stereocilia. Scale bar: 10 μm.

apparently do not contact, Hensen's stripe, a ridge that protrudes from the underside of the tectorial membrane (Fig. 8.1D).

8.2 **Mechanotransduction**

When the cochlea is stimulated by sound, the basilar membrane is deflected by pressure changes in cochlear fluids, causing the tectorial membrane to shear radially over the IHCs and OHCs,

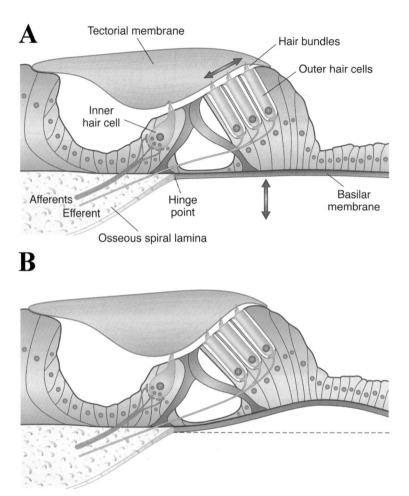

Fig. 8.2 (A) Transverse section through a middle turn of the cochlea, showing the organ of Corti, an assembly of intricately shaped supporting cells and inner and outer hair cells supported by the flexible basilar membrane. The organ of Corti is ~150 μm wide. (B) Upwards displacement of the basilar membrane stimulates the hair cells by bending their stereociliary bundles against the acellular tectorial membrane. Because of the point about which the basilar membrane hinges, the inner hair cells (IHCs) must be stimulated mainly by motion of the tectorial membrane but are thought to be stimulated indirectly by the flow of endolymph past their hair bundles. Signals from each IHC are relayed to the brain via 10–20 afferent fibres of the VIIIth cranial nerve. Outer hair cells have both sensory and motor capabilities and possess electromotility that underlies the cochlear amplifier. They have a sparse afferent innervation (not shown) and are contacted mainly by efferent nerves, which regulate the electromotility and influence cochlear sensitivity.
Reproduced with permission from Fettiplace and Hackney (2006).

deflecting the stereocilia. Deflection toward the tallest row of stereocilia opens the MET channels in the stereociliary bundle while deflection toward the shortest row closes them (Fig. 8.2). Because the driving force on potassium and calcium is inwards from the endolymphatic fluid, opening of cation-permeant MET channels allows an influx of these ions into the hair cell (Fig. 8.3). The MET channels in non-mammalian and mammalian hair cells are remarkable for their large

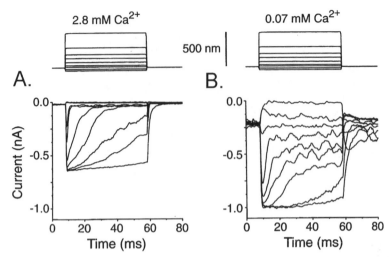

Fig. 8.3 Mechanotransducer currents recorded from patch-clamped turtle cochlear hair cells bathed in high (left) and low (right) extracellular calcium ion concentrations. The upper traces indicate the stepwise mechanical deflections of the hair bundle, the lower traces indicate the resultant mechanotransducer currents. Note that in both conditions, the current is on at rest but that this is greater in the low calcium condition. The rapid onset of the current indicates the direct mechanical gating of the mechanotransducer channel with more current flowing in the low calcium condition. Adaptation can be seen in both conditions as calcium ions block the channel, the time course of which is slower when the calcium concentration is low.
Reproduced with permission from Ricci *et al.* (1998). *J. Neurosci.* 18:8261. © *The Journal of Neuroscience.*

conductance (~50–300 pS) and permeability to calcium (Ricci *et al.*, 2003; Beurg *et al.*, 2006). The inward cationic transduction current depolarizes the hair cell, opening voltage-gated calcium channels, thereby causing an increase in the release of neurotransmitter from the afferent synapses at the base of the cell (Chapter 9). As will be explained further, calcium influx through the MET channels underlies rapid and slower phases of transducer adaptation.

Initial descriptions of hair cell mechanotransduction were obtained from various *in vitro* preparations from cold-blooded vertebrates, especially the bullfrog sacculus (Corey & Hudspeth 1979, 1983) and the turtle auditory end-organ, the basilar papilla (Crawford & Fettiplace, 1981). Among a host of findings, these studies showed the directionality of mechanotransduction (Shotwell *et al.*, 1981), initial estimates of dynamic range and sensitivity, and the first hints that active mechanical processes contribute to transduction (Crawford & Fettiplace, 1985). The most revealing studies use voltage-clamp recording from the hair cell during controlled deflection of the hair bundle (Fig. 8.3). Inward currents (by convention downward-going or negative) result from the influx of cations when MET channels are opened. The complex form of those inward currents will be further explored in a following section on adaptation.

Perhaps the biggest surprise was that several experimental approaches all located the MET channels near the tips of the stereocilia (Hudspeth, 1982; Jaramillo & Hudspeth, 1991; Denk *et al.*, 1995; Lumpkin & Hudspeth, 1995), rather than at their 'ankles' as seems logical (the point of maximal torque as the rigid hairs bend about their insertions). This tip location was complemented by the description of 'tip-links' (Pickles *et al.*, 1984), extracellular strands running from the tops of shorter stereocilia to the sides of adjacent taller ones (Fig. 8.4). Like mechanotransduction,

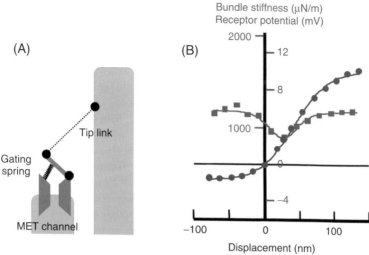

Bundle stiffness (μN/m)
Receptor potential (mV)

Fig. 8.4 The gating-spring model of mechanotransduction. (A) Mechanotransducer channels (METs) reside near the top of each stereocilium near the insertion point of tip links that extend to the next tallest stereocilium. It is postulated that lateral shear between stereocilia pulls the tip link, acting against the closing force of a spring-like gating element of the MET. The disposition of links, gates, and springs shown here is hypothetical. (B) Evidence for a 'gating-spring' is derived in part from measurements of hair bundle stiffness. These show that the measured stiffness (in red) is minimal at the midpoint of the activation curve (receptor potential in blue), corresponding to a displacement where half the MET channels are open. Stiffness is higher when all the channels are closed, or all open. Thus channel gating alters hair bundle stiffness. In the absence of external displacement, the intrinsic bundle tension acts to hold a minor fraction of MET channels open.
Figure 8.4B redrawn with permission from Howard and Hudspeth (1988).

tip-links only occur along the axis of bilateral symmetry of the hair bundle. Exposure to strong extracellular calcium buffer (BAPTA) breaks the tip links and eliminates mechanotransduction (Assad *et al.*, 1991). It has been shown that parallel recovery of tip-link structure and transducer function occurs in cultured chicken hair cells previously exposed to BAPTA (Zhao *et al.*, 1996).

8.3 The gating-spring hypothesis

Later experiments characterized the mechanical properties of the hair bundles in both cold- and warm-blooded vertebrates (Howard *et al.*, 1988; Géléoc & Holt, 2003; Kennedy *et al.*, 2003). This required optical techniques for rapidly capturing submicrometre motions of the hair bundle. To produce 'force steps', flexible glass probes of known stiffness were used to deflect hair bundles, providing estimates of bundle stiffness by the principle of reciprocity (Crawford & Fettiplace, 1985). From these efforts the 'passive' stiffness and gating compliance of hair bundles were obtained. These features of mechanotransduction are summarized in the 'gating-spring' hypothesis which posits that hair bundle motion transmits energy to the MET channel through a spring-like element (Fig. 8.4A). Critical support for this model was provided by the observation that hair bundle stiffness decreases (compliance increases) over the range of motion in which MET channels gate (Fig. 8.4B), that is, movement of the channel gate relieves some of the gating-spring's stiffness, requiring direct coupling between channel and gating spring (Howard & Hudspeth, 1988). Direct mechanical coupling also accords with the speed of MET gating. As noted above, some hair cells signal in the 100 kHz range, thus requiring microsecond gating kinetics and making any type of enzymatic interactions highly unlikely (Ricci *et al.*, 2006). It is important to note that the gating-spring model does not identify molecular mechanisms. In particular, the spring-like property could reside in the channel or any mechanically connected proteins. In fact, the current evidence suggests that the tip link itself is probably too stiff to serve as the gating spring but rather acts as a simple tether (Kachar *et al.*, 2000, and see below), requiring that 'springiness' resides elsewhere.

Nonetheless, experimental results can be interpreted in the light of the gating-spring model. So for example, assuming parallel activation of MET channels, the force required to deflect the hair bundle implies that the single channel gating force is ~0.3 pN (Howard *et al.*, 1988; van Netten & Kros, 2000), of the same order of magnitude as the forces estimated for other voltage or ligand-mediated molecular conformational changes (Ricci *et al.*, 2002). In fact, technical limitations of these measurements may make this an underestimate. More recent experiments from mammalian cochlear hair cells imply much larger gating forces (Kennedy *et al.*, 2003), supporting a role for active mechanical feedback during sensory transduction (see below).

The gating compliance is only a fraction of the total bundle stiffness, which also includes passive components such as the stiffness of the stereocilia and their rootlets (Crawford & Fettiplace, 1985), the structures in the 'ankle' region of the stereocilia about which they pivot, and the extracellular cross-links between stereocilia (see later for detailed descriptions of these structures). If the gating compliance and passive stiffness are of comparable magnitude, the hair bundle can become unstable and undergo low-frequency oscillatory motions up to 20 nm in extent, as observed in frog saccular hair cells (Martin *et al.*, 2000) (Fig. 8.5A, B). In turtle auditory hair cells spontaneous hair bundle oscillations can occur at the characteristic frequency of the cell (Crawford & Fettiplace, 1985). Such observations show clearly that active processes are involved in mechanotransduction and that biological energy must contribute to sensitivity and tuning. Indeed, continued study has revealed surprising complexity in hair bundle motion during imposed displacements (Ricci *et al.*, 2006), including that of hair cells in the mammalian cochlea (Kennedy *et al.*, 2005). In mammalian cochlear hair cells however, the speed of those reactive motions, and the calculated forces, are much greater than those obtained from non-mammalian hair cells, suggesting as yet undefined additional active processes (Fettiplace, 2006). The reactive motions of the hair bundle occur in both positive and negative directions, with rapid and slow kinetics. This active bundle motion is calcium dependent and may contribute to cochlear amplification (Chan & Hudspeth, 2005). How this occurs and how such amplification might interact with the amplification based on somatic motility in OHCs is presently uncertain, but there is evidence for anatomical connections between the hair bundle and the basolateral membrane via the stereociliary rootlets (Furness *et al.*, 2008b), which could allow for some interaction. Although much remains to be learned, some of these active motions also seem to be related to processes of rapid and slow adaptation.

8.4 Adaptation of mechanotransduction

During a sustained deflection of the hair bundle, MET channels open but then close again, so that the inward current decays over a complex time course (see Fig. 8.3). This process differs from voltage-dependent inactivation or ligand-dependent desensitization of ion channels. In contrast to those states that are at least temporarily irreversible, the adapted MET channels can be reopened simply by increasing hair bundle deflection. Indeed, hair bundle adaptation is equivalent to a linear shift of the mechanosensor along the displacement/response axis (Fig. 8.6B). The displacement sensitivity and maximum response remain essentially the same. Studies in hair cells from various vertebrate species have revealed that adaptation occurs along two distinct time

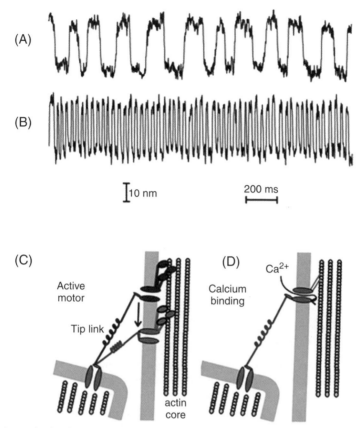

Fig. 8.5 Active and adaptive properties of MET channels. (A) Spontaneous oscillations (6 Hz, 18 nm rms) of the hair bundle in the frog's sacculus. (B) Higher-frequency (27 Hz, 18 nm rms) oscillations of a different hair bundle. (C) Slow adaptation could be mediated by myosin-based adaptation motors that tension the MET by pulling along the stereocilia's actin core. (D) More rapid adaptation may occur at the MET itself. Both slow and fast adaptation are calcium dependent
Figure 8.5B reproduced with permission from Martin *et al.* (2003), *J. Neurosci.* 23:4533–48. © *The Journal of Neuroscience.* Figure 8.5C reproduced with permission from Holt and Corey (2000), *Proc Natl Acad Sci U S A.* 97:11730–5. © (2000) National Academy of Sciences, U.S.A.

courses, both of which are calcium dependent (Fig. 8.5C, D). The slower component, with time constants on the order of 100 ms, is thought to result from the contribution of myosin motors that produce tension on the MET channel by pulling against the actin core of the stereocilium (see review by Gillespie & Cyr, 2004). Evidence in support of myosin-dependent adaptation is provided by experiments on transgenic mice in which the putative adaptation motor, myosin 1c, is made sensitive to an experimental ligand that reversibly eliminates slow adaptation (Holt *et al.*, 2002). A more rapid component of adaptation (time constants ~1–10 ms) may result from direct feedback of calcium onto the MET channel (Fig. 8.5D), reducing its open probability (Crawford *et al.*, 1989; Benser *et al.*, 1996; Ricci *et al.*, 2000). However, it has been shown that functional myosin 1c also is required for rapid adaptation in mouse vestibular hair cells (Stauffer *et al.*, 2005), implicating a short-lived, calcium-dependent effect of myosin on MET open probability. Adaptation 'motors' may contribute to active hair bundle mechanics. This suggestion is supported

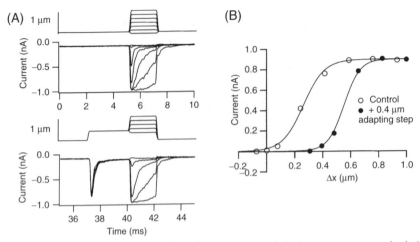

Fig. 8.6 Adaptation in rat cochlear hair cells. (A) A succession of displacement steps to the hair bundle caused successively larger, adapting inward currents. After a 0.4 μm adapting step, the stimulus paradigm was repeated. (B) Peak currents produced under the two conditions show that adaptation caused a shift in the displacement-response curve nearly equivalent to the adapting step.
Reproduced with permission from Fettiplace (2006).

by the correlation between hair bundle adaptation rate and characteristic frequency along the tonotopic axis in both the turtle (Ricci *et al.*, 2000) and the rat auditory epithelium (Ricci *et al.*, 2005). In the rat hair cells adaptation rates as brief as 100 μs have been observed.

The calcium dependence of MET adaptation has important consequences (Holt & Corey, 2000). When the hair bundle is bathed by endolymph-like concentrations of calcium (as would exist *in vivo*), adaptation is reduced and slowed. Consequently, the resting open probability of the MET channels is raised (Fig. 8.3). The effects of external calcium depend on the magnitude of the MET current and the level of cytoplasmic calcium buffer, both of which vary along the tonotopic axis. Finally, calcium dependent MET adaptation in hair cells is further modulated by cyclic nucleotides (Ricci & Fettiplace, 1997; Martin *et al.*, 2003). Mechanotransduction in hair cells is subject then to multiple levels of regulation. The expression of calcium buffers and pumps will be considered further in a later section.

8.5 Organization and maintenance of the cytoskeleton of the hair cell apex

Since hair cells have to detect, and therefore withstand, mechanical energy, a primary requirement of the mechanosensory hair bundle and the apical region into which it is anchored is that they should both have strength and stability. Accordingly, the stereocilia that form the bundle and the apical filamentous raft, the cuticular plate, into which they are rooted, are filled with cytoskeletal proteins. The predominant cytoskeletal protein is actin, which forms at least three distinct networks, the core of the stereocilia, the matrix of the cuticular plate, and an apical peripheral ring (Drenckhahn *et al.*, 1991). Each network appears to contain a different structural organization of actin filaments and associated proteins.

The actin is present in two forms, β-cytoplasmic actin and non-muscle γ-actin (Fig. 8.7). Quantitative immunocytochemistry suggests that stereocilia and cuticular plate contain different

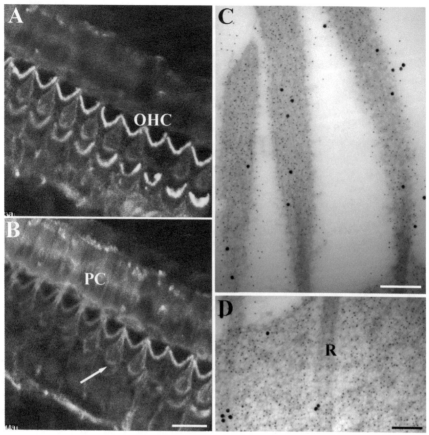

Fig. 8.7 Immunolabelling of guinea pig cochlea for γ- (green fluorescence and 15 nm gold particles) and β-actin (red fluorescence and 30 nm gold particles). (A, B) The OHC stereocilia are clearly labelled for γ-actin at their apices; towards their bases, there is more evidence of β-actin. Supporting cells, especially the heads of the rod-like pillar cells (PC) that lie between IHC and OHC rows and the ends of the outer pillar cell processes between OHCs of the first row (arrow), label for β-actin. Scale bar for A and B: 10 μm. (C) Immunogold labelling of stereocilia. Note that the densities of the gold particles do not represent the relative concentrations of the two types of actin as the two antibodies used are of different sensitivities. However, the double labelling suggests that both are present in the stereocilia. Scale bar: 250 nm. (D) Both the cuticular plate and rootlet are labelled for γ-actin but the roolets (R) are also labelled for β-actin. Scale bar: 200 nm.

relative amounts of these two isoforms, consistent with the suggestion that these are distinct networks (Furness *et al.*, 2005). Overall, there seems to be more γ-actin than β-actin in the hair cell apex (Hofer & Drenckhahn, 1997) in contrast to the adjacent supporting cells of the cochlea (Fig. 8.7; Furness *et al.*, 2005). This may result in different mechanical properties in these two types of cell.

As well as actin, the stereocilia and cuticular plate contain several forms of non-muscle myosin and a range of proteins associated with development and maintenance of the structures of the apex. The growth and maintenance of stereocilia have received attention because most genetic defects that disturb the organization of the bundle lead to hearing loss. Phenotypic alterations caused by mutations in genes coding for cytoskeletal proteins have allowed molecules crucial to

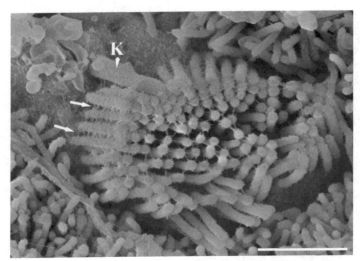

Fig. 8.8 Scanning electron micrograph of a mouse IHC hair bundle at postnatal day 0. Note the extensive hexagonally arranged cross-linking between the stereocilia including the links towards the base of the stereocilia (arrows) and along their lengths, and multiple links around the tops. Extracellular links can also be seen between the kinocilium (K) and the adjacent stereocilia. Scale bar: 1 μm.

hair bundle development to be identified, as well as explaining several types of inherited deafness.

In immature hair cells, the bundle first appears to consist of a disorganized cluster of stereocilia of equal length (Fig. 8.8). Gradually, some of the stereocilia increase differentially in length while others are reabsorbed to create the polarized hair bundle with its precise staircase arrangement (see, for example, Furness *et al.*, 1989). In adult hair cell stereocilia, the actin of the core is arranged in a bundle of parallel actin filaments of the same polarity, some of which penetrate through into the cuticular plate to form, in mammals, a narrow rootlet, associated with dense material (Itoh, 1982). The actin filaments are regularly cross-linked by bridges composed of fimbrin (plastin) (Tilney *et al.*, 1989) and espin (Zheng *et al.*, 2000). The tight packing and regular cross-linking of the actin filaments in the bundle (see Fig. 8.9B below) gives the core of the stereocilium a paracrystalline organization (Tilney *et al.*, 1980) which is presumed to contribute to its stiffness. The precise length of this core, and thus the stereocilia, must be specified during growth in order to produce the different heights of stereocilia within the bundle to create the staircase. Moreover, the staircase shows tonotopically organized changes in length which hint at a complex control mechanism for stereociliary growth along the cochlea, the basis of which is not yet understood.

Genetic defects and developmental studies suggest that espins (Rzadzinska *et al.*, 2005) and plastins (Daudet & Lebart, 2002) are involved in the growth and maintenance of the actin core. The espin deficient jerker mouse has abnormalities in the hair bundles that cause deafness and balance disorders (Zheng *et al.*, 2000). Although only I-plastin is found in adults, the T-plastin isoform appears transiently in developing stereocilia, suggesting that the latter has a developmental role (Daudet & Lebart, 2002).

Another major protein critical for the elongation of the stereocilia is myosin XVa (Belyantseva *et al.*, 2005), lack of which occurs in shaker 2 mice (Stepanyan *et al.*, 2006). The amount of myosin XVa at the stereociliary tip, as determined by its fluorescent intensity after immunolabelling, appears to correlate with the length of the stereocilium (Rzadzinska *et al.*, 2004). Although it seems to be involved in development and maintenance of the core and is apparently essential for normal hearing (Liburd *et al.*, 2001), recent studies indicate that absence of myosin XVa does not appear to affect the physiological properties of transduction, including adaptation, in relatively young hair cells (rat P3-P7) (Stepanyan *et al.*, 2006). Thus myosin XVa does not seem to be an essential part of the MET apparatus nor does it assist in its initial assembly and function. At later ages, myosin XVa deficient hair bundles show obvious defects in organization. Myosin XVa appears to be necessary for the targeting of whirlin to the stereociliary tips, defects in which underlie the phenotype of the whirler mouse (Kikkawa *et al.*, 2005). Whirlin is a PDZ protein that appears transiently in stereocilia during development in a systematic pattern which crosses the bundle in a way that suggests this protein is associated with growth of the different lengths of the rows of stereocilia in the staircase. This idea is supported by the fact that whirler mutants display shorter stereocilia (Belyantseva *et al.*, 2005; Møgensen *et al.*, 2007).

In early postnatal mouse cultures, β-cytoplasmic actin has been shown to be incorporated at the tips of the stereocilia and to travel down the core (Rzadzinska *et al.*, 2004). The rate of addition of subunits depends on the lengths of the stereocilia in a way that ensures that actin in the hair bundle turns over simultaneously. Espin incorporation takes place at a similar rate and in a similar sequence, indicating that formation of espin cross-bridges only occurs as the actin is polymerized (Rzadzinska *et al.*, 2005). Taken together, these data suggest that establishment of the actin core requires a temporally and spatially sensitive combination of elongation cues, such as the rate of actin polymerization, and the concentrations of whirlin, myosin XVa, plastins, and espins, to enable them to grow to the correct length.

Genes mutated in both syndromic and non-syndromic forms of deafness in humans, and their mouse homologues, encode a number of other proteins likely to be involved in the development of the hair bundle and the apical supporting structures. An example of this is protocadherin 15, a putative component of the filamentous cross-links between stereocilia. Abnormalities in this protein result in disorganized hair bundles and changes within the cuticular plate, specifically rotations or misalignments of the hair bundle and stereociliary rootlets (Pawlowski *et al.*, 2006). Other proteins that are associated with the Usher complex are myosin VIIa, cadherin 23, harmonin and SANs, a scaffolding protein (see review by El-Amraoui & Petit, 2005). Myosin VIIa is localized to the shaft of the stereocilia (Rzadzinska *et al.*, 2004), where it may form links between the actin core and the membrane, and cadherin 23, like protocadherin 15, could be part of a macromolecular assembly that anchors the links between stereocilia. Cadherin 23 also binds with another protein, harmonin, which may also, therefore, form part of the cross-links between stereocilia (Siemens *et al.*, 2002) and which associates with catenin-cadherin complexes (Küssel-Andermann *et al.*, 2000). The two other proteins that also bind to myosin VIIa and which are found in stereocilia and are believed to belong to this link-anchoring complex, are vezatin (an ubiquitous protein of adhesion junctions) and PHR1, a putative integral membrane protein (Küssel-Andermann *et al.*, 2000; Etournay *et al.*, 2005).

Defects in myosin VIIa affect bundle formation and cause disorganization of the stereocilia. They result in lower sensitivity to deflection and increased rate of adaptation (Kros *et al.*, 2002) suggesting that myosin VIIa could be a component of the MET apparatus and thus involved in the processes of mechanotransduction and adaptation. The ankle membrane of the stereocilia contains radixin (Pataky *et al.*, 2003), one of the ezrin-radixin-moesin (ERM) family of proteins associated with membrane-cytoskeleton interactions. Radixin interacts with myosin VIIa and myosin XVa, indicating possible formation of complexes between these proteins, binding actin to the membrane. Radixin deficiency does not prevent stereociliary formation but in the cochleae of adult radixin-deficient mice, stereocilia degenerate whereas in the vestibular system they do not, indicating a complex behaviour in stereociliary maintenance (Kitajiri *et al.*, 2004). Radixin may be associated with the chloride channel CLIC5, which also has been found in stereocilia in similar locations (Gagnon *et al.*, 2006).

Another unconventional myosin, myosin 1c has been more directly linked to adaptation (Stauffer *et al.*, 2005). Binding studies indicate that this protein associates with cadherin 23 at the tips of stereocilia. Both proteins are thought to be crucial components of the MET apparatus, and their roles are discussed further below in relation to the interstereociliary links and mechanotransduction. Myosin VI has also been found in hair cells (Hasson *et al.*, 1997). In zebra fish, it is localized to the ankle regions of stereocilia. Zebra fish defective for Myo6 show loss of MET (Kappler *et al.*, 2004). In Snell's waltzer mice, which also have a defective Myo6 gene, stereocilia become fused (Self *et al.*, 1999). It has been suggested that myosin VI is involved in anchoring the stereociliary membrane (Kappler *et al.*, 2004).

8.6 **Structure and function of the extracellular linkages**

As noted above, the stereocilia are connected together by various forms of extracellular filaments (Fig. 8.9). The precise appearance and organization of these filaments depends firstly on how the tissue is prepared, and secondly on the type and origin of the hair cells. Addition of tannic acid and cationic dyes such as cuprolinic blue (Tsuprun & Santi, 2002), Alcian blue, and ruthenium red (Santi & Anderson, 1987) to fixatives enhance the appearance and increase the visible extent of these links. Hair cells from different auditory and vestibular organs show various patterns of linkages and have subsets of the linkages that are compositionally distinct (Goodyear & Richardson, 1994; see review by Nayak *et al.*, 2007).

A particular interest in the cross-links between stereocilia stems from suggestions by Thurm (1981) and Hudspeth (1982) that physical links could represent the gating spring discussed earlier, that is, the gating springs of the MET channels would be represented by a visible, morphological element. The hypothesis is that the gating spring is an extracellular link that attaches to the gate of the channels and, during deflection of the bundle, pulls on them. Thus, excitatory deflections of the bundle would stretch the spring, pulling the channel open, like a bath plug on a chain, thus depolarizing the hair cell, whereas inhibitory deflections would relax the spring allowing the channels to close, hyperpolarizing the cell.

The search for these gating springs was assisted by the development of high resolution scanning electron microscopy (SEM), which enabled detailed three-dimensional imaging of hair bundles at magnifications that show the cross-links relatively clearly (Fig. 8.9A). Studies by both SEM and transmission electron microscopy (TEM) revealed the tip link which connects the tips of shorter stereocilia to the sides of the taller stereocilia (Pickles *et al.*, 1984). The tip link appears to be in an ideal location to represent a gating spring, provided the MET channels are located near one or the other (or both) ends of the link. Determining the location of the channels is therefore crucial to identifying the gating spring from the various other extracellular links.

The tip link consists of a strand running from the tip of all except the tallest stereocilia in a bundle that projects obliquely towards the sides of the taller stereocilia in the adjacent row (Fig. 8.9C). A number of studies suggest that the tip link bifurcates part way along so that two strands connect to the membrane of the taller stereocilia (Hackney & Furness, 1995; Kachar *et al.*, 2000). The bifurcation has been observed in all vertebrate classes except fish hair cells (Furness & Hackney, 2006). A report based on TEM tomography suggests that one branch of the fork might be an auxiliary structure rather than part of the main link (Auer *et al.*, 2008). This discrepancy between the electron tomography and other methodologies has yet to be resolved. At both the lower and upper terminations of the tip link are dense patches beneath the membrane (Furness & Hackney, 1985; Little & Neugebauer, 1985) which probably contain myosins and potentially

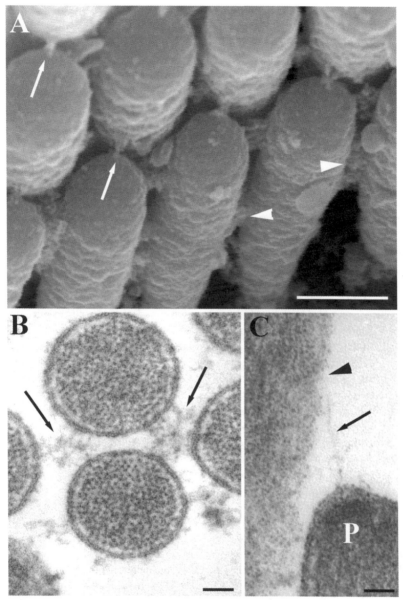

Fig. 8.9 (A) Scanning and (B, C) transmission electron micrographs showing further details of the extracellular linkages between the stereocilia. (A) Tip links (arrows) and lateral linkages (arrowheads) connect the serried rows of stereocilia. Scale bar: 250 nm. (B) Cross-section of six stereocilia; the actin filaments that they contain can be seen within each stereociliary profile. Extracellular lateral linkages (see, for example, arrows) with a central denser region can be seen to run between the stereocilia. Scale bar: 50 nm. (C) A tip link (arrow) extends between a shorter and a taller stereocilium. It is attached to the side of the taller stereocilium (arrowhead). An electron dense region (P) underlies its attachment to the shorter stereocilium, the plasma membrane of which appears to be under tension ('tenting') at the point at which the link is attached. Scale bar: 50 nm.

harmonin-b; the tip patch is likely to contain whirlin and myosin XVa (see earlier discussion) while the patch at the upper end of the tip link is thought to contain myosin 1c (Steyger et al., 1998). Both regions are enriched in calmodulin which could be associated with these myosins and modulate their activity in way that is associated with calcium binding (Furness et al., 2002).

The tip links appear to be refined developmentally from a more extensive set of multiple links around the stereociliary tips (Fig. 8.8; Furness et al., 1989). In vestibular organs, multiple tip links can still be observed in some adult hair cells (Furness & Hackney, 2006), making individual tip links difficult to identify. Evidence from immunocytochemistry, mutations and knockouts suggest that cadherin 23 (Söllner et al., 2004) and protocadherin 15 (Ahmed et al., 2006) interact to form the tip links, cadherin 23 forming the upper, frequently branched, portion of the tip link while protocadherin 15 forms the lower part (Kazmierczak et al., 2007). Information about the dimensions of the tip links and the effects of various levels of extracellular calcium are consistent with this suggestion (Furness et al., 2008a). Further evidence that cadherin 23 forms at least part of the tip link comes from experiments showing that the membrane-associated guanylate kinase protein, MAGI-1, binds to cadherin 23 and is localized in a punctate staining pattern on the stereocilia during development and in adults (Xu et al., 2008).

It has also been shown that myosin VIIa, harmonin-b, cadherin 23, and protocadherin 15 are concentrated in the stereociliary tips of developing hair bundles of mice. Soon after birth, results from immunofluorescence and confocal microscopy suggest that harmonin-b relocates to the position of the upper end of the tip link, a change which does not occur in mice deficient in harmonin-b or protocadherin 15 (Lefèvre et al., 2008).

Myosin 1c in the stereocilia also disappears in the absence of cadherin 23, and after calcium chelation (Phillips et al., 2006), which is known to destroy the tip links and eliminate transduction (Assad et al., 1991). The direct association between the tip links and MET channels, however, remains uncertain; observations of the structure by freeze fracture, deep etch electron microscopy suggests that the tip link is composed of a braided macromolecule that is likely to be insufficiently elastic to be the gating spring (Kachar et al., 2000), an observation supported by studies using different electron microscopic techniques (Tsuprun & Santi, 2000; Furness et al., 2008a). So far, no unambiguous anatomical or electrophysiological localization of the MET channels has been achieved with sufficient resolution to place the channels at the end(s) of the tip link. However, there is evidence that clearly defined tip links appear during development concurrently with the ability of hair cells to transduce (Géléoc & Holt, 2003).

In addition to the tip links, there are various kinds of horizontal cross-links or lateral links between the shafts of the stereocilia (Fig. 8.9A, B). Such links project in all directions, attaching the nearest neighbours (Pickles et al., 1984; Furness & Hackney, 1985). Links occur at various points along the shafts. There appears to be a particular band of horizontal connections just below the tips of shorter stereocilia (top connectors), close to the tip link insertions, and lower down, lateral links with a medial stripe (Fig. 8.9B) consisting of globular structures (Tsuprun & Santi, 2002), which couple stereocilia both between rows and within rows (Furness & Hackney, 1985). In some non-mammalian vertebrates a category of ankle links has also been described (Goodyear & Richardson, 1999) and links in similar locations can be observed in immature cochlear hair bundles (Fig. 8.8).

The lateral links may be anchored to the stereocilia via the harmonin-vezatin-catenin complexes discussed earlier and may be important in stereociliary development. The harmonin complex proteins also interact with myosin VIIa that occurs along the stereociliary shaft. An interaction between protocadherin 15 and myosin VIIa is also necessary during bundle development (Senften et al., 2006). There is also a report that a set of lateral links containing cadherin 23 is transiently present (Michel et al., 2005). Another recently discovered component of ankle links, the very large

G-protein-coupled receptor (VLGR1; McGee *et al.*, 2006), and the transmembrane protein, usherin (Michalski *et al.*, 2007), also seem to be involved in bundle development. All of these molecules may take part in the process that culminates in proper targeting of the different categories of cross-link to the correct places in the stereocilia. How the development of the links occurs is uncertain but one possible regulator is transient receptor potential mucolipin 3, TRPML3 (a member of the TRP ion channel protein family), loss of which in the varitint-waddler mouse causes stereociliary splaying (Atiba-Davies & Noben-Trauth, 2007).

While there is good evidence that the different categories of these lateral links have distinct composition, they are not morphologically consistent across all hair cells in different vertebrate classes to the same extent as the tip link. Their precise contribution to hair bundle function, other than development and maintenance, remains speculative. It is likely that they tie the bundle of stereocilia together to enable it to act as a unit and they prevent it from splaying. Measurements of bundle motion imply that the stereocilia are tightly constrained so that there is little lag between the motion of stereocilia on either side of the bundle and they all move coherently resulting in maximally efficient gating of the MET channels (Kozlov *et al.*, 2007). Whether the lateral links contribute to transduction more directly remains to be determined but there is some evidence that the channels may be associated with horizontal connections near the tips of shorter stereocilia (Hackney *et al.*, 1992).

8.7 Location, identity, and function of the mechanotransducer channels

The precise location and identity of the MET channels themselves remain controversial. It seems well established that the channel is located in the hair bundle near the stereociliary tips (see review by Furness & Hackney, 2006), but as noted above, their association with the tip links has yet to be determined unequivocally. The main reason for this is that an irreversible electron microscopic marker for the channel has yet to be identified. Physiological measurements suggest that there are only about 100 or so functional channels per hair cell and hair cell epithelia contain only a few thousand hair cells, so it is possible that there are too few copies of the channel molecule to permit purification of the protein and then raise antibodies to it.

Earlier attempts to localize the channels at the electron microscopic level were made with antibodies against an epithelial sodium channel on the basis that both shared an amiloride-binding site that might be antigenically similar. This approach yielded the interesting but controversial result of consistent immunogold labelling near the tips of the stereocilia at the site of the contact region, a zone of close approach between the tips of the shorter stereocilia and the sides of the taller stereocilia (Hackney *et al.*, 1991, 1992), about 50–200 nm below the tip-link insertion into the shorter stereocilium (Fig. 8.10). This location could be influenced by the tip link pulling on the plasma membrane at the stereociliary tip and it also contains a region of horizontal connections between the stereocilia which might represent alternative gating structures. The binding of the antibodies to this location was inhibited by the MET channel blocker dihydrostreptomycin and the binding site could also be protected from trypsinization by another blocker, amiloride (Furness *et al.*, 1996). Kinematic analysis has shown that links at this site would be efficient in detecting shear between stereocilia (Furness *et al.*, 1997). Another antibody, an anti-idiotypic monoclonal antibody to amiloride-binding sites, also interferes with transduction but is unfortunately not a good marker at the electron microscopic level probably as a result of its epitopic binding site being sensitive to fixation (Schulte *et al.*, 2002). Other attempts to show that the tip link is synonymous with the gating spring have been based on chemical interference with transduction or using calcium-sensitive dyes to localize calcium influx through the channel.

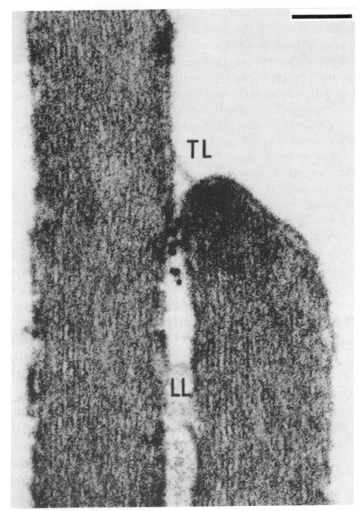

Fig. 8.10 Transmission electron micrograph of guinea pig stereocilia immunolabelled with an antibody for the amiloride-binding site of the epithelial sodium channel. A tip link (TL) and lateral links (LL) can be seen connecting the two stereocilia. The labelling, which is indicated by gold particles (black spheres) is, however, seen at the point where the two stereociliary membranes come into the closest contact. Scale bar: 100 nm.
Modified with permission from Hackney and Furness (1995).

The former suffer from having potential consequences that could secondarily affect transduction or the tip link so the data are indirect or ambiguous; the latter are visualized light microscopically with insufficient resolution to observe the links or distinguish the site of the tip links from the contact region.

Examples of chemical interference with transduction include the use of low calcium buffers, achieved by applying a calcium chelator, BAPTA, which causes disruption of the tip links and loss of transduction (Assad *et al.*, 1991). This effect is reversible *in vitro* over a period of 24 hours, in which the tip links and transduction reappear simultaneously (Zhao *et al.*, 1996), as noted earlier. Enzymatic destruction using elastase also causes loss of tip links and normal mechanotransduction, but in some studies the channels appear to remain open after both BAPTA and elastase, and are blockable with the MET channel blocker dihydrostreptomycin (Meyer *et al.*, 1998). The latter result is difficult to explain if tip-link tension opens the channels. The possibility remains therefore that the tip link does not gate the channel directly.

Calcium-sensitive dyes show calcium influx near the tips of the stereocilia (Lumpkin & Hudspeth, 1995) and have been used to assess whether all stereociliary rows contain MET channels (Denk *et al.*, 1995). In the latter study, all rows of stereocilia in a bundle appeared to display calcium influx suggesting that if channels do occur at the tip-link attachment sites, they are at both ends. However, this assumes that calcium influx into the stereocilia only occurs through the MET channels. Another type of channel found in stereocilia is the ATP-gated $P2X_2$ channels (Housley *et al.*, 1999). $P2X_2$ channels also permit the entry of calcium (Egan & Khakh, 2004) and so calcium influx could reflect entry through these channels.

Recent findings also suggest that the stereocilia may contain acid-sensing channels (ASIC), in particular, isoform ASIC1b (Ugawa *et al.*, 2006). The ASICs are proton-gated sodium channels of the mammalian degenerin (MDEG) family, which includes the amiloride-sensitive epithelial sodium channel (ENaC), and are also partially permeable to calcium (Waldmann *et al.*, 1997); thus if all stereocilia contain these channels, calcium influx may not provide a specific indication of MET channel location. The ASICs have been localized to the ankle region of the stereocilia. These channels may therefore explain an earlier finding that calcium-induced FURA-2 fluorescence could be quenched by manganese entry in the ankle region (Ohmori, 1988).

Since the identity of the MET channel is unknown, but it has sensitivity to amiloride, it is possible that it could be related in some way to the MDEG or ASIC channel family or to the ATP-gated purinoceptors. As described earlier, investigations of the MET channel properties show that it has a large unitary conductance that varies between 50 pS and 300 pS (from chick, mouse, and turtle data *in vitro*) and increases along the tonotopic axis from low to high frequency (Ricci *et al.*, 2003; Beurg *et al.*, 2006). In the presence of low (50 μM) calcium (a permeant blocker) the single-channel conductance is 300 pS. The pore size is of the order of 1.26 nm (Farris *et al.*, 2004). As well as dihydrostreptomycin, amiloride and its derivative benzamil, and calcium ions, the MET channel can be blocked by other cations such as magnesium, gadolinium, and lanthanum (see review by Fettiplace & Ricci, 2006). Estimates of the number of functional channels per stereocilium indicate that there may be only one or two (Beurg *et al.*, 2006), although this does not preclude the possibility that there could be non-functional channels or subunits en route through the hair cell or stereocilia (see for instance, Hackney *et al.*, 1992).

There are a number of mechanosensory and other channels to consider as candidates. As noted above, channels of the MDEG-ENaC superfamily are blocked by amiloride but at substantially lower concentrations than the MET channel, and their unitary conductance is smaller. ATP-gated $P2X_2$ channels have a pore diameter of about 2 nm, and a conductance of around 60 pS. They are equally permeable to Na^+ and K^+, and are blocked by Ca^{2+} to which they are only weakly permeable (Ding & Sachs, 2000). The ATP and MET channels show differential sensitivity to D-tubocurarine and combined stimulation of hair bundles with ATP and mechanical stimuli produces an additive current, suggesting that the two channels are independent (Glowatzki *et al.*, 1997). Another possible channel type is the cyclic-nucleotide-gated channel (CNG). These are similar to the MET with respect to amiloride sensitivity and calcium block but have a low unitary conductance (Farris *et al.*, 2004).

Attention has also been drawn to the transient receptor potential (TRP) channels. Studies of *Drosophila* revealed that no mechanoreceptor potential C (nompC), a relative of the TRP channel OSM-9 (osmotic avoidance abnormal 9), was involved in mechanosensory bristles (Walker *et al.*, 2000) and recent studies of zebrafish using antisense oligonucleotides to knock down channel function produced initial deafness and imbalance (Sidi *et al.*, 2003). nompC does not occur in mammalian hair cells although another TRP channel, TRPA1, also has been suggested to be present. Antibodies to this channel label the stereocilia, and small interfering (si)RNA for TRPA1 introduced into hair cells *in vitro* prevented transduction (Corey *et al.*, 2004). However, knock-out mice lacking TRPA1 appear to retain normal auditory function (Bautista *et al.*, 2006; Kwan *et al.*, 2006).

The mRNA for at least three other types of TRP channel, TRPV4, TRPML3, and TRPP has been found in an organ of Corti library (Cuajungco *et al.*, 2007). As for TRPA1, TRPV4 knock-outs show no evidence of auditory deficit (Liedtke & Friedman 2003; Tabuchi *et al.*, 2005) so neither of these are critical independent components of the MET channel. Although TRPML3 is localized to the hair cell and its mutation causes delayed onset deafness, the channel conductance is substantially smaller than that of the MET (Nagata *et al.*, 2008). Only TRPP (also known as PKD) channels, mechanoreceptors in the kidney and heart, have comparable properties with large unitary conductance and high calcium permeability relative to that of sodium (Volk *et al.*, 2003; Owsianik *et al.*, 2006) and both PKD2 and PKD2L1 have amiloride half-blocking concentrations comparable with those of the MET. Thus although the identity of the elusive MET channel still remains to be determined, there are a number of possible candidates.

Despite the uncertainties, the scenario for mechanotransduction that is most commonly accepted at present is that the tip link gates the MET channel by tension. The channel closes rapidly, resulting in the fast phase of adaptation, followed by slipping of the upper tip-link attachment down the stereociliary core, which produces the slow phase of adaptation. Both processes are modulated by calcium, changes in which have been demonstrated physiologically to affect channel gating and adaptation. This model suggests that myosin 1c in the upper dense patch

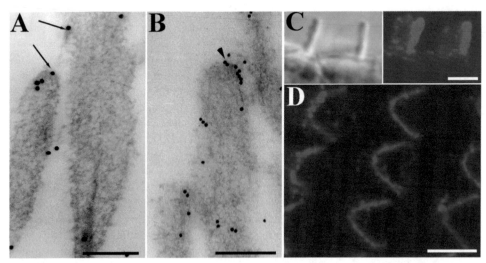

Fig. 8.11 (A, B) Electron and (C, D) light microscopic immunolabelling of guinea pig cochlear hair cells for calmodulin and plasma membrane calcium-ATPases (PMCAs). (A, B) Post-embedding immunogold labelling for calmodulin indicates that it occurs at either end (arrows) of the tip link. It is also concentrated at the region of closest contact between the short and tall stereocilia (arrowhead). Scale bar: 250 nm. (C, D). Light microscopic images of outer hair cell (OHC) bundles to show PMCAs. (C) OHC bundle bright field (left panel) and immunofluorescence (right panel). (D) Top view of OHC bundles. The images suggest that PMCA is concentrated in the stereociliary bundles. Scale bars in both: 5 μm.

forms an adaptation motor responsible for the slow phase of adaptation (Gillespie & Cyr, 2004). Recently, it has been shown that lack of myosin 1c also eliminates fast adaptation (Stauffer *et al.*, 2005) although an enzyme-based interaction would be too slow to provide fast adaptation directly and it is possible that in the absence of myosin 1c, other components of the transducer apparatus itself are not fully formed or functional.

8.8 Calcium handling mechanisms in the hair bundle

The calcium sensitivity of transduction and its role in adaptation mean that the transducer apparatus also needs calcium regulating and sensing proteins. Calmodulin is enriched at the tips of the stereocilia at both ends of the tip link as well as in the stereociliary contact region (Fig. 8.11A, B; Furness *et al.*, 2002). In these locations, calmodulin could be an integral component of the MET

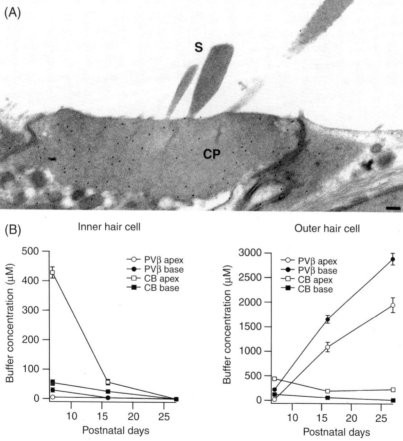

Fig. 8.12 (A) Apex of a rat hair cell labelled for calbindin. There is labelling in the cuticular plate (CP) and cell body but very little in the stereocilia (S). Scale bar: 150 nm. (B, C) Graphs showing the buffer concentration of parvalbumin-β and calbindin-D-28K at various postnatal developmental stages in rat at the cochlear apex and base. In the IHCs, there is a large decline in the level of the major calcium buffers that appears to coincide with the onset of hearing (postnatal day 12) whereas in the OHCs there is a rapid increase in the amount of parvalbumin-β.
Modified with permission from Hackney *et al.* (2005), © *The Journal of Neuroscience*.

channel itself, allowing calcium to have a direct influence on channel gating. However, myosin molecules bind calmodulin, so this may reflect an interaction with myosin 1c or myosin VIIa, representing the 'slow' adaptation motor, or myosin XVa. In mammals, calmodulin also occurs along the lateral wall of the stereocilia where myosin VIIa is found.

Plasma membrane calcium-ATPases (pumps – PMCAs) also occur at high density in the vicinity of the transducer apparatus. These work together with calcium buffers, such as calbindin, to exercise fine control over calcium concentration and thus regulate its effects on the MET channel. PMCAs have been immunolocalized in both adult frog sacculus and mammalian cochlear hair bundles (Fig. 8.11C, D). The different isoforms of PMCA show distinct distributions; the stereocilia contain predominantly or exclusively PMCA2 (Dumont *et al.*, 2001) and there is evidence of rapid turnover of this protein in the stereociliary membrane (Grati *et al.*, 2006). A mouse mutant lacking PMCA (the deafwaddler mouse) and PMCA2 knock-outs become deaf and display vestibular dysfunction (Kozel *et al.*, 1998; Street *et al.*, 1998).

A number of diffusible calcium buffers have been detected in hair cells (Fig. 8.12). These include parvalbumin-3 (Heller *et al.*, 2002), calbindin-D28K, parvalbumin-α, parvalbumin-β (oncomodulin) and calretinin (Hackney *et al.*, 2003, 2005; see also Ricci *et al.*, 1998 for the physiological basis of this research), some of which may be involved in control of local calcium concentrations in the bundle associated with the modulation of mechanotransduction. In the mouse, calretinin is present developmentally in hair cells but at least in OHCs, it disappears by

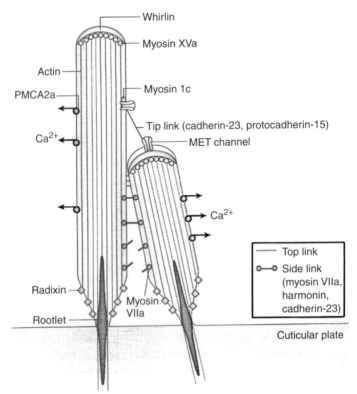

Fig. 8.13 Schematic drawing of stereocilia indicating candidate proteins contributing to structure and function of the mechanosensitive hair bundle.

postnatal day 22 (Dechesne *et al.*, 1994). In rats, the level of endogenous calcium buffering reduces markedly in the IHCs at the onset of hearing, and it increases to muscle-like levels in the OHCs (Fig. 8.9B). This observation supports the hypothesis that the two different hair cell types in mammals have different roles in hearing – the IHCs being mainly sensory whereas the OHCs are involved in cochlear amplification.

8.9 Concluding remarks

A summary of some of the structural and compositional features of the bundle is shown in Figure 8.13, incorporating recent findings from molecular biology and human genetics. These findings have led to a significant expansion in our knowledge and understanding of normal hearing and hearing impairment. A major challenge now is in understanding the difference between the genes that are involved in the development of the inner ear and those that are involved in its maintenance as a terminally differentiated sensory system.

Acknowledgements

Our work has been supported mainly by grants from the Wellcome Trust and Deafness Research UK. Our thanks are also due to the University of Wisconsin-Madison and R Fettiplace for providing additional funding for CMH. Thanks are due also to P Fuchs and R Fettiplace for their comments on and additions to this chapter.

References

Auer M, Koster AJ, Ziese U, Bajaj C, Volkmann N, Wang da N & Hudspeth AJ. (2008) Three-dimensional architecture of hair-bundle linkages revealed by electron-microscopic tomography. *J Assoc Res Otolaryngol* 9: 215–24.

Ahmed ZM, Goodyear R, Riazuddin S, Lagziel A, Legan PK, Behra M, Burgess SM, Lilley KS, Wilcox ER, Riazuddin S, Griffith AJ, Frolenkov GI, Belyantseva IA, Richardson GP & Friedman TB. (2006) The tip-link antigen, a protein associated with the transduction complex of sensory hair cells, is protocadherin-15. *J Neurosci* 26: 7022–34.

Assad JA, Shepherd GM & Corey DP. (1991) Tip-link integrity and mechanical transduction in vertebrate hair cells. *Neuron* 7: 985–94.

Atiba-Davies M & Noben-Trauth K. (2007) TRPML3 and hearing loss in the varitint-waddler mouse. *Biochim Biophys Acta* 1772: 1028–31.

Bautista DM, Jordt SE, Nikai T, Tsuruda PR, Read AJ, Poblete J, Yamoah EN, Basbaum AI & Julius D. (2006) TRPA1 mediates the inflammatory actions of environmental irritants and proalgesic agents. *Cell* 124: 1269–82.

Belyantseva IA, Boger ET, Naz S, Frolenkov GI, Sellers JR, Ahmed ZM, Griffith AJ & Friedman TB. (2005) Myosin-XVa is required for tip localization of whirlin and differential elongation of hair-cell stereocilia. *Nat Cell Biol* 7: 148–56.

Benser ME, Marquis RE & Hudspeth AJ. (1996) Rapid, active hair bundle movements in hair cells from the bullfrog's sacculus. *J Neurosci* 16: 5629–43.

Beurg M, Evans MG, Hackney CM & Fettiplace R. (2006) A large-conductance calcium-selective mechanotransducer channel in mammalian cochlear hair cells. *J Neurosci* 26: 10992–1000.

Brown AM & Pye JD. (1975) Auditory sensitivity at high frequencies in mammals. *Adv Comp Physiol Biochem* 6: 1–73.

Chan DK & Hudspeth AJ. (2005) Mechanical responses of the organ of Corti to acoustic and electrical stimulation in vitro. *Biophys J* 89: 4382–95.

Corey DP & Hudspeth AJ. (1979) Response latency of vertebrate hair cells. *Biophys J* 26: 499–506.

Corey DP & Hudspeth AJ. (1983) Kinetics of the receptor current in bullfrog saccular hair cells. *J Neurosci* 3: 962–76.

Corey DP, Garcia-Anoveros J, Holt JR, Kwan KY, Lin SY, Vollrath MA, Amalfitano A, Cheung EL, Derfler BH, Duggan A, Géléoc GS, Gray PA, Hoffman MP, Rehm HL, Tamasauskas D & Zhang DS. (2004) TRPA1 is a candidate for the mechanosensitive transduction channel of vertebrate hair cells. *Nature* 432: 723–30.

Crawford AC & Fettiplace R. (1981) An electrical tuning mechanism in turtle cochlear hair cells. *J Physiol* 312: 377–412.

Crawford AC & Fettiplace R. (1985) The mechanical properties of ciliary bundles of turtle cochlear hair cells. *J Physiol* 364: 359–79.

Crawford AC, Evans MG & Fettiplace R. (1989) Activation and adaptation of transducer currents in turtle hair cells. *J Physiol* 419: 405–34.

Cuajungco MP, Grimm C & Heller S. (2007) TRP channels as candidates for hearing and balance abnormalities in vertebrates. *Biochim Biophys Acta* 1772: 1022–7.

Daudet N & Lebart MC. (2002) Transient expression of the T-isoform of plastins/fimbrin in the stereocilia of developing auditory hair cells. *Cell Motil Cytoskeleton* 53: 326–36.

Dechesne CJ, Rabejac D & Desmadryl G. (1994) Development of calretinin immunoreactivity in the mouse inner ear. *J Comp Neurol* 346: 517–29.

Denk W, Holt JR, Shepherd GM & Corey DP. (1995) Calcium imaging of single stereocilia in hair cells: localization of transduction channels at both ends of tip links. *Neuron* 15: 1311–21.

Ding S & Sachs F. (2000) Ion permeation and block of P2X(2) purinoceptors: single channel recordings. *J Membr Biol* 172: 215–23.

Drenckhahn D, Engel K, Hofer D, Merte C, Tilney L & Tilney M. (1991) Three different actin filament assemblies occur in every hair cell: each contains a specific actin cross-linking protein. *J Cell Biol* 112: 641–51.

Dumont RA, Lins U, Filoteo AG, Penniston JT, Kachar B & Gillespie PG. (2001) Plasma membrane Ca^{2+}-ATPase isoform 2a is the PMCA of hair bundles. *J Neurosci* 21: 5066–78.

Egan TM & Khakh BS. (2004) Contribution of calcium ions to P2X channel responses. *J Neurosci* 24: 3413–20.

El-Amraoui A & Petit C. (2005) Usher I syndrome: unravelling the mechanisms that underlie the cohesion of the growing hair bundle in inner ear sensory cells. *J Cell Sci* 118: 4593–603.

Etournay R, El-Amraoui A, Bahloul A, Blanchard S, Roux I, Pézeron G, Michalski N, Daviet L, Hardelin J-P, Legrain P & Petit C. (2005) PHR1, an integral membrane protein of the inner ear sensory cells, directly interacts with myosin 1c and myosin VIIa. *J Cell Sci* 118: 2891–9.

Farris HE, LeBlanc CL, Goswami J & Ricci AJ. (2004) Probing the pore of the auditory hair cell mechanotransducer channel in turtle. *J Physiol* 558: 769–92.

Fettiplace R. (2006) Active hair bundle movements in auditory hair cells. *J Physiol* 576: 29–36.

Fettiplace R & Hackney CM. (2006) The sensory and motor roles of auditory hair cells. *Nat Rev Neurosci* 7: 19–29.

Fettiplace R & Ricci AJ. (2006) Mechanoelectrical transduction in auditory hair cells. In: Eatock RA, Fay RR & Popper AN, eds. *Vertebrate Hair Cells*. Springer, New York, pp. 154–203.

Furness DN & Hackney CM. (1985) Cross-links between stereocilia in the guinea-pig cochlea. *Hear Res* 18: 177–88.

Furness DN & Hackney CM. (2006) The structure and composition of the stereociliary bundle of vertebrate hair cells. In: Eatock RA, Fay RR & Popper AN, eds. *Vertebrate Hair Cells*. Springer, New York, pp 95–153.

Furness DN, Richardson GP & Russell IJ. (1989) Stereociliary bundle morphology in organotypic cultures of the mouse cochlea. *Hear Res* 38: 95–109.

Furness DN, Hackney CM & Benos DJ. (1996) The binding site on cochlear stereocilia for antisera raised against renal Na+ channels is blocked by amiloride and dihydrostreptomycin. *Hear Res* 93: 136–46.

Furness DN, Zetes DE, Hackney CM & Steele CR. (1997) Kinematic analysis of shear displacement as a means for operating mechanotransduction channels in the contact region between adjacent stereocilia of mammalian cochlear hair cells. *Proc R Soc Lond B Biol Sci* **264**: 45–51.

Furness DN, Karkanevatos A, West B & Hackney CM. (2002) An immunogold investigation of the distribution of calmodulin in the apex of cochlear hair cells. *Hear Res* **173**: 10–20.

Furness DN, Katori Y, Mahendrasingam S & Hackney CM. (2005) Differential distribution of beta- and gamma-actin in guinea-pig cochlear sensory and supporting cells. *Hear Res* **207**: 22–34.

Furness DN, Katori Y, Kumar BN & Hackney CM. (2008a) The dimensions and structural attachments of tip links in mammalian cochlear hair cells and the effects of exposure to different levels of extracellular calcium. *Neuroscience* **154**: 10–21.

Furness DN, Mahendrasingam S, Ohashi M, Fettiplace R & Hackney CM. (2008b) The dimensions and composition of stereociliary rootlets in mammalian cochlear hair cells: comparison between high- and low-frequency cells and evidence for a connection to the lateral membrane. *J Neurosci* **28**: 6342–53.

Gagnon LH, Longo-Guess CM, Berryman M, Shin JB, Saylor KW, Yu H, Gillespie PG & Johnson KR. (2006) The chloride intracellular channel protein CLIC5 is expressed at high levels in hair cell stereocilia and is essential for normal inner ear function. *J Neurosci* **26**: 10188–98.

Géléoc GS & Holt JR. (2003) Developmental acquisition of sensory transduction in hair cells of the mouse inner ear. *Nat Neurosci* **6**: 1019–20.

Gillespie PG & Cyr JL. (2004) Myosin-1C, the hair cell's adaptation motor. *Annu Rev Physiol* **66**: 521–45.

Glowatzki E, Ruppersberg JP, Zenner HP & Rusch A. (1997) Mechanically and ATP-induced currents of mouse outer hair cells are independent and differentially blocked by d-tubocurarine. *Neuropharmacology* **36**: 1269–75.

Goodyear R & Richardson G. (1994) Differential glycosylation of auditory and vestibular hair bundle proteins revealed by peanut agglutinin. *J Comp Neurol* **345**: 267–78.

Goodyear R & Richardson G. (1999) The ankle-link antigen: an epitope sensitive to calcium chelation associated with the hair-cell surface and the calyceal processes of photoreceptors. *J Neurosci* **19**: 3761–72.

Grati M, Schneider ME, Lipkow K, Strehler EE, Wenthold RJ & Kachar B. (2006) Rapid turnover of stereocilia membrane proteins: evidence from the trafficking and mobility of plasma membrane $Ca^{(2+)}$-ATPase 2. *J Neurosci* **26**: 6386–95.

Hackney CM & Furness DN. (1995) Mechanotransduction in vertebrate hair cells: structure and function of the stereociliary bundle. *Am J Physiol* **268**: C1–13.

Hackney CM, Furness DN & Benos DJ. (1991) Localisation of putative mechanoelectrical transducer channels in cochlear hair cells by immunoelectron microscopy. *Scanning Microsc* **5**: 741–5.

Hackney CM, Furness DN, Benos DJ, Woodley JF & Barratt J. (1992) Putative immunolocalization of the mechanoelectrical transduction channels in mammalian cochlear hair cells. *Proc R Soc Lond B Biol Sci* **248**: 215–21.

Hackney CM, Mahendrasingam S, Jones EMC & Fettiplace R. (2003) The distribution of calcium buffering proteins in the turtle cochlea. *J Neurosci* **23**: 4577–89.

Hackney CM, Mahendrasingam S, Penn A & Fettiplace R. (2005) The concentrations of calcium buffering proteins in mammalian cochlear hair cells. *J Neurosci* **25**: 7867–86.

Hasson T, Gillespie PG, Garcia JA, MacDonald RB, Zhao Y, Yee AG, Mooseker MS & Corey DP. (1997) Unconventional myosins in inner-ear sensory epithelia. *J Cell Biol* **137**: 1287–307.

Heller S, Bell AM, Denis CS, Choe Y & Hudspeth AJ. (2002) Parvalbumin 3 is an abundant Ca^{2+} buffer in hair cells. *J Assoc Res Otolaryngol* **3**: 488–98.

Hofer DW & Drenckhahn D. (1997) Sorting of actin isoforms in chicken auditory hair cells. *J Cell Sci* **110**: 765–70.

Holt JR & Corey DP. (2000) Two mechanisms for transducer adaptation in vertebrate hair cells. *Proc Natl Acad Sci U S A* **97**: 11730–5.

Holt JR, Gillespie SK, Provance DW, Shah K, Shokat KM, Corey DP, Mercer JA & Gillespie PG. (2002) A chemical-genetic strategy implicates myosin-1c in adaptation by hair cells. *Cell* 108: 371–81.

Housley GD, Kanjhan R, Raybould NP, Greenwood D, Salih SG, Jarlebark L, Burton LD, Setz VC, Cannell MB, Soeller C, Christie DL, Usami S, Matsubara A, Yoshie H, Ryan AF & Thorne PR. (1999) Expression of the P2X(2) receptor subunit of the ATP-gated ion channel in the cochlea: implications for sound transduction and auditory neurotransmission. *J Neurosci* 19: 8377–88.

Howard J & Hudspeth AJ. (1988) Compliance of the hair bundle mediates adaptation in mechanoelectrical transduction by the bullfrog's saccular hair cell. *Neuron* 1: 189–99.

Howard J, Roberts WM & Hudspeth AJ. (1988) Mechanoelectrical transduction by hair cells. *Annu Rev Biophys Biophys Chem* 17: 99–124.

Hudspeth AJ. (1982) Extracellular current flow and the site of transduction by vertebrate hair cells. *J Neurosci* 2: 1–10.

Itoh M. (1982) Preservation and visualization of actin-containing filaments in the apical zone of cochlear sensory cells. *Hear Res* 6: 277–89.

Jaramillo F & Hudspeth AJ. (1991) Localization of the hair cell's transduction channels at the hair bundle's top by iontophoretic application of a channel blocker. *Neuron* 7: 409–20.

Kachar B, Parakkal M, Kurc M, Zhao Y & Gillespie PG. (2000) High-resolution structure of hair-cell tip links. *Proc Natl Acad Sci U S A* 97: 13336–41.

Kappler JA, Starr CJ, Chan DK, Kollmar R & Hudspeth AJ. (2004) A nonsense mutation in the gene encoding a zebra fish myosin VI isoform causes defects in hair-cell mechanotransduction. *Proc Natl Acad Sci U S A* 101: 13056–61.

Kazmierczak P, Sakaguchi H, Tokita J, Wilson-Kubalek EM, Milligan RA, Muller U & Kachar B. (2007) Cadherin 23 and protocadherin 15 interact to form tip-link filaments in sensory hair cells. *Nature* 449: 87–92.

Kennedy HJ, Evans MG, Crawford AC & Fettiplace R. (2003) Fast adaptation of mechanoelectrical transducer channels in mammalian cochlear hair cells. *Nat Neurosci* 6: 832–6.

Kennedy HJ, Crawford AC & Fettiplace R. (2005) Force generation by mammalian hair bundles supports a role in cochlear amplification. *Nature* 433: 880–3.

Kikkawa Y, Mburu P, Morse S, Kominami R, Townsend S & Brown SD. (2005) Mutant analysis reveals whirlin as a dynamic organizer in the growing hair cell stereocilium. *Hum Mol Genet* 14: 391–400.

Kitajiri S, Fukumoto K, Hata M, Sasaki H, Katsuno T, Nakagawa T, Ito J, Tsukita S & Tsukita S. (2004) Radixin deficiency causes deafness associated with progressive degeneration of cochlear stereocilia. *J Cell Biol* 166: 559–70.

Kozel PJ, Friedman RA, Erway LC, Yamoah EN, Liu LH, Riddle T, Duffy JJ, Doetschman T, Miller ML, Cardell EL & Shull GE. (1998) Balance and hearing deficits in mice with a null mutation in the gene encoding plasma membrane Ca^{2+}-ATPase isoform 2. *J Biol Chem* 273: 18693–6.

Kozlov AS, Risler T & Hudspeth AJ. (2007) Coherent motion of stereocilia assures the concerted gating of hair-cell transduction channels. *Nat Neurosci* 10: 87–92.

Kros CJ, Marcotti W, van Netten SM, Self TJ, Libby RT, Brown SD, Richardson GP & Steel KP. (2002) Reduced climbing and increased slipping adaptation in cochlear hair cells of mice with Myo7a mutations. *Nat Neurosci* 5: 41–7.

Küssel-Andermann P, El-Amraoui A, Safieddine S, Nouaille S, Perfettini I, Lecuit M, Cossart P, Wolfrum U & Petit C. (2000) Vezatin, a novel transmembrane protein, bridges myosin VIIA to the cadherin-catenins complex. *EMBO J* 19: 6020–9.

Kwan KY, Allchorne AJ, Vollrath MA, Christensen AP, Zhang DS, Woolf CJ & Corey DP. (2006) TRPA1 contributes to cold, mechanical, and chemical nociception but is not essential for hair-cell transduction. *Neuron* 50: 277–89.

Lefèvre G, Michel V, Weil D, Lepelletier L, Bizard E, Wolfrum U, Hardelin JP & Petit C. (2008) A core cochlear phenotype in USH1 mouse mutants implicates fibrous links of the hair bundle in its cohesion, orientation and differential growth. *Development* 135: 1427–37.

Liburd N, Ghosh M, Riazuddin S, Naz S, Khan S, Ahmed Z, Riazuddin S, Liang Y, Menon PS, Smith T, Smith AC, Chen KS, Lupski JR, Wilcox ER, Potocki L & Friedman TB. (2001) Novel mutations of MYO15A associated with profound deafness in consanguineous families and moderately severe hearing loss in a patient with Smith-Magenis syndrome. *Hum Genet* **109**: 535–41.

Little KF & Neugebauer D-Ch. (1985) Interconnections between the stereovilli of the fish inner ear. II. Systematic investigation of saccular hair bundles from Rutilus rutilus (Teleostei). *Cell Tissue Res* **242**: 427–32.

Liedtke W & Friedman JM. (2003) Abnormal osmotic regulation in trpv4-/- mice. *Proc Natl Acad Sci U S A* **100**: 13698–703.

Lumpkin EA & Hudspeth AJ. (1995) Detection of Ca^{2+} entry through mechanosensitive channels localizes the site of mechanoelectrical transduction in hair cells. *Proc Natl Acad Sci U S A* **92**: 10297–301.

Martin P, Mehta AD & Hudspeth AJ. (2000) Negative hair-bundle stiffness betrays a mechanism for mechanical amplification by the hair cell. *Proc Natl Acad Sci U S A* **97**: 12026–31.

Martin P, Bozovic D, Choe Y & Hudspeth AJ. (2003) Spontaneous oscillation by hair bundles of the bullfrog's sacculus. *J Neurosci* **23**: 4533–48.

Meyer J, Furness DN, Zenner HP Hackney CM & Gummer AW. (1998) Evidence for opening of hair-cell transducer channels after tip-link loss. *J Neurosci* **18**: 6748–56.

McGee J, Goodyear RJ, McMillan DR, Stauffer EA, Holt JR, Locke KG, Birch DG, Legan PK, White PC, Walsh EJ & Richardson GP. (2006) The very large G-protein-coupled receptor VLGR1: a component of the ankle link complex required for the normal development of auditory hair bundles. *J Neurosci* **26**: 6543–53.

Michalski N, Michel V, Bahloul A, Lefèvre G, Barral J, Yagi H, Chardenoux S, Weil D, Martin P, Hardelin JP, Sato M & Petit C. (2007) Molecular characterization of the ankle-link complex in cochlear hair cells and its role in the hair bundle functioning. *J Neurosci* **27**: 6478–88.

Michel V, Goodyear RJ, Weil D, Marcotti W, Perfettini I, Wolfrum U, Kros CJ, Richardson GP & Petit C. (2005) Cadherin 23 is a component of the transient lateral links in the developing hair bundles of cochlear sensory cells. *Dev Biol* **280**: 281–94.

Møgensen MM, Rzadzinska A & Steel KP. (2007) The deaf mouse mutant whirler suggests a role for whirlin in actin filament dynamics and stereocilia development. *Cell Motil Cytoskeleton* **64**: 496–508.

Nagata K, Zheng L, Madathany T, Castiglioni AJ, Bartles JR & García-Añoveros J. (2008) The varitint-waddler (Va) deafness mutation in TRPML3 generates constitutive, inward rectifying currents and causes cell degeneration. *Proc Natl Acad Sci U S A* **105**: 353–8.

Nayak GD, Ratnayaka HS, Goodyear RJ & Richardson GP. (2007) Development of the hair bundle and mechanotransduction. *Int J Dev Biol* **51**: 597–608.

Ohmori H. (1988) Mechanical stimulation and Fura-2 fluorescence in the hair bundle of dissociated hair cells of the chick. *J Physiol* **399**: 115–37.

Owsianik G, Talavera K, Voets T & Nilius B. (2006) Permeation and selectivity of TRP channels. *Annu Rev Physiol* **68**: 685–717.

Pataky F, Pironkova R & Hudspeth AJ. (2003) Radixin is a constituent of stereocilia in hair cells. *Proc Natl Acad Sci U S A* **101**: 2601–06.

Pawlowski KS, Kikkawa YS, Wright CG & Alagramam KN. (2006) Progression of inner ear pathology in Ames waltzer mice and the role of protocadherin 15 in hair cell development. *J Assoc Res Otolaryngol* **7**: 83–94.

Phillips KR, Tong S, Goodyear R, Richardson GP & Cyr JL. (2006) Stereociliary myosin-1c receptors are sensitive to calcium chelation and absent from cadherin 23 mutant mice. *J Neurosci* **26**: 10777–88.

Phillips KR, Biswas A & Cyr JL. (2008) How hair cells hear: the molecular basis of hair-cell mechanotransduction. *Curr Opin Otolaryngol Head Neck Surg* **16**: 445–51.

Pickles JO, Comis SD & Osborne MP. (1984) Cross-links between stereocilia in the guinea pig organ of Corti, and their possible relation to sensory transduction. *Hear Res* **15**: 103–12.

Ricci AJ & Fettiplace R. (1997) The effects of calcium buffering and cyclic AMP on mechano-electrical transduction in turtle auditory hair cells. *J Physiol* **501**: 111–24.

Ricci AJ, Wu Y-C & Fettiplace R. (1998) The endogenous calcium buffer and the time course of transducer adaptation in auditory hair cells. *J Neurosci* **18**: 8261–77.

Ricci AJ, Crawford AC & Fettiplace R. (2000) Active hair bundle motion linked to fast transducer adaptation in auditory hair cells. *J Neurosci* **20**: 7131–42.

Ricci AJ, Crawford AC & Fettiplace R. (2002) Mechanisms of active hair bundle motion in auditory hair cells. *J Neurosci* **22**: 44–52.

Ricci AJ, Crawford AC & Fettiplace R. (2003) Tonotopic variation in the conductance of the hair cell mechanotransducer channel. *Neuron* **40**: 983–90.

Ricci AJ, Kennedy HJ, Crawford AC & Fettiplace R. (2005) The transduction channel filter in auditory hair cells. *J Neurosci* **5**: 7831–9.

Ricci AJ, Kachar B, Gale J & Van Netten SM. (2006) Mechano-electrical transduction: New insights into old ideas. *J Membr Biol* **209**: 71–88.

Rzadzinska AK, Schneider ME, Davies C, Riordan GP & Kachar B. (2004) An actin molecular treadmill and myosins maintain stereocilia functional architecture and self-renewal. *J Cell Biol* **164**: 887–97.

Rzadzinska A, Schneider M, Noben-Trauth K, Bartles JR & Kachar B. (2005) Balanced levels of espin are critical for stereociliary growth and length maintenance. *Cell Motil Cytoskeleton* **62**: 157–65.

Santi PA & Anderson CB. (1987) A newly identified surface coat on cochlear hair cells. *Hear Res* **27**: 47–65.

Schulte C, Meyer J, Furness DN, Hackney CM, Kleyman TR & Gummer AW. (2002) An antibody to amiloride-binding sites blocks mechanoelectrical transduction in outer hair cells. *Hear Res* **164**: 190–205.

Self T, Sobe T, Copeland NG, Jenkins NA, Avraham KB & Steel KP. (1999) Role of myosin VI in the differentiation of cochlear hair cells. *Dev Biol* **214**: 331–41.

Senften M, Schwander M, Kazmierczak P, Lillo C, Shin JB, Hasson T, Géléoc GS, Gillespie PG, Williams D, Holt JR & Muller U. (2006) Physical and functional interaction between protocadherin 15 and myosin VIIa in mechanosensory hair cells. *J Neurosci* **26**: 2060–71.

Shotwell SL, Jacobs R & Hudspeth AJ. (1981) Directional sensitivity of individual vertebrate hair cells to controlled deflection of their hair bundles. *Ann N Y Acad Sci* **374**: 1–10.

Sidi S, Friedrich RW & Nicolson T. (2003) NompC TRP channel required for vertebrate sensory hair cell mechanotransduction. *Science* **301**: 96–9.

Siemens J, Kazmierczak P, Reynolds A, Sticker M, Littlewood-Evans A & Muller U. (2002) The Usher syndrome proteins cadherin 23 and harmonin form a complex by means of PDZ-domain interactions. *Proc Natl Acad Sci U S A* **99**: 14946–51.

Söllner C, Rauch GJ, Siemens J, Geisler R, Schuster SC, Muller U & Nicolson T; Tubingen 2000 Screen Consortium. (2004) Mutations in cadherin 23 affect tip links in zebra fish sensory hair cells. *Nature* **428**: 955–9.

Stauffer EA, Scarborough JD, Hirono M, Miller ED, Shah K, Mercer JA, Holt JR & Gillespie PG. (2005) Fast adaptation in vestibular hair cells requires myosin-1c activity. *Neuron* **47**: 541–53.

Stepanyan R, Belyantseva IA, Griffith AJ, Friedman TB & Frolenkov GI. (2006) Auditory mechanotransduction in the absence of functional myosin-XVa. *J Physiol* **576**: 801–8.

Steyger PS, Gillespie PG & Baird RA. (1998) Myosin I beta is located at tip link anchors in vestibular hair bundles. *J Neurosci* **18**: 4603–15.

Street VA, McKee-Johnson JW, Fonseca RC, Tempel BL & Noben-Trauth K. (1998) Mutations in a plasma membrane Ca^{2+}-ATPase gene cause deafness in deafwaddler mice. *Nat Genet* **19**: 390–4.

Tabuchi K, Suzuki M, Mizuno A & Hara A. (2005) Hearing impairment in TRPV4 knockout mice. *Neurosci Lett* **382**: 304–8.

Thurm U. (1981) Mechano-electric transduction. *Biophys Struct Mech* **7**: 245–6.

Tilney LG, Derosier DJ & Mulroy MJ. (1980) The organization of actin filaments in the stereocilia of cochlear hair cells. *J Cell Biol* **86**: 244–59.

Tilney MS, Tilney LG, Stephens RE, Merte C, Drenckhahn D, Cotanche DA & Bretscher A. (1989) Preliminary biochemical characterization of the stereocilia and cuticular plate of hair cells of the chick cochlea. *J Cell Biol* **109**: 1711–23.

Tsuprun V & Santi P. (2000) Helical structure of hair cell stereocilia tip links in the chinchilla cochlea. *J Assoc Res Otolaryngol* **1**: 224–31.

Tsuprun V & Santi P. (2002) Structure of outer hair cell stereocilia side and attachment links in the chinchilla cochlea. *J Histochem Cytochem* **50**: 493–502.

Ugawa S, Inagaki A, Yamamura H, Ueda T, Ishida Y, Kajita K, Shimizu H & Shimada S. (2006) Acid-sensing ion channel-1b in the stereocilia of mammalian cochlear hair cells. *Neuroreport* **17**: 1235–39.

van Netten SM & Kros CJ. (2000) Gating energies and forces of the mammalian hair cell transducer channel and related hair bundle mechanics. *Proc Biol Sci* **267**: 1915–23.

Volk T, Schwoerer AP, Thiessen S, Schultz JH & Ehmke H. (2003) A polycystin-2-like large conductance cation channel in rat left ventricular myocytes. *Cardiovasc Res* **58**: 76–88.

Vollrath MA, Kwan KY & Corey DP. (2007) The micromachinery of mechanotransduction in hair cells. *Annu Rev Neurosci* **30**: 339–65.

Waldmann R, Champigny G, Bassilana F, Heurteaux C & Lazdunski M. (1997) A proton-gated cation channel involved in acid-sensing. *Nature* **386**: 173–7.

Walker R.G, Willingham AT & Zuker CS. (2000) A Drosophila mechanosensory transduction channel. *Science* **287**: 2229–34.

Xu Z, Peng AW, Oshima K & Heller S. (2008) MAGI-1, a candidate stereociliary scaffolding protein, associates with the tip-link component cadherin 23. *J Neurosci* **28**: 11269–76.

Zhao Y, Yamoah EN & Gillespie PG. (1996) Regeneration of broken tip links and restoration of mechanical transduction in hair cells. *Proc Natl Acad Sci U S A* **93**: 15469–74.

Zheng L, Sekerkova G, Vranich K, Tilney LG, Mugnaini E & Bartles JR. (2000) The deaf jerker mouse has a mutation in the gene encoding the espin actin-bundling proteins of hair cell stereocilia and lacks espins. *Cell* **102**: 377–85.

Chapter 9

The afferent synapse

Jonathan Ashmore

9.1 Introduction

The auditory synapse is the first relay point for the input of sound into the nervous system and the properties of this synapse determine how well a signal from the hair cells is relayed up the auditory brainstem. The information in the sound signal entering the ear includes information about:

* frequency content of the sound
* relative phases between the time varying signals
* amplitudes of the constituent sounds.

This information needs to be re-encoded as a pattern in the auditory nerve for subsequent analysis by the brain. The frequency content of the sound is encoded by the pattern of the whole population of nerve fibres, with individual fibres carrying information about only a specific narrow frequency band. The phase and amplitude of the component sound frequency is information which could easily be degraded by poor transmission from the hair cell (as the detector) to the nerve (as the communication channel). The design of the afferent synapse ensures that the information content is not degraded and is a principle which will be developed here. Few signals in a biological sound are stationary in time (a situation which only occurs in an experimental sound), and so one of the main functions of the hair cell synapse is to convey the information in a way that captures small temporal changes, that is, the rise and fall of the signal, in a reliable way.

The purpose of this chapter is to introduce a number of critical features of the afferent synapse with particular reference to mammalian hearing. As will be clear, however, it is sometimes necessary to extrapolate from non-mammalian systems. A number of excellent reviews have recently been published providing further pointers to the primary literature (Glowatzki & Fuchs, 2002; Fuchs *et al.*, 2003; Moser *et al.*, 2006; Glowatzki *et al.*, 2008).

9.2 The response of the auditory nerve

The classical era of cochlear physiology developed the techniques for recording from single auditory nerve fibres. The array of myelinated fibres terminates for the most part on the inner hair cells (IHCs). Extracellular recordings from the afferent nerve fibres in anaesthetized mammalian species have showed that each fibre responded to a very narrow range of sound frequencies centred on its optimal or characteristic frequency (CF). It is now known that such properties are essentially determined by the mechanics of the cochlea so that each fibre has a particular CF depending on its site of cochlear origin. In addition, fibres in the nerve have been shown to be spontaneously active (sometimes showing resting activity rates above 100 spikes/s) (Kiang *et al.*, 1967; Evans, 1972; Liberman, 1982). It was found that they could respond to sound intensity above threshold by increasing their firing rate to up to many hundreds of spikes per second.

In each fibre, the initial rate is not maintained (that is fibres 'adapt'). Within a few tens of milliseconds, the fibres adopt a new and lower firing rate which is subsequently maintained for sustained periods. We shall see that this phenomenon has an explanation in the cellular structure and physiology of the synapse. Auditory nerve fibres also exhibit 'phase locking' to the stimulus: the action potentials tend to fire, although not necessarily with certainty, at a particular phase of the cyclical pressure changes. Phase locking can occur up to relatively high frequencies. In guinea pig, selected fibres can synchronize their firing to sounds over 1 kHz in frequency and this synchronization only falls to random firing at around 3.5 kHz (Palmer & Russell, 1986). In the cat auditory nerve, fibres phase lock up to frequencies an octave higher.

These two auditory nerve fibre properties, sustained operation and phase locking, point to highly specialized properties of the synapse between the hair cell and the auditory nerve, unlike many neuronal synapses that can only operate at much lower information transmission rates. On this basis the hair cell synapse ranks as an ultrafast synapse.

9.3 Structure of the synapse

The typical hair cell afferent contact, as found in mammalian vestibular end-organs and all non-mammalian hair cell organs, involves not a single synapse but a cluster of contact points, 10 or more, between the hair cell and the auditory nerve dendrite (Fig. 9.1). The mammalian cochlea, however, presents a special case in which the afferent neurones, whose cell bodies form the spiral ganglion in the central modiolus of the cochlea, extend a single dendrite to end opposite a single presynaptic specialization of an inner hair cell. Typically 20–30 afferent neurones contact one IHC, although the number of contacts varies slightly depending on cochlear position. The maximum

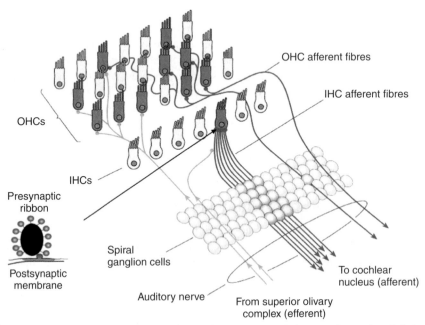

Fig. 9.1 The organization of the cochlear inner and outer hair cells (IHCs and OHCs) and their innervation. The inset shows the schematic profile of the ribbon found at each afferent contact between the hair cells and the potsynaptic afferent terminal.
Adapted with permission from Hackney, Ch3 in Signals and Perception, OU (2002).

number of contacts generally occurs on cells half way along the cochlea (Moser *et al.*, 2006). Such afferent fibres form the population of myelinated type I fibres of the auditory nerve. Their pattern of activity will be described in detail in Volume 2 of this series (*The Auditory Brain*). The population is characterized physiologically as a set of fibres showing a range of spontaneous activities, with high spontaneous rates correlating with a high sensitivity to sound levels and lower spontaneous rates correlating with fibres with much higher thresholds.

9.3.1 Inner versus outer hair cell synapses

Although the emphasis in this chapter is on the IHC synapse and its type I afferents, outer hair cells (OHCs) also possess an afferent synapse. This is much less obvious than the IHC synapse but nevertheless is assumed to be responsible for transmission of information to a subpopulation of fibres of the auditory nerve, termed type II afferents. To date only one anatomically confirmed type II fibre has been identified (Robertson, 1984); like other candidate fibres (Robertson *et al.*, 1999) it had no spontaneous activity and did not respond to sound. It is presumed that type II fibres are likely to be broadly tuned, reflecting the convergence of multiple OHCs onto a single fibre. The precise information that these fibres carry to the central nervous system (CNS) is not known but may be critical in setting the overall gain of the auditory system.

9.3.2 The ribbon synapse and its proteins

The synapse of cochlear hair cells differs in structure from the synapses found between most neurones. It is a 'ribbon' synapse. Similar types of synapse are found also in photoreceptors and bipolar cells in the retina as well as in some cells in the pineal organ. The name 'ribbon' synapse derives from the appearance in electron micrographs (Fig. 9.2) of a dense body near the presynaptic membrane around which the vesicles cluster. The vesicles have a diameter of about 35 nm and cluster around a dense core (as it appears in the electron microscope) so that the overall structure is about 0.5–1 μm in size. In many species, the precise numbers of ribbons per cell have not been determined although specific markers for the ribbons are now available. It is worth noting that the cochlea is not unique in employing ribbon synapses: the hair cells of the vestibular system also use ribbon systems at the contacts with the vestibular nerve endings. At vestibular sensory cells, the afferent terminals are themselves specialized (into boutons or into enveloping calyceal endings) depending on the type of sensory hair cells and the position in each epithelium.

Ribbon synapses differ in structure in different cells. While serial reconstruction reveals the hair cell ribbons to be approximately spherical, at least in the case of amphibian synapses where they have been thoroughly investigated (Lenzi *et al.*, 1999), in the photoreceptors the name more truly reflects the morphology, and the structure is a flat plate, ~30 nm wide and extending ~150 nm from the ridge of the presynaptic membrane. However, there may be considerable variation in the size and number of the dense structures between different species and hair cell types. The shape of the ribbon structure also may change as the synapse matures. In immature IHCs it starts as a spherical structure about 200–400 nm in diameter, sometimes present as multiple densities facing a single afferent terminal, but then develops into a more ellipsoidal structure. In mature OHCs it reported to be more elongated and 100–200 nm in length (Moser *et al.*, 2006).

Synaptic vesicles cluster around the ribbon. Those in the immediate vicinity of the presynaptic membrane are thought to constitute a pool of vesicles that can be released in a short period (within the first 20 ms). Around each ribbon there are about 350 vesicles, a number determined both by serial reconstruction in frog saccular hair cells (Lenzi *et al.*, 1999) or by using functional measures (capacitance measurements) of exocytosis which will be described below (Beutner *et al.*, 2001).

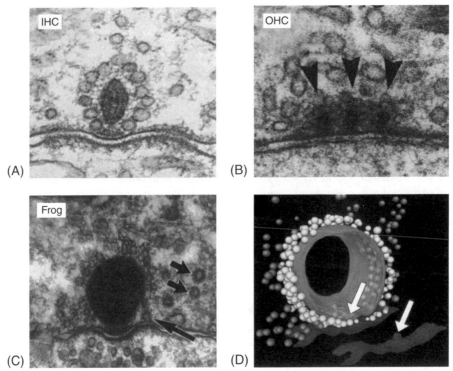

Fig. 9.2 Ribbon structure in electron microscopy. (A) Inner hair cell (IHC) ribbon from guinea pig middle turn, with vesicles clustered around core. (B) Out hair cell (OHC) taken from cat apical turn. In all cases the clustered vesicles have a diameter of approximately 35 nm. (C) Ribbon synapse from a bullfrog saccular hair cell. The ribbon core is more spherical and slightly larger than in mammals. Arrowed is a structure which may represent an endocytotic even and (with short arrows) vesicles surrounded by a clathrin network as if endocytosed. (D) Electron tomographical reconstruction of the ribbon, showing (blue) the outer surface of the ribbon core, (white) vesicles associated with the ribbon, and (grey) vesicles not tightly associated with the ribbon. Arrowed is a possible endocytotic event.

Figure 9.2A reproduced with permission from Saito (1980). Figure 9.2B reproduced with permission from Liberman *et al.* (1990). Figure 9.2C, D reproduced with permission from Lenzi *et al.* (1999).

The total number of vesicles corresponds to the number of vesicles which can readily be assembled around the ribbon. This number includes about 40 vesicles directly attached to the ribbon core and a further 300 or so more loosely associated with the ribbon by what resemble a 'tether'. This population of vesicles form what has been called the 'readily releasable pool' (RRP) or, more familiarly a 'vesicular vending machine' (Fuchs *et al.*, 2003). There is an additional population of vesicles further from the presynaptic release zone and it is thought that they can be released but may take longer to be mobilized. This population is termed the 'releasable pool' (RP) of vesicles, and may be much larger in number. The RP size may be around 40 000 vesicles if estimated from physiological release experiments.

The molecular structure of the ribbon and its tethering proteins remains relatively poorly determined (Fig. 9.3). The models for the ribbon are informed strongly by structures in the retina where there is much more material for study. A core protein forming the ribbon density is RIBEYE (Schmitz, 2000). This protein, a splice variant of the c-terminal binding protein CtBP2

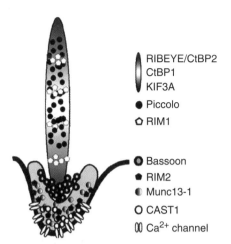

Fig. 9.3 Summary of component elements of the ribbon and its attachment to the presynaptic membrane. The molecular components of the ribbon showing the differential distribution of some of the known proteins defining two compartment of the ribbon. The ribbon associated complex and the arciform density includes the protein RIM2. The protein bassoon is localized at the border between the two compartments.
From Tom *et al.* (2005) with permission.

(a transcriptional repressor), has self-aggregating properties, and was identified as the major component of the photoreceptor ribbon structure. Antibodies raised against RIBEYE domains produce staining patterns that line up opposite the afferent terminals (Khimich *et al.*, 2005). A further two large structural proteins, bassoon and piccolo, are present as scaffolding proteins and are present in photoreceptors (Brandstatter *et al.*, 1999). These proteins appear to be critical for the correct functioning of hair cell and photoreceptor synapses. Mice with the Bassoon gene deleted have ribbon structures that float freely in the cytoplasm and, while able to release transmitter, can only do so slowly, being not able to mobilize and release transmitter rapidly (i.e. within the first 50 ms after the stimulus onset). Other proteins implicated in photoreceptor ribbon synapses have yet to be described fully in the hair cell system. This list includes a ribeye homologue, the transcriptional repressor protein CtBP1, the kinesin motor protein KIF3A, and several secretion-associated proteins including RIM2, MUNC13–1 (Dick *et al.*, 2001). The names of these proteins owe more to the history of their discovery than their molecular function.

The ribbon structure plays a role that allows rapid delivery of vesicles to a site where they can be fused to the membrane. It is known that, within a hair cell, vesicles are loaded by a specific vesicular glutamate transporter transporter, VGLUT3, with the neurotransmitter glutamate (Seal *et al.*, 2008). On fusion, vesicles release their cargo of neurotransmitter into the synaptic cleft. The protein machinery that facilitates the fusion process has been intensively studied but the molecular details are still not fully resolved. The synaptic vesicle (Fig. 9.4), although only 35 nm in diameter, can itself be considered an intracellular organelle and a near-complete inventory of its associated proteins has recently been published (Takamori *et al.*, 2006). In brief, fusion of a synaptic vesicle with the membrane is thought to arise from the formation of the SNARE complex, which squeezes the vesicular membrane down onto the presynaptic membrane. The formation of the SNARE complex is controlled at most exocytotic membranes by proteins of the synaptotagmin family. This family of proteins, characterized by two calcium-binding domains, or calcium sensors, contain two members, synaptogamins I and II, which have been implicated in the fast

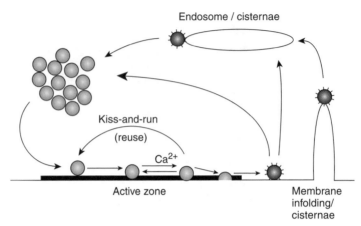

Fig. 9.4 The cycle of events in the life of a synaptic vesicle. The diagram show classical exocytosis and clathrin-dependent endocytosis. In addition, a more rapid mode is possible, kiss and run, where vesicle collapse does not occur but after discharge of the neurotransmitter the vesicle is rapidly returned to the pool for rapid release
From Harata *et al.* (2006) with permission.

release of vesicles at almost all neuronal synapses (Sudhof, 2002). Very surprisingly, these two specific synaptotagmins are absent from adult hair cells (Safieddine & Wenthold, 1999), leaving open the question of which protein regulates vesicular fusion in hair cells. As will be seen below, another protein, otoferlin, also possessing calcium-binding domains, has been proposed to fill the role. Most of the other vesicle-related proteins and SNARE complex proteins found in neurones can be identified in hair cells. There are two exceptions: synaptophysin, a glycoprotein present on the vesicle surface, and synapsin, a protein that is thought to be involved in the regulation of vesicle numbers, at least in conventional neuronal synapses. Both of these proteins are also absent from hair cells.

9.4 **Physiological properties of the synapse**

9.4.1 **Techniques**

There is now a wide range of techniques for physiologically recording the properties of the living hair cell synapse. In some systems, such as in fish saccular afferents (Furukawa *et al.*, 1978), and in turtle vestibular afferents (Holt *et al.*, 2006), the postsynaptic terminals are sufficiently large for a microelectrode to be inserted into the ending where excitatory postsynaptic potentials (EPSPs) can be recorded. More recently it has proved possible to study the synapse by directly patch-clamping both pre and post synaptically at the same time (Glowatzki & Fuchs, 2002; Keen & Hudspeth, 2006; Goutman & Glowatzki, 2007) (Fig. 9.5). These methods, so far used in relatively few laboratories, allow experiments that measure the transfer of information directly at a single ribbon synapse.

The detailed biophysics of the exocytotic process at the synapse is best studied by investigating the changes in the hair cell area as vesicles fuse to the presynaptic membrane (Fig. 9.6) (e.g Parsons *et al.*, 1994; Moser & Beutner, 2000). The principle underlying these measurements is that the membrane capacitance of a cell is linearly proportional to membrane area and thus vesicle fusion can be measured by making accurate measurements of the cell capacitance using patch-clamp techniques. In practice, the highest resolution measurements have not, so far, been made from hair cells even though single vesicle fusions can be detected as capacitance steps in

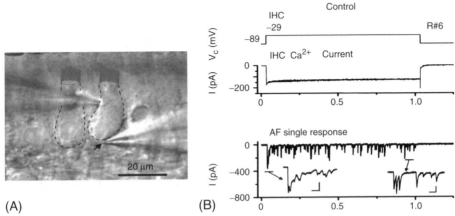

(A) (B)

Fig. 9.5 Electrophysiological recording from the afferent synapse using patch-clamp recording of both postsynaptic and presynaptic sites. (A) Both presynaptic and postsynaptic patch pipettes are placed under visual control. (B) Top panel: The inward calcium current in the inner hair cell (IHC) is observed when the cell is depolarized from –89 mV to –29 mV. It is maintained for the duration of the step as a consequence of the L-type calcium channel activated. Bottom panel: Simultaneous recordings from the postsynaptic afferent terminal show evoked excitatory postsynaptic currents, with an initial high rate of release
Reproduced with permission from Goutman and Glowatzki (2007).

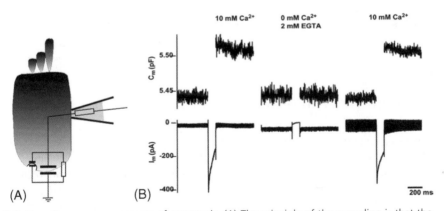

(A) (B)

Fig. 9.6 Capacitance measurements of exocytosis. (A) The principle of the recording is that the additional membrane resulting from exocytosis increases the membrane capacitance of the cell, and this increase can be detected using patch-clamp recording methods. (B) The capacitance jumps (0.160 pF in this experiment), which occurs following a voltage step command of the presynaptic IHC, can be recorded when calcium enters the cell. The main source of calcium is from the extracellular medium, so that the reduction of external calcium reduces the inwards calcium current to zero (leaving only a small outwards current present) and eliminates exocytosis.
Reproduced from Beutner et al. (2001).

chromaffin cells, with much larger, dense-core vesicles (Albillos *et al.*, 1997), or at some specialized synaptic membranes such as the calyx of Held (He *et al.*, 2006). This patch-clamp method gives information about the balance between exocytosis and endocytosis from all the synaptic release sites in a single cell.

Imaging methods have recently provided information about vesicle fusion and the reuptake of membrane. By labelling the vesicles with a fluorescent tag, single release sites can be visualized and studied dynamically. A number of fluorescent markers of membrane have been developed. One of these is a styryl dye, FM1-43; it has been used extensively to study vesicle dynamics at a variety of different synapses (Betz *et al.*, 1992). The spatial resolution of current optical microscope technologies is not yet at the point to detect single vesicles in cochlear tissue, but on the other hand the fusion of groups of vesicles can be followed with millisecond time resolution at all stages of release. In hair cells, single release sites can be marked by this dye (Griesinger *et al.*, 2005) and the results of these experiments will be discussed briefly below.

Some genetically encoded markers of synaptic vesicles have been developed which can be applied to study exocytosis. Those that offer considerable promise include the pH-sensitive fluorescent proteins (pHluorins) that can be linked to vesicle-associated proteins such as synaptobrevin. These protein–probe combinations can be expressed by transient transfection or used to construct transgenic animals. With suitable promoters, the proteins can be expressed in a variety of tissues. The resulting construct monitors the luminal pH of a vesicle (Miesenbock *et al.*, 1998). When the vesicle fuses, the pH rises from the normally acidic levels (pH 5–6) in the vesicle interior to physiological levels, and a flash of fluorescence is seen at the release site.

9.5 Presynaptic mechanisms

The synaptic region of a hair cell is relatively easy to identify by light microscopy. As the hair cells lie in a line in the tissue and the afferents approach them directly, the sites of contact are delineated. In addition, the postsynaptic terminals are 1–2 μm in diameter. They may swell when the membrane becomes permeable (for example, as a result of ischaemia or when glutamate is continuously released onto the terminal). In this pathological condition, the terminals then become so large that they fill the space below the IHC body (Puel *et al.*, 1994). Such excitotoxicity is regarded as one of the sequelae of noise exposure.

9.5.1 Ionic currents and the control of neurotransmitter release

When hair cells are activated by sound they become depolarized since the transducer channels' mean open-time increases. At low frequencies the potential change in the cell follows the deflection of the stereocilia. As the frequency increases, the membrane time constant filters out the phasic component (the 'AC' component) leaving only a tonic depolarizing receptor potential (the 'DC' component) (Pickles, 1988). The precise form of the receptor potential is determined by the potassium channels that are expressed in the basolateral membrane of the hair cell. The reported types of K+ channels found in different hair cells are quite diverse. Their main function, however, is to keep the cell hyperpolarized while permitting the potassium entering through the transducer channels from the scala media to exit from the basolateral membrane. For example, one type found in mammalian IHCs is the large-conductance calcium-activated (BK) potassium channel and the resulting current is responsible for the high fidelity of afferent firing by keeping the IHC time constant small (Oliver *et al.*, 2006). However, the BK channel is found in many other hair cell systems where its role can be different (see below). The range of K channels has an expression pattern that can depend as well on the cell's position along the cochlea and the developmental stage of the animal (Marcotti *et al.*, 2003).

The membrane depolarization needs to be sufficient to activate an L-type calcium channel, which unlike many neuronal calcium channels does not undergo substantial inactivation. The calcium channel type in hair cells, characterized by its α-subunit, is mainly of the $Ca_v1.3$-type and has a relatively low threshold. Mutations in the defining α-subunit of the channel lead to a failure of transmission and thus deafness (Platzer *et al.*, 2000). In the IHC, calcium continues to enter the cell during a sustained tone and leads to the exocytosis of the neurotransmitter at the synapse. Although additional calcium channel types may be present in hair cells in variety of different species, $Ca_v1.3$ is definitively the dominant Ca entry pathway at the mammalian IHC synapse and is the source of the calcium around the individual ribbon release sites (Brandt *et al.*, 2003).

It is not known in detail how the calcium channels are distributed around the release zone. Electron microscopy strongly hints that the calcium channels are in close proximity to the ribbon. Frog saccular hair cells and turtle papillar hair cells exhibit an intrinsic electrical tuning unlike mammalian hair cells. Thus in these cases calcium channels may even be shared for two functions, for the triggering of release of neurotransmitter at the synapse and for activating calcium-dependent (BK) potassium channels responsible for electrical oscillations in the membrane (Roberts *et al.*, 1990; Tucker & Fettiplace, 1995). There are two competing hypotheses of the importance of calcium channels being clustered at the active zone of a single ribbon. It seems clear from electrical recording and immunolocalization studies that calcium channels are clustered in domains of less than about 200 nm in diameter, the resolution limit of these methods (Wu *et al.*, 1996). To be more precise about the distribution of calcium entering through the channels requires recourse to models of calcium dynamics with additional assumptions about the cell structure (e.g. Bortolozzi *et al.*, 2008). It has been proposed that calcium channels form *microdomains*, so that activation of the channels (estimated to be about 80 at a mammalian ribbon synapse (Brandt *et al.*, 2005)) flood the release zone with calcium to drive exocytosis. It also has been proposed that calcium channels are further clustered within the region of the active zone into *nanodomains*, each channel closely associated with a vesicle fusion site. In the case of a microdomain, the elevation of calcium will depend on the average open probability of the calcium channels and the cooperativity of the calcium dependence of release. In the case of a nanodomain structure, the release of vesicles would be controlled by the stochastic opening and closing of the calcium channels, as a single channel opening would lead inevitably to vesicle release. In the former case, variability arises from the release process itself. In the latter case, it could well be the statistics of opening and closing of single calcium channels that determine the release statistics.

In vivo, resting but unstimulated IHCs are slightly depolarized with a resting potential near −50 mV, close to the threshold for activation of the calcium channels. As a result there is a small level of transmitter release and it seems probable that this is the origin of spontaneous activity in fibres of the nerve (Robertson & Paki, 2002). This conclusion has implications for a longstanding problem in the encoding of sound intensity. Measured in the auditory nerve, the intensity of a sound is coded as a spike rate from auditory threshold to over 80 dB SPL, or 10 000 times, in input sound pressure level. How this comes about, given that individual nerve fibres appear to saturate in their firing rate within about 40 dB of their threshold, is known as the *dynamic range problem*.

One possible solution is that, within the auditory nerve, there are subpopulations of nerve fibres that segregate the intensity range into different response bands. Thus the population of fibres includes those that have a high resting spontaneous rate (50–150 spikes/second) but respond to low levels of sound; and those that have a much lower spontaneous rate and might require a stimulus of 60 dB SPL before they respond (Sachs & Abbas, 1974). There is some evidence from the cat cochlea (Fig. 9.7) that fibres with different spontaneous rates make contact with different parts of the basolateral membrane of the IHC (Liberman, 1982). Intracellular marking, recovery,

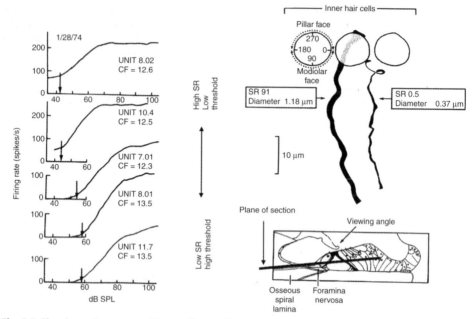

Fig. 9.7 The dynamic range problem. Afferent fibres exhibit a range of sound intensity response characteristics. (A) Low-threshold fibres are associated with high spontaneous rates, high-threshold fibres with low spontaneous rates. (B) The two different fibres types may be associated with different synaptic contact sites on the IHC, with the high spontaneous rate fibres being larger in diameter and associated with the abneural surface of the cell. Data from cat recordings.
Figure 9.7B upper panel is reproduced with permission from Sachs and Abbas (1974) and the lower panel from Liberman (1982).

and tracing of recorded fibres indicate that fibres with a high spontaneous rate and low threshold contact the abneural surface of the IHC whereas fibres with a low spontaneous rate and high threshold contact more modiolar regions of the IHC basolateral surface. Although it is not known currently whether there are differences between the postsynaptic membranes that might account for some of the differences between fibres, these classic observations imply that the presynaptic release sites of IHCs may themselves constitute a heterogeneous population with different basal release rates of transmitter, and different sensitivities to depolarization. The problem needs to be further explored.

9.5.2 Synaptic vesicle exocytosis at the inner hair cell synapse

The sequence of events that follows depolarization of the IHC consists of activation of the calcium channels around the synaptic sites, a local increase of intracellular calcium at this release site and subsequent fusion of synaptic vesicles to release their neurotransmitter contents into the synaptic cleft. How release occurs and how it is regulated at many neuronal synapses is a hotly contested research field (Chapman, 2002; Lisman et al., 2007). In the case of the ribbon synapse in cochlear hair cells there are additional questions, yet to be answered: how is a high release rate possible at this synapse? and how is the excess membrane recovered (Wu et al., 2007)?

The classical sequence of events is that vesicles overcome an energy barrier to fuse to the membrane, initially forming a pore that then continues to open fully. From the moment of fusion there can be continuity between the vesicle interior and the extracellular space. In such full fusion events, the vesicles exocytose their contents into the cleft. In exceptional circumstances the synaptic vesicle can be caught in the process of fusing (Heuser *et al.*, 1979). Subsequently, after the vesicle membrane is added to the plasma membrane, membrane is taken up by a process of endocytosis and recycled around via the endoplasmic reticulum to become new releasable vesicles. Since each vesicle is a sphere of membrane about 35 nm in diameter, it is associated with area of 0.0040 μm^2. The complete fusion of 300 vesicles, the estimated number of vesicles released from just one ribbon per second (see below Beutner *et al.*, 2001; Goutman & Glowatzki, 2007), would be the equivalent of adding about 0.1% of the surface area of membrane to an IHC. Thus there has to be some mechanism for taking up the excess membrane and to prevent the cell swelling indefinitely.

The process of endocytosis, particularly if it clathrin dependent, is both rate-limiting and energy-demanding (Harata *et al.*, 2006). It is rate-limiting unless there is such a large population of vesicles that the supply never runs out under normal conditions, even though it takes time to replenish the stores. It has been an attractive idea, therefore, and one originally emerging from the electron microscope images, that there is not complete fusion of vesicle membrane and release of transmitter but that a mechanism of partial fusion occurs, and this is followed by immediate reformation of internalized vesicles (Fesce *et al.*, 1994). This mechanism of 'kiss and run' kinetics is attractive as, in principle, it allows for much faster recycling of transmitter vesicles and is much less energy demanding: the machinery of endocytosis is not required (see Fig. 9.4). The evidence for any kiss-and-run mechanism is circumstantial and the case for this so-called 'non-classical' release may vary from synapse to synapse (Harata *et al.*, 2006). The other contentious issue, even if both 'classical' and 'non-classical' mechanisms exist, is how much each process contributes to the transmission at the synapse (He & Wu, 2007). This is a quantitative question. At the calyx of Held, for example, there are kiss-and-run events that can be detected by high-resolution capacitance measurements, but they comprise only 3% of all the vesicle fusions measured at the presynaptic membrane (He *et al.*, 2006).

Do single vesicles fuse at the IHC ribbon synapse? Detecting the fusion of a single vesicle is beyond the limit of current technologies: in capacitance measurements there is a trade-off between time and amplitude resolution and thus the ability to see single fusion events. Fusion of a single vesicle with a diameter of 35 nm would increase the membrane capacitance by about 40 aF (1 aF = 10^{-18}F). Whole cell capacitance methods measure the fusion of vesicles to the entire cell membrane, which in hair cells equates to about 10 pF (1 pF = 10^{-12}F) and thus the technical challenge is to resolve single events as a change of this much larger value. Although it may prove possible to measure single events in a cell-attached mode, where the pipette restricts the area of membrane recorded this has so far not been reported in hair cells. As an alternative, it might be possible to investigate fluctuations in membrane capacitance using methods of noise analysis familiar from its use in ionic channel analysis. This has indeed been carried out in mouse IHCs (Neef *et al.*, 2007) To vary the mean level of the capacitance, the events arising during the run-down of a releasable pool of exocytosing synaptic vesicles were followed. By measuring the excess fluctuations in capacitance after a stimulus, the analysis of capacitance variance suggested that there is an underlying elementary fusion event of around 95 aF in amplitude in mature synapses. This value is about *twice* what would be expected for the fusion of a single vesicle (30–40 aF). There appeared to be no spurious coordination of release by additional calcium from cytoplasmic stores as the vesicle size estimate was not affected by application of ryanodine.

The above data therefore suggest that there is coordinated release of synaptic vesicles at the presynaptic membrane. If so, the mechanisms are unknown but include the possibilities that:

♦ a single calcium channel may be coordinating two vesicle fusion events (consistent with a nanodomain explanation)

- vesicle fusion events may be occurring presynaptically before exocytosis
- vesicles may fuse as they exocytose.

All these possibilities have been suggested in the exocytosis literature but have yet to be established for any synapses, including ribbons. Nevertheless there is still a mismatch between the degree of coordination of vesicle release and the estimates derived from the size of the elementary excitatory postsynaptic current (EPSC) observed post synaptically in the afferent terminals (Glowatzki & Fuchs, 2002; Keen & Hudspeth, 2006). In the case of the IHC, a quantal analysis of the distribution of evoked EPSC amplitudes (Neef *et al.*, 2007) suggests that best fit can be obtained with a distribution where the mean is about four rather than two times the size of the elementary vesicular event (estimated from Glowatzki & Fuchs (2002) as 30–36 pA when measured in the afferent terminal).

9.5.3 Synaptic membrane endocytosis at the IHC synapse

As already indicated there are good theoretical arguments that endocytosis does occur at cochlear afferent synapses. Experimentally it has been found that horseradish peroxidase, injected into the scala tympani, is taken up from the basolateral surface (Siegel & Brownell, 1986). The electron micrographs indicate that endocytosis occurs via clathrin-coated pits, for pits can be observed at the basal surface of both IHCs and, to a lesser extent (which reflects a lower level of afferent activity), at OHCs. In these experiments, labelled synaptic vesicles were often found associated with presynaptic bodies of IHCs (and OHCs). This result suggests that at least some synaptic vesicle membrane is retrieved from the plasmalemma by endocytosis.

Two other types of measurement also indicate that endocytosis in hair cells occurs. Capacitance measurements to determine the IHC membrane area show a reduction in area following an exocytotic event which can be interpreted as due to membrane uptake by endocytosis (Parsons *et al.*, 1994; Beutner *et al.*, 2001). Experiments on IHCs have used flash photolysis of caged calcium to raise the intracellular calcium rapidly. These experiments reveal two kinetically distinct types of endocytosis: one with an exponential time constant of ~15 s when Ca_i was increased up to 15 µM; and a much faster component characterized by an exponential time constant of about 300 ms when Ca_i levels exceeded 10 µM. These increases in intracellular calcium produced large capacitance steps (typically 2–3 pF) which, when translated into synaptic vesicle numbers, corresponded to a fusion pool of ~40 000 vesicles or about 2000 vesicles per ribbon synapse. These values are about an order of magnitude higher than is found in other neuronal presynaptic terminals that have been studied in the same way.

Endocytosis of basolateral membrane also can be demonstrated using the endocytosis marker FM1-43. This amphiphilic dye is believed not to cross membranes although it may permeate some cation channels (Meyers *et al.*, 2003). When applied extracellularly to the basolateral membrane, fluorescence spreads from the base towards the apex of the cell. The fluorescence was interpreted as basal endocytosis with a transport of vesicles up to the apical endosomal structures (Griesinger *et al.*, 2002). The apparent uptake rate cannot be quantified as precisely as in the capacitance measurements although the uptake time constant to equilibrium was approximately 50 s.

9.5.4 Imaging synaptic release

Whole cell current recordings from hair cells measure trigger parameters of the synapse. These include the calcium current that activates the synapse and the other basolateral membrane currents (mainly potassium currents) that shape the response of the cell to hair bundle deflection. Capacitance measurements, carried out with the same patch-clamp technology, measure the difference between exocytosis and endocytosis, but with the technical limitation that capacitance measurements cannot be made during the stimulus pulse. For this reason it has proved helpful to turn to imaging methods which can visualize changes in the synaptic vesicle population during the stimulus. The two optical methods mentioned above use fluorescent markers of endocytosed membrane (the FM family of dyes) or genetically encoded fluorescent protein tags (GFP, EGFP, DsRed, etc.) which can be linked to proteins associated with the synaptic membrane. Coupled with physiological stimulation and multiphoton microscopy to enhance image quality, in order to provide quantification and to look deeper into the tissues, it has proved possible to measure the time course of vesicle fusion events at single ribbon synapses.

Synaptic vesicle populations can be loaded with FM dyes by endocytosis across the cell's *apical* membrane (Griesinger *et al.*, 2005; Kaneko *et al.*, 2006). Both IHCs and OHCs load in this way although it seems likely that the FM cationic dyes can also enter through the transduction channel or other activated apical membrane channels. This pathway represents a parallel route of entry (Gale *et al.*, 2001) which can label the cytoplasmic rather than the luminal membrane of the vesicle. The dye is trafficked intracellularly to the basolateral membrane where it concentrates in 'hotspots', which can be recognized as ribbon release sites (Fig. 9.8). These regions appear to be 0.6–1.0 μm in diameter, matching the electron micrographic measurements. By converting the fluorescence intensity into a vesicle count, the number of vesicles aggregated at the hotspot was found to about 400. This is close to that estimated for the RRP. It is also close to the number estimated, using very different techniques, at the mossy-fibre granule cell synapse of the cerebellum (Saviane & Silver, 2006), also a fast synapse specialized for high fidelity transmission of sensory information (Rancz *et al.*, 2007). Membrane polarization by extrinsic current, or by extracellular K^+, leads to a destaining of the hotspot/ribbon. The destaining is interpreted as a fusion of vesicles to the presynaptic region with resulting washout of the luminal FM1-43. The values found for the release rates, converted to vesicle counts, are about 3 vesicles/ribbon-ms, close to the estimates inferred from capacitance measurements once the values for the aggregate of all ~20 ribbons in the cell are included (Moser & Beutner, 2000).

After the cessation of the depolarizing stimulus, the rate of recovery of the fluorescence at the hotspot has two components. One component is relatively fast at 2 vesicles/ribbon-ms. The second component is slower, with a time course that may take 20 seconds to complete. This latter process can restore the fluorescence intensity at the hotspot to its original brightness. These values are compatible with other measures of ribbon function. The additional advantage of this imaging technique it allows much faster screening of multiple ribbons in intact tissues. In principle, it also has the potential for conducting experiments where several synaptic proteins labelled with distinct fluorophores are simultaneously tracked.

9.6 **Postsynaptic mechanisms**

9.6.1 **Postsynaptic EPSPs and EPSCs**

Although the first recordings of EPSPs were made using microelectrodes from afferent terminals in the goldfish (Furukawa *et al.*, 1978) and from turtles (Crawford & Fettiplace, 1980), high-resolution records of EPSCs awaited patch-clamp recording from the afferent boutons with relatively small diameter pipettes (Glowatzki & Fuchs, 2002). Spontaneously occurring EPSCs were reported to be quite variable in amplitude. In the recording conditions used, EPSCs have varied from 15 pA to 800 pA in amplitude, even at a single bouton. Some of these events must therefore be due to multivesicular release of neurotransmitter from the presynaptic cells, although not necessarily all synchronized in time. At room temperature, the EPSC rise time was than 0.5 ms, while it decayed exponentially with a time constant of about 1.1 ms (Glowatzki and Fuchs, 2002).

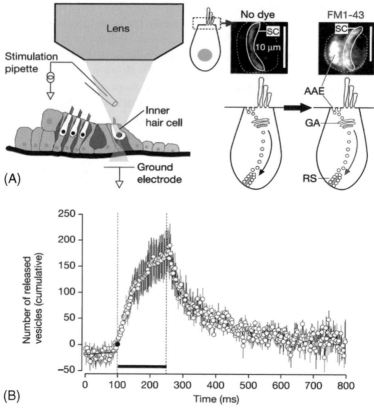

Fig. 9.8 Imaging synaptic vesicle release in inner hair cells. (A) The principle of FM1-43 dye loading is shown: the dye is taken up by the apical membrane and is then trafficked to the basolateral membrane via the apical endosomal structures. The dye-loaded clusters of vesicles can be detected by two photon-confocal microscopy when they lie in an imaging plane that intersects the whole organ of Corti. (B) Release of vesicles from a single fluorescent 'hot spot' in the basolateral membrane corresponding to a ribbon site. The degree of destaining can be converted numerically into a vesicle count and shows rapid release (in the first 50 ms), followed by slower release and subsequent recovery when the depolarization ceases.
Reproduced with permission from Griesinger et al. (2005).

In such experiments 40 mM K^+ was used to depolarize the IHC (although not measured directly) and it produced a significant increase in spontaneous rates but little change in the amplitude distribution of the events.

Unlike the classical analysis of the endplate potential at the neuromuscular junction, where EPSPs (strictly endplate potentials, EPPs) are multiples of a fundamental or miniature EPP (Fatt & Katz, 1951), the amplitude distribution of EPSCs at the IHC bouton does not show multiple modes. Instead, the EPSC distribution in the neonatal IHC bouton is highly skewed. Interval analysis showed that two exponentials are required to fit that distribution. Such a departure from a simple Poisson distribution is consistent with a mechanism of multivesicular release, a conclusion also suggested by the analysis resulting from high-resolution capacitance measurements (Neef et al., 2007). The unique mode of the spontaneous EPSC distribution is about 36 pA, which would be equivalent to a conductance of 400 pS, or the opening of about 50 α-amino-5-hydroxy-3-methyl-4-isoxazole propionic acid (AMPA)-gated channels in the postsynaptic bouton.

Given reasonable estimates of the input resistance of the afferent bouton (1–2 Gohms), it appears that the elementary quantum would be capable of producing a sufficiently large postsynaptic depolarization (35–70 mV) to initiate an action potential in the terminal neurite. That still larger EPSCs are observed thus suggests that the safety factor for transmission is considerable. This could serve to enhance temporal fidelity. This result therefore might be construed as a consequence of the design of the ribbon synapse.

9.6.2 Clearance of neurotransmitter from the cleft

When a vesicle fuses with the hair cell membrane and releases its contents into the cleft, the neurotransmitter diffuses across the gap and acts on the receptors in the postsynaptic membrane of the afferent terminal. There is now much evidence that these receptors are glutamate receptors of the AMPA variety, both in mammals (Glowatzki & Fuchs, 2002) as well as in frog hair cells (Keen & Hudspeth, 2006). Under some circumstances, such as following excess glutamate release there is evidence from *in vivo* experiments that N-methyl-D-aspartate (NMDA) receptors also are present and it has been suggested that these may perform a neurotrophic role (Ruel *et al.*, 2000). Nevertheless the clearest experiments, from recordings of the postsynaptic afferent terminals, do suggest that the overwhelming majority of receptors are AMPA receptors: they are characteristically blocked by the receptor antagonist 6-cyano-7-nitroquinoxaline-2,3-dione (CNQX) at 10–50 µM concentrations. In addition, the decay time of the responses is slowed fourfold by cyclothiazide, a drug that reduces AMPA receptor desensitization (Glowatzki & Fuchs, 2002). When these AMPA receptors are blocked, there is virtually a complete reduction in the afferent firing rate. Chronic blockade of all the AMPA receptors also leads to degeneration of the nerve.

At neuronal synapses the neurotransmitter has to be cleared after binding with the postsynaptic receptors. This prevents continued activation of the receptors and problems associated with excitoxicity where permeation of the ions and elevated intracellular calcium can lead to cell death. At the inner hair cell synapse this is a particular problem as the release rates can be high. In addition, it is important for faithful transmission that successive EPSPs should not be blurred together by residual levels of the neurotransmitter. In the cochlea the clearance of glutamate is specifically carried out by the glutamate transporter GLAST (glutamate-aspartate transporter). GLAST is also found in astroglia, which also often contain other glutamate transporters such as GLT-1, although in the cochlea there is little evidence for this latter transporter. GLAST uses sodium and proton gradients to carry in the amino acid with small participation of anions (Marcaggi *et al.*, 2005).

GLAST is distributed all around the IHC afferent terminals and in particularly high levels on the membranes of the inner phalangeal cells (Furness & Lehre, 1997; Glowatzki *et al.*, 2006). This electrogenic transporter takes up the glutamate into the border cells for subsequent recycling by the afferent terminals of the IHCs. Experimentally, the ability to use aspartate as the substrate has the experimental consequence that the transporter can be studied in the tissue without activating the glutamate receptors at the afferent terminals (Glowatzki *et al.*, 2006). Patch-clamp recordings have been made in the cochlea of young mice where rapid uptake of D-aspartate and L-glutamate can be observed and confirm the immunohistochemical observations. In mice where the *GLAST* gene has been deleted there is a considerably reduced glutamate uptake. In contrast, at the OHC synapse, the (much smaller) levels of glutamate are also removed by GLAST associated with Deiters' cells around the afferent terminal (Furness *et al.*, 2002). So far the transporter function at the OHC synapse has not been studied as explicitly as at the IHC synapse.

9.6.3 Paired presynaptic and postsynaptic responses

Continuous activation of the hair cell, for example by a long burst of sound, leads to a rapid decline of firing rate in the afferent fibres. It is not immediately clear whether this is due to postsynaptic adaptation of the nerve (for example, by desensitization of the postsynaptic neurotransmitter receptor, or activation of an outward rectifier leading to relative refractoriness of the nerve) or is due to presynaptic mechanisms. Although there is longstanding evidence that hair cell adaptive mechanisms are probably presynaptic (Furukawa *et al.*, 1978), some recent data clearly point to a rundown of release at single presynaptic sites both in hair cells of the frog amphibian papilla (Keen & Hudspeth, 2006) and in terminals of rat IHCs (Fig. 9.6) (Goutman & Glowatzki, 2007). In these latter remarkable experiments, simultaneous presynaptic and postsynaptic recordings have been made using fine recording pipettes which could be directed to specific sites in the cochlea of young rats. By depolarizing the IHC with a prolonged voltage command, an inward presynaptic calcium current was recorded which showed a minimal degree of inactivation (Goutman & Glowatzki, 2007). This is the expected signature of an L-type calcium current. The postsynaptic activity in the terminal was a series of randomly occurring inward currents, EPSCs, which rapidly decreased in frequency over the first 10 ms and more slowly over the subsequent 200 ms to reach a steady state which was about 6% of the initial peak. This pattern of adaptation is very similar to that described in earlier auditory nerve recordings. The adaptation cannot be explained by a decline in calcium current (shown to be minimal) or by postsynaptic receptor desensitization (for 100 μM cyclothiazide reduces receptor desensitization but does not alter adaptation). It is therefore is a property of the presynaptic release mechanism. By identifying the individual EPSCs in the response, a one-second IHC stimulation producing the largest calcium current produced about 70 EPSCs; 12 of these were activated during the initial 10 ms fast component. The numbers are consistent with the numbers of vesicles docked by a single ribbon seen by electron microscopy as well as with the numbers released from all 10–20 ribbons in whole hair cell measured by capacitance.

The other data obtainable from these simultaneous recordings are transfer functions. A transfer function indicates how well presynaptic depolarization is encoded as postsynaptic activity. This information will be used below. In both frog and rat hair cells the postsynaptic response was found to be essentially proportional to the hair cell depolarization *for potentials in the physiological range*. In this range, despite voltage non-linearities of calcium channel gating, the effect is a linear transfer of signal, converting a voltage change into a rate code. The models of release at the presynaptic membrane which best fit this linear result are those that propose 'nanodomains' of calcium channels, where a single presynaptic channel activates only a small number of local vesicles. In this situation the released vesicles count only the small numbers of activated calcium channels, and this number is itself linearly dependent on presynaptic potential.

However, at depolarized potentials beyond the physiological range, the input-output function is measurably non-linear. The experiments are more difficult to interpret although one explanation is that in these conditions the non-linearity of the calcium sensor is being revealed, showing a cooperative binding of three to five Ca^{2+} ions at the calcium sensor.

9.7 Functional consequences of synaptic processing

9.7.1 The minimum hair cell signal for transmission

Hair cells produce graded potential responses to deflection of their stereocilia. In the mammalian cochlea the sharp tuning of the basilar membrane ensures that at low sound levels only a few hair cells are stimulated at levels above the thermal noise floor. As realized many years ago, the mechanoelectrical transducer channel strictly has no absolute threshold (Pickles, 1988) although a 'thought-experiment' suggests that absolute threshold must be set by a displacement which opens a single mechanoelectrical channel. The threshold stimulus is one which causes one extra postsynaptic action potential in the associated nerve, or in a small population of fibres. The question,

'What is the minimum signal in the hair cell?' is instead partially answered by measurements from the afferent bouton (Glowatzki & Fuchs, 2002), which show that the single postsynaptic quantal event possibly arising from the release of two or three vesicles can generate an action potential. An upper bound for the hair cell receptor potential that leads to this event can be determined from the synaptic transfer function (postsynaptic current change/presynaptic potential change) measured in simultaneous presynaptic and postsynaptic recordings independent of the input resistance of the IHC. An upper bound for the slope of the transfer function at physiological potentials is about 40 pA /mV (Goutman & Glowatzki, 2007). A smaller value for the slope is found from paired recordings from frog hair cells in the amphibian papilla (Keen & Hudspeth, 2006). Hence, where a single contact point is involved in signal transmission, a minimum signal of about 1 mV would be required in the IHC.

The data for these transfer functions are obtained by averaging the response over long steps. For much shorter steps the postsynaptic response is considerably enhanced but then desensitizes (adapts) to around 10% of the initial peak. It has been suggested above that this is primarily a consequence of depletion of the readily releasable pool at the presynaptic ribbon. If a correction for adaptation is applied to the hair cell transfer response, a short presynaptic signal of 100 μV would produce the necessary postsynaptic event for a spike in a single bouton.

Finally, it is necessary to consider the problem faced by the central nervous system in detecting this additional spike in the presence of variability of the responses in the individual nerve dendrites. The stochastic transmission across a noisy synapse degrades the signal. It has been known by signal engineers for over 80 years that sending the same information along multiple channels reduces degradation due to noisy transmission lines. Referred to as the 'multiline trick' by John von Neumann, the founder of the theory of neural computation, the principle applies with equal force to the N = 10–30 auditory nerve fibres associated with each IHC. As a result the signal-to-noise ratio for transmission from a single hair cell should be increased by a factor $N^{1/2}$. With N = 16, it might be deduced that the minimum detectable change in signal in a mammalian hair cell is around 100 μV/4 = 25 μV.

9.7.2 Synaptic adaptation and noise

The correct functioning of the hair cell afferent synapse is important for theories of audition. The perception of complex sounds over a wide range of sound intensities almost certainly involves adaptation in the rate of firing of the nerve fibre when presented with a continuous tone. In an attempt to provide a physiological underpinning for psychoacoustic data, models of the IHC have been constructed that include the effects of variability in synaptic transmission as well as the effects of adaptation.

An analysis of spike timing has been carried out recently for the auditory nerve of the chick which gives some idea of the way in which underlying physiological properties of the synapse affect the signal encoding (Avissar et al., 2007). Recordings from single nerve fibres show that there is some phase jitter (i.e. spike initiation is not precisely synchronized to a particular phase of the sound pressure cycle). The variability decreases, or equivalently, timing precision increases, with increasing fibre CF up to the highest CF measured (3 kHz). These measurements show that temporal jitter does not change during the initial or the adapted periods. Nevertheless the variance relative to the mean number of the spikes (the Fano factor = variance/mean) does increase during short-term adaptation, so that, with sustained stimulation, the signal-to-noise ratio in a single afferent declines. This may be another reason why having multiple afferent synapses on single hair cells (i.e. the 'multiline' trick) is a good design principle in a system where there is a trade-off between high temporal fidelity and the demands of sustained release.

Trying to understand some of these interacting features of synaptic afferent transmission means that mathematical models are often helpful. At the cellular level there are detailed models of vesicle dynamics that show that temporal precision is greatly enhanced if the vesicles can undergo coordinated release from an active zone immediately adjacent to the ribbon (Wittig & Parsons, 2008). Whatever detailed assumptions are made, even the simplest models can provide an important underpinning for psychoacoustical results where there are questions about the response to complex patterns of sound. The situation up to 1995 is summarized by Mountain and Hubbard (1995) and it is clear that quite simple physiological assumptions, such as pool depletion and clearance of neurotransmitter from the cleft can account broadly for the properties of adaptation and timing in postsynaptic spike rate. In some cases mathematical models can be constructed that provide a reasonable fit to the experimental data. The conclusions are qualitatively robust against parameter variation although the physiological data on synaptic release depend upon parameters unknown at the time. The advantage of such models is that the population behaviour of such synapses can be computationally predicted.

9.8 **The genetics of the synapse**

Several forms of deafness have been associated with abnormalities of the inner hair cell synapse. Although many, but not all, of the genes associated with hereditary deafness have been linked to alteration of the hair cell transduction complex, genes associated with auditory neuropathies are beginning to be identified. These genes, which cause a failure of the hair cell to signal to the nerve and higher brainstem nuclei, will also be classified as genes of functional deafness. Of particular importance for our understanding are those cases where there is a disturbed auditory brainstem response (ABR) but other functions of the cochlea (such as OHC responses measured in the ear canal as distortion products – see Chapter 4) appear to be unimpaired. Some of these candidate genes are listed in Table 9.1.

Table 9.1 Summary of some of the genes known to affect transmission at the afferent synapse. The human gene locus is given where appropriate, but in many cases the data are derived from transgenic mouse models

Gene	Human locus	Protein description	Function	Reference
Cav1.3	(Mouse only)	α-subunit of calcium channel	Controls Ca entry to IHC	Platzer et al. (2000)
OTOF	DFNB9	Otoferlin	Possible calcium release sensor	Roux et al. (2006)
TMC1	DFNB7	Trans-membrane protein	Unknown function	Marcotti et al. (2006)
Pax8	(Mouse only)	Transcription factor	Controls multiple developmental programmes	Knipper et al. (2000); Brandt et al. (2007)
PJVK	DFNB59	Pejvakin	Possible auditory pathway determinant	Delmaghani et al. (2006)
RIBEYE/CtBP2	(Mouse only)	Ribbon protein	Determines ribbon assembly	Tom et al. (2005)
Bassoon	(Mouse only)	Ribbon protein	Determines size of RRP	Khimich et al. (2005)
SLC17A8	DFNA25	Vglut3	Vesicular glutamate transporter	Ruel et al. (2008); Seal et al. (2008)
Prosaposin	(Mouse only)	Inner hair cell protein	Innervation pattern control	Akil et al. (2006)

◆ **Calcium channel Ca$_v$1.3** (Platzer *et al.*, 2000): The synapse depends on a reliable calcium influx to initiate exocytosis, and the physiology of that requirement can be studied in mouse models. Mutations in the α-subunit (α1-D) of this calcium channel leads to deafness (the mouse with the gene deleted is deaf). The knock-out has virtually no ABR and an IHC calcium current reduced by over 90% compared with the wild-type. In mice with a Ca$_v$1.3 deletion there also is a reduction of the Ca-activated pottassium currents in the cells and slowing in the development of the adult innervation pattern. It can be argued that a secondary function of the calcium channel is the stabilization of the hair cell and the synapse (Nemzou *et al.*, 2006).

◆ **Otoferlin** (Yasunaga *et al.*, 1999; Roux *et al.*, 2006): Otoferlin is a protein with six calcium binding motifs that is found in hair cells. Mutations in the otoferlin gene (*OTOF*) lead to (recessive) deafness mutations in human populations at locus DFNB9. In mouse hair cells, it is localized in hair cells in a developmental pattern that corresponds to the maturation of the IHC synapse, with relatively little expression in the OHCs. Mice with the gene deleted have a marked reduction in the exocytosis associated with the readily releasable pool of vesicles. Since otoferlin binds to the SNARE complex in a calcium-dependent manner, it has been proposed that otoferlin is the ribbon synapse calcium sensor, replacing the missing synaptotagmins.

◆ **Transmembrane channel 1 (TMC1)** (Marcotti *et al.*, 2006): The protein TMC1 was identified in a mouse screen for deafness and underlies profound congenital deafness (DFNB7/B11) and progressive hearing loss (DFNA36) in human populations. The precise role of this protein, which contains 6–11 transmembrane domains, is not known, but in the mouse mutants there are abnormalities in the development of the hair cells and the exocytosis at the synapse related to incomplete maturation of the hair cell. At a stage when hair cells should have reached the adult form, the cells in the mutant begin to deteriorate. It is thought that TMC1 may be a trafficking molecule involved in the maturation of the synapse.

◆ **Pax8 and Thyroid hormone deficiency**: A number of synaptic defects have been associated with alterations of thyroid metabolism. It has been known for a long time that hypothyroidism is often associated with deafness. In animals lacking the transcription factor Pax8, the thyroid follicular cells fail to form and thyroid hormones are not produced (Sendin *et al.*, 2007). It is clear that there are several windows in cochlear development that are dependent on activation of appropriate thyroid receptors without which potassium currents in IHCs and features of OHCs fail to mature (Knipper *et al.*, 2000). However, thyroid hormones also regulate synaptic development in IHCs so that hypothyroid rodents have an extended period where the synapse fails to reach its adult function (Brandt *et al.*, 2007). In this case there is a prolonged period where the cell exhibits calcium spiking characteristic of immature cells (Chapter 12) and the exocytosis pattern resembles that of an immature hair cell. Although there is an elevated calcium current in hypothyroid hair cells, the synaptic efficiency (defined as exocytosis per unit calcium entry) is less, especially for short (<50 ms) pulses. Otoferlin expression is also reduced. These results point to the late maturation of the RRP of the synapse in this system.

◆ **Pejvakin**: Finally, it is worth noting that there are genes which may encode connectivity and function specifically in the auditory system. As a result, mutations produce deafness resembling the synaptic neuropathies where no ABRs are measurable. One of these genes is responsible for recessive deafnesses at locus DFNB59 (Delmaghani *et al.*, 2006). In mouse models, the protein pejvakin is expressed in the spiral ganglion cells although other isoforms may be expressed in OHCs (Schwander *et al.*, 2007). The precise function of the protein is not currently known. Mice with a mutant copy of the gene knocked in show a compromised ABR, but the cochlear phenotype is variable and depends on the isoform of the expressed protein.

9.9 **Future prospects and unsolved problems**

The hair cell synapse is an elegant and complex piece of machinery. In comparing what we now know with a review of synaptic transmission in the cochlea made just over a decade ago (Tom et al., 2005) it can be seen that we have made major strides as a consequence of new imaging methods, high-resolution electrophysiology, and the ubiquitous arrival of molecular biology tools into virtually every laboratory. However, the detailed structure of the synapse is still not understood: it awaits the new generation of computer tomographic reconstructions which might allow us to understand the relationships of the structures and proteins contributing to synaptic release. We still do not understand how the machinery can release neurotransmitter packets reliably, and how precisely the underlying mechanism of multivesicular release might occur. As we have seen, the debate about the mechanism of fusion is still not resolved for a wide range of synapses. Is there any non-classical 'kiss-and-run' release at the IHC ribbon synapse and if so what is the balance between that mode and classical fusion and release? Some of these questions may be resolved if single fusion or partial fusion events during hair cell synaptic activity can be measured.

Some of these questions can also be answered if the difficulties of recording signals from mature hair cells can be overcome. At present many facets of our understanding of hair cells and their synapses are derived from relatively immature hair cells, as it has proved easier to maintain such systems under experimental conditions. Since many animal models, particularly mouse and rat models, exhibit postnatal development even after the onset of hearing (Fig. 9.9), the danger of confusing development with adult function is always present. Conversely, and equally importantly, we do not know the sequence of events that allow a highly ordered and reliable piece

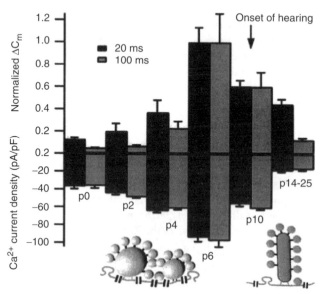

Fig. 9.9 The development of exocytosis during maturation of the mouse cochlea. Both the calcium current in the IHC and the efficiency of release (measured by capacitance change per unit calcium entry) change during the development of the cochlea and before the behavioural onset of hearing. In mice, these changes occur before postnatal day 14 (P14). Schematic ribbon morphology changes shown below.
Reproduced with permission from Beutner and Moser (2001).

of machinery, the hair cell's ribbon synapse, to be constructed and to endure for the lifetime of the cell.

But these are problems for the future.

Acknowledgements

This work was carried out during the award of Chaire Blaise Pascal (Île de France) and supported by EU FP6 grant 'EuroHear'. I thank Paul Fuchs, Saaid Saffiedine, and colleagues at the Institut Pasteur for many helpful comments.

References

Akil O, Chang J, Hiel H, Kong JH, Yi E, Glowatzki E & Lustig LR. (2006) Progressive deafness and altered cochlear innervation in knock-out mice lacking prosaposin. *J Neurosci* **26**: 13076–88.

Albillos A, Dernick G, Horstmann H, Almers W, varez de TG & Lindau M. (1997) The exocytotic event in chromaffin cells revealed by patch amperometry. *Nature* **389**: 509–12.

Avissar M, Furman AC, Saunders JC & Parsons TD. (2007) Adaptation reduces spike-count reliability, but not spike-timing precision, of auditory nerve responses. *J Neurosci* **27**: 6461–72.

Betz WJ, Mao F & Bewick GS. (1992) Activity-dependent fluorescent staining and destaining of living vertebrate motor nerve terminals. *J Neurosci* **12**: 363–75.

Beutner D & Moser T. (2001) The presynaptic function of mouse cochlear inner hair cells during development of hearing. *J Neurosci* **21**: 4593–9.

Beutner D, Voets T, Neher E & Moser T. (2001) Calcium dependence of exocytosis and endocytosis at the cochlear inner hair cellafferent synapse. *Neuron* **29**: 681–90.

Bortolozzi M, Lelli A & Mammano F. (2008) Calcium microdomains at presynaptic active zones of vertebrate hair cells unmasked by stochastic deconvolution. *Cell Calcium* **44**: 158–68.

Brandstatter JH, Fletcher EL, Garner CC, Gundelfinger ED & Wassle H. (1999) Differential expression of the presynaptic cytomatrix protein bassoon among ribbon synapses in the mammalian retina. *Eur J Neurosci* **11**: 3683–93.

Brandt A, Striessnig J & Moser T. (2003) CaV1.3 channels are essential for development and presynaptic activity of cochlear inner hair cells. *J Neurosci* **23**: 10832–40.

Brandt A, Khimich D & Moser T. (2005) Few CaV1.3 channels regulate the exocytosis of a synaptic vesicle at the hair cell ribbon synapse. *J Neurosci* **25**: 11577–85.

Brandt N, Kuhn S, Munkner S, Braig C, Winter H, Blin N, Vonthein R, Knipper M & Engel J. (2007) Thyroid hormone deficiency affects postnatal spiking activity and expression of Ca^{2+} and K^+ channels in rodent inner hair cells. *J Neurosci* **27**: 3174–86.

Chapman ER. (2002) Synaptotagmin: a Ca(2+) sensor that triggers exocytosis? *Nat Rev Mol Cell Biol* **3**: 498–508.

Crawford AC & Fettiplace R. (1980) The frequency selectivity of auditory nerve fibres and hair cells in the cochlea of the turtle. *J Physiol* **306**: 79–125.

Delmaghani S, del Castillo FJ, Michel V, Leibovici M, Aghaie A, Ron U, Van LL, Ben-Tal N, Van CG, Weil D, Langa F, Lathrop M, Avan P & Petit C. (2006) Mutations in the gene encoding pejvakin, a newly identified protein of the afferent auditory pathway, cause DFNB59 auditory neuropathy. *Nat Genet* **38**: 770–8.

Dick O, Hack I, Altrock WD, Garner CC, Gundelfinger ED & Brandstatter JH. (2001) Localization of the presynaptic cytomatrix protein Piccolo at ribbon and conventional synapses in the rat retina: comparison with Bassoon. *J Comp Neurol* **439**: 224–34.

Evans EF. (1972) The frequency response and other properties of single fibres in the guinea-pig cochlear nerve. *J Physiol* **226**: 263–87.

Fatt P & Katz B. (1951) An analysis of the end-plate potential recorded with an intracellular electrode. *J Physiol* **115**: 320–70.

Fesce R, Grohovaz F, Valtorta F & Meldolesi J. (1994) Neurotransmitter release: fusion or 'kiss-and-run'? *Trends Cell Biol* **4**: 1–4.

Fuchs PA, Glowatzki E & Moser T. (2003) The afferent synapse of cochlear hair cells. *Curr Opin Neurobiol* **13**: 452–8.

Furness DN & Lehre KP. (1997) Immunocytochemical localization of a high-affinity glutamate-aspartate transporter, GLAST, in. *Eur J Neurosci* **9**: 1961–9.

Furness DN, Hulme JA, Lawton DM & Hackney CM. (2002) Distribution of the glutamate/aspartate transporter GLAST in relation to the afferent synapses of outer hair cells in the guinea pig cochlea. *J Assoc Res Otolaryngol* **3**: 234–47.

Furukawa T, Hayashida Y & Matsuura S. (1978) Quantal analysis of the size of excitatory post-synaptic potentials at synapses between hair cells and afferent nerve fibres in goldfish. *J Physiol* **276**: 211–26.

Gale JE, Marcotti W, Kennedy HJ, Kros CJ & Richardson GP. (2001) FM1–43 dye behaves as a permeant blocker of the hair-cell mechanotransducer channel. *J Neurosci* **21**: 7013–25.

Glowatzki E & Fuchs PA. (2002) Transmitter release at the hair cell ribbon synapse. *Nat Neurosci* **5**: 147–54.

Glowatzki E, Cheng N, Hiel H, Yi E, Tanaka K, Ellis-Davies GC, Rothstein JD & Bergles DE. (2006) The glutamate-aspartate transporter GLAST mediates glutamate uptake at inner hair cell afferent synapses in the mammalian cochlea. *J Neurosci* **26**: 7659–64.

Glowatzki E, Grant L & Fuchs P. (2008) Hair cell afferent synapses. *Curr Opin Neurobiol* **18**: 389–95.

Goutman JD & Glowatzki E. (2007) Time course and calcium dependence of transmitter release at a single ribbon synapse. *Proc Natl Acad Sci U S A* **104**: 16341–6.

Griesinger CB, Richards CD & Ashmore JF. (2002) FM1-43 reveals membrane recycling in adult inner hair cells of the mammalian cochlea. *J Neurosci* **22**: 3939–52.

Griesinger CB, Richards CD & Ashmore JF. (2005) Fast vesicle replenishment allows indefatigable signalling at the first auditory synapse. *Nature* **435**: 212–5.

Harata NC, Aravanis AM & Tsien RW. (2006) Kiss-and-run and full-collapse fusion as modes of exo-endocytosis in neurosecretion. *J Neurochem* **97**: 1546–70.

He L & Wu LG. (2007) The debate on the kiss-and-run fusion at synapses. *Trends Neurosci* **30**: 447–55.

He L, Wu XS, Mohan R & Wu LG. (2006) Two modes of fusion pore opening revealed by cell-attached recordings at a synapse. *Nature* **444**: 102–5.

Heuser JE, Reese TS, Dennis MJ, Jan Y, Jan L & Evans L. (1979) Synaptic vesicle exocytosis captured by quick freezing and correlated with quantal transmitter release. *J Cell Biol* **81**: 275–300.

Holt JC, Xue JT, Brichta AM & Goldberg JM. (2006) Transmission between type II hair cells and bouton afferents in the turtle posterior crista. *J Neurophysiol* **95**: 428–52.

Kaneko T, Harasztosi C, Mack AF & Gummer AW. (2006) Membrane traffic in outer hair cells of the adult mammalian cochlea. *Eur J Neurosci* **23**: 2712–22.

Keen EC & Hudspeth AJ. (2006) Transfer characteristics of the hair cell's afferent synapse. *Proc Natl Acad Sci U S A* **103**: 5537–42.

Khimich D, Nouvian R, Pujol R, Tom DS, Egner A, Gundelfinger ED & Moser T. (2005) Hair cell synaptic ribbons are essential for synchronous auditory signalling. *Nature* **434**: 889–94.

Kiang NY, Sachs MB & Peake WT. (1967) Shapes of tuning curves for single auditory-nerve fibers. *J Acoust Soc Am* **42**: 1341–2.

Knipper M, Zinn C, Maier H, Praetorius M, Rohbock K, Kopschall I & Zimmermann U. (2000) Thyroid hormone deficiency before the onset of hearing causes irreversible damage to peripheral and central auditory systems. *J Neurophysiol* **83**: 3101–12.

Lenzi D, Runyeon JW, Crum J, Ellisman MH & Roberts WM. (1999) Synaptic vesicle populations in saccular hair cells reconstructed by. *J Neurosci* **19**: 119–32.

Liberman MC. (1982) Single-neuron labeling in the cat auditory nerve. *Science* **216**: 1239–41.

Liberman MC, Dodds LW & Pierce S. (1990) Afferent and efferent innervation of the cat cochlea: quantitative analysis with light and electron microscopy. *J Comp Neurol* **301**: 443–60.

Lisman JE, Raghavachari S & Tsien RW. (2007) The sequence of events that underlie quantal transmission at central glutamatergic synapses. *Nat Rev Neurosci* **8**: 597–609.

Marcaggi P, Hirji N & Attwell D. (2005) Release of L-aspartate by reversal of glutamate transporters. *Neuropharmacology* **49**: 843–9.

Marcotti W, Johnson SL, Holley MC & Kros CJ. (2003) Developmental changes in the expression of potassium currents of embryonic, neonatal and mature mouse inner hair cells. *J Physiol* **548**: 383–400.

Marcotti W, Erven A, Johnson SL, Steel KP & Kros CJ. (2006) Tmc1 is necessary for normal functional maturation and survival of inner and outer hair cells in the mouse cochlea. *J Physiol* **574**: 677–98.

Meyers JR, MacDonald RB, Duggan A, Lenzi D, Standaert DG, Corwin JT & Corey DP. (2003) Lighting up the senses: FM1–43 loading of sensory cells through nonselective ion channels. *J Neurosci* **23**: 4054–65.

Miesenbock G, De Angelis DA & Rothman JE. (1998) Visualizing secretion and synaptic transmission with pH-sensitive green fluorescent proteins. *Nature* **394**: 192–5.

Moser T & Beutner D. (2000) Kinetics of exocytosis and endocytosis at the cochlear inner hair cell afferent synapse of the mouse. *Proc Natl Acad Sci USA* **97**: 883–8.

Moser T, Brandt A & Lysakowski A. (2006) Hair cell ribbon synapses. *Cell Tissue Res* **326**: 347–59.

Mountain D & Hubbard A. (1995) Computational analysis of hair cell and auditory nerve processes. In: Hawkins H, McMullan T, Popper AN & Fay R, eds. *Auditory Computation.* Springewr, New York, pp. 121–56.

Neef A, Khimich D, Pirih P, Riedel D, Wolf F & Moser T. (2007) Probing the mechanism of exocytosis at the hair cell ribbon synapse. *J Neurosci* **27**: 12933–44.

Nemzou NR, Bulankina AV, Khimich D, Giese A & Moser T. (2006) Synaptic organization in cochlear inner hair cells deficient for the CaV1.3 (alpha1D) subunit of L-type Ca^{2+} channels. *Neuroscience* **141**: 1849–60.

Oliver D, Taberner AM, Thurm H, Sausbier M, Arntz C, Ruth P, Fakler B & Liberman MC. (2006) The role of BKCa channels in electrical signal encoding in the mammalian auditory periphery. *J Neurosci* **26**: 6181–9.

Palmer AR & Russell IJ. (1986) Phase-locking in the cochlear nerve of the guinea-pig and its relation to the receptor potential of inner hair-cells. *Hear Res* **24**: 1–15.

Parsons TD, Lenzi D, Almers W & Roberts WM. (1994) Calcium-triggered exocytosis and endocytosis in an isolated presynaptic cell: capacitance measurements in saccular hair cells. *Neuron* **13**: 875–83.

Pickles JO. (1988) *An Introduction to the Physiology of Hearing.* Academic Press, London.

Platzer J, Engel J, Schrott-Fischer A, Stephan K, Bova S, Chen H, Zheng H & Striessnig J. (2000) Congenital deafness and sinoatrial node dysfunction in mice lacking class D L-type Ca^{2+} channels. *Cell* **102**: 89–97.

Puel JL, Pujol R, Tribillac F, Ladrech S & Eybalin M. (1994) Excitatory amino acid antagonists protect cochlear auditory neurons from excitotoxicity. *J Comp Neurol* **341**: 241–56.

Rancz EA, Ishikawa T, Duguid I, Chadderton P, Mahon S & Hausser M. (2007) High-fidelity transmission of sensory information by single cerebellar mossy fibre boutons. *Nature* **450**: 1245–8.

Roberts WM, Jacobs RA & Hudspeth AJ. (1990) Colocalization of ion channels involved in frequency selectivity and synaptictransmission at presynaptic active zones of hair cells. *J Neurosci* **10**: 3664–84.

Robertson D. (1984) Horseradish peroxidase injection of physiologically characterized afferent and efferent neurones in the guinea pig spiral ganglion. *Hear Res* **15**: 113–21.

Robertson D & Paki B. (2002) Role of L-type Ca^{2+} channels in transmitter release from mammalian inner hair cells, II. Single-neuron activity. *J Neurophysiol* **87**: 2734–40.

Robertson D, Sellick PM & Patuzzi R. (1999) The continuing search for outer hair cell afferents in the guinea pig spiral ganglion. *Hear Res* **136**: 151–8.

Roux I, Safieddine S, Nouvian R, Grati M, Simmler MC, Bahloul A, Perfettini I, Le GM, Rostaing P, Hamard G, Triller A, Avan P, Moser T & Petit C. (2006) Otoferlin, defective in a human deafness form, is essential for exocytosis at the auditory ribbon synapse. *Cell* **127**: 277–89.

Ruel J, Bobbin RP, Vidal D, Pujol R & Puel JL. (2000) The selective AMPAreceptor antagonist GYKI 53784 blocks action potential generation and excitotoxicity in the guinea pig cochlea. *Neuropharmacology* **39**: 1959–73.

Ruel J, Emery S, Nouvian R, Bersot T, Amilhon B, Van Rybroek JM, Rebillard G, Lenoir M, Eybalin M, Delprat B, Sivakumaran TA, Giros B, El MS, Moser T, Smith RJ, Lesperance MM & Puel JL. (2008) Impairment of SLC17A8 encoding vesicular glutamate transporter-3, VGLUT3, underlies nonsyndromic deafness DFNA25 and inner hair cell dysfunction in null mice. *Am J Hum Genet* **83**: 278–92.

Sachs MB & Abbas PJ. (1974) Rate versus level functions for auditory-nerve fibers in cats: tone-burst stimuli. *J Acoust Soc Am* **56**: 1835–47.

Safieddine S & Wenthold RJ. (1999) SNARE complex at the ribbon synapses of cochlear hair cells: analysis of synaptic vesicleand synaptic membrane-associated proteins. *Eur J Neurosci* **11**: 803–12.

Saviane C & Silver RA. (2006) Fast vesicle reloading and a large pool sustain high bandwidth transmission at a central synapse. *Nature* **439**: 983–7.

Schmitz F, Konigstorfer A & Sudhof TC. (2000) RIBEYE, a component of synaptic ribbons: a protein's journey through evolution. *Neuron* **28**: 857–72.

Schwander M, Sczaniecka A, Grillet N, Bailey JS, Avenarius M, Najmabadi H, Steffy BM, Federe GC, Lagler EA, Banan R, Hice R, Grabowski-Boase L, Keithley EM, Ryan AF, Housley GD, Wiltshire T, Smith RJ, Tarantino LM & Muller U. (2007) A forward genetics screen in mice identifies recessive deafness traits and reveals that pejvakin is essential for outer hair cell function. *J Neurosci* **27**: 2163–75.

Seal RP, Akil O, Yi E, Weber CM, Grant L, Yoo J, Clause A, Kandler K, Noebels JL, Glowatzki E, Lustig LR & Edwards RH. (2008) Sensorineural deafness and seizures in mice lacking vesicular glutamate transporter 3. *Neuron* **57**: 263–75.

Sendin G, Bulankina AV, Riedel D & Moser T. (2007) Maturation of ribbon synapses in hair cells is driven by thyroid hormone. *J Neurosci* **27**: 3163–73.

Siegel JH & Brownell WE. (1986) Synaptic and Golgi membrane recycling in cochlear hair cells. *J Neurocytol* **15**: 311–28.

Sudhof TC. (2002) Synaptotagmins: why so many? *J Biol Chem* **277**: 7629–32.

Takamori S, Holt M, Stenius K, Lemke EA, Gronborg M, Riedel D, Urlaub H, Schenck S, Brugger B, Ringler P, Muller SA, Rammner B, Grater F, Hub JS, De Groot BL, Mieskes G, Moriyama Y, Klingauf J, Grubmuller H, Heuser J, Wieland F & Jahn R. (2006) Molecular anatomy of a trafficking organelle. *Cell* **127**: 831–46.

Tom DS, Altrock WD, Kessels MM, Qualmann B, Regus H, Brauner D, Fejtova A, Bracko O, Gundelfinger ED & Brandstatter JH. (2005) Molecular dissection of the photoreceptor ribbon synapse: physical interaction of Bassoon and RIBEYE is essential for the assembly of the ribbon complex. *J Cell Biol* **168**: 825–36.

Tucker T & Fettiplace R. (1995) Confocal imaging of calcium microdomains and calcium extrusion in turtle hair cells. *Neuron* **15**: 1323–35.

Wittig JH Jr & Parsons TD. (2008) Synaptic ribbon enables temporal precision of hair cell afferent synapse by increasing the number of readily releasable vesicles: a modeling study. *J Neurophysiol* **100**: 1724–39.

Wu LG, Ryan TA & Lagnado L. (2007) Modes of vesicle retrieval at ribbon synapses, calyx-type synapses, and small central synapses. *J Neurosci* **27**: 11793–802.

Wu YC, Tucker T & Fettiplace R. (1996) A theoretical study of calcium microdomains in turtle hair cells. *Biophys J* **71**: 2256–75.

Yasunaga S, Grati M, Cohen-Salmon M, El-Amraoui A, Mustapha M, Salem N, El-Zir E, Loiselet J & Petit C. (1999) A mutation in OTOF, encoding otoferlin, a FER-1-like protein, causes DFNB9, a nonsyndromic form of deafness. *Nat Genet* **21**: 363–9.

Chapter 10

Efferent innervation and function

A Belén Elgoyhen and Paul A Fuchs

10.1 Introduction

Mechanosensory hair cells of the organ of Corti and vestibular end-organs transmit information regarding either sound or body position and motion to the central nervous system by way of peripheral afferent neurons. In return, the central nervous system provides feedback and modulates the afferent stream of information through efferent neurons. The octavo-lateralis efferent system receives input from ascending sensory fibers in the hindbrain and projects centrally to first-order sensory nuclei and peripherally to mechanoreceptive end-organs of the inner ear (cochlea, otolith macula, and semicircular canal cristae). Efferent activity inhibits auditory end-organs, but provides a mixture of excitation and inhibition to the vestibular periphery of most vertebrates. This chapter is focused on auditory signaling and so will touch only incidentally on efferents in vestibular end-organs. The interested reader is referred to reviews of the vestibular innervation, for example Guth *et al.* (1998).

Stimulation of the olivocochlear axons causes a reduction in amplitude of the compound action potential (CAP) recorded extracellularly from the VIIIth nerve in response to an acoustic click or brief tone burst (Galambos, 1956). This inhibitory effect in the mammalian cochlea is now known to result from inhibition of the active electromotile response of outer hair cells (OHCs). The resolution of this effect was an important motivator in solving the functional role of OHCs in cochlear sensitivity and tuning. However, our understanding of that synaptic mechanism derived in large part from studies in non-mammalian hair cells in which electromotility is not an issue. In this chapter we will concentrate on a description of efferent inhibition in the mammalian cochlea. Exploration of cellular mechanisms, in particular, will depend on comparative studies, and the strong conservation of molecular mechanisms of inhibition among vertebrates.

10.2 Efferent innervation of the mammalian cochlea

In mammals, inner ear efferent neurons are located in the superior olivary complex of the brainstem and project to the cochlea. Olivocochlear efferent neurons permit the central nervous system to control the way that sounds are processed in the auditory periphery, offering the potential to improve the detection of signals in background noise, to selectively attend to particular signals, and to protect the periphery from damage caused by overly loud sounds (Guinan, 1996). A first subdivision of the efferent pathway came from the pioneering work of Rasmussen (1946), who originally divided the efferent fibers into the uncrossed and crossed olivocochlear bundles; the latter crossing the midline near the floor of the fourth ventricle. Warr and Guinan (1979) later used tract-tracing experiments to classify the olivocochlear efferents into the two subsystems that we know today: lateral and medial. Lateral olivocochlear (LOC) efferents originate from small neurons in or around the lateral superior olivary nucleus and project predominately to the region near the inner hair cells (IHCs) in the ipsilateral cochlea (Fig. 10.1). These lateral efferents have

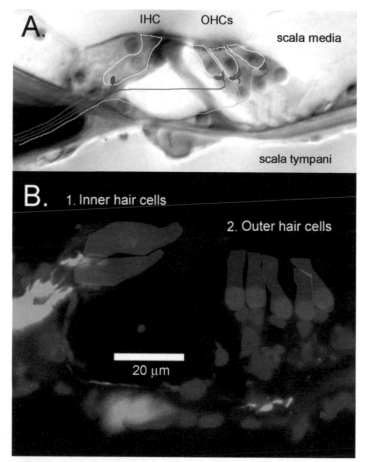

Fig. 10.1 Schematic efferent innervation of the mammalian organ of Corti. (A) Medial olivocochlear efferents (in red) innervate outer hair cells (OHCs), along with type II afferents (turquoise). Lateral olivocochlear efferents (fuchsia) contact type I afferents (blue) beneath the inner hair cells (IHCs) in the adult cochlea. Neurons drawn onto histological section of the middle turn of the mouse cochlea provided by J Taranda, University of Buenos Aires. (B) Cholinergic efferent innervation labeled by antibody to choline acetyltransferase (ChAT – red). Large terminals are seen beneath OHCs. ChAT immunoreactivity intermingles with afferent innervation (green label of NF200 antibody) beneath IHCs. Cell nuclei are labeled blue (DAPI). The approximate outlines of several inner and outer hair cells are indicated by opaque overlay.
Figure 10.1 B is a cryo-section from a P21 mouse cochlea courtesy of J-H Kong, Johns Hopkins University School of Medicine.

unmyelinated fibers that terminate on the radial dendrites of type I auditory afferents postsynaptic to the IHCs. Medial olivocochlear (MOC) efferents originate from larger neurons located ventral, medial, and anterior to the medial superior olivary nucleus and project mostly contralaterally via myelinated fibers to make synaptic contacts directly onto the OHCs. The OHC possesses a near-membrane endoplasmic cistern that is co-extensive with the efferent contact (Fig. 10.2). Postsynaptic cisterns also occur where MOC efferents transiently innervate IHCs prior to the onset of hearing (see Section 10.4).

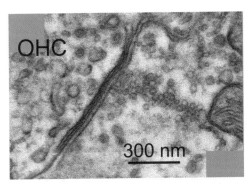

Fig. 10.2 Efferent synaptic structure. Transmission electron micrograph of a medial olivocochlear efferent ending on an outer hair cell (OHC) in the middle turn of a P21 mouse cochlea. Synaptic vesicles occasionally form discrete clusters in the efferent terminal. A near-membrane synaptic cistern in the OHC parallels the efferent contact. This cistern lies within 20 nm of the plasma membrane, and has a narrow lumen that usually expands somewhat at its margins.
Image courtesy of Dr M Lehar, Johns Hopkins University School of Medicine.

Although this summary view is correct in major outline, the original anterograde tracer experiments suggested minor projections of LOC neurons to the OHC regions and of MOC neurons to
the IHC region (Guinan *et al.*, 1983). Definitive evidence for the projection patterns of MOC
neurons came from intracellular labeling experiments in which single neurons were traced from
the brainstem to peripheral terminals in the organ of Corti. Such intracellularly labeled fibers
were always myelinated, always originated from the MOC cell group, always projected to OHCs,
and never sent branches to the IHC area (Brown, 1987). A larger body of data from extracellularly
labeled cochlear neurons has supported the view that the myelinated (thus presumably MOC)
efferent fiber population never gives rise to branches or *en passant* endings in the IHC area
(Brown, 1987).

In contrast, the idea that a subset of LOC neurons may project to the OHC area, especially in
the apical half of the cochlea, has received indirect support from a number of studies. First,
immunolabeling for vesicle-associated proteins (i.e. synaptophysin) visualized a significant population of thin, beaded fibers in the apical half of the cat cochlea giving rise to small terminal and
en passant swellings among the OHCs (Liberman *et al.*, 1990). Such beaded fiber morphology
is characteristic of the LOC system and distinctly different from the larger, non-beaded MOC
processes. Second, a comprehensive immunolabeling study of the olivocochlear system in the rat
showed significant populations of calcitonin gene-related peptide (CGRP)- and γ-aminobutyric
acid (GABA)-containing terminals on OHCs, whereas immunolabeling of brainstem sections
showed evidence of GABA or CGRP only in LOC neurons (identified via retrograde tracers in the
cochlea (Vetter *et al.*, 1991)). Third, a number of studies have suggested that some OHC terminals are positive for opioid peptides such as Met-enkephalin, yet studies of the olivary complex
have suggested that only the LOC neurons show immunoreactivity to Met-enkephalin. More
recent studies have shifted to the mouse, due to the possibility of obtaining genetically modified
specimens. In this species, efferent endings in the vicinity of the IHCs arise almost exclusively
from the LOC system (Maison *et al.*, 2003a). Therefore, while the possibility remains that the
LOC system also sends some projections to the OHCs, the segregation of LOC and MOC targets
appears to be the predominant pattern.

Lateral and medial efferent innervation patterns differ along the length of the cochlea. In cat
and guinea pig, the distribution of vesiculated terminals on OHCs peaks in the upper basal turn,

with considerably lower innervation densities toward the basal and apical extremes. In the mouse, the longitudinal gradient of efferent terminals peaks in the middle of the cochlear spiral. Such a tonotopic focus is consistent with electrophysiological studies of the MOC system in the mouse, where electrical stimulation of the MOCs produces peak inhibition near the 10 kHz region (Maison et al., 2003a). In contrast, LOC inputs spread more widely. In the IHC area of the mouse, guinea pig, and rat the rich plexus of nerve fibers and terminals in the inner spiral bundle extends throughout the length of the cochlea (Vetter et al., 1991; Maison et al., 2003a).

The most striking difference between the olivocochlear innervation pattern in the mouse and that of other mammalian species examined to date is in the relative innervation density on the three OHC rows. In cat and guinea pig, where the best quantitative information is available, there is a steep radial gradient in the distribution of vesiculated terminals on the OHCs. In cats, for example, at the cochlear region of peak OHC innervation density, the mean olivocochlear terminal area for first row OHCs is more than four times greater than that for the third row (Liberman et al., 1990). In contrast, mouse data show no radial gradient in innervation density across the three rows of OHCs.

An important difference between medial and lateral cochlear efferents is that medial efferents are myelinated, but lateral efferents are not. The larger myelinated fibers have a lower threshold for extracellular current stimulation than do the smaller unmyelinated fibers. Further, the MOC axons travel nearer the floor of the fourth ventricle, where stimulating electrodes are usually placed, giving a still larger threshold advantage. Taken together, these observations imply that electrical stimulation excites medial but not lateral efferents, and therefore essentially all efferent effects that have been demonstrated so far by electrical stimulation are attributed to the MOC system (Guinan, 1996).

10.3 Efferent neurotransmitters

10.3.1 Acetylcholine

Acetylcholine (ACh) has been known to be an efferent neurotransmitter since 1959. At that time Schuknecht et al. (1959) reported that the histochemical reaction for acetylcholinesterase (AChE) labeled processes in the intact cochlea, but failed to do so in those that had been surgically de-efferented. During the following years, biochemical and immunohistochemical studies supported the hypothesis that ACh is the main neurotransmitter of the MOC system (Eybalin, 1993). These included the demonstration of choline acetyltransferase (ChAT) and AChE in cochleas from various species. Also, ChAT-immunoreactive neurons as well as AChE-positive neurons were detected in the nuclei containing the cell bodies of origin of the MOC axons. Similarly, both enzymes could be localized in the organ of Corti itself. Both the ChAT-like immunolabel and the AChE histochemical reaction product were present in fibers crossing the tunnel of Corti in an upper position to form patches below the OHCs. At the electron microscopic level, these ChAT-like immunolabeled patches were shown to correspond to large axosomatic synapses on the OHCs, nearly all of which were immunolabeled for ChAT. Moreover, lesions of part or all of the efferent cochlear supply strongly decreased the activity of ChAT (Eybalin, 1993).

Throughout the 1970s, cholinergic agonists were tested for their ability to alter extracellular potentials recorded from the cochleas of cats and guinea pigs. These physiological experiments often used electrical shocks applied to the floor of the fourth ventricle. As noted above, this kind of stimulation should activate only the myelinated fibers of the crossed component of the medial efferent system. It would have left unaffected the small population of unmyelinated fibers forming the crossed component of the lateral efferent system, since unmyelinated fibers would have higher thresholds and reduced responses to electrical stimulation at high rates. Consequently, it is most likely that these various physiological experiments addressed the cholinergic nature of the medial efferents (Guinan, 1996). As described in the following sections, the 1990s also witnessed the description by electrophysiological techniques of the direct effects of ACh on isolated hair cells (Housley & Ashmore, 1991; Shigemoto & Ohmori, 1991; Fuchs & Murrow, 1992b; Sugai *et al.*, 1992; Erostegui *et al.*, 1994; Dulon & Lenoir, 1996; Evans, 1996; He & Dallos, 1999), leading to the identification and cloning of the subunits that compose the hair cell cholinergic receptor (Elgoyhen *et al.*, 1994, 2001) and to the generation of the first genetically modified mice with alterations in medial olivocochlear efferent activity (Vetter *et al.*, 1999, 2007).

While the biochemical, physiological and electrophysiological approaches successfully established the cholinergic nature of the medial efferent neurons, these approaches did not resolve whether ACh also served as a neurotransmitter for the LOC. It was only with the advent of reliable chemical neuroanatomy techniques, particularly ChAT immunocytochemistry, that supporting data concerning this lateral efferent system were gained (Eybalin, 1993; Simmons, 2002). Antibodies against ChAT showed immunolabel in the rat and guinea pig inner spiral bundles, the pathway for LOCs. At the ultrastructural level, two populations of ChAT-like immunoreactive fibers were identified within the rat inner spiral bundle. The first one consisted of unvesiculated fibers, mostly present in the lower part of the bundle, and the second of varicosities that were mostly found in its upper part. This second population, which accounted for approximately one-half of the efferent varicosities in the bundle, made synaptic contact with the radial dendrites of type I cochlear afferents beneath the IHCs. These vesiculated endings were proposed to belong to the lateral efferent system. In support of this conclusion, ChAT-like immunoreactivity also was detected in neurons of the lateral superior olive in rats and guinea pigs, or just peripheral to it in cats, squirrel monkeys, and humans. In the rat lateral superior olive, ChAT-like immunoreactivity co-localized with a retrograde label transported from the cochlea (the fluorescent compound Fast Blue). This co-localization showed that all the ChAT-like immunolabeled neurons in the lateral superior olive constituted a subpopulation of the lateral efferents innervating the cochlea.

Due to the predominance of cholinergic innervation to the cochlea, and the lower threshold to shock of MOC axons, it is likely that the effects of brainstem electrical stimulation are due to ACh released by medial efferents. The best known cochlear effects of activation of the olivocochlear bundle are the suppression of cochlear responses such as CAPs or distortion product otoacoustic emissions (DPOAEs). These classic olivocochlear effects have long been thought to arise from cholinergic effects of the MOC synapses on OHCs (Guinan, 1996). This has been confirmed by the recent demonstration that all such effects of olivocochlear stimulation on CAPs and DPOAEs are absent in mice lacking the nicotinic cholinergic receptor subunits expressed by OHCs (Vetter *et al.*, 1999, 2007).

10.3.2 GABA

Acetylcholine is not the only possible efferent neurotransmitter within the cochlea. Antibodies made directly against either GABA or its synthesizing enzyme, glutamate decarboxylase (GAD), show immunoreactivity in cell bodies located in the superior olivary complex and in terminals located below hair cells, suggesting GABA as a second neurotransmitter of the efferent system (Eybalin, 1993). Consistent with such a role, cochlear efferent terminals demonstrate GABA uptake. Electron microscopic studies show that GABA/GAD-like immunoreactive fibers form two separate populations. The varicose fibers in the inner spiral bundle and in the tunnel spiral bundle would likely belong to the lateral efferent innervation, while the fibers forming large axosomatic synapses with the OHCs would belong to the medial efferent system (Eybalin & Altschuler, 1990).

The presence of GABA and GAD immunoreactive fibers and terminals below the IHC region and OHCs has led some to propose GABA as a neurotransmitter for both medial and lateral olivoco-chlear neurons. However, the presence of GABA- and GAD-immunoreactive cell bodies is not very well established in rat periolivary regions containing medial olivocochlear neurons, but these are clearly observed in the lateral superior olive by combinations of retrograde labeling and immunocytochemistry. This observation originally raised some doubt as to the MOC origin of GABAergic innervation to the OHCs (Vetter *et al.*, 1991). However, still more recent studies in mice provide good evidence that virtually all olivocochlear innervation of OHCs, including cholinergic and GABAergic projections, arise from the MOC system; whereas endings in the IHC area arise almost exclusively from the LOC system (Maison *et al.*, 2003a). The longitudinal distribution of GABAergic terminals beneath OHCs appears to vary from species to species (and among investigators examining a single species). In guinea pig, GABAergic innervation of OHCs is restricted to the apical half of the cochlea. Some investigators have described a similar pattern in rat. In the squirrel monkey, GABAergic terminals are distributed throughout the entire length of the organ of Corti. In the mouse, GAD immunostaining labels terminals on OHCs throughout the cochlea.

10.3.3 Dopamine

Immunocytochemical studies have suggested that catecholamines may function as efferent neurotransmitters or neuromodulators in the organ of Corti, specifically for the lateral efferent system (Darrow *et al.*, 2006). A tyrosine hydroxylase-like immunoreactivity was reported in the inner spiral and tunnel spiral bundles, as well as in neurons of the lateral superior olive. Both the inner spiral bundle and the tunnel spiral bundle are not immunoreactive to either dopamine β-hydroxylase or to phenylethanolamine *N*-methyltransferase. Similarly, neurons of the lateral superior olive are not immunoreactive to dopamine β-hydroxylase, suggesting that these lateral efferent neurons synthesize dihydroxyphenylalanine and/or dopamine but not norepinephrine and epinephrine. Dopamine could be detected in rat cochlear homogenates and chinchilla cochlear perilymph using high-performance liquid chromatography (HPLC), supporting its identity as a possible efferent neurotransmitter. The hypothesis of a neurotransmitter or neuromodulator function for dopamine within lateral efferents was further supported by immunolabeling of varicosities synapsing with radial afferent dendrites using antibodies to enzymes contributing to the synthesis of dopamine: tyrosine hydroxylase and aromatic amino acid decarboxylase (Eybalin *et al.*, 1993). Using direct cochlear perfusion, it has been shown that dopamine can inhibit transmission between the IHCs and the dendrites of the type I primary auditory neurons (Ruel *et al.*, 2001). Finally, an interesting approach in support of this proposal is based on the observation that metabolic or loud sound damage leads to temporary swelling of afferent terminals beneath IHCs, a form of transient excitotoxicity. Cochlear perfusion with dopamine receptor inhibitors causes these same excitotoxic changes, as although lateral efferents provide tonic, dopaminergic inhibition that normally prevents afferent activity from becoming pathological (Ruel *et al.*, 2001).

10.3.4 Neuropeptides

A number of neuropeptides have been identified in the cochlea, including: calcitonin gene-related peptide (CGRP), enkephalins, dynorphins, and urocortin (Fex & Altschuler, 1981; Altschuler *et al.*, 1983, 1984, 1985; Kuriyama *et al.*, 1990; Tohyama *et al.*, 1990; Vetter *et al.*, 2002). Based largely on chemical neuroanatomical studies, the peptide calcitonin gene-related protein (CGRP) has been proposed as a neurotransmitter or neuromodulator in the auditory system, in particular with respect to efferents innervating the cochlea (Kuriyama *et al.*, 1990; Tohyama *et al.*, 1990).

Correspondingly, mRNAs coding for CGRP have been detected in the superior olivary complex, and CGRP-like immunolabeled neurons have been localized in the lateral superior olive and periolivary neurons, particularly in the ventral and lateral nuclei of the trapezoid body. At the light microscopic level, CGRP-like immunolabel is found in the inner spiral and tunnel spiral bundles and, in most experiments, at the basal pole of the OHCs. The CGRP-like immunolabel disappeared after section of the efferent axons just medial to the principal sensory trigeminal nucleus. CGRP-containing terminals have been identified both in radial afferents beneath IHCs and most medial efferent synapses with OHCs (Kuriyama *et al.*, 1990; Tohyama *et al.*, 1990; Saffieddine & Eybalin, 1992; Cabanillas & Luebke, 2002; Maison *et al.*, 2003a).

The first evidence favoring the presence of a prodynorphin-related peptide (dynorphin B) in olivocochlear efferents came from radioimmunoassay in the guinea pig, later duplicated in the rat (Hoffman *et al.*, 1985). The association with the olivocochlear system was further supported by the localization of dynorphin β-like and α-neoendorphin-like immunoreactivities within fibers of the inner spiral bundle and tunnel spiral bundle in the guinea pig cochlea, strongly suggesting a lateral efferent origin of these immunoreactive fibers (Altschuler *et al.*, 1985). This was confirmed by a combined retrograde tract-tracing and immunofluorescence study in rats. Dynorphin-like immunoreactive perikarya were also found within the lateral superior olive in the guinea pig.

Met- and Leu-enkephalin-like immunoreactivities have been reported in bundles containing efferent fibers: outside the organ of Corti, within the intraganglionic spiral bundle and within the organ of Corti, in the inner spiral bundle, and tunnel spiral bundle (Fex & Altschuler, 1981). Proenkephalin-derived peptides were found in lateral efferent varicosities in the inner spiral bundle and tunnel spiral bundle. In the inner bundle, these varicosities were seen establishing synapses with radial afferent dendrites. Their efferent nature was also indicated by the strong reduction of the Met- and Leu-enkephalin immunoreactivities after sectioning of the inferior branch of the vestibular nerve in which cochlear efferents run (Altschuler *et al.*, 1984). Of the various subdivisions of the rat and guinea pig superior olivary complex, only the lateral superior olive displayed perikarya immunolabeled for Met-enkephalin. There is evidence that Met-enkephalin could be released under noisy conditions.

Finally, urocortin has been shown to be expressed in the lateral superior olivary system. Moreover, urocortin reactive fibers and synaptic terminals have been detected in the IHC cell – but not the OHC – region of the cochlea, suggesting a role for urocortin in the lateral efferent innervation (Vetter *et al.*, 2002).

10.3.5 Co-localization of neurotransmitters within efferent neurons

The idea that cytochemical subgroups might exist within the MOC or LOC subsystem has long been an intriguing possibility, given the multitude of neurotransmitters and neuromodulators that appear to be expressed in the cochlear terminals of these fiber systems. Despite the importance of this question to understanding olivocochlear function, relatively few direct studies have been published, because the experiments are technically challenging. To address the question rigorously in the brainstem, retrograde transport from the cochlea (to identify the small number of olivocochlear neurons from the large number of other neurons in the olivary complex and periolivary nuclei) must be coupled with double immunolabeling. One study in rats has taken this rigorous approach: the authors concluded that MOC neurons comprise a homogeneous group of cholinergic neurons, whereas LOC neurons could be split into a cholinergic group that co-expresses CGRP and a separate and distinct GABAergic group (Vetter *et al.*, 1991). Another co-localization study of olivocochlear neurons relied on brainstem location in rats and guinea pigs and immunolabeling for cholinergic markers to identify the MOC and LOC cells. The researchers concluded that there is only one population of LOC neurons, with more than 80% of cholinergic LOC cells co-expressing CGRP and Met-enkephalin; no GABAergic markers were investigated (Saffiedine & Eybalin, 1992). As for putative MOC cells, there is evidence that a small subpopulation of the cholinergic cells co-express CGRP, whereas none express Met-enkephalins. A more recent study in mice suggests the complete congruence of GABAergic and cholinergic markers in the IHC and OHC areas (Maison et al., 2003a). The differences between studies could be due to species differences but most likely relates to differences in detection threshold coupled with differential longitudinal gradients for GABAergic and cholinergic markers. Evidence for similarity, rather than disparity, between the rat and mouse come from immunoelectron microscopy studies, which provided strong evidence for ChAT and GAD co-localization in efferent terminals on OHCs throughout the rat cochlea (Dannhof et al., 1991). The idea that GABA and ACh are co-localized within the same terminal, although not commonly reported in the nervous system, is not without precedent (Kosaka et al., 1988).

10.4 Development of efferent innervation

Most investigations of the efferent innervation of the mammalian cochlea have assumed that efferent projections to IHCs originate from lateral olivocochlear neurons whereas efferent projections to OHCs originate from medial olivocochlear neurons. Although this dichotomy is probably true in the adult cochlea, cholinergic efferent terminals also synapse with IHCs in the first ~ two weeks of life, prior to the onset of hearing (Simmons, 2002). In rodents, behavioral hearing begins in the second postnatal week. Nonetheless, neonatal and even embryonic hair cells have functional transduction channels and a number of voltage-gated ion channels. Together these channels generate Ca^{2+} action potentials, a characteristic of immature IHCs, which may drive rhythmic or bursting activity of neurons at higher levels of the auditory pathway (Eatock & Hurley, 2003). This electrical activity of immature hair cells may influence afferent synaptogenesis. With maturation, a number of changes combine to reduce IHC spiking, including a drop in the number of voltage-gated calcium channels, and the onset of a large, rapidly voltage-gated potassium conductance (Eatock & Hurley, 2003; Marcotti et al., 2003). These changes signal the transformation from a developing epithelium with active formation of synaptic contacts to a sensing epithelium where receptor potentials represent and transmit the mechanical input in a graded fashion, and whose synaptic contacts have stabilized. The stabilization of synaptic contacts includes a profound change to the efferent innervation of IHCs. Cholinergic inhibitory inputs that are reliably found on neonatal IHCs rapidly disappear at the onset of hearing in rats (Katz et al., 2004). Anatomical studies in the hamster and rat support the idea of an initial transient innervation of IHCs by medial olivocochlear terminals (Simmons, 2002). Anterograde labeling of the crossed olivocochlear projections in the neonatal animals results in labeled efferent axons terminating first in the greater epithelial ridge region of the organ of Corti, and then beneath the IHCs. This period when medial olivocochlear axons accumulate below the IHCs is reminiscent of a developmental waiting period. Such 'waiting periods' have been studied extensively during the development of thalamocortical projections (Molnar & Blakemore, 1995).

A characteristic of the immature IHC efferent innervation is the surprisingly high number of direct contacts between synaptic endings and the IHC itself, most of them showing typical synaptic differentiations such as a postsynaptic cistern in the IHC (Pujol et al., 1998). These efferent axosomatic synapses with immature IHC are supposed to have a functional importance since, first, the efferent synapse on immature IHCs is functional (Glowatzki & Fuchs, 2000) and second axosomatic synapses reappear transiently in adulthood after the IHC has been disconnected from auditory dendrites by excitotoxic injury (Puel et al., 1995). One possibility is that they play a role in the rhythmic firing of immature auditory afferents. Clearly they can suppress the excitability of the IHCs, and presumably prevent evoked and spontaneous transmitter release from ribbon synapses known to be functional at this stage (Glowatzki & Fuchs, 2000, 2002). Some studies have suggested that this transient efferent innervation may play a role in the ultimate functional maturation of cochlear hair cells (Simmons, 2002). Most impressively, surgical lesion of the efferent nerve supply causes kittens to fail to develop normal hearing (Walsh *et al.*, 1998).

10.5 **Hair cell responses**

As with other aspects of hair cell physiology, initial progress in defining cellular mechanisms came from studies of efferent inhibition in hair cells of non-mammalian vertebrates. Later studies in mammals consolidated the view that the fundamental mechanisms of hair cell inhibition have been well-conserved among vertebrates, as indeed are the known molecular constituents. Intracellular recordings showed that efferent activity caused longlasting hyperpolarizing inhibitory postsynaptic potentials (IPSPs) in hair cells of the fish lateral line (Flock & Russell, 1973). Similar IPSPs have been observed in hair cells of frogs (Ashmore & Russell, 1983; Sugai *et al.*, 1992), reptiles (Art *et al.*, 1984) and birds (Shigemoto & Ohmori, 1991; Fuchs & Murrow, 1992b) and consist of a brief depolarization preceding a much larger, longer-lasting hyperpolarization. The advent of the *ex vivo* organ of Corti preparation has made it possible to observe essentially identical efferent synaptic effects with intracellular recordings from mammalian cochlear hair cells (Fig. 10.3C, D) (Glowatzki & Fuchs, 2000; Oliver *et al.*, 2000; Katz *et al.*, 2004; Lioudyno *et al.*, 2004; Gomez-Casati *et al.*, 2005; Goutman *et al.*, 2005).

Whether by spontaneous or electrically evoked release from efferent axons, or by direct application, ACh causes a biphasic change in the membrane conductance of mammalian cochlear hair cells. This has been shown both for neonatal IHCs that receive efferent synapses prior to the onset of hearing (Glowatzki & Fuchs, 2000; Katz *et al.*, 2004; Gomez-Casati *et al.*, 2005; Goutman *et al.*, 2005) and in older OHCs (Oliver *et al.*, 2000; Lioudyno *et al.*, 2004) in the mammalian cochlea. In all vertebrate hair cells examined to date, the efferent neurotransmitter ACh opens ligand-gated cation channels (the α9α10-containing nicotinic ACh receptor (nAChR)) through which calcium and sodium enter the hair cell, followed by activation of calcium-sensitive potassium channels. These are encoded by the *SK2* (*Kcnn*) gene in mammals (Dulon *et al.*, 1998; Marcotti *et al.*, 2004) and birds (Yuhas & Fuchs, 1999; Matthews *et al.*, 2005). The relatively rapid coupling between these two ionic fluxes, their voltage-dependence (Fig. 10.4), as well as sensitivity to strong calcium buffering has led to the assumption of direct activation of SK (small or slow potassium) channels by calcium influx through the nAChR (Fuchs & Murrow, 1992a; Martin & Fuchs, 1992; Oliver *et al.*, 2000) (Fig. 10.5). Other lines of evidence suggest that release of calcium from an internal store, perhaps the nearby synaptic cistern (Shigemoto & Ohmori, 1991; Kakehata *et al.*, 1993; Yoshida *et al.*, 1994; Lioudyno *et al.*, 2004), contributes to activation of the SK channels. This latter hypothesis will be examined further below.

Current through the non-selective nAChR can be carried by a combination of sodium, potassium and calcium. At negative membrane potentials inward current is carried by sodium and calcium influx. Measurements of the relative divalent permeability (p_{Ca}/p_{Na}) of α9α10-containing nAChRs expressed in *Xenopus* oocytes give a permeability ratio of ~10.0 (Weisstaub *et al.*, 2002) and in hair cells 8.0 (McNiven *et al.*, 1996; Gomez-Casati *et al.*, 2005). To date only limited single channel data have been collected from α9α10 receptors expressed in *Xenopus* oocytes. These give a single channel conductance near 100 pS (with very low external calcium) and open time distributions with components at 90 μs and 320 μs at room temperature (Plazas *et al.*, 2005a). The single channel conductance in hair cells is likely to be smaller due to block by physiological levels of

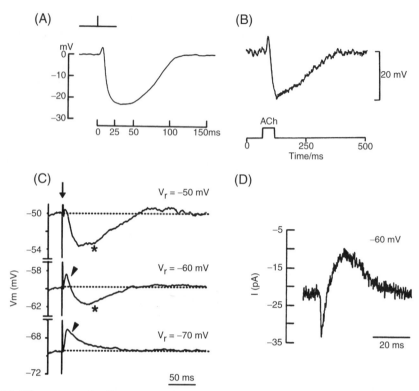

Fig. 10.3 Efferent synaptic effects on vertebrate hair cells. (A) A single shock to the efferent nerve supply (vertical tick) produced an inhibitory postsynaptic potential (IPSP) in a turtle hair cell (averaged record at −45 mV). (B) Voltage response of isolated chicken hair cell to 'puff' of 100 μM acetylcholine (ACh), membrane potential −50 mV. (C) Electrical shocks to the efferent nerve supply produced IPSPs in a neonatal rat inner hair cell (IHC). Current injection was used to change the membrane potential and demonstrate reversal of the biphasic waveform near −60 mV.
(D) Spontaneous ACh release from the efferent terminal produced a biphasic membrane current at −60 mV in neonatal rat IHCs.
Figure 10.3B reproduced with permission from Figure 1, Fuchs and Murrow (1992).
Figure 10.3C reproduced with permission from Figure 1, Goutman et al. (2005). Figure 10.3D courtesy of E Glowatzki, Johns Hopkins University School of Medicine, Baltimore, USA.

external calcium. With allowances for differences in recording conditions, one can estimate that ACh (bath application) activates a maximum of 100–200 nAChRs in individual hair cells, and that ACh released by a single efferent action potential activates approximately one-tenth that number.

The SK2 channel has a small conductance (10 pS), is half-activated by 0.6 μM calcium and is voltage-insensitive (Kohler et al., 1996). The single channel conductance leads one to estimate that ACh released by a single efferent action potential can activate ~100 SK channels, while application of exogenous ACh maximally activates 1000 or more.

10.5.1 Synaptic currents activated by release of ACh

Spontaneous efferent synaptic currents have been observed in neonatal IHCs and older OHCs (Glowatzki & Fuchs, 2000; Oliver et al., 2000; Katz et al., 2004; Lioudyno et al., 2004; Gomez-Casati et al., 2005; Goutman et al., 2005). For the most part these synaptic currents are quite

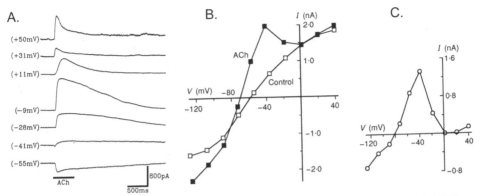

Fig. 10.4 Membrane currents evoked in guinea pig outer hair cells by acetylcholine (ACh). (A) The evoked membrane current changed polarity, amplitude, and waveform as the membrane potential was varied in the voltage clamp. Application of ACh is indicated by the horizontal bar. (B) Peak membrane current as a function of membrane potential at indicated membrane potentials with (filled squares) varies as a function of membrane potential, and ACh-dependent current is lost at positive Vm. Membrane current in the absence of ACh is shown by open squares. (C) ACh-dependent current obtained by subtraction of control from ACh data in (B). ACh-evoked current reverses at −80 mV (near the potassium equilibrium potential), peaks at −40 mV, and diminishes at positive voltages. This pattern reflects the calcium-dependence of ACh-evoked potassium current, falling with calcium driving force at positive membrane potential.
Reprinted with permission from Figures 2b and 2c, Evans (1994).

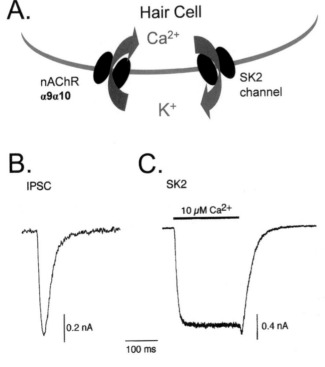

Fig. 10.5 Calcium-activated, SK, potassium channels in hair cells. (A) Acetylcholine (ACh) opens ligand-gated α9α10-containing nAChR. Inward current includes calcium that results in activation of calcium-dependent SK channels. (B) Spontaneous synaptic current through SK channels in rat outer hair cell (potassium driving force inward) activates and deactivates rapidly. (C) Rapid application of calcium to membrane patches activates heterologously expressed SK channels (*Xenopus* oocytes). Onset and decay times similar to those found in hair cells, suggesting that SK channel kinetics determine postsynaptic time course. Figures 10.5B, C reproduced with permission from Figure 3, Oliver *et al.* (2000).

similar in waveform; that is, biphasic at membrane potentials positive to E_K and negative to E_{cation} (often these are recorded in high potassium saline to accelerate the frequency of release from efferent endings). The kinetically dominant outward SK component has a decay time constant of 30–50 ms (at room temperature), while inward current through the nAChR (isolated by strong calcium buffering) decays ~ three- to fivefold faster. Thus the elementary synaptic events have a relatively rapid time-course, consistent with tight coupling between nAChRs activated by brief efferent transmitter release, and localized activation of hair cell SK channels. It is of interest, however, that when efferents are activated by a train of shocks, transmitter release facilitates, as seen in the turtle ear (Art & Fettiplace, 1984; Art et al., 1984), producing substantially stronger inhibition (Goutman et al., 2005). Moreover, the time constant of decay of that inhibition becomes greatly prolonged, as though additional, slower processes were recruited, giving a time course more like that of efferent effects in vivo (see below). One mechanism that could lengthen the duration of efferent effects is calcium-induced calcium release (CICR) from the associated synaptic cistern.

10.5.2 Calcium stores and cholinergic inhibition

Various features of the hair cell's efferent synapse suggest that internal calcium stores might participate. Leading the way is the physical presence of the synaptic cistern (see Fig. 10.2), a near-membrane (within 20 nm) endoplasmic reticulum that is co-extensive with the efferent synaptic contact (Gulley & Reese, 1977; Hirokawa, 1978; Saito, 1980). The resemblance of similar structures in neurons to the sarcoplasmic reticulum of muscle was recognized early on (Gulley & Reese, 1977). Initial reports on cholinergic effects in isolated hair cells raised the possibility that release from internal calcium stores might underlie the seconds-long time course of potassium current activation seen in those experimental conditions (Housley et al., 1990; Shigemoto & Ohmori, 1990, 1991; Kakehata et al., 1993; Yoshida et al., 1994). Later work found evidence that ryanodine-sensitive calcium stores enhanced SK currents produced by exogenous or synaptically released ACh (Lioudyno et al., 2004). The most parsimonious interpretation of the present literature is that influx through the nAChR can lead to CICR from the synaptic cistern. During prolonged efferent stimulation, calcium may build up in the subcisternal space so that CICR becomes semi-regenerative. The irregular, highly variable waveform observed during prolonged ACh application (Fig. 10.6) would be consistent with some form of sporadic calcium release from the synaptic cistern. Studies of efferent inhibition in the intact ear have added further weight to a potential role for hair cell calcium stores in cholinergic inhibition, as will be discussed below.

10.6 Efferent effects on cochlear output

Efferent inhibition can be activated by sound presented to the contralateral ear (Kujawa et al., 1993; Kujawa et al., 1994). However, physiological studies of efferent inhibition have relied almost exclusively on electrical stimulation of efferent axons to produce effects in the cochlea (Fig. 10.7A, B). This method activates the medial, but not lateral, olivocochlear fibers and exploits the strong facilitation of transmitter release that can be produced with repetitive stimulation (Rajan & Johnstone, 1988; Goutman et al., 2005) to cause maximal efferent effects. Electrical stimulation in the floor of the fourth ventricle activates contra- and ipsilateral axons of the MOC efferents to reduce the amplitude of the compound action potential ('N1') produced by a brief acoustic stimulus (Galambos, 1956), especially at low sound levels. Since medial olivocochlear efferents innervate OHCs, this observation requires that OHC inhibition be communicated to the IHC/afferent fiber pathway that generates afferent action potentials. This conundrum of efferent inhibition was a strong motivator for the proposed 'motor' function of OHCs. Indeed, the elegant

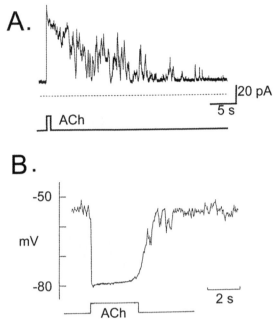

Fig. 10.6 Release from calcium stores may prolong the response to acetylcholine (ACh). (A) A one-second long 'puff' of ACh produced a prolonged outward current with prominent fluctuations in a frog saccular hair cell. Such transient currents may reflect pulsatile release of stored calcium. B. Seconds-long application of ACh hyperpolarized a chicken hair cell. Note slow voltage fluctuations during recovery. Figure 10.6A reproduced with permission from Yoshida *et al.* (1994). Figure 10.6B repro- duced with permission from Figure 1, Shigemoto and Ohmori (1991).

model of OHC electromotility (Chapter 6) ideally complements efferent inhibition, since the efferent synaptic conductance change and hyperpolarization will serve to suppress voltage-dependent motility of OHCs that is required for the IHC's sensitive response. Intracellular record-ings from IHCs during acoustic and efferent stimulation have confirmed this interpretation (Fig. 10.7C) (Brown & Nuttal, 1984). The IHC receptor potential produced by a tone burst was reduced in amplitude by efferent stimulation, but no synaptic conductance change was seen. As also predicted by this hypothesis, basilar membrane motion is diminished by efferent activity (Murugasu & Russell, 1996; Dolan *et al.*, 1997; Russell & Murugasu, 1997) (see Fig. 10.9A below), as though the motor output of OHCs was reduced. Unfortunately, it has not yet proved possible to record intracellularly from OHCs during acoustic stimulation and efferent inhibition in the intact cochlea. However, much has been learned using extracellular signals such as the action potentials of afferent neurons or DPOAEs generated by OHCs (see Chapter 4).

10.6.1 Efferent inhibition of cochlear tuning

The functional effects of efferent inhibition have been detailed in the acoustic response of audi-tory nerve fibers. Efferent activity suppressed the response of a single auditory nerve fiber such that a louder tone was required to produce a threshold response (Wiederhold & Kiang, 1970; Gifford & Guinan, 1987). This threshold shift could reach 20 dB at the fiber's characteristic fre-quency (CF), but was smaller for frequencies above and below CF (at least for fibers tuned to higher frequencies); resulting in a broader tuning curve, that is, diminished frequency selectivity, for the individual afferent neuron (Fig. 10.8A). Thus, efferent inhibition not only desensitizes the cochlea, but also affects the cochlear tuning mechanism. Again, this outcome is consistent with the hypothesis that OHC activity normally enhances basilar membrane tuning (Chapter 5), which is then diminished by efferent inhibition of OHCs.

Interestingly, similar effects were seen in the turtle inner ear where efferent inhibition also desensitizes and 'de-tunes' the acoustic response of individual afferent fibers (Fig. 10.8B) (Art &

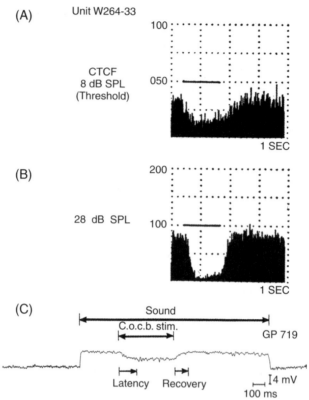

Fig. 10.7 Inhibition of afferent fibers and inner hair cells (IHCs) in the mammalian cochlea. (A, B) Afferent spike histograms during continuous tones (sound intensity indicated beside each panel), and electrical stimulation of efferent axons (dark bar indicates timing of efferent shocks). Compiled from 100 repetitions of tones and efferent shock trains. (C) Intracellular recording from a guinea pig IHC during presentation of a continuous tone (timing indicated by upper, longer bar), and with electrical stimulation of efferent axons (timing indicated by lower, shorter bar).
Figures 10.7A, B reused with permission from Wiederhold ML and Kiang NYS (1970) *J Acoust Soc Am* **48**: 950. © 1970, Acoustical Society of America. Figure 7 reproduced with permission from Figure 10.7, Brown and Nuttall (1984).

Fettiplace, 1984). Here, however, efferent inhibition shunts and dampens the electrical tuning mechanism that confers frequency selectivity onto turtle hair cells. Nonetheless, this similarity in effect suggests an underlying functional role for efferent feedback, that is, to adjust auditory tuning. Because sharply tuned filters 'ring' to transient stimuli and broad filters less so, it could be beneficial to suppress tuning as needed to improve temporal resolution – to locate sounds, for example. Although the underlying cellular mechanisms of tuning can differ, efferent inhibition may be providing the same functional utility in quite different vertebrate ears. As noted elsewhere in this chapter, it remains to be determined whether particular refinements were required to encompass the expanded frequency range of mammalian hearing.

10.6.2 Time course of inhibition in the cochlea

The time course of efferent inhibition in the intact cochlea has been examined by combining various measurements of the sound response with brainstem electrical stimulation of MOC fibers.

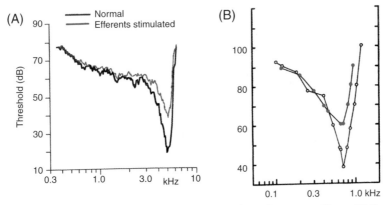

Fig. 10.8 Effect of inhibition on frequency selectivity of single auditory nerve fibers. (A) Tuning curve of single auditory nerve fiber in the cat VIIIth nerve. Sound pressure to achieve criterion response plotted as a function of frequency. During electrical shocks to efferent axons in the brainstem, sensitivity at characteristic frequency (CF) was suppressed most strongly (red curve). (B) Efferent inhibition 'de-tuned' a single auditory nerve fiber in the turtle inner ear (open circles, control tuning curve, red circles during train of shocks to efferent axons).
Figure 10.8A adapted with permission from Figure 1, Guinan and Gifford (1988). Figure 10.8B adapted with permission from Figure 7, Art and Fettiplace (1984).

The activity of single auditory nerve fibers is suppressed and recovers with time constants of approximately 100 ms (Wiederhold & Kiang, 1970). However, when inhibition was prolonged for several seconds, a small component of inhibition of compound action potentials was observed that decayed thousands of times more slowly (Sridhar *et al.*, 1995). This slow suppression was more prominent for high frequency acoustic stimuli, and was blocked by antagonists of the hair cell nAChR. The magnitude of the slow effect was enhanced by ryanodine and cyclopiazonic acid, compounds that alter the efficacy of calcium release from internal stores (Sridhar *et al.*, 1997). It remains unknown whether fast and slow effects of inhibition result entirely from changes in membrane potassium conductance as have been observed in hair cell recordings from various species. It is also possible that, especially for the slow effect, prolonged efferent activation leads to enzymatic/metabolic changes that alter OHC mechanics directly. Prolonged application of ACh to OHCs isolated from the guinea pig cochlea resulted, after a delay of several seconds, in enhanced electromotility that lasted for tens of seconds (Fig. 10.9B) (Dallos *et al.*, 1997). This was shown to be due to reduced axial stiffness of the OHC, and was accompanied by a rise of intracellular calcium. It is unknown how this mechanical effect would relate to the reduction in basilar membrane motion observed in the presence of ACh (Fig. 10.9A) (Murugasu & Russell, 1996; Dolan *et al.*, 1997; Russell & Murugasu, 1997).

10.6.3 Inhibition of DPOAEs

An important measure of efferent inhibition is the suppression of DPOAEs. These low energy signals are recorded with a sensitive microphone in the external canal when combination tones are presented to the ear, and are thought to result from the active contributions of OHC electromotility (see Chapter 4). The $2f_1 - f_2$ ($f_1 < f_2$) distortion product is most commonly used; its amplitude is reduced during efferent stimulation (Mountain *et al.*, 1980). Since DPOAEs can be recorded non-invasively in the ear canal, they provide a means to study cochlear mechanisms in human subjects (Moulin *et al.*, 1993). Further, efferent inhibition can be assessed by the

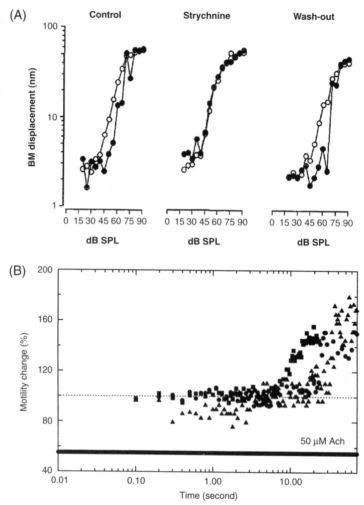

Fig. 10.9 Effects of acetylcholine (ACh) on cochlear mechanics. (A) Basilar membrane motion with (filled symbols) and without (open symbols) electrical stimulation of efferent axons. During efferent activity basilar membrane motion was reduced in amplitude. This effect was blocked reversibly by strychnine, an antagonist of the α9α10-containing nAChR of the OHCs. (B) Application of ACh to the OHCs isolated from the guinea pig cochlea gradually enhanced the extent of electromotility over tens of seconds. Motility of isolated OHCs was evoked and monitored with the 'microchamber' method.

Figure 10.9A reproduced with permission from Figure 5, Murugasu and Russell (1996). Figure 10.9B reproduced with permission from Figure 7, Dallos et al. (1997).

suppression of DPOAEs via contralateral sound that activates crossed MOC efferent fibers (Williams et al., 1994).

There is compelling evidence that DPOAE suppression results from activation of the cholinergic MOC efferents. Cochlear perfusion with antagonists of the hair cell α9α10-containing nAChR prevents efferent suppression of DPOAEs produced by contralateral sound (Kujawa et al., 1994). Also, efferent suppression of DPOAEs is completely absent in mice lacking the α9 or α10 subunits of the hair cell nAChR (Vetter et al., 1999, 2007).

10.7 **Hair cell 'nicotinic' receptors**

Considerable progress towards defining the molecular components that underlie mammalian hair cell hyperpolarization has been achieved via combined pharmacological, neuroanatomical, electrophysiological, and molecular studies. Acetylcholine is the principal neurotransmitter released by MOC efferent axons. Throughout the nervous system, ACh signals through two pharmacologically, structurally, and genetically distinct receptor types, namely the muscarinic and the nicotinic receptors. Metabotropic muscarinic receptors are linked to second messenger systems, while the ionotropic nicotinic receptors are ligand-gated ion channels. While both muscarinic and nicotinic receptors have been proposed to mediate the effects of ACh in the cochlea, extant pharmacological and electrophysiological data suggest a central role for an atypical, nicotinic cholinergic receptor located at the synapse between efferent fibers and vertebrate outer and developing inner hair cells (Fuchs, 1996). Current data support a model in which hair cell inhibition results from a small, transient, ACh-gated depolarization followed by activation of calcium-activated potassium channels and consequent hair cell hyperpolarization (see above).

The hair cell cholinergic receptor exhibits a baroque pharmacological profile with atropine, nicotine, strychnine, α-bungarotoxin, *d*-tubocurarine, and bicuculline acting as antagonists (Fuchs, 1996). It was not until the cloning of the α9 nicotinic cholinergic receptor subunit that the molecular nature of the hair cell cholinergic receptor began to be deciphered and the ionotropic nature and inclusion within the nicotinic family of cholinergic receptor subunits was established (Elgoyhen *et al.*, 1994). Characterization of the rat α9 nAChR subunit revealed that it formed homomeric, calcium-permeable, ACh-gated channels in *Xenopus laevis* oocytes with pharmacological properties largely indistinguishable from those reported for the native hair cholinergic receptor. Moreover, a combination of *in situ* hybridization and reverse transcription (RT)-polymerase chain reaction (PCR) experiments has shown α9 transcripts in cochlear and vestibular hair cells of several vertebrate species.

nAChRs are members of the 'Cys-loop' family of neurotransmitter-gated ion channels that also includes $GABA_A$, $GABA_C$, glycine and 5-hydroxytryptamine-3 ($5HT_3$) receptors as well as some invertebrate anionic glutamate receptors (Karlin, 2002). Receptors in the family are formed by five homologous subunits oriented around a central ion-conducting pore. The subunits of these receptors have similar sequences and distributions of hydrophobic, membrane-spanning segments. Each subunit contains, in its ligand-binding, amino-terminal half, two (presumably disulfide-linked) cysteine residues separated by 13 other residues, thus giving this family the name of the Cys-loop receptors. A diversity of nicotinic receptor subunits have been cloned in recent years. The nicotinic receptor at the neuromuscular junction mediates fast synaptic transmission and is thought to have a $(\alpha 1)_2\beta 1\gamma\delta$ stoichiometry. Ten genes that encode neuronal nicotinic subunits have been identified in the vertebrate central or peripheral nervous system: α2–α8 and β2–β4. In heterologous expression systems, the neuronal subunits α2, α3, α4, and α6 lead to the assembly of functional nicotinic receptors in combination with either β2 or β4. They preserve the structural motif of muscle nicotinic receptors with a pentameric structure that includes two α and three β subunits. The α7 and α8 subunits form part of a different group within the neuronal nAChR, because they can assemble into functional receptors in the absence of any other subunit and α7 receptors account for the α-bungarotoxin-binding sites in the central nervous system.

Until recently, a longstanding pharmacological distinction between the nicotinic and muscarinic receptors remained intact. However, the cloning of the α9 subunit added a peculiar member to the nicotinic family of receptor subunits. When expressed in *Xenopus laevis* oocytes, α9 forms a homomeric receptor-channel complex that is activated by ACh, but displays a very distinct pharmacological profile. This matches neither the nicotinic nor the muscarinic subdivision of the pharmacological scheme of cholinergic receptors and in addition has sensitivities in common with $GABA_A$, glycine and $5HT_3$ receptors (Rothlin et al., 1999). On the other hand, whereas neuronal nicotinic α subunits and the muscle α1 subunit share sequence homologies ranging from 48% to 70%, the sequence identity between α9 and all known nicotinic subunits is less than 39%. This, taken together with the fact that the structure of the gene that encodes the α9 nAChR subunit differs from that of all known genes coding for nicotinic receptor subunits (Elgoyhen et al., 1994), indicates that α9 represents an early divergent branch closer to the ancestor that gave rise to the nicotinic gene family.

After the cloning of α9, the working hypothesis was that the α9 nicotinic subunit, functioning as a homopentameric acetylcholine-gated channel, was the native hair cell cholinergic receptor. However, three features remained at odds with this hypothesis: the current-voltage relationship, the Ca^{2+} sensitivity, and the desensitization properties of homomeric α9 receptors did not match those seen in isolated hair cells (Blanchet et al., 1996; Dulon & Lenoir, 1996; McNiven et al., 1996). With the cloning of the α10 nAChR from cochlear libraries and the expression of both α9 and α10 in Xenopus laevis oocytes it was demonstrated that the α9 α10 receptor recapitulates the pharmacological and biophysical properties of hair cell receptors (Elgoyhen et al., 2001). It is now believed that the hair cell cholinergic receptor that mediates synaptic transmission between efferent olivocochlear fibers and hair cells of the cochlea, is formed by both α9 and α10 subunits, in a pentameric structure with a $(\alpha 9)_2 (\alpha 10)_3$ stoichiometry (Elgoyhen et al., 1994, 2001; Plazas et al., 2005b).

An interesting feature of the α9 and α10 nAChR subunits is their evolutionary history (Franchini & Elgoyhen, 2006). The introduction of a descending fiber pathway to the inner ear occurred early in evolution, predating the emergence of terrestrial life. Since cholinergic efferent feedback to hair cells is a common feature among all vertebrates (Guinan, 1996), it would be expected that the evolutionary history of the genes coding for the α9 (Chrna9) and the α10 (Chrna10) subunits would look similar along all vertebrate lineages. Intriguingly, while Chrna9 has been under strong purifying pressure throughout vertebrates, Chrna10 shows signs of positive Darwinian selection only along the lineage leading to mammals. This suggests that mammalian nicotinic receptors acquired a novel function for this subunit that evolved in conjunction with properties specific to mammalian hearing. Co-varying with the evolutionary history of Chrna10 is prestin, the protein responsible for somatic electromotility of mammalian OHCs, which has also been under positive selection pressure only in mammals (Franchini & Elgoyhen, 2006). Thus, it is tempting to speculate that Chrna10 has evolved to give the mammalian auditory system feedback control of prestin-driven somatic electromotility, a capacity that is not required in non-mammalian species.

10.7.1 Insights from genetically modified mice

The generation of mice carrying a null mutation for Chrna9 has demonstrated that this subunit is a main component of the native OHC cholinergic receptor (Vetter et al., 1999). Chrna9 knock-out mice fail to show suppression of cochlear responses (DPOAEs and CAP) during efferent fiber activation, demonstrating the key role α9 receptors play in mediating the known effects of the olivocochlear system. Moreover, in the null mutant mice most OHC are innervated by one large terminal instead of multiple smaller terminals as in wild-types, suggesting that the α9 nAChR subunit also plays some role in normal synapse formation between efferent fibers and hair cells. Further behavioral studies on this α9 knock-out demonstrated no decrease in tone detection and intensity discrimination in quiet and continuous background noise, as has been shown for mice with olivocochlear pathway lesions, suggesting that central efferent pathways might work in combination with the peripheral olivocochlear system to enhance hearing in noise (May *et al.*, 2002). Additional studies have shown that cochlear sensitivity, based on CAP thresholds, is similar for homozygous mutant and wild-type mice, and that electromotility is also present in OHCs, independent of whether the α9 subunit is present or absent (He *et al.*, 2004).

A transgenic mouse overexpressing the nAChR α9 subunit also has been developed. These mice demonstrate markedly reduced acoustic injury from exposures causing either temporary or permanent threshold shifts, without changing pre-exposure cochlear sensitivity to low- or moderate-level sound (Maison *et al.*, 2002). These data demonstrate that efferent protection is at least in part mediated via the α9 nAChR in the OHCs and further support the notion that olivocochlear efferents play an important role in protecting the cochlea from traumatic sound.

The generation of *Chrna10* null mutant mice has indicated that, while functional homomeric α9 channels are present in OHCs of these genetically modified mice, they are insufficient to drive normal olivocochlear efferent inhibition to the cochlea, demonstrating that the α10 subunit is also an essential component of the hair cell nAChR (Vetter *et al.*, 2007).

Mice carrying deletions of GABA$_A$ receptor subunits have provided some evidence towards the role of the GABAergic efferent innervation to hair cells. Rather than subserving an independent action on OHC motility, GABA at the OHC/efferent synapse could modulate cholinergic effects. Indeed, reduction in electrically evoked efferent suppression in β2 nulls has been reported. However, histological analysis revealed a reduction in density of OHC efferents. Thus, a GABAergic role in maintenance of the efferent innervation rather than in the phasic modulation of their peripheral effects has been proposed (Maison *et al.*, 2006). In the case of CGRP, a strain of mice carrying a null mutation of the gene coding for the αCGRP has suggested a postsynaptic effect on cochlear afferent neurons via release of the neuropeptide from lateral olivocochlear terminals rather than an effect on the MOC system (Maison *et al.*, 2003b).

10.8 Summary and conclusion

Efferent innervation of the vertebrate inner ear is provided by neurons found near the superior olivary complex. MOC neurons have larger axons innervating OHCs in the functionally mature cochlea (i.e. after the onset of hearing). Prior to the onset of hearing MOC neurons synapse with IHCs. While there is evidence that GABA might be a neurotransmitter in some MOCs, functional studies to date have only shown that ACh is released to inhibit IHCs or OHCs. LOC neurons innervate type I afferent neurons beneath IHCs. These too are positive for cholinergic markers such as ChAT, but GABA, dopamine, and a variety of peptides also have been suggested as possible neurotransmitters. Little is known conclusively regarding lateral efferent function. The hair cell's response to ACh released from MOCs is mediated by two genetically distant members of the nicotinic AChR family, α9 and α10. These combine to form a non-selective cation channel with a high permeability to calcium. The resulting rise in cytoplasmic calcium activates SK2 channels through which potassium flows to hyperpolarize the cell.

While good progress has been made in identifying the ionic channels that contribute to the hair cell's cholinergic response, a variety of questions remain for future study. The roles played by intracellular calcium stores and enzymatic signaling pathways have been hinted at, but not yet fully delineated. In particular, the influence of cholinergic input on the mechanical properties of OHCs is suspected but far from understood. New, targeted genetic manipulations of the cholinergic pathway will help to unravel these mysteries. Also, comparative studies of efferent function and cellular mechanisms among different vertebrate species will continue to enlighten our understanding of inhibitory feedback to the ear.

References

Altschuler RA, Parakkal MH & Fex J. (1983) Localization of enkephalin-like immunoreactivity in acetylcholinesterase-positive cells in the guinea-pig lateral superior olivary complex that project to the cochlea. *Neuroscience* **9**: 621–30.

Altschuler RA, Parakkal MH, Rubio JA, Hoffman DW & Fex J. (1984) Enkephalin-like immunoreactivity in the guinea pig organ of Corti: ultrastructural and lesion studies. *Hear Res* **16**: 17–31.

Altschuler RA, Hoffman DW, Reeks KA & Fex J. (1985) Localization of dynorphin B-like and alpha-neoendorphin-like immunoreactivities in the guinea pig organ of Corti. *Hear Res* **17**: 249–58.

Art J, Fettiplace R & Fuchs P. (1984) Synaptic hyperpolarization and inhibition of turtle cochlear hair cells. *J Physiol* **365**: 525–50.

Art JJ & Fettiplace R. (1984) Efferent desensitization of auditory nerve fibre responses in the cochlea of the turtle Pseudemys scripta elegans. *J Physiol* **356**: 507–23.

Ashmore JF & Russell IJ. (1983) Sensory and effector functions of vertebrate hair cells. *J Submicrosc Cytol* **15**: 163–6.

Blanchet C, Erostegui C, Sugasawa M & Dulon D. (1996) Acetylcholine-induced potassium current of guinea pig outer hair cells: its dependence on a calcium influx through nicotinic-like receptors. *J Neurosci* **16**: 2574–84.

Brown MC. (1987) Morphology of labeled efferent fibers in the guinea pig cochlea. *J Comp Neurol* **260**: 605–18.

Brown MC & Nuttal AL. (1984) Efferent control of cochlear inner hair cell responses in guinea-pig. *J Physiol* **354**: 625–46.

Cabanillas LA & Luebke AE. (2002) CGRP- and cholinergic-containing fibers project to guinea pig outer hair cells. *Hear Res* **172**: 14–7.

Dallos P, He DZ, Lin X, Sziklai I, Mehta S & Evans BN. (1997) Acetylcholine, outer hair cell electromotility, and the cochlear amplifier. *J Neurosci* **17**: 2212–26.

Dannhof BJ, Roth B & Bruns V. (1991) Anatomical mapping of choline acetyltransferase (ChAT)-like and glutamate decarboxylase (GAD)-like immunoreactivity in outer hair cell efferents in adult rats. *Cell Tissue Res* **266**: 89–95.

Darrow KN, Simons EJ, Dodds L & Liberman MC. (2006) Dopaminergic innervation of the mouse inner ear: evidence for a separate cytochemical group of cochlear efferent fibers. *J Comp Neurol* **498**: 403–14.

Dolan DF, Guo MH & Nuttall AL. (1997) Frequency-dependent enhancement of basilar membrane velocity during olivocochlear bundle stimulation. *J Acoust Soc Am* **102**: 3587–96.

Dulon D & Lenoir M. (1996) Cholinergic responses in developing outer hair cells of the rat cochlea. *Eur J Neurosci* **8**: 1945–52.

Dulon D, Luo L, Zhang C & Ryan AF. (1998) Expression of small-conductance calcium-activated potassium channels (SK) in outer hair cells of the rat cochlea. *Eur J Neurosci* **10**: 907–15.

Eatock RA & Hurley KM. (2003) Functional development of hair cells. *Curr Top Dev Biol* **57**: 389–448.

Elgoyhen AB, Johnson DS, Boulter J, Vetter DE & Heinemann S. (1994) Alpha9: an acetylcholine receptor with novel pharmacological properties expressed in rat cochlear hair cells. *Cell* **79**: 705–15.

Elgoyhen AB, Vetter D, Katz E, Rothlin C, Heinemann S & Boulter J. (2001) Alpha 10: A determinant of nicotinic cholinergic receptor function in mammalian vestibular and cochlear mechanosensory hair cells. *Proc Natl Acad Sci U S A* **98**: 3501–6.

Erostegui C, Norris CH & Bobbin RP. (1994) In vitro characterization of a cholinergic receptor on outer hair cells. *Hear Res* **74**: 135–47.

Evans M. (1996) Acetylcholine activates two currents in guinea-pig outer hair cells. *J Physiol* **491**: 563–78.

Eybalin M. (1993) Neurotransmitters and neuromodulators of the mammalian cochlea. *Physiol Rev* **73**: 309–73.

Eybalin M & Altschuler RA. (1990) Immunoelectron microscopic localization of neurotransmitters in the cochlea. *J Electron Microsc Tech* **15**: 209–24.

Eybalin M, Charachon G & Renard N. (1993) Dopaminergic lateral efferent innervation of the guinea-pig cochlea: immunoelectron microscopy of catecholamine-synthesizing enzymes and effect of 6-hydroxydopamine. *Neuroscience* **54**: 133–42.

Fex J & Altschuler RA. (1981) Enkephalin-like immunoreactivity of olivocochlear nerve fibers in cochlea of guinea pig and cat. *Proc Natl Acad Sci U S A* **78**: 1255–9.

Flock A & Russell I. (1973) Efferent nerve fibres: postsynaptic action on hair cells. *Nat New Biol* **243**: 89–91.

Franchini LF & Elgoyhen AB. (2006) Adaptive evolution in mammalian proteins involved in cochlear outer hair cell electromotility. *Mol Phylogenet Evol* **41**: 622–35.

Fuchs P. (1996) Synaptic transmission at vertebrate hair cells. *Curr Opin Neurobiol* **6**: 514–9.

Fuchs PA & Murrow BW. (1992a) Cholinergic inhibition of short (outer) hair cells of the chick's cochlea. *J Neurosci* **12**: 800–9.

Fuchs PA & Murrow BW. (1992b) A novel cholinergic receptor mediates inhibition of chick cochlear hair cells. *Proc R Soc Lond B Proc Biol Sci* **248**: 35–40.

Galambos R. (1956) Suppression of auditory nerve activity by stimulation of afferent fibers to the cochlea. *J Neurophysiol* **19**: 424–37.

Gifford ML & Guinan JJ Jr. (1987) Effects of electrical stimulation of medial olivocochlear neurons on ipsilateral and contralateral cochlear responses. *Hear Res* **29**: 179–94.

Glowatzki E & Fuchs P. (2000) Cholinergic synaptic inhibition of inner hair cells in the neonatal mammalian cochlea. *Science* **288**: 2366–8.

Glowatzki E & Fuchs P. (2002) Transmitter release at the hair cell ribbon synapse. *Nat Nerosci* **5**: 147–54.

Gomez-Casati ME, Fuchs PA, Elgoyhen AB & Katz E. (2005) Biophysical and pharmacological characterization of nicotinic cholinergic receptors in cochlear inner hair cells. *J Physiol* **566**: 103–18.

Goutman JD, Fuchs PA & Glowatzki E. (2005) Facilitating efferent inhibition of inner hair cells in the cochlea of the neonatal rat. *J Physiol* **566**: 49–59.

Guinan JJ. (1996) Physiology of olivocochlear efferents. In: Dallos P, Popper AN & Fay RF, eds. *The Cochlea*. Springer-Verlag, New York, pp. 435–502.

Guinan JJ, Warr WB & Norris BE. (1983) Differential olivocochlear projections from lateral vs medial zones of the superior olivary complex. *J Comp Neurol* **221**: 358–70.

Gulley RL & Reese TS. (1977) Freeze-fracture studies on the synapses in the organ of Corti. *J Comp Neurol l* **171**: 517–43.

Guth PS, Perin P, Norris CH & Valli P. (1998) The vestibular hair cells: post-transductional signal processing. *Prog Neurobiol* **54**: 193–274.

He DZ & Dallos P. (1999) Development of acetylcholine-induced responses in neonatal gerbil outer hair cells. *J Neurophysiol* **81**: 1162–70.

He DZ, Cheatham MA, Pearce M & Vetter DE. (2004) Mouse outer hair cells lacking the alpha9 ACh receptor are motile. *Brain Res Dev Brain Res* **148**: 19–25.

Hirokawa N. (1978) The ultrastructure of the basilar papilla of the chick. *J Comp Neurol* **181**: 361–74.

Hoffman DW, Zamir N, Rubio JA, Altschuler RA & Fex J. (1985) Proenkephalin and prodynorphin related neuropeptides in the cochlea. *Hear Res* **17**: 47–50.

Housley GD & Ashmore JF. (1991) Direct measurement of the action of acetylcholine on isolated outer hair cells of the guinea pig cochlea. *Proc R Soc Lond B Proc Biol Sci* **244**: 161–7.

Housley GD, Norris CH & Guth PS. (1990) Cholinergically-induced changes in outward currents in hair cells isolated from the semicircular canal of the frog. *Hear Res* **43**: 121–33.

Kakehata S, Nakagawa T, Takasaka T & Akaike N. (1993) Cellular mechanism of acetylcholine-induced response in dissociated outer hair cells of guinea-pig cochlea. *J Physiol* **463**: 227–44.

Karlin A. (2002) Ion channel structure: emerging structure of the nicotinic acetylcholine receptors. *Nat Rev Neurosci* **3**: 102–14.

Katz E, Elgoyhen AB, Gomez-Casati ME, Knipper M, Vetter DE, Fuchs PA & Glowatzki E. (2004) Developmental regulation of nicotinic synapses on cochlear inner hair cells. *J Neurosci* **24**: 7814–20.

Kohler M, Hirschberg B, Bond CT, Kinzie JM, Marrion NV, Maylie J & Adelman JP. (1996) Small-conductance, calcium-activated potassium channels from mammalian brain. *Science* 273: 1709–14.

Kosaka T, Tauchi M & Dahl JL. (1988) Cholinergic neurons containing GABA-like and/or glutamic acid decarboxylase-like immunoreactivities in various brain regions of the rat. *Exp Brain Res* 70: 605–17.

Kujawa SG, Glattke TJ, Fallon M & Bobbin RP. (1993) Contralateral sound suppresses distortion product otoacoustic emissions through cholinergic mechanisms. *Hear Res* 68: 97–106.

Kujawa SG, Glattke TJ, Fallon M & Bobbin R. (1994) A nicotinic-like receptor mediates suppression of distortion product otoacustic emissions by contralateral sound. *Hear Res* 74: 122–34.

Kuriyama H, Shiosaka S, Sekitani M, Tohyama Y, Kitajiri M, Yamashita T, Kumazawa T & Tohyama M. (1990) Electron microscopic observation of calcitonin gene-related peptide-like immunoreactivity in the organ of Corti of the rat. *Brain Res* 517: 76–80.

Liberman MC, Dodds LW & Pierce S. (1990) Afferent and efferent innervation of the cat cochlea: quantitative analysis with light and electron microscopy. *J Comp Neurol* 301: 443–60.

Lioudyno M, Hiel H, Kong JH, Katz E, Waldman E, Parameshwaran-Iyer S, Glowatzki E & Fuchs PA. (2004) A 'synaptoplasmic cistern' mediates rapid inhibition of cochlear hair cells. *J Neurosci* 24: 11160–4.

Maison SF, Luebke AE, Liberman MC & Zuo J. (2002) Efferent protection from acoustic injury is mediated via alpha9 nicotinic acetylcholine receptors on outer hair cells. *J Neurosci* 22: 10838–46.

Maison SF, Adams JC & Liberman MC. (2003a) Olivocochlear innervation in the mouse: immunocytochemical maps, crossed versus uncrossed contributions, and transmitter colocalization. *J Comp Neurol* 455: 406–16.

Maison SF, Emeson RB, Adams JC, Luebke AE & Liberman MC. (2003b) Loss of alpha CGRP reduces sound-evoked activity in the cochlear nerve. *J Neurophysiol* 90: 2941–9.

Maison SF, Rosahl TW, Homanics GE & Liberman MC. (2006) Functional role of GABAergic innervation of the cochlea: phenotypic analysis of mice lacking GABA(A) receptor subunits alpha 1, alpha 2, alpha 5, alpha 6, beta 2, beta 3, or delta. *J Neurosci* 26: 10315–26.

Marcotti W, Johnson SL, Holley MC & Kros CJ. (2003) Developmental changes in the expression of potassium currents of embryonic, neonatal and mature mouse inner hair cells. *J Physiol* 548: 383–400.

Marcotti W, Johnson SL & Kros CJ. (2004) A transiently expressed SK current sustains and modulates action potential activity in immature mouse inner hair cells. *J Physiol* 560: 691–708.

Martin AR & Fuchs PA. (1992) The dependence of calcium-activated potassium currents on membrane potential. *Proc Biol Sci* 250: 71–6.

Matthews TM, Duncan RK, Zidanic M, Michael TH & Fuchs PA. (2005) Cloning and characterization of SK2 channel from chicken short hair cells. *J Comp Physiol A Neuroethol Sens Neural Behav Physiol* 191: 491–503.

May BJ, Prosen CA, Weiss D & Vetter D. (2002) Behavioral investigation of some possible effects of the central olivocochlear pathways in transgenic mice. *Hear Res* 171: 142–57.

McNiven AI, Yuhas WA & Fuchs PA. (1996) Ionic dependence and agonist preference of an acetylcholine receptor in hair cells. *Aud Neurosci* 2: 63–77.

Molnar Z & Blakemore C. (1995) How do thalamic axons find their way to the cortex?. *Trends Neurosci* 18: 389–97.

Moulin A, Collet L & Duclaux R. (1993) Contralateral auditory stimulation alters acoustic distortion products in humans. *Hear Res* 65: 193–210.

Mountain DC, Geisler CD & Hubbard AE. (1980) Stimulation of efferents alters the cochlear microphonic and the sound-induced resistance changes measured in scale media of the guinea pig. *Hear Res* 3: 231–40.

Murugasu E & Russell IJ. (1996) The effect of efferent stimulation on basilar membrane displacement in the basal turn of the guinea pig cochlea. *J Neurosci* 16: 325–32.

Oliver D, Klocker N, Schuck J, Baukrowitz T, Ruppersberg JP & Fakler B. (2000) Gating of Ca^{2+}-activated K^+ channels controls fast inhibitory synaptic transmission at auditory outer hair cells. *Neuron* 26: 595–601.

Plazas PV, De Rosa MJ, Gomez-Casati ME, Verbitsky M, Weisstaub N, Katz E, Bouzat C & Elgoyhen AB. (2005a) Key roles of hydrophobic rings of TM2 in gating of the alpha9alpha10 nicotinic cholinergic receptor. *Br J Pharmacol* **145**: 963–74.

Plazas PV, Katz E, Gomez-Casati ME, Bouzat C & Elgoyhen AB. (2005b) Stoichiometry of the $\alpha 9 \alpha 10$ Nicotinic Cholinergic Receptor. *J Neurosci* **25**: 10905–12.

Puel J, Safieddine S, Gervais d'Àldin C & Pujol R. (1995) Synaptic regeneration and functional recovery after excitotoxicity injury in the guinea pig cochlea. *C R Acad Sci III* **318**: 67–75.

Pujol R, Lavigne-Revillard M & Lenoir M. (1998) Development of sensory and neural structures in the mammalian cochlea. In: Rubel E, Popper A & Fay R, eds. *Development of the Auditory System*. Springer, New York, pp. 146–92.

Rajan R & Johnstone BM. (1988) Binaural acoustic stimulation exercises protective effects at the cochlea that mimic the effects of electrical stimulation of an auditory efferent pathway. *Brain Res* **458**: 241–55.

Rasmussen GL. (1946) The olivary peduncle and other fiber projections of the superior olivary complex. *J Comp Neurol* **84**: 141–219.

Rothlin C, Verbitsky M, Katz E & Elgoyhen A. (1999) The $\alpha 9$ nicotinic acetylcholine receptor shares pharmacological properties with type A γ-aminobutyric acid, glycine and type 3 serotonin receptors. *Mol Pharmacol* **55**: 248–54.

Ruel J, Nouvian R, Gervais d'Aldin C, Pujol R, Eybalin M & Puel JL. (2001) Dopamine inhibition of auditory nerve activity in the adult mammalian cochlea. *Eur J Neurosci* **14**: 977–86.

Russell IJ & Murugasu E. (1997) Medial efferent inhibition suppresses basilar membrane responses to near characteristic frequency tones of moderate to high intensities. *J Acoust Soc Am* **102**: 1734–8.

Saffiedine S & Eybalin M. (1992) Triple immunofluorescence evidence for the coexistence of acetylcholine, enkephalins and calcitonin gene-related peptide within efferent (olivocochlear) neurons of rats and guinea pigs. *Eur J Neurosci* **4**: 981–92.

Saito K. (1980) Fine structure of the sensory epithelium of the guinea pig organ of Corti: afferent and efferent synapses of hair cells. *J Ultrastruct Res* **71**: 222–32.

Schuknecht HF, Churchill JA & Doran R. (1959) The localization of acetylcholinesterase in the cochlea. *AMA Arch Otolaryngol* **69**: 549–59.

Shigemoto T & Ohmori H. (1990) Muscarinic agonists and ATP increase the intracellular Ca2+ concentration in chick cochlear hair cells. *J Physiol* **420**: 127–48.

Shigemoto T & Ohmori H. (1991) Muscarinic receptor hyperpolarizes cochlear hair cells of chick by activating Ca(2+)-activated K+ channels. *J Physiol* **442**: 669–90.

Simmons DD. (2002) Development of the inner ear efferent system across vertebrate species. *J Neurobiol* **53**: 228–50.

Sridhar TS, Liberman MC, Brown MC & Sewell WF. (1995) A novel cholinergic 'slow effect' of efferent stimulation on cochlear potentials in the guinea pig. *J Neurosci* **15**: 3667–78.

Sridhar TS, Brown MC & Sewell WF. (1997) Unique postsynaptic signaling at the hair cell efferent synapse permits calcium to evoke changes on two time scales. *J Neurosci* **17**: 428–37.

Sugai T, Yano J, Sugitani M & Ooyama H. (1992) Actions of cholinergic agonists and antagonists on the efferent synapse in the frog sacculus. *Hear Res* **61**: 56–64.

Tohyama Y, Senba E, Yamashita T, Kitajiri M, Kuriyama M, Kumazawa T, Ohata K & Tohyama M. (1990) Coexistence of calcitonin gene-related peptide and enkephalin in single neurons of the lateral superior olivary nucleus of the guinea pig that project to the cochlea as lateral olivocochlear system. *Brain Res* **515**: 312–14.

Vetter D, Lieberman M, Mann J, Barhanin J, Boulter J, Brown MC, Saffiote-Kolman J, Heinemann SF & Elgoyhen AB. (1999) Role of a9 nicotinic ACh receptor subunits in the development and function of cochlear efferent innervation. *Neuron* **23**: 93–103.

Vetter DE, Adams JC & Mugnani E. (1991) Chemically distinct rat olivocochlear neurons. *Synapse* **7**: 21–43.

Vetter DE, Li C, Zhao L, Contarino A, Liberman MC, Smith GW, Marchuk Y, Koob GF, Heinemann SF, Vale W & Lee KF. (2002) Urocortin-deficient mice show hearing impairment and increased anxiety-like behavior. *Nat Genet* **31**: 363–9.

Vetter DE, Katz E, Maison SF, Taranda J, Turcan S, Ballestero J, Liberman MC, Elgoyhen AB & Boulter J. (2007) The alpha10 nicotinic acetylcholine receptor subunit is required for normal synaptic function and integrity of the olivocochlear system. *Proc Natl Acad Sci U S A* **104**: 20594–9.

Walsh E, McGee J, McFadden S & Liberman M. (1998) Long-term effects of sectioning the olivocochlear bundle in neonatal cats. *J Neurosci* **18**: 3859–69.

Warr WB & Guinan JJ Jr. (1979) Efferent innervation of the organ of Corti: two separate systems. *Brain Res* **173**: 152–5.

Weisstaub N, Vetter D, Elgoyhen A & Katz E. (2002) The alpha9/alpha10 nicotinic acetylcholine receptor is permeable to and is modulated by divalent cations. *Hear Res* **167**: 122–35.

Wiederhold ML & Kiang NYS. (1970) Effects of electrical stimulation of the crossed olivocochlear bundle on cat single auditory nerve fibres. *J Acoust Soc Am* **48**: 950–65.

Williams EA, Brookes GB & Prasher DK. (1994) Effects of olivocochlear bundle section on otoacoustic emissions in humans: efferent effects in comparison with control subjects. *Acta Otolaryngologica* **114**: 121–9.

Yoshida N, Shigemoto T, Sugai T & Ohmori H. (1994) The role of inositol triphosphate on ACh-induced outward currents in bullfrog saccular hair cells. *Brain Res* **644**: 90–100.

Yuhas WA & Fuchs PA. (1999) Apamin-sensitive, small-conductance, calcium-activated potassium channels mediate cholinergic inhibition of chick auditory hair cells. *J Comp Physiol A* **185**: 455–62.

Chapter 11

Cochlear supporting cells

Jonathan Gale and Daniel Jagger

11.1 Introduction

The sensory epithelia of the inner ears of all animals are made up of two main cell types: sensory receptor hair cells and supporting cells. The sensory epithelium of the mammalian cochlea, the organ of Corti is unique among the organs of the auditory and vestibular systems in that it contains highly differentiated and functionally distinct supporting cells. This review is focused on the anatomy of cochlear supporting cell types, their molecular specializations, and their functional or physiological roles during normal hearing and during damage or overstimulation.

11.2 Cellular organization of the cochlea

11.2.1 Supporting cell types in the mature organ of Corti

The organ of Corti is the only hair cell epithelium that contains supporting cells that are sufficiently differentiated to discriminate different cell types in the population. This high degree of differentiation reflects the specific functional roles of those different supporting cells during normal hearing. The organ of Corti houses two subtypes of sensory hair cells (Fig. 11.1A, B), the inner and the outer hair cells, organized in what can be considered to be two compartments of supporting cells. These compartments are delineated by the tunnel of Corti, which is itself formed by the interlocked pillar cells. The inner hair cells are located in the 'medial compartment' of the organ of Corti, which develops from a region known as the greater epithelial ridge, and the outer hair cells are found in the 'lateral compartment' derived from the lesser epithelial ridge during development (see Kelley, 2007 and Chapter 12).

Here we will outline the major supporting cell subtypes based on their localization within the organ of Corti. For a comprehensive description of the anatomy of supporting cell subtypes see the thorough review by Slepecky (1996). The major individual cell types are shown in Figure 11.1. At the medial edge of the mature organ of Corti (Fig. 11.1A, B) is a single layer of *inner sulcus cells*, which have basally located nuclei and elongated apical phalangeal processes. On the medial face of the inner hair cell's basolateral membrane is the *inner border cell*, and on the lateral face is the *inner phalangeal cell*. These two cell types have basally located nuclei and fine phalangeal processes. These processes form a calyx-like structure that completely surrounds the inner hair cell and its afferent nerve fibres. The inner phalangeal cell abuts the medial face of the *inner pillar cell* phalange or rod.

The other wall of the tunnel of Corti is formed by the *outer pillar cell*, and lateral to that are three *Deiters' cells*. Deiters' cells, like pillar cells, but unlike hair cells, are attached to the basilar membrane at their basal pole. The basolateral membrane of each outer hair cell is supported in the 'cup region' at the top of the cell body of the underlying Deiters' cells, and each outer hair cell apical pole (at the level of the cuticular plate) interlocks with the phalangeal processes of several Deiters' cells at the epithelial surface, the reticular lamina (Slepecky, 1996). Lateral to the third

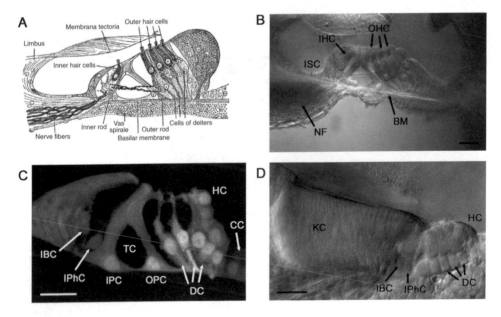

Fig. 11.1 Supporting cell types in the cochlea. (A) Drawing by Gustaf Retzius (1842–1919), describing the cell types found in the human cochlea. (B) Differential interference contrast (DIC) micrograph of the mid-turn region of the P15 rat cochlea. (C) Gap junctional dye-coupling between epithelial supporting cells in the P8 rat organ of Corti, reveals the major cell types in a mature-like arrangement. (D) DIC micrograph showing the basal turn region of the P0 rat cochlea. Kölliker's cells (KC) lie medial to the inner hair cell in Kölliker's organ. The organ of Corti is relatively compact, lacking the fluid-filled spaces observed in (B) and (C). Scale bars 20 μm. IHC, inner hair cell; OHC, outer hair cell; BM, basilar membrane; NF, nerve fibres; CC, Claudius' cells; DC, Deiters' cells; HC, Hensen's cells; IBC, inner border cell; IPC, inner pillar cell; IPhC, inner phalangeal cell; ISC, inner sulcus cell; OPC, outer pillar cell; TC, tunnel of Corti.

row of Deiters' cells are *Hensen's cells*. These can often be identified by large intracellular lipid-filled vacuoles and they have no clear contact with the basilar membrane. The lateral edge of the organ of Corti is bounded by *Claudius' cells*, squamous epithelial cells attached to the basilar membrane and extending to the outer sulcus.

11.2.2 Changes during cochlear development

The rodent cochlea has been used extensively as a model for the study of the development of mammalian hearing. Embryonic development of the cochlea has been reviewed recently (Kelley, 2007 and see Chapter 12), and thus we will limit this part of the review to the postnatal period. Rats and mice are born with an immature auditory system and are unable to hear for approximately the first two postnatal weeks. During that two-week period, both hair cells and supporting cells undergo considerable development up to, but also beyond, the onset of hearing, which occurs at around postnatal day 12.

At birth most of the cell types found in the adult cochlea are already recognizable (Fig. 11.1D). At this developmental stage, however, the inner sulcus cells are not seen. Instead, there is a transient structure termed Kölliker's organ, a thickened epithelium that stretches from the modiolar edge of the cochlear duct to the inner border cells. Kölliker's organ, the major constituent of an

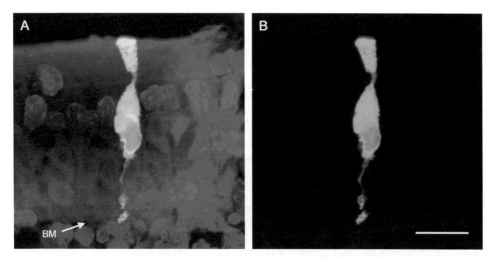

Fig. 11.2 Cytoarchitecture of Kölliker's cells. (A) A confocal z-stack projection showing localization of fluorescent dyes injected during a whole cell patch-clamp recording in Kölliker's organ. Neurobiotin (red) transferred from the injected cell to all others in the organ, via gap junctional intercellular coupling. Fluorescein-dextran (10 kDa, green) was too large to pass through gap junctions and remained in the injected cell. Nuclei were labelled with DAPI (blue).
(B) Fluorescein-dextran fluorescence reveals the distinct apico-basal organization of a single Kölliker's cell. At the basal end of the cell is a fine process and a 'foot' structure attaching the cell to the basilar membrane. The cell spans the whole extent of the organ, with a 'head' structure at the organ's apical surface. Scale bar 10 μm. BM, basilar membrane.

embryonic structure termed the greater epithelial ridge (see Chapter 12) consists of a wide expanse of tightly packed columnar-shaped supporting cells (Fig. 11.2). *Kölliker's cells* (KC) are thought to undergo extensive reorganization and/or cell death before eventually forming the population of cells that are later described as inner sulcus cells. The precise roles that Kölliker's cells may play remain undefined, but recent work has suggested that they are directly responsible for the spontaneous activity that has been observed in the immature cochlea, before the onset of hearing (Tritsch *et al.*, 2007). It remains to be shown whether Kölliker's cells are essential for the appropriate development of neural connections in the auditory pathway.

11.2.3 Supporting cells in non-mammalian hearing organs and vestibular systems

Supporting cells in all hair cell epithelia perform basic, yet essential functions: maintenance of the epithelial barrier, ion homeostasis, and trophic support. The latter role, in particular, is somewhat undefined and warrants further scrutiny. Unlike cochlear supporting cells, supporting cells in other hair cell epithelia appear to be a homogenous population as there is little to distinguish them. The caveat, of course, is that without specific molecular markers and knowledge of those cells we may not have been looking with the appropriate tools. It could be argued that the spectacular array of supporting cells in the organ of Corti is far more striking than any differences in the hair cells. One clear difference is that given the appropriate stimulus, supporting cells in all other hair cell epithelia can *either* re-enter the cell cycle, divide, and make new hair cells and supporting cells *or* they can undergo direct phenotypic conversion or transdifferentiation into hair cells (see Chapter 13). Supporting cells from the mature cochlea do not have this capacity and may lose that capacity during the postnatal developmental period (White *et al.*, 2006). These findings implicate the highly differentiated state of cochlear supporting cells in their lack of ability to de-differentiate and either re-enter the cell cycle or convert their phenotype.

11.3 Functional roles of supporting cells

11.3.1 Homeostasis in the cochlea

Barrier function and adherence

Normal hearing relies on a barrier that separates the endolymph from the perilymph, thereby maintaining the endocochlear potential and the high K^+ concentration of endolymph (see Chapter 7). The mosaic of supporting cells and hair cells form a tight neuroepithelium that plays an essential role in this function. To enable this barrier/separation function, supporting cells and hair cells are interconnected via unique 'tight-type' tight junctions (Jahnke, 1975). The tight junctions also allow the supporting cells and hair cells to display an apico-basal polarization, with distinct basolateral (perilymph-facing) and apical (endolymph-facing) specializations of the cell membrane kept separate. These specializations include a polarized expression of various ion channels and transporters, and membrane specializations such as micro-villi and, for example, in the case of outer hair cells, prestin (see Chapter 6). The apical part of all tight junctions in the reticular lamina is composed of multiple parallel protein strands (Jahnke, 1975; Gulley & Reese, 1976). The lower part of the tight junctions between supporting cells and hair cells is formed of a labyrinth of shorter irregular strands. The cochlear partition is subject to unique mechanical stresses, and accordingly, between adjacent supporting cells there is an additional adherens junction, or *fasciae occludentes*, that adds to the mechanical stability of the junction. The adherens junction is also the site of polarized association with the intracellular cytoskeleton (Fanning *et al.*, 2002).

The restriction of solute movement through paracellular spaces is known as the 'barrier function' of tight junctions. Experimental evidence suggests that the barrier function of individual tissues is determined by specific complexes of proteins. Occludin is an integral part of cochlear tight junctions (Kitajiri *et al.*, 2004; Nunes *et al.*, 2006), and associates with zona occludens (ZO) family members (Riazuddin *et al.*, 2006), and multiple claudin family members (Kitajiri *et al.*, 2004). Claudins form the major barrier to solute movements at tight junctions, and claudin-14 has been identified specifically at the apical portion of junctions between Deiters' cells and outer hair cells. The essential nature of these junctions is strongly supported by the finding that mutations of claudin-14 cause deafness in humans (*DFNB29*) and mice (Wilcox *et al.*, 2001; Ben-Yosef *et al.*, 2003). At the adherens junctions there is dense expression of multiple cadherin types (Mahendrasingam *et al.*, 1997; Nunes *et al.*, 2006), as well as claudin-6, claudin-9, and p120[ctn] (Nunes *et al.*, 2006). Tricellulin is expressed in the tight junctions formed where three cells meet, so called 'tri-cellular junctions', (Ikenouchi *et al.*, 2005, Riazuddin *et al.*, 2006). Mutations of tricellulin cause deafness in humans (*DFNB49*), most likely caused by the mutant, truncated forms of tricellulin being unable to bind to ZO-1 and occludin.

Gap junctions and connexins in the organ of Corti

Gap junctions are intercellular channels that control the transfer of certain ions and molecules between adjacent cells. The mammalian cochlear duct possesses two gap junction networks, one within the epithelial tissue, formed by supporting cells, and one within the connective tissue (Wangemann, 2002; Zhao *et al.*, 2006). The connective tissue network associated with the cochlear lateral wall is discussed elsewhere in this volume (Chapter 7). The epithelial gap junction system connects the supporting cells of the organ of Corti and bordering epithelial cells (Jagger & Forge, 2006).

There is no clear evidence in support of gap junctions between mammalian hair cells and supporting cells. The continuity of gap junction networks in the epithelial and connective tissues of the cochlea has supported a theory of K^+ recirculation within the cochlea. In this theoretical model, K^+ ions that enter hair cells during auditory transduction and exit their basolateral membrane via voltage-gated ion channels are then siphoned from the extracellular perilymph by proteins in the membrane of supporting cells. The K^+ions are then transferred via the intercellular epithelial gap junction network to the connective tissue gap junction network. This model is derived largely from indirect evidence, mostly in the form of protein expression data, and awaits unequivocal physiological evidence to support it. The extensive volume of the cell network or syncytium may, however, also act as a K^+ sink that allows the redistribution of the K^+ ions to regions of relative inactivity (Jagger & Forge, 2006). A similar mechanism of spatial buffering has been suggested as the dominant mechanism of K^+ management in glial cell networks of the brain (Karwoski et al., 1989).

Freeze fracture experiments reveal that the subcellular distribution of supporting cell gap junctions is comparable between different auditory and vestibular organs, and between species (Forge et al., 2003). Small gap junction plaques are found just beneath adherence junctions at the apex of supporting cells, and larger ones are located along the membrane of the cell body, where they constitute up to 25% of the total cell membrane area. The gap junction plaques found between supporting cells are possibly the largest in any tissues of the body, those between Deiters' cells contain as many as 100 000 channels. The gap junction plaques are distributed in such a way that suggests there is radial connectivity not only between supporting cells, but also longitudinally along the cochlear partition.

Experimental evidence has suggested that the supporting cell–epithelial gap junction system may itself be subdivided into separate compartments. Cells that lie medial to the inner hair cell show extensive expression of ion transport proteins that could manage K^+ following its gap-junction-mediated exit from the inner phalangeal cells and inner border cells (Spicer & Schulte, 1998). This suggests a system for the management of K^+ derived from inner hair cell activity, distinct from that for outer hair cell derived K^+. In support of this medial buffering compartment theory, small dye molecules injected into functionally mature supporting cells around inner hair cells are not detected in supporting cells around outer hair cells, and vice versa. This suggests that these compartments may be functionally separate (Fig. 11.3). This spatially restriction pattern of gap junction coupling is developed during the first two postnatal weeks (Jagger & Forge, 2006).

K^+ and neurotransmitter clearance: glial cells of the organ of Corti

The close anatomical apposition of the basolateral membranes of inner hair cells and supporting cells reveals a close functional interrelationship between these contrasting cell types. During auditory transduction, the mechanoelectrical depolarization and subsequent repolarization activity of hair cells results in a net efflux of K^+ ions and a potential excess of exocytosed neurotransmitter. Neurotransmitter is released from the basolateral membrane and into the synapse between the hair cell and afferent neurites. Applying a model taken from the function of glial cells in the brain, we assume that supporting cells play a vital homeostatic role by (i) clearing the excess neurotransmitter and K^+ ions, thereby (ii) terminating the neurochemical signal, and (iii) maintaining low K^+ concentration of the perilymph. These actions prevent excitotoxicity of sensory cells caused by excess activation via neurotransmitter, and depolarization caused by raised K^+ concentration.

Protein localization and functional evidence suggest that supporting cells carry out neurotransmitter clearance via transporter-mediated uptake. The glutamate/aspartate transporter (GLAST) has been immuno-localized to inner phalangeal cells and inner border cells surrounding inner hair cells (Furness & Lehre, 1997; Hakuba et al., 2000; Furness & Lawton, 2003; Glowatzki et al., 2006).

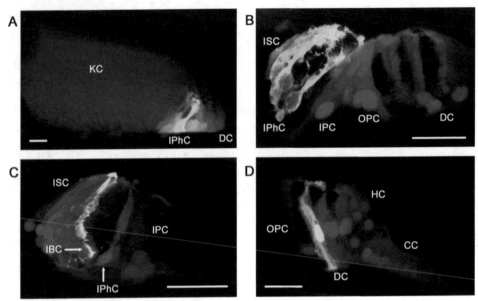

Fig. 11.3 Developmental changes of gap junctional dye-coupling between cochlear supporting cells. (A) Basal turn region of the P2 rat cochlea. During a whole cell patch-clamp recording, neurobiotin (red) and Lucifer yellow (green) injected into a single inner phalangeal cell (IPhC) transfer to surrounding supporting cells, but not into hair cells. Neurobiotin spreads noticeably further, including to Deiters' cells (DC), and throughout Kölliker's cells (KC), note this is a projection of a confocal z series. (B) Apical turn region of the P8 cochlea. As at P2, neurobiotin and Lucifer yellow transfer from a single IPhC to adjacent supporting cells, but not into hair cells. By this age there is more extensive spread of neurobiotin via the inner pillar cells (IPC) and outer pillar cells (OPC) to the lateral supporting cells, including Deiters' cells and Hensen's cells (HC). (C) By P13 (after the onset of hearing), Lucifer yellow transfer from a basal turn inner border cell is more restricted, and neurobiotin no longer transfers via inner pillar cells to outer pillar cells. (D) The reciprocal pattern of dye transfer is seen from a basal turn P12 Deiters' cell. Neurobiotin spreads relatively freely between Claudius' cells (CC) but not across the tunnel of Corti past the outer pillar cell. Scale bars 20 μm. ISC, inner sulcus cell.

GLAST transports glutamate and aspartate into the supporting cell in an electrogenic fashion, by coupling transport to the electrochemical gradient for Na^+, and as a result is also associated with an anion conductance (Danbolt, 2001). There is only limited expression of GLAST in the membrane of Deiters' cells (Furness *et al.*, 2002), consistent with the paucity of afferent innervation to outer hair cells (Jagger & Housley, 2003). Acoustic overstimulation of mice lacking GLAST results in raised perilymphatic concentrations of glutamate and exacerbated hearing loss (Hakuba *et al.*, 2000). Elegant patch-clamp experiments directly demonstrated GLAST activity in postnatal (5–15 days) inner phalangeal cells and, as there was no detectable neurotransmitter uptake at the presynaptic (inner hair cell) or postsynaptic (spiral ganglion cell) membranes, suggested that supporting cells alone are responsible for glutamate clearance from around the hair cells (Glowatzki *et al.*, 2006).

K$^+$ clearance or 'siphoning' by supporting cells has been suggested to occur via members of the K/Cl co-transporter (KCC) family. These electro-neutral transporters contribute to cell volume regulation, transepithelial transport, and intracellular Cl⁻ concentration regulation (Mount *et al.*, 1999). KCC4 has been immuno-localized to Deiters' cells and inner phalangeal cells in the mouse organ of Corti, and although KCC4-deficient mice have normal thresholds at hearing onset they display rapid-onset hearing loss due to hair cell death (Boettger *et al.*, 2002). KCC3-deficient mice also display hearing loss, but this occurs over a much longer timescale (Boettger *et al.*, 2003). As hearing thresholds are initially normal in both these mutant mice, it suggests that the KCC transporters are not essential for normal hearing *per se*, and thus other mechanisms must contribute to K⁺ siphoning. It is worth reiterating that to date there is no direct, functional evidence of K⁺ clearance or 'siphoning' by supporting cells and so further work is critical here.

Osmotic and pH balance in supporting cells

There are considerable fluxes of ions during auditory transduction. As a consequence compensatory mechanisms are required to ensure the osmotic balance of the supporting cell cytoplasm and these are also likely to contribute to the osmotic balance of the cochlear fluids. Failure to regulate osmotic balance has been implicated in Ménière's disease. One mechanism contributing to normal osmotic homeostasis is the expression of aquaporin (AQP) molecules by supporting cells. These 'water channels' allow the transport of water across osmotically active tissues. Using reverse transcription (RT)-polymerase chain reaction (PCR) techniques the mRNA of several aquaporin (AQP) subtypes have been detected in inner ear tissue (Huang *et al.*, 2002). AQP4 has been immuno-localized in Hensen's cells, Claudius' cells, and inner sulcus cells (Takumi *et al.*, 1998), whereas AQP7 has been detected in Deiters' cells (Huang *et al.*, 2002). This cell-specific expression suggests that AQP subtypes play particular roles in normal osmotic homeostasis in the organ of Corti. The detection of the Cl⁻/HCO$_3$⁻ exchanger and the H⁺-ATPase in supporting cells (Stankovic *et al.*, 1997) also suggests that the pH of the intracellular milieu of these cells and/or the extracellular milieu is highly regulated.

Epithelial repair: a response to trauma

When the cochlea is subjected to any kind of trauma the cells that appear to be most sensitive are the sensory hair cells. A considerable amount of work has been focused on how hair cells respond to trauma. As a result we know much less about how supporting cells respond during hair cell damage and death. Supporting cells do play a fundamental role in the repair process that occurs in damaged hair cell epithelia (Raphael, 2002). When an outer hair cell is damaged either by noise trauma or ototoxicity, the apical surfaces of Deiters' cells expand, join together and form new tight junctions in what has been termed a 'scar' (Forge 1985; Raphael & Altschuler 1991; Leonova & Raphael 1997; Lenoir *et al.*, 1999). In this way, Deiters' cells are thought to re-seal the epithelium thereby minimizing any loss of ionic composition or endocochlear potential and preventing any further cell loss due to K⁺ overload. Definitive evidence of the rapidity and effectiveness of this wound healing process is lacking. The repair process appears to be conserved and highly energetic, involving both actin and myosin. Similar 'scar' structures (Steyger *et al.*, 1997; Hordichok & Steyger 2007) and actin-cable structures (Gale *et al.*, 2002) are observed in lower vertebrate species. Furthermore, it has also been suggested that cochlear supporting cells can phagocytose dead hair cells, although the extent to which this is occurring and the timing of this process is far from clear (Forge, 1985; Abrashkin *et al.*, 2006). Novel dynamic experimental approaches are required to understand the contribution of supporting cells in this regard. Whether supporting cells also play a role in hair cell death, rather then being simply the 'cleaners' is not clear. We have recently shown that during neomycin treatment of hair cells in cochlear explant cultures, there is activation of the extracellular regulated kinases 1 and 2 (ERK1/2), members of the mitogen-activated protein kinase (MAPK) family, in phalangeal cells surrounding hair cells (see 11.5.2).

Activation of this pathway may play a role in inner hair cell death, implicating those supporting cells as potential mediators of hair cell death (Lahne & Gale, 2008). These results are important because they suggest that supporting cells themselves could be a target for potential therapies aimed at preventing hair cell loss. Thus further work on the role of supporting cells in hair cell pathophysiology is anticipated.

11.3.2 Structural support/mechanics

Tectorial membrane

The tectorial membrane is an essential component of transduction (Legan *et al.*, 2000). It is an extracellular matrix gel composed of molecules that are manufactured and secreted by supporting cells. In the developing cochlea, Kölliker's, border, inner phalangeal, pillar, Deiters', and Hensen's cells express mRNA for both α- and β-tectorins (Legan *et al.*, 1997; Rau *et al.*, 1999), which are critical components of the tectorial membrane. Other components of the tectorial membrane, for example collagen (Thalmann *et al.*, 1986) and otogelin (Cohen-Salmon *et al.*, 1997) also appear to be produced and secreted by supporting cells.

Reticular lamina

The surface of the organ of Corti is known as the reticular lamina. Along with hair cells, supporting cells contribute to the structure of the reticular lamina which forms part of the impermeable epithelial barrier and acts as a fundamental structural support system for the apices of hair cells. Cochlear mechanics require the precise coordination of movements and transfer of mechanical energy between the basilar membrane and the tectorial membrane/hair bundle/reticular lamina complex (see Chapters 5 and 8). It is the phalangeal supporting cells, Deiters', and the pillar cells that are thought to perform the main structural role in this system. There is some experimental evidence and also modelling data that supporting cells, in particular the pillar and Deiters' cells, contribute significantly to the control of hearing sensitivity and cochlear micromechanics (Laffon & Angelini, 1996; Flock *et al.*, 1999). Suffice it to say that the micromechanics of a cochlea lacking either Deiters' cells or pillar cells are likely to be severely disrupted.

Supporting cell innervation

There is a limited amount of evidence that supporting cells may play a more sophisticated role during normal hearing. Anatomical tracing techniques have revealed a complex innervation of Hensen's cells and Deiters' cells, particularly at the low frequency end of the cochlea (Fechner *et al.*, 2001). The overwhelming majority of these synaptic contacts could be identified as branches from type II spiral ganglion neurones, the afferent neurones of outer hair cells, although there was also a contribution from the olivocochlear efferent fibres. In addition, individually traced type II spiral ganglion neurones have been seen to contact supporting cells (Jagger & Housley, 2003). At present, however, a sensory role for supporting cells remains highly speculative in the absence of physiological evidence of sensory transduction mechanisms in these cells. During cellular damage, supporting cells do contribute to Ca^{2+} waves by releasing ATP via connexin hemichannels (Gale *et al.*, 2004). ATP released in the vicinity of type II nerve fibres could act as a signal trigger, hence the supporting cells could contribute to 'damage sensation'. It should also be noted that the physiological role of type II spiral ganglion neurones remains unclear, although their membrane characteristics and innervation pattern are consistent with a role in the coding of information with low spatial and temporal resolution.

11.4 Molecular specializations of supporting cells

11.4.1 Development of the supporting cell cytoskeleton

The critical structural roles played by cochlear supporting cells during the normal hearing process rely on specialized cytoskeletal elements within those cells. Some supporting cells are uniquely endowed with specialized microtubules. The microtubule arrays are stabilized by various accessory proteins such as actin, providing a characteristic stiffness that contributes to the overall mechanical properties of the cochlear partition (Tolomeo & Holley, 1997; Robles & Ruggero, 2001).

In newborn altricial rodents such as rats, mice, and gerbils, the organ of Corti appears relatively undifferentiated with supporting cells and hair cells closely compacted (see Fig. 11.1D). Over the subsequent 7–10 days of development all cells undergo significant morphological alterations. One of the most dramatic is the growth of large apico-basal arrays of tubulin-based microtubules in inner and outer pillar cells and Deiters' cells (Hallworth et al., 2000). The mechanism of microtubule growth is closely regulated by nucleating sites, referred to as microtubule-organizing centres (MTOC), under the control of various anchoring and transport proteins (Mogensen et al., 1997; Mogensen, 1999).

11.4.2 Mature arrangement of the cytoskeleton

In the functionally mature organ of Corti there are obvious distinctions between the cytoskeletal elements of supporting cells and hair cells (Fig. 11.4). Although tubulins are highly concentrated in both cell types, certain post-translational modifications are seen exclusively in supporting cells (Bane et al., 2002). Thus there appears to be a dichotomy in the function of the cytoskeleton in cochlear cells; dynamic microtubules are present in hair cells, but more stable microtubules are necessary in supporting cells. Microtubule array stability is enhanced by anchorage at the apex and base of pillar cells and Deiters' cells. Filamentous meshworks of actin, keratin and vimentin act to attach the arrays to supporting cell adherens junctions (Schulte & Adams, 1989; Mogensen et al., 1998) which would add to the overall stability of the reticular lamina and organ of Corti.

11.4.3 Connexins and gap junctions

An earlier section discussed the function of gap junctions in K^+ recycling. Here we review other aspects of connexins and gap junctions in supporting cells. The voltage-dependence and gating properties of gap junction channels in native cochlear tissue have been determined using patch-clamp techniques. The voltage-dependence of gap junctions in Hensen's cells has been divided into four groups (Zhao & Santos-Sacchi, 2000). These responses showed varying degrees of electrical rectification. The observation of such asymmetrical voltage gating suggests a complexity in gap junctional coupling, and argues in favour of multiple channel types composed of non-homotypic connexin types (see below). Channels between adjacent Deiters' cells also display rectification. These channels can be modulated by physiological factors such as nitric oxide (Blasits et al., 2000). The biophysical properties of any gap junction channels depend on their subunit composition. Multiple lines of evidence point to cochlear gap junction channels consisting of varying combinations of connexin 26 (Cx26) and Cx30.

Experimental evidence suggests that there are variations in the molecular selectivity of cochlear gap junctions, depending on cellular localization and developmental age. Gap junction channels allow the intercellular flux of the second messenger molecule inositol 1,4,5-trisphosphate (IP_3) between Hensen's cells (Beltramello et al., 2005). Data from dye transfer experiments in cochlear slices suggest that the transfer of large anionic molecules such as IP_3 would be limited between

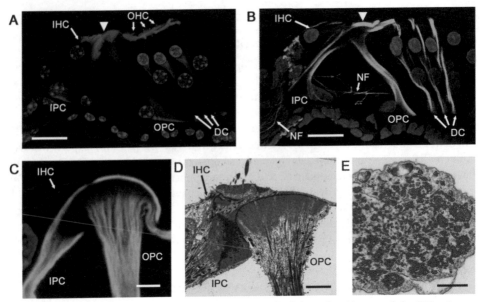

Fig. 11.4 Cytoskeletal elements in cochlear supporting cells. (A) Confocal image of the P21 rat organ of Corti showing localization of actin (red, phalloidin). Actin is localized to the apical pole of outer hair cells (OHCs) and inner hair cells (IHCs), at the cuticular plate, and the stereociliary bundle. In inner pillar cells (IPCs) and outer pillar cells (OPCs) there is dense actin expression where the head regions meet (denoted by arrowhead), and at the feet of these cells. Actin is seen in the cup region of Deiters' cells (DC), just beneath the outer hair cells. Nuclei are stained with DAPI (blue). (B) In a similar section, an anti-acetylated tubulin antibody (green) localizes to bundles of microtubules in supporting cells, especially in pillar cells and in Deiters' cells. Antibody labelling is also evident in nerve fibres (NF) at the base of IHCs and crossing the tunnel of Corti. (C) In a similar section, high magnification of the pillar cell head region shows individual microtubule bundles. (D) Transmission electron micrograph (TEM) of the pillar cell head region shows microtubule bundles (dark fibre-like structures) inserting into the actin-containing meshwork (homogeneous grey areas). E, TEM cross-section of the outer pillar cell stalk, revealing numerous bundles of microtubules. Scale bars: (A, B) 20 μm; (C, D) 5 μm. E, 1 μm.
Figures 11.4D, E were kindly provided by Andy Forge (UCL Ear Institute).

certain supporting cell types. As in some other tissues, gap junction channels between Deiters' cells have the ability to select between molecules of different molecular weight and/or charge (Jagger & Forge, 2006). They show a preference for positively charged species over negatively charged ones, and restrict the movement of molecules with a high molecular weight. This ability is likely to reflect a higher expression of Cx30 in Deiters' cells, compared with Hensen's cells, in which Cx26 expression appears to be more prevalent.

The predominant connexins in the mammalian inner ear are Cx26 and Cx30 (see Fig. 11.5), which are present in all cells comprising the epithelial and connective tissue gap junction systems of the cochlea and vestibule (Lautermann *et al.*, 1998; Forge *et al.*, 2003; Jagger & Forge, 2006). However, within the organ of Corti there are variations in the relative expression of Cx26 and Cx30 (Zhang *et al.*, 2005; Jagger & Forge, 2006). In Hensen's cells Cx26 expression is relatively stronger than Cx30 whereas in Deiters' cells the opposite is seen. This may explain the range of

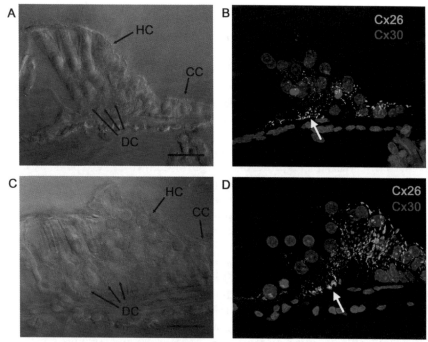

Fig. 11.5 Connexin expression in the mature cochlea. (A) Mid-apical turn region of the P28 rat cochlea. (B) Confocal immunofluorescence reveals connexin 26 (Cx26, green) and Cx30 (red) expressed in discrete puncta between supporting cells. At the base of Deiters' cells there are double-labelled puncta (white arrow), suggesting co-expression of Cx26 and Cx30. Cx26-only puncta are seen in Hensen's cells and Claudius' cells. Labelling is absent from outer hair cells. (C) Mid-basal turn region of the same cochlea. In the basal region of the rat cochlea there is a noticeably larger mass of lateral supporting cells such as Hensen's cells. (D) Cx26/Cx30 immunofluorescence reveals more numerous puncta in the basal than in the mid-apical region (B), and noticeably larger double-labelled gap junction plaques (white arrow) between Deiters' cells. Plaques labelled by Cx26 only are evident in the lateral supporting cell mass. Scale bars 20 μm. CC, Claudius' cells; DC, Deiters' cells; HC, Hensen's cells.

biophysical properties of gap junctions between different supporting cell types (see above). In most cells though, Cx26 and Cx30 can be co-localized within individual gap junction plaques in the inner ear, and they can be co-immunoprecipitated (Forge *et al.*, 2003). This raises the likelihood that some cochlear gap junctions incorporate oligomers of Cx26 and Cx30. In the avian inner ear, the chicken orthologues of mammalian Cx30, Cx26, and Cx43 have been identified as major connexin isoforms. Chicken Cx30 is exclusively expressed in inner ear tissues and is present in all cells comprising the gap junction networks of the sensory and ion transporting epithelia of the cochlear duct and utricle (Nickel *et al.*, 2006).

There is a growing body of evidence that connexin hemichannels, unpaired connexons, may play crucial roles during tissue development (Dale, 2008). The contribution of connexins to gap junctional communication has been studied extensively in the cochlea. A description of potential roles for hemichannel activity during cochlear development and damage is discussed below.

11.4.4 **Purinergic receptors**

The role of purinergic signalling in normal hearing

Extracellular nucleotides such as ATP, ADP, and UTP are recognized as important signalling molecules in many tissues. Purinergic receptors are widely expressed in cochlear tissues and are thought to play a number of roles in cochlear development and normal hearing (Housley et al., 2002). P2X receptors (ligand-gated ion channels) have been immuno-localized to the luminal (scala media facing) surfaces of supporting cells and hair cells (Housley et al., 1999), and it has been hypothesized that ATP released into the endolymph can activate these receptors to activate a shunt conductance that decreases hearing sensitivity (Munoz et al., 1999). In addition, ATP may regulate the micromechanical properties of the organ of Corti via P2X receptors (Skellett et al., 1997). The widespread expression of extracellular nucleotide-metabolizing enzymes increases the likelihood that nucleotides are endogenous signalling molecules in the organ of Corti (Vlajkovic et al., 2002). These endonucleotidases regulate the levels of active nucleotides in the cochlear fluids, and so restrict or terminate purinergic signalling.

P2Y (G protein-coupled) receptors have been implicated in supporting cell Ca^{2+} signalling (Lagostena et al., 2001; Gale et al., 2004; Piazza et al., 2007) and have been hypothesized to play a role in the management of K^+ during normal hearing (Bruzzone & Cohen-Salmon, 2005). This idea is based on the observation that ATP is released from cochlear supporting cells as part of the intercellular spread of damage-induced calcium waves in neonatal cochlear cultures (Gale et al., 2004). ATP acts as a paracrine signalling agent, stimulating purinergic receptors in adjacent cells resulting in further IP_3 generation, calcium changes, ATP release, and continued signal propagation. The mechanism by which ATP is released by undamaged cells remains to be resolved, although the suggestion is that it occurs via connexin hemichannels. The consequences of damage-induced Ca^{2+} waves are discussed elsewhere in this chapter.

A combination of molecular and electrophysiological techniques have determined that a predominant P2X subtype in the organ of Corti is $P2X_2$ (Housley et al., 1998; Chen et al., 2000), and in particular a slowly-desensitizing splice variant $P2X_{2-1}$ (Housley et al., 1999). The expression of slowly-desensitizing $P2X_2$ receptors has been confirmed by pharmacological and electrophysiological dissection of purinergic currents in isolated Deiters' cells (Chen & Bobbin, 1998; Kanjhan et al., 2003). It has been suggested that purinoreceptor signalling could alter the mechanical compliance of Deiters' cells. In various preparations of Hensen's cells and Deiters' cells, exogenously applied ATP has revealed complex signalling mechanisms and osmotic effects. ATP application activates a biphasic current (Sugasawa et al., 1996; Lagostena et al., 2001), primarily a P2X-gated fast inward current, and a subsequent slow current. The secondary response has been attributed to a calcium activated Cl^- current, activation of which is linked to P2Y-mediated intracellular Ca^{2+} release from IP_3-gated stores (Lagostena et al., 2001). ATP-mediated increases of intracellular Ca^{2+} concentration may also inhibit intercellular communication and signalling due to the effect of raised intracellular Ca^{2+} on gap junction permeability. Persistent questions are whether, during normal physiological function in the mature cochlea, ATP is released in sufficient quantity to activate such signals, which cells release it and via what mechanism?

Role of purinergic signalling in development

The extensive expression of purinergic receptors in supporting cells, hair cells, and afferent neurons prior to the onset of hearing has led to recent studies probing the role of purinergic signalling in cochlear development. Recent findings have implicated supporting cells of Kölliker's organ, the Kölliker's cells as fundamental players in the development of neuronal activity, patterning and possibly synaptic connection remodeling (Tritsch et al., 2007 and see Chapter 12). An array of techniques showed that the spontaneous activity observed in hair cells and the primary afferent nerve fibres originated from cells in Kölliker's organ. Pharmacological inhibition indicated release of ATP from the Kölliker's cells as a central mechanism. This spontaneous release of ATP triggered intercellular calcium waves and large inward currents that propagated through many cells due to the extensive gap junction coupling between the cells. The purinergic-dependent currents recorded from Kölliker's cells had complex characteristics, probably due to the network properties imposed by the gap-junctional coupling observed in these cells (Jagger & Forge, 2006). When the spontaneous activity was local enough the released ATP activated purinergic receptors on the surface of inner hair cells, thereby driving excitatory activity in those cells in the absence of auditory stimuli. The resulting neurotransmitter released from inner hair cells stimulated the sensory neurites of developing spiral ganglion neurones (Tritsch et al., 2007). The innervation of hair cells undergoes dramatic changes during the period just prior to the onset of hearing in rodents (Huang et al., 2007) and purinergic receptors, acting either directly or indirectly, have been implicated in the process of ganglion cell outgrowth (Greenwood et al., 2007). Spiral ganglion neurones innervating either inner hair cells or outer hair cells are known to be responsive to exogenous purinergic agonists during this critical developmental window (Jagger & Housley, 2003). The kinetics and pharmacological profile of inward currents activated in neonatal spiral ganglion cells indicate that they result from the activation of unique heteromultimeric P2X receptors (Salih et al., 2002). Together, these recent studies point towards a critical role for supporting cell-derived purinergic signalling in the postnatal development and fine-tuning of sensory elements in the cochlea. Whether there is a fundamental role for purinergic signalling during earlier embryonic cochlear development, as there is in retinal development (Dale, 2008) remains to be determined.

11.4.5 Other ion channels

As described previously, cochlear supporting cells are responsible for the management of K^+ following auditory transduction. Movements of K^+ ions during extended periods of sound stimulation are likely to be important. Consequently it would be expected that supporting cells (especially the phalangeal cells adjacent to hair cells) should possess specialized membrane-derived mechanisms that would allow them to maintain an appropriate intracellular electrolyte balance. Deiters' cells isolated from the adult guinea pig cochlea possess large outwardly rectifying K^+ currents (Nenov et al., 1998). The commonly used K^+ channel blockers tetra-ethyl ammonium (TEA) and 4-amino pyridine (4-AP) have differential effects on these K^+ currents, suggesting there may be multiple types of ion channels responsible. A rigorous molecular analysis of the ion channel types in Deiters' cells has yet to be carried out. Outwardly rectifying currents have also been observed in neonatal inner phalangeal cells (Glowatzki et al., 2006). Ca^{2+}-activated Cl^- currents have been observed in guinea pig Hensen's cells (Lagostena et al., 2001), and Cl^- channels have been detected using immunohistochemical methods (Qu et al., 2006) but Cl^- currents have not been studied in cochlear supporting cells. Similarly, there are no published reports of voltage-gated Ca^{2+} channels in these cells.

11.5 Functions of cochlear supporting cells during development, damage, repair and regeneration

11.5.1 Development

Cochlear development and the patterning of cells in the organ of Corti are covered in Chapter 12 and recently by Kelley (2007). In the previous section we described the role of purinergic signalling in regulating spontaneous activity in the cochlea prior to hearing onset, and the involvement of a particular cochlear supporting cell found in Kölliker's organ. During embryonic, and in altricial animals, early postnatal development, there are numerous tall columnar cells at the medial side of the sensory patch that will become the hair cell region. These cells form a structure called Kölliker's organ and the cells themselves have been termed Kölliker's cells (Mogensen *et al.*, 1997). Until recently little function could be ascribed to these cells although they appear to be a pool of cells that, given the appropriate cues, for example the transcription factor Atoh1, can develop as prosensory cells and be pushed towards a hair cell fate (Kelley, 2007). As described earlier it is now thought that Kölliker's cells spontaneously release ATP onto inner hair cells causing them to depolarize and fire Ca^{2+} action potentials, leading to the release of glutamate and excitation of afferent nerve fibres. Thus in the developing cochlea it appears to be the supporting cells that effectively initiate electrical activity in auditory nerves in the absence of sound and they do this via an ATP release-based mechanism (Tritsch *et al.*, 2007). A surprising finding was that the spontaneous electrical activity was highly correlated with waves of activity that could simply be observed as changes in the transmittance of the epithelium viewed using differential interference contrast transmitted light imaging. The change in transmittance, most likely due to some cell shrinkage, was concomitant with or was preceded by spontaneous increases in cytoplasmic Ca^{2+} that propagated between cells as intercellular Ca^{2+} waves. The spontaneous activity is not restricted to the developing rat cochlea, as similar intercellular calcium waves followed by changes in the light transmitting properties of the tissue are observed in the immature mouse cochlea (Fig. 11.6). The changes in intracellular calcium could drive the ATP release, via connexin hemichannels; the electrophysiological changes in the supporting cells, by activating Ca-activated Cl⁻ currents; and due to the latter, the apparent cell shrinkage observed optically. The spontaneous activity results in the coordinated firing of hair cells and their afferent fibres that are located close to one another (91% of activity recorded from inner hair cell pairs was synchronized in cells located within 70 μm of one another). Such a mechanism could contribute to the generation of the tonotopic map in the auditory pathway, although this hypothesis remains to be tested.

Despite the continued expression of purinergic receptors by hair cells and supporting cells (Housley *et al.*, 2002) the ATP-dependent spontaneous activity ceases abruptly after the onset of hearing (Tritsch *et al.*, 2007). Future work is required to determine the nature of the molecular changes that underlie this cessation of activity. It is also important to know whether the reactivation of such ATP-dependent activity in situations of noise damage, where ATP is likely to be released, could result in the inappropriate firing of spiral ganglion neurones. Such activity, could in the acute phase contribute to the initiation of a tinnitus percept and in the longer term contribute to the generation of longer lasting centrally derived tinnitus.

11.5.2 Damage signalling, epithelial repair, and hair cell death

As described earlier supporting cells play a key role in the repair of the cochlear epithelium after damage. Perhaps unsurprisingly, supporting cells are extremely sensitive to damage in the inner ear. Damage to a single hair cell in immature cochlear explants elicits an intercellular wave of cytosolic calcium that can spread through supporting cells to distant sites (Gale *et al.*, 2004; Piazza *et al.*, 2007). Spread of the calcium wave over long distances requires the repetitive or regenerative release of ATP by the supporting cells. Thus the signalling is again dependent upon extracellular ATP, on the expression of sensitive purinoreceptor in considerable amounts and on the release of ATP by the supporting cells. The damage-induced intercellular calcium waves appear to be relatively independent of gap junctions but may well require functional connexins in the form of hemichannels (Gale *et al.*, 2004; Mammano *et al.*, 2007). This intercellular calcium wave activity is highly reminiscent of waves observed in glial cells, particularly astrocytes (Newman, 2001).

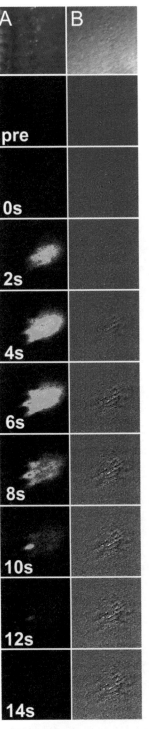

Fig. 11.6 Spontaneous calcium waves and optical changes in the Kölliker's organ of the immature mouse cochlea. (A) Sequence of images showing changes in cytoplasmic calcium measured on a laser scanning confocal microscope using Fluo4. First image is the raw Fluo4 (F0) signal from the left hand edge showing a row of outer hair cells and then a row of inner hair cells. Pseudocolour images show the change in calcium obtained by subtracting subsequent images from the first image (F-F0 images). Warmer colours represent increases in cytoplasmic calcium. (B) Sequence of simultaneously recorded brightfield images showing changes in the refractivity of Kölliker's organ that correspond spatially and follow temporally the changes in cytoplasmic calcium. Time indicated on left for both A and B. Scale bar 10 μm (also see Tritsch et al., 2007).

We thank Guy Richardson for providing the neonatal mouse cochlear cultures.

In glial cells damage signalling can be conferred via members of the MAPK family, in particular ERK1/2. Recent work in our lab using immature cochlear explants (Lahne & Gale, 2008) has shown that damage-induced activation of ERK1/2 occurs specifically in the supporting cells that surround hair cells, the Deiters', and inner phalangeal cells with little or no ERK1/2 activation occurring in the hair cells (Fig. 11.7). This suggests two main possibilities: either those phalangeal cells express the appropriate receptors to respond to the damage stimulus or the hair cells release a factor that acts locally to activate only their immediate neighbours. Exogenous application of ATP can replicate this activation pattern remarkably well, suggesting that the former explanation is the most likely and that the appropriate receptors are purinergic. As described earlier there is good evidence for the expression of many purinergic receptors by supporting cells, although the

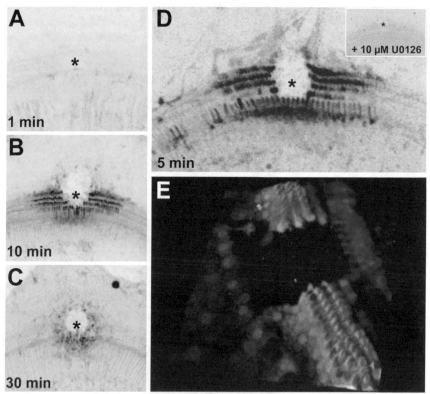

Fig. 11.7 Damage-induced ERK activation in the mammalian cochlea is specific to supporting cells. Coarse mechanical damage to the organ of Corti (*) in immature cochlear explants (from 1–2-day-old rats) triggers the activation of ERK1/2 (stained with a phospho-specific antibody) in phalangeal cells ten minutes after damage (B). One minute after damage, there is no activation, acting as a control for the antibody. After 30 minutes the activation has declined, although some cells close to the damage site are still activated. (D) The mechanical damage activates ERK1/2 via the MEK1/2 pathway as the addition of U0126 prevents activation (inset). (E) Three-dimensional reconstruction of confocal sections of activated ERK1/2 labelling in the organ of Corti shows the specificity of activation, with strong signal being observed in the phalangeal cells surrounding the hair cells. We thank Manuela Lahne for the images.

actual molecular nature of those native receptors is far from clear. In cochlear explant preparations aminoglycoside treatment resulted in similar activation of ERK1/2 in supporting cells surrounding damaged hair cells and when the activation of ERK1/2 was prevented by pharmacological manipulation this rescued hair cells from neomycin toxicity (Lahne & Gale, 2008). Further work will clarify how critical this signalling pathway is to the process of cochlear damage and repair in the mature and even ageing cochlea and whether supporting cells are implicated in the death of hair cells in the adult cochlea and/or other hair cell epithelia.

11.5.3 Regeneration: supporting cells as progenitor cells

Our current understanding of hair cell regeneration places the supporting cells in critical roles either as progenitor cells that re-enter the cell cycle, divide, and make new hair cells and/or supporting cells *or* as a supply of cells that can convert into hair cells given the appropriate triggers (usually the loss of surrounding hair cells). Recent research in avian auditory hair cell regeneration has suggested that there is a greater contribution from the latter mode of replacement than originally thought (Chapter 13) and also the mode of recovery depends upon the position of the cells in the organ, either abneural, for direct transdifferentiation or neural, for mitosis (Cafaro *et al.*, 2007). However, in the mature mammalian cochlea neither of these modes of regeneration occurs naturally and hearing loss is therefore permanent.

The present chapter is devoted to specializations of mammalian supporting cells. It is possible that it is exactly because of the extensive specializations that are required for these cells to perform such vital roles that their innate ability to de-differentiate and/or re-enter the cell cycle has been lost. Despite this, viral transduction of the basic helix-loop-helix (bHLH) transcription factor Atoh1 in mature cochlear supporting cells appears to be able to re-specify those cells to become hair cells, particularly when the therapy occurs immediately after hair cell loss, that is, in damaged cochleae, (Kawamoto *et al.*, 2003; Izumikawa *et al.*, 2005).

11.6 What is in the future for cochlear supporting cells?

For many years the supporting cells in hair cell epithelia have played second fiddle to the sensory receptor hair cells. In the cochlea, supporting cells, as well as performing their supporting role, have well-defined roles that are indicated by their highly differentiated state. The availability of mutant and transgenic animal models for genes expressed either exclusively or highly by supporting cells has provided evidence in favour of these cells performing essential roles for both the structure and function of the cochlea. Recent functional data has also implicated supporting cell subtypes in critical roles in both cochlear development and maturation and in repair after damage. Furthermore, supporting cells are now targets for therapeutic strategies aimed at regenerating hair cells in deafened ears. Research into the function of supporting cells in the normal, damaged, and ageing ear will take us closer to understanding cochlear physiology and the possibility of alleviating cochlear pathophysiology.

Acknowledgements

We thank Manuela Lahne, Jonathan Bird, Andy Forge, Dwight Bergles and Nic Tritsch for helpful discussions.

References

Abrashkin K, Izumikawa M, Miyazawa T, Wang C, Crumling M, Swiderski D, Beyer L, Gong T & Raphael Y. (2006) The fate of outer hair cells after acoustic or ototoxic insults. *Hear Res* **218**: 20–9.

Bane BC, MacRae TH, Xiang H, Bateman J & Slepecky NB. (2002) Microtubule cold stability in supporting cells of the gerbil auditory sensory epithelium: correlation with tubulin post-translational modifications. *Cell Tissue Res* **307**: 57–67.

Beltramello M, Piazza V, Bukauskas FF, Pozzan T & Mammano F. (2005) Impaired permeability to Ins(1,4,5)P3 in a mutant connexin underlies recessive hereditary deafness. *Nat Cell Biol* **7**: 63–9.

Ben-Yosef T, Belyantseva IA, Saunders TL, Hughes ED, Kawamoto K, Van Itallie CM, Beyer LA, Halsey K, Gardner DJ, Wilcox ER, Rasmussen J, Anderson JM, Dolan DF, Forge A, Raphael Y, Camper SA & Friedman TB. (2003) Claudin 14 knockout mice, a model for autosomal recessive deafness DFNB29, are deaf due to cochlear hair cell degeneration. *Hum Mol Genet* **12**: 2049–61.

Blasits S, Maune S & Santos-Sacchi J. (2000) Nitric oxide uncouples gap junctions of supporting Deiters cells from Corti's organ. *Pflugers Arch* **440**: 710–2.

Boettger T, Hubner CA, Maier H, Rust MB, Beck FX & Jentsch TJ. (2002) Deafness and renal tubular acidosis in mice lacking the K-Cl co-transporter Kcc4. *Nature* **416**: 874–8.

Boettger T, Rust MB, Maier H, Seidenbecher T, Schweizer M, Keating DJ, Faulhaber J, Ehmke H, Pfeffer C, Scheel O, Lemcke B, Horst J, Leuwer R, Pape HC, Volkl H, Hubner CA & Jentsch TJ. (2003) Loss of K-Cl co-transporter KCC3 causes deafness, neurodegeneration and reduced seizure threshold. *Embo J* **22**: 5422–34.

Bruzzone R & Cohen-Salmon M. (2005) Hearing the messenger: Ins(1,4,5)P3 and deafness. *Nat Cell Biol* **7**: 14–6.

Cafaro J, Lee G & Stone J. (2007) Atoh1 expression defines activated progenitors and differentiating hair cells during avian hair cell regeneration. *Dev Dyn* **236**: 156–70.

Chen C & Bobbin RP. (1998) P2X receptors in cochlear Deiters' cells. *Br J Pharmacol* **124**: 337–44.

Chen C, Parker MS, Barnes AP, Deininger P & Bobbin RP. (2000) Functional expression of three P2X(2) receptor splice variants from guinea pig cochlea. *J Neurophysiol* **83**: 1502–9.

Cohen-Salmon M, El-Amraoui A, Leibovici M & Petit C. (1997) Otogelin: a glycoprotein specific to the acellular membranes of the inner ear. *Proc Natl Acad Sci U S A* **94**: 14450–5.

Dale N. (2008) Dynamic ATP signalling and neural development. *J Physiol* **586**: 2429–36.

Danbolt NC. (2001) Glutamate uptake. *Prog Neurobiol* **65**: 1–105.

Fanning AS, Ma TY & Anderson JM. (2002) Isolation and functional characterization of the actin binding region in the tight junction protein ZO-1. *Faseb J* **16**: 1835–7.

Fechner FP, Nadol JJ, Burgess BJ & Brown MC. (2001) Innervation of supporting cells in the apical turns of the guinea pig cochlea is from type II afferent fibers. *J Comp Neurol* **429**: 289–98.

Flock A, Flock B, Fridberger A, Scarfone E & Ulfendahl M. (1999) Supporting cells contribute to control of hearing sensitivity. *J Neurosci* **19**: 4498–507.

Forge A. (1985) Outer hair cell loss and supporting cell expansion following chronic gentamicin treatment. *Hear Res* **19**: 171–82.

Forge A, Marziano NK, Casalotti SO, Becker DL & Jagger D. (2003) The inner ear contains heteromeric channels composed of cx26 and cx30 and deafness-related mutations in cx26 have a dominant negative effect on cx30. *Cell Commun Adhes* **10**: 341–6.

Furness DN & Lehre KP. (1997) Immunocytochemical localization of a high-affinity glutamate-aspartate transporter, GLAST, in the rat and guinea-pig cochlea. *Eur J Neurosci* **9**: 1961–9.

Furness DN & Lawton DM. (2003) Comparative distribution of glutamate transporters and receptors in relation to afferent innervation density in the mammalian cochlea. *J Neurosci* **23**: 11296–304.

Furness DN, Hulme JA, Lawton DM & Hackney CM. (2002) Distribution of the glutamate/aspartate transporter GLAST in relation to the afferent synapses of outer hair cells in the guinea pig cochlea. *J Assoc Res Otolaryngol* **3**: 234–47.

Gale J, Meyers J, Periasamy A & Corwin J. (2002) Survival of bundleless hair cells and subsequent bundle replacement in the bullfrog's saccule. *J Neurobiol* **50**: 81–92.

Gale JE, Piazza V, Ciubotaru CD & Mammano F. (2004) A mechanism for sensing noise damage in the inner ear. *Curr Biol* **14**: 526–9.

Glowatzki E, Cheng N, Hiel H, Yi E, Tanaka K, Ellis-Davies GC, Rothstein JD & Bergles DE. (2006) The glutamate-aspartate transporter GLAST mediates glutamate uptake at inner hair cell afferent synapses in the mammalian cochlea. *J Neurosci* **26**: 7659–64.

Greenwood D, Jagger DJ, Huang LC, Hoya N, Thorne PR, Wildman SS, King BF, Pak K, Ryan AF & Housley GD. (2007) P2X receptor signaling inhibits BDNF-mediated spiral ganglion neuron development in the neonatal rat cochlea. *Development* **134**: 1407–17.

Gulley RL & Reese TS. (1976) Intercellular junctions in the reticular lamina of the organ of Corti. *J Neurocytol* **5**: 479–507.

Hakuba N, Koga K, Gyo K, Usami SI & Tanaka K. (2000) Exacerbation of noise-induced hearing loss in mice lacking the glutamate transporter GLAST. *J Neurosci* **20**: 8750–3.

Hallworth R, McCoy M & Polan-Curtain J. (2000) Tubulin expression in the developing and adult gerbil organ of Corti. *Hear Res* **139**: 31–41.

Hordichok A & Steyger P. (2007) Closure of supporting cell scar formations requires dynamic actin mechanisms. *Hear Res* **232**: 1–19.

Housley GD, Luo L & Ryan AF. (1998) Localization of mRNA encoding the P2X2 receptor subunit of the adenosine 5'-triphosphate-gated ion channel in the adult and developing rat inner ear by *in situ* hybridization. *J Comp Neurol* **393**: 403–14.

Housley GD, Kanjhan R, Raybould NP, Greenwood D, Salih SG, Jarlebark L, Burton LD, Setz VC, Cannell MB, Soeller C, Christie DL, Usami S, Matsubara A, Yoshie H, Ryan AF & Thorne PR. (1999) Expression of the P2X(2) receptor subunit of the ATP-gated ion channel in the cochlea: implications for sound transduction and auditory neurotransmission. *J Neurosci* **19**: 8377–88.

Housley GD, Jagger DJ, Greenwood D, Raybould NP, Salih SG, Jarlebark LE, Vlajkovic SM, Kanjhan R, Nikolic P, Munoz DJ & Thorne PR. (2002) Purinergic regulation of sound transduction and auditory neurotransmission. *Audiol Neurootol* **7**: 55–61.

Huang D, Chen P, Chen S, Nagura M, Lim DJ & Lin X. (2002) Expression patterns of aquaporins in the inner ear: evidence for concerted actions of multiple types of aquaporins to facilitate water transport in the cochlea. *Hear Res* **165**: 85–95.

Huang LC, Thorne PR, Housley GD & Montgomery JM. (2007) Spatiotemporal definition of neurite outgrowth, refinement and retraction in the developing mouse cochlea. *Development* **134**: 2925–33.

Ikenouchi J, Furuse M, Furuse K, Sasaki H & Tsukita S. (2005) Tricellulin constitutes a novel barrier at tricellular contacts of epithelial cells. *J Cell Biol* **171**: 939–45.

Izumikawa M, Minoda R, Kawamoto K, Abrashkin K, Swiderski D, Dolan D, Brough D & Raphael Y. (2005) Auditory hair cell replacement and hearing improvement by Atoh1 gene therapy in deaf mammals. *Nat Med* **11**: 271–6.

Jagger DJ & Housley GD. (2003) Membrane properties of type II spiral ganglion neurones identified in a neonatal rat cochlear slice. *J Physiol* **552**: 525–33.

Jagger DJ & Forge A. (2006) Compartmentalized and signal-selective gap junctional coupling in the hearing cochlea. *J Neurosci* **26**: 1260–8.

Jahnke K. (1975) The fine structure of freeze-fractured intercellular junctions in the guinea pig inner ear. *Acta Otolaryngol* **336 (Suppl)**: 1–40.

Kanjhan R, Raybould NP, Jagger DJ, Greenwood D & Housley GD. (2003) Allosteric modulation of native cochlear P2X receptors: insights from comparison with recombinant P2X2 receptors. *Audiol Neurootol* **8**: 115–28.

Karwoski C, Lu H & Newman E. (1989) Spatial buffering of light-evoked potassium increases by retinal Müller (glial) cells. *Science* **244**: 578–80

Kawamoto K, Ishimoto S, Minoda R, Brough D & Raphael Y. (2003) Math1 gene transfer generates new cochlear hair cells in mature guinea pigs *in vivo*. *J Neurosci* **23**: 4395–400.

Kelley MW. (2007) Cellular commitment and differentiation in the organ of Corti. *Int J Dev Biol* **51**: 571–83.

Kitajiri SI, Furuse M, Morita K, Saishin-Kiuchi Y, Kido H, Ito J & Tsukita S. (2004) Expression patterns of claudins, tight junction adhesion molecules, in the inner ear. *Hear Res* **187**: 25–34.

Laffon E & Angelini E. (1996) On the Deiters cell contribution to the micromechanics of the organ of Corti. *Hear Res* **99**: 106–9.

Lagostena L, Ashmore JF, Kachar B & Mammano F. (2001) Purinergic control of intercellular communication between Hensen's cells of the guinea-pig cochlea. *J Physiol* **531**: 693–706.

Lahne M & Gale J. (2008) Damage-induced activation of ERK1/2 in cochlear supporting cells is a hair cell death-promoting signal that depends on extracellular ATP and calcium. *J Neurosci* **28**: 4918–28.

Lautermann J, ten Cate WJ, Altenhoff P, Grummer R, Traub O, Frank H, Jahnke K & Winterhager E. (1998) Expression of the gap-junction connexins 26 and 30 in the rat cochlea. *Cell Tissue Res* **294**: 415–20.

Legan P, Rau A, Keen J & Richardson G. (1997) The mouse tectorins. Modular matrix proteins of the inner ear homologous to components of the sperm-egg adhesion system. *J Biol Chem* **272**: 8791–801.

Legan P, Lukashkina V, Goodyear R, Kossi M, Russell I & Richardson G. (2000) A targeted deletion in alpha-tectorin reveals that the tectorial membrane is required for the gain and timing of cochlear feedback. *Neuron* **28**: 273–85.

Lenoir M, Daudet N, Humbert G, Renard N, Gallego M, Pujol R, Eybalin M & Vago P. (1999) Morphological and molecular changes in the inner hair cell region of the rat cochlea after amikacin treatment. *J Neurocytol* **28**: 925–37.

Leonova E & Raphael Y. (1997) Organization of cell junctions and cytoskeleton in the reticular lamina in normal and ototoxically damaged organ of Corti. *Hear Res* **113**: 14–28.

Mahendrasingam S, Katori Y, Furness DN & Hackney CM. (1997) Ultrastructural localization of cadherin in the adult guinea-pig organ of Corti. *Hear Res* **111**: 85–92.

Mammano F, Bortolozzi M, Ortolano S & Anselmi F. (2007) Ca2+ signaling in the inner ear. *Physiology (Bethesda)* **22**: 131–44.

Mogensen MM. (1999) Microtubule release and capture in epithelial cells. *Biol Cell* **91**: 331–41.

Mogensen MM, Mackie JB, Doxsey SJ, Stearns T & Tucker JB. (1997) Centrosomal deployment of gamma-tubulin and pericentrin: evidence for a microtubule-nucleating domain and a minus-end docking domain in certain mouse epithelial cells. *Cell Motil Cytoskeleton* **36**: 276–90.

Mogensen MM, Henderson CG, Mackie JB, Lane EB, Garrod DR & Tucker JB. (1998) Keratin filament deployment and cytoskeletal networking in a sensory epithelium that vibrates during hearing. *Cell Motil Cytoskeleton* **41**: 138–53.

Mount DB, Mercado A, Song L, Xu J, George AL Jr., Delpire E & Gamba G. (1999) Cloning and characterization of KCC3 and KCC4, new members of the cation-chloride cotransporter gene family. *J Biol Chem* **274**: 16355–62.

Munoz DJ, Thorne PR & Housley GD. (1999) P2X receptor-mediated changes in cochlear potentials arising from exogenous adenosine 5'-triphosphate in endolymph. *Hear Res* **138**: 56–64.

Nenov AP, Chen C & Bobbin RP. (1998) Outward rectifying potassium currents are the dominant voltage activated currents present in Deiters' cells. *Hear Res* **123**: 168–82.

Newman E. (2001) Propagation of intercellular calcium waves in retinal astrocytes and M?cells. *J Neurosci* **21**: 2215–23.

Nickel R, Becker D & Forge A, (2006) Molecular and functional characterization of gap junctions in the avian inner ear. *J Neurosci* **26**: 6190–9.

Nunes FD, Lopez LN, Lin HW, Davies C, Azevedo RB, Gow A & Kachar B. (2006) Distinct subdomain organization and molecular composition of a tight junction with adherens junction features. *J Cell Sci* **119**: 4819–27.

Piazza V, Ciubotaru CD, Gale JE & Mammano F. (2007) Purinergic signalling and intercellular Ca2+ wave propagation in the organ of Corti. *Cell Calcium* **41**: 77–86.

Qu C, Liang F, Hu W, Shen Z, Spicer SS & Schulte BA. (2006) Expression of CLC-K chloride channels in the rat cochlea. *Hear Res* **213**: 79–87.

Raphael Y. (2002) Cochlear pathology, sensory cell death and regeneration. *Br Med Bull* **63**: 25–38.

Raphael Y & Altschuler R. (1991) Scar formation after drug-induced cochlear insult. *Hear Res* **51**: 173–83.

Rau A, Legan P & Richardson G. (1999) Tectorin mRNA expression is spatially and temporally restricted during mouse inner ear development. *J Comp Neurol* **405**: 271–80.

Riazuddin S, Ahmed ZM, Fanning AS, Lagziel A, Kitajiri S, Ramzan K, Khan SN, Chattaraj P, Friedman PL, Anderson JM, Belyantseva IA, Forge A & Friedman TB. (2006) Tricellulin is a tight-junction protein necessary for hearing. *Am J Hum Genet* **79**: 1040–51.

Robles L & Ruggero MA. (2001) Mechanics of the mammalian cochlea. *Physiol Rev* **81**: 1305–52.

Salih SG, Jagger DJ & Housley GD. (2002) ATP-gated currents in rat primary auditory neurones *in situ* arise from a heteromultimetric P2X receptor subunit assembly. *Neuropharmacology* **42**: 386–95.

Schulte BA & Adams JC. (1989) Immunohistochemical localization of vimentin in the gerbil inner ear. *J Histochem Cytochem* **37**: 1787–97.

Skellett RA, Chen C, Fallon M, Nenov AP & Bobbin RP. (1997) Pharmacological evidence that endogenous ATP modulates cochlear mechanics. *Hear Res* **111**: 42–54.

Slepecky NB. (1996) Structure of the mammalian cochlea. In: Dallos P, Popper AN & Fay RR, eds. *The Cochlea*. Springer, New York, 1996, pp. 44–129.

Spicer SS & Schulte BA. (1998) Evidence for a medial K+ recycling pathway from inner hair cells. *Hear Res* **118**: 1–12.

Stankovic KM, Brown D, Alper SL & Adams JC. (1997) Localization of pH regulating proteins H+ATPase and Cl-/HCO3- exchanger in the guinea pig inner ear. *Hear Res* **114**: 21–34.

Steyger PS, Burton M, Hawkins JR, Schuff NR & Baird RA. (1997) Calbindin and parvalbumin are early markers of non-mitotically regenerating hair cells in the bullfrog vestibular otolith organs. *Int J Dev Neurosci* **15**: 417–32.

Sugasawa M, Erostegui C, Blanchet C & Dulon D. (1996) ATP activates a cation conductance and Ca(2+)-dependent Cl- conductance in Hensen cells of guinea pig cochlea. *Am J Physiol* **271**: C1817–27.

Takumi Y, Nagelhus EA, Eidet J, Matsubara A, Usami S, Shinkawa H, Nielsen S & Ottersen OP. (1998) Select types of supporting cell in the inner ear express aquaporin-4 water channel protein. *Eur J Neurosci* **10**: 3584–95.

Thalmann I, Thallinger G, Comegys T & Thalmann R. (1986) Collagen – the predominant protein of the tectorial membrane. *ORL J Otorhinolaryngol Relat Spec* **48**: 107–15.

Tolomeo JA & Holley MC. (1997) Mechanics of microtubule bundles in pillar cells from the inner ear. *Biophys J* **73**: 2241–7.

Tritsch NX, Yi E, Gale JE, Glowatzki E & Bergles DE. (2007) The origin of spontaneous activity in the developing auditory system. *Nature* **450**: 50–5.

Vlajkovic SM, Thorne PR, Sevigny J, Robson SC & Housley GD. (2002) Distribution of ectonucleoside triphosphate diphosphohydrolases 1 and 2 in rat cochlea. *Hear Res* **170**: 127–38.

Wangemann P. (2002) K(+) cycling and its regulation in the cochlea and the vestibular labyrinth. *Audiol Neurootol* **7**: 199–205.

Wilcox ER, Burton QL, Naz S, Riazuddin S, Smith TN, Ploplis B, Belyantseva I, Ben-Yosef T, Liburd NA, Morell RJ, Kachar B, Wu DK, Griffith AJ & Friedman TB. (2001) Mutations in the gene encoding tight junction claudin-14 cause autosomal recessive deafness DFNB29. *Cell* **104**: 165–72.

White P, Doetzlhofer A, Lee Y, Groves A & Segil N. (2006) Mammalian cochlear supporting cells can divide and trans-differentiate into hair cells. *Nature* **441**: 984–7.

Zhang Y, Tang W, Ahmad S, Sipp JA, Chen P & Lin X. (2005) Gap junction-mediated intercellular biochemical coupling in cochlear supporting cells is required for normal cochlear functions. *Proc Natl Acad Sci U S A* **102**: 15201–6.

Zhao HB & Santos-Sacchi J. (2000) Voltage gating of gap junctions in cochlear supporting cells: evidence for nonhomotypic channels. *J Membr Biol* **175**: 17–24.

Zhao HB, Kikuchi T, Ngezahayo A & White TW. (2006) Gap junctions and cochlear homeostasis. *J Membr Biol* **209**: 177–86.

Chapter 12

Development of the inner ear

Lynne M Bianchi and Paul A Fuchs

12.1 Introduction

As described in earlier chapters, the adult inner ear is a very small, yet highly complex structure. In cross-section, the spiral-shaped cochlea is seen to include three fluid-filled chambers, or scalae. A specialized epithelium, the organ of Corti, rests on the basilar membrane separating the scala tympani from the scala media (Fig. 12.1). The organ of Corti is the sensory region of the cochlea, and contains a variety of distinct supporting cells, as well as the sensory hair cells that convey information to the brainstem via the bipolar spiral ganglion neurons (SGNs) located within the modiolus. Both the sensory epithelium and the SGNs are organized in a precise, tonotopic pattern to relay frequency information to the central auditory pathway. Yet, in contrast to the highly complex structure of the adult inner ear, the early embryonic inner ear appears remarkably simple, consisting of a single hollow ball of cells. Some of the most intriguing questions in embryogenesis relate to the mechanisms that govern the transformation of this simple otic vesicle into the highly complex, and exquisitely organized, inner ear (compare Figs 12.2–12.4). Developmental auditory scientists often cite a quote from Swanson *et al.* (1990) that refers to the development of the inner ear as 'one of the most remarkable displays of precision microengineering in the vertebrate body'. The more one learns about the many detailed and specific mechanisms of inner ear development, the more one grows to appreciate this statement.

A vast number of precisely timed and complex cellular and molecular events must occur in order for the final anatomical organization to be recognized. First, embryonic cells must become specified as the cochlear tissue. The cells must then proliferate to ensure a sufficiently large population of each cellular subtype. These progenitor cells, which apparently have the capacity to give rise to all the cells of the cochlea, begin to differentiate into distinct cell types such as sensory hair cells and the various supporting cells. Further patterning and alignment must take place in order to attain the final geometric organization that is the hallmark of the mammalian cochlea. This chapter will focus primarily on the development of mammalian cochlear structures, particularly the mouse cochlea, as it is a frequently studied animal model. The major developmental events, however, appear similar across mammalian species, to the best of our current knowledge.

12.1.1 Gross differentiation of cochlear structures

The inner ear first forms alongside the rhombencephalon (hindbrain) adjacent to rhombomeres 5 and 6. The inner ear arises from a thickened patch of ectoderm, the otic placode. This otic placode then invaginates to form the otic pit. The pit closes off below the surface ectoderm and forms the hollow ball known as the otic vesicle, or otocyst. In human embryos, the otic placode invaginates at the fourth week post conception (reviewed by Lim & Rueda, 1992). In the mouse embryo, the forming otic vesicle is first detected at embryonic day 9 (E9; Morsli *et al.*, 1998) and the closed otocyst is easily observable by E11 (Sher, 1971). The development of the cochlea is dependent,

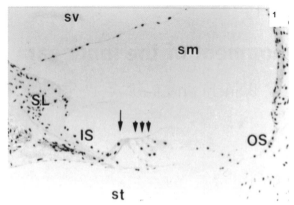

Fig. 12.1 Cross-section through the adult cochlea identifying some major structural regions. The sensory hair cells of the organ of Corti rest on the basilar membrane (arrow: inner hair cell; arrowheads: outer hair cells). The three fluid-filled chambers, the scala vestibuli (sv), scale tympani (st), and scala media (sm), surround the cellular regions. The spiral limbus (SL) and inner sulcus (IS) are at the modiolar edge, whereas the outer sulcus (OS) is located at the strial edge of the cochlea.

at the earliest stages, on interactions between the rhombencephalon, and slightly later, the surrounding periotic mesenchyme (reviewed by Barald & Kelley, 2004). Induction of the otic tissues involves a number of molecules, including members of the fibroblast growth factor family (i.e. FGF3, FGF8, FGF10; Table 12.1) and wnt family. These molecules originate in the hindbrain or periotic mesenchyme and have either direct or indirect effects on otocyst induction (Barald & Kelley, 2004).

As noted above, the otocyst will ultimately give rise to all of the sensory hair cells, and nearly all of the supporting cells and neurons associated with both cochlear and vestibular sections of the inner ear. It is important to note that both cochlear and vestibular regions develop simultaneously from this otocyst. Only a population of Schwann cells, found in the auditory and vestibular ganglia, the melanocytes of the stria vascularis, and perhaps some vestibular neurons, derive from neural crest cells that arise outside the otocyst (D'Amico-Martel, 1982; D'Amico-Martel & Noden, 1983).

Although seemingly homogeneous in appearance, even at these early stages of otocyst formation the developing inner ear tissues segregate into cellular regions that will give rise to specific

Fig. 12.2 At mid-embryonic stages, the inner ear consists of a coiled cochlear duct. As seen in this cross-section, each duct consists of a region of developing, columnar epithelium (arrow). The scalae are not yet present. The cochlear ganglion cells are located adjacent to the differentiating cochlear ducts (arrowhead).

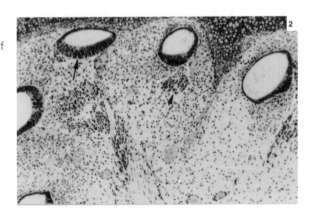

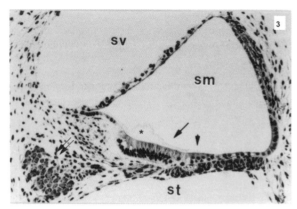

Fig. 12.3 The cochlea remains immature at birth in rodents. The inner hair cell (arrow) and outer hair cell (arrowhead) regions are identifiable and correspond to the regions of the greater and lesser epithelia ridges, respectively. The three scalae are present (sv, scala vestibuli; st, scale tympani; sm, scala media). The tectorial membrane (*) is not fully formed but is seen extending over the region of the greater epithelial ridge. The cochlear ganglion neurons are located adjacent to the sensory epithelium (double arrows).

inner ear structures. One of the first observable patterning events that occurs is the establishment of anteroposterior and dorsoventral axes that will set the stage for organization of future inner ear regions. Members of the bone morphogenetic protein family (BMPs), and molecules that antagonize the BMPs, help establish this early patterning (Barald & Kelley, 2004).

The ventral region of the otocyst gives rise to auditory (cochlear) regions of the inner ear, whereas the dorsal region will give rise to the vestibular structures (Fig. 12.4). A number of genes have been identified that either directly influence normal development of ventral (cochlear)

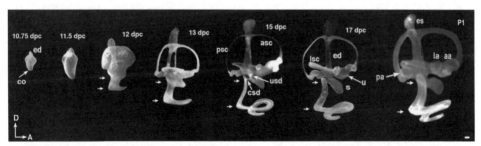

Fig. 12.4 Gross maturation of the mouse inner ear. A latex paint solution was used to fill the membranous labyrinths of mouse inner ears (from 10.75 days post coitum [dpc] through postnatal day 1 [P1]). The figure shows lateral views of the cochlear and vestibular regions of the inner ear. The cochlear region (co) begins to protrude from the ventral portion at 10.75 dpc and cochlear coiling is evident by 15 dpc. By 17 dpc, the gross anatomy of the mouse inner ear appears mature. The short arrows indicate the proximal region of the cochlea. Scale bar $=100 \mu m$. Ducts and sac: csd, cochleosaccular duct; ed, endolymphatic duct; usd, utriculosaccular duct; es, endolymphatic sac. Vestibular structures: aa, anterior ampulla; asc, anterior semicircular canal; la, lateral ampulla; lsc, lateral semicircular canal; pa, posterior ampulla; psc, posterior semicircular canal; s, saccule; u, utricle.
Adapted with permission from Cantos et al. (2000) © 2000, National Academy of Sciences, USA.

Table 12.1 Otic induction and differentiation of epithelium: molecules identified to date that are associated with initial formation of the otocyst and differentiation of sensory epithelia and associated structures. (The order of molecules in the table is consistent with the sequence discussed in the text)

Molecules in inner ear development	Identified role in inner ear development
Fibroblast growth factors (FGF proteins)	Otic induction, pillar cell formation
Bone morphogenetic proteins (BMP proteins)	Otic axis patterning
Sox2 (transcription factor)	Development of prosensory epithelium
p27^{kip1} (kinase inhibitor)	Regulation of mitosis, regulation of hair cell number
Atonal (Math1) (transcription factor)	Hair cell formation
Jagged/delta (ligand protein)	Inhibition of hair cell formation in Notch-expressing cells
Notch (receptor protein)	Cells expressing notch adopt support cell fate
Hes 1, Hes 5 (transcription factors)	Prevent hair cell formation in presumptive support cells
Pou4f3 (Brn3.1/Brn3c) (transcription factor)	Hair cell differentiation/survival
Retinoic acid (protein)	Regulation of hair cell number
Thyroid hormone	Differentiation of hair cells, maturation of organ of Corti, tectorial membrane formation, regulation of efferent innervation
Tectorin (protein)	Tectorial membrane formation
Otogelin (protein)	Tectorial membrane formation

structures, or regulate expression of other molecules needed for formation of ventral structures. Among the genes necessary for early specification and formation of auditory regions of the inner ear are *Six1* and sonic hedgehog (*Shh*). Deletion of either of these genes leads to a loss of cochlear sensory regions (Barald & Kelley, 2004).

The cochlea itself arises as a tubular extension, or outpocketing, from the ventromedial portion of the otocyst (Fig. 12.4, reviewed by Fritzsch *et al.*, 1998). As the cochlear duct elongates, it begins to spiral into the coiled cochlea (i.e. by E15 in the mouse, Cantos *et al.*, 2000; and by E16 in the rat, Nikolic *et al.*, 2000). The number of turns of the cochlear spiral will vary with species (for example: human, just over 2.5 turns; guinea pig, 4.5 turns). In the mouse, the cochlear duct begins to elongate at embryonic day (E) 12.5 and forms the final 1.5 turns by E17.5 (Lim & Anniko, 1985; Cantos *et al.*, 2000). In cross-section, the cochlear duct appears as a single chamber at each turn (Fig. 12.2). During this cochlear duct phase of development, the scala tympani and scala vestibuli have not yet opened. At approximately E18–19 in the rat, the scala vestibuli and scala tympani begin to open into the perilymphatic spaces, following a basal to apical gradient (Nikolic *et al.*, 2000), and are fully present by birth in rodents (Fig. 12.3).

The developing epithelium within the cochlear duct also begins patterning into specific cellular types shortly after otocyst formation (E12.5 in the mouse, Lim & Anniko, 1985; eight weeks post conception in human; reviewed in Lim & Rueda, 1992). Initially the ventral wall is two to three cell layers in thickness whereas the dorsal wall is six cell layers thick. The dorsal wall of the cochlear duct will give rise to the inner sulcus, spiral limbus, and organ of Corti (Fig. 12.1). Within the developing organ of Corti, two general developmental patterning gradients are observed. The mechanisms of such patterning will be discussed in more detail below. In general, there is a longitudinal basal to apical gradient of cellular differentiation (that begins in the mid-basal turn), and a neural (modiolar) to abneural (strial) gradient in which inner hair cells (IHCs) differentiate prior to each row of outer hair cells (OHCs). For example, in the human cochlea, the IHCs are detected prior to the OHCs, beginning ten to 11 weeks post conception. Mature OHCs and the surrounding Deiters' cells are not observed until approximately 30 weeks post conception in humans (Lavigne-Rebillard & Pujol, 1986)

As development proceeds (i.e. by E16 in the mouse), the epithelium of the dorsal wall of the cochlear duct differentiates further and is characterized by the greater (inner) and lesser (outer) epithelial ridges (GER and LER, respectively; Fig. 12.5). Cells from the GER will differentiate into the inner sulcus, spiral limbus, and probably the IHCs (reviewed by Kelley & Bianchi, 2001). The LER in contrast, will differentiate into OHCs, Deiters' cells, Claudius' cells, Hensen's cells, and Boettcher's cells (Fig. 12.5). The pillar cells form at the boundary between the GER and LER (Kelley & Bianchi, 2001). Together the pillar cells and basement membrane will form the border of the triangular shaped tunnel of Corti that arises later in development.

The inner sulcus forms as the GER recedes (Fig. 12.5). This occurs during the first postnatal week of development in rodents. Areas of cell death (apoptosis) are noted in the GER beginning at postnatal day 7 (P7) in the rat (Kamiya et al., 2001). The inner sulcus attains a mature state of formation by approximately P12 in mouse (Lim & Rueda, 1992). This is also the stage when the tunnel of Corti begins to form, attaining final maturation by P16 in mouse. In contrast, the

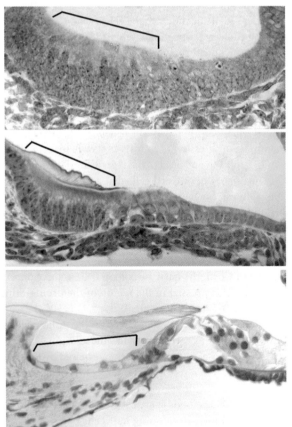

Fig. 12.5 Maturation of epithelial ridges. The brackets in the upper and middle panels mark the general region of the undifferentiated epithelium of the greater epithelial ridge (GER). (top panel, mouse, E14.5). In the middle panel, the future inner sulcus is seen below the developing tectorial membrane (mouse, P0). In the lower panel, the bracket outlines the inner sulcus of the adult inner ear.

spaces of Nuel, which surround OHC, do not reach mature form until P20, the stage when the mouse organ of Corti reaches its structural maturity (Lim & Rueda, 1992).

12.1.2 Hair cell differentiation

Cells in the cochlear duct proliferate to ensure that a sufficient pool of progenitor cells is obtained. These cells then differentiate into specific sensory or supporting cell types. Although the cells forming the floor of the cochlear duct appear homogeneous early in development (i.e. E12 in mouse), they already express markers that indicate they will give rise to sensory epithelium. For example, the transcription factor Sox2 is detected in the E12 mouse inner ear in the cells that will later give rise to the organ of Corti (Kiernan et al., 2005). Thus, this region is often called the 'prosensory region'. Hair cell development itself begins shortly after that (around E13 in mouse cochlea; see Figs 12.2, 12.5; reviewed by Kelley, 2006; Shim, 2006).

The cells of the cochlea proliferate in an orderly sequence. In the 1960s, Ruben (1967) determined the general pattern of proliferation and terminal mitosis in the mouse inner ear through a series of tritiated thymidine experiments. Using this marker, it was possible to establish that terminal mitosis of the various cell types occurred between E12 and E16 in an apical to basal gradient, that is, the majority of cells that are postmitotic at E12 were found in the cochlear apex, and those that were postmitotic at E16 were located in the base of the cochlea (Ruben, 1967). In most developing systems, cells undergo terminal mitosis, after which they begin to differentiate and take on specific phenotypic characteristics. In the organ of Corti, however, the cells differentiate in a basal to apical gradient, opposite to the gradient noted for terminal mitosis. The first cells that develop characteristics necessary for clear identification are the IHCs. The IHCs in mouse are recognized in the mid-basal turn of the cochlea at approximately E15. In contrast to the mid-basal region, cellular differentiation of the apical region does not occur until E18 in mouse (reviewed by Kelley & Bianchi, 2001). This means that in the apical region of the developing cochlea cells undergo terminal mitosis at E12, then 'wait' for approximately six days before undergoing differentiation.

The proliferating cells of the cochlear duct must exit the cell cycle in order to undergo final differentiation into hair or supporting cell types. $p27^{kip1}$ is a cyclin-dependent kinase inhibitor that induces exit from the cell cycle by stopping progression of mitosis (Kelley & Bianchi, 2001). It is expressed in the mouse cochlea from E12 to 14 in an apical to basal gradient (Chen & Segil, 1999; Lowenheim et al., 1999). By E14, all future organ of Corti cells that are Sox2 positive are also $p27^{kip1}$ positive (Kiernan et al., 2005). In mice lacking $p27^{kip1}$, there is an extended period of proliferation, yet eventually terminal mitosis and differentiation occur, which results in an overproduction of hair and supporting cells within the organ of Corti (Chen & Segil, 1999; Lowenheim et al., 1999). Thus, $p27^{kip1}$ is required for regulating the final number of cells that comprise the progenitor pool for the organ of Corti.

As terminal mitosis ends in the organ of Corti, the basic helix loop helix transcription factor Atonal1 (Atoh1, previously called Math1) is expressed in the region of the proliferating cells (Bermingham et al., 1999; Lanford et al., 2000; Chen et al., 2002, Woods et al., 2004). Expression of Atoh1 is dependent on Sox2 expression (Kiernan et al., 2005). atoh1 is the earliest gene shown to be sufficient for hair cell formation, possibly as early as E11 in mouse. Atoh1 expression is clearly detectable by E13 and extends along a basal to apical gradient (reviewed by Kelley, 2006). Deletion of atoh1 leads to loss of all hair cells and a secondary, indirect loss of supporting cells (Bermingham et al., 1999; Woods et al., 2004). Conversely, overexpression of atoh1 leads to induction of extra hair cells (Zheng & Gao, 2000; Woods et al., 2004; Jones et al., 2006).

As specification of the hair cell fate continues, developing hair cells begin to express the ligands Jagged2 (Jag2) and Delta 1 (Dll 1), both of which bind and activate the Notch receptors.

This pathway helps to regulate the number of cells that will develop as hair cells by inhibiting adjacent notch receptor-expressing cells from becoming hair cells and thereby causing them to adopt a supporting cell fate. The Notch1 receptor is first expressed in the developing cochlear duct at E12 in the mouse. This expression continues until early postnatal stages (at least P3 in mouse; Lewis et al., 1998; Lanford et al., 1999). Expression of the ligands Jag2 and Dll 2 begins slightly later at E13–14 in the mouse (Lanford et al., 1999; Morrison et al., 1999), prior to the stage when hair cell types are clearly distinguishable (E17 in mouse). Disruption of the Notch pathway leads to an increase in hair cells, particularly IHCs, which form a nearly complete second row in some mutations (Lanford et al., 1999; Zheng & Gao, 2000; Zine et al., 2001; Kiernan et al., 2005).

Hes1 and Hes5 are downstream targets of Notch signaling that are localized to supporting cells. Hes1 and Hes5 expression appears to be regulated by the Notch ligands. HES genes may lead to inhibition or downregulation of atoh1 to prevent formation of the hair cell phenotype in the cells that ultimately become supporting cells (reviewed by Kelley 2006; Shim, 2006).

12.1.3 Regulation of hair cell survival, number and patterning

Once cells are committed to a particular fate and begin to differentiate into a hair cell or supporting cell subtype, the cells come to rely on other factors to maintain survival. The transcription factors Pou4f3 (also previously identified as Brn3.1 or Brn3c), Gfi1and Barhl1 have all been implicated in maintaining hair cell survival. Comparisons of various mouse mutations suggests that Barhl1 is likely involved only in hair cell survival, whereas Pou4f3 and Gfi1 may regulate both differentiation and survival of hair cells (Kelley, 2006). Pou4f3 is one of the first genes detected in cells that become hair cells. Expression begins in the basal turns of the cochlea (i.e. E13.5 in mouse) and extends apically. In mice, the lack of Pou4f3 leads to a complete loss of hair cells by the early postnatal stages of development. These cells appear to go through the first stages of development before degenerating, suggesting that Pou4f3 must act at a specific, later, developmental point in the differentiation of hair cells (Erkman et al., 1996; Xiang et al., 1997, 1998).

Several proteins have been shown to regulate the number of hair cells produced. Among the proteins studied in most detail is retinoic acid (RA). RA is synthesized from vitamin A and plays numerous roles in different systems throughout embryonic development. Both RA and its receptors (RXR and RAR) are present in the developing organ of Corti (Kelley & Bianchi, 2001). Experimental preparations have demonstrated the importance of RA in regulating hair cell number. Exposure to RA increased the number of hair cells in cultured organ of Corti preparations. In contrast, antagonists to RA receptors inhibited hair cell formation. Such effects were greatest at E13–15 in mouse, corresponding to the period of hair cell differentiation (Kelley et al., 1993; Raz & Kelley, 1999). In addition to these in vitro studies, the role of RA receptors has been demonstrated in vivo. In mice lacking the genes for both RAR α and γ, formation of the spiral ganglion and organ of Corti failed to occur (reviewed by Mullen & Ryan, 2001). Thus, RA appears necessary for proper formation of cells within the organ of Corti.

Thyroid hormone also has been shown to be necessary for formation of cochlear structures and may influence the differentiation of hair cells (Table 12.1). In hypothyroid mice, which produce too little thyroid hormone, a variety of defects is noted. Similar defects are noted in mice lacking the thyroid receptor required for thyroid hormone signaling. These defects typically include: incomplete maturation of the organ of Corti, degeneration of at least some OHC, defects in tectorial membrane formation, alteration in the expression of voltage-gated ion channels, and defects in innervation to the cochlea from the efferent fibers (reviewed by Kelley & Bianchi, 2001; Walsh & McGee, 2001). In both humans and mice the effects of hypothyroidism tend to be highly variable and not all of the above defects will be noted in any one case (Kelley & Bianchi, 2001;

Walsh & McGee, 2001). One hypothesis is that thyroid hormone plays a role in regulating the rate of cellular differentiation. Any alteration in the timing of cellular differentiation would lead to defects in the final structural organization of the organ of Corti.

Changes in supporting cell development will also change the final structure of the organ of Corti, disrupting normal cochlear function. Members of the FGF family of proteins are known to influence a number of events in inner ear development. One function appears to be to regulate formation of the pillar cells. In mice lacking FGF3 for example, there is a loss of pillar cells. In contrast, when excess FGF3 was applied to organ of Corti cultures, an overproduction of pillar cells was observed (Colvin et al., 1996; Mueller et al., 2002). Further, in mice lacking the sprouty 2 (spry2) gene, which antagonizes FGF signaling, there is an increase in pillar cells and the formation of an ectopic tunnel of Corti (Shim et al., 2005). When the FGF receptor 1 gene (Fgfr1) is deleted in mice, there is a disruption of patterning such that small areas of sensory cells are found separated by large areas of unpatterned cells. It has been suggested that lack of FGF signaling leads to a decrease in the progenitor pool of cells needed to pattern the cochlear sensory epithelium (Pirvola et al., 2002; Barald & Kelley, 2004). Thus, FGFs may be involved in proliferation, differentiation and patterning of sensory and supporting cells in the organ of Corti.

Once specified, the cells of the sensory epithelium also appear to use migratory mechanisms to reach their final position. Ruben (1967) proposed a 'proliferative center' near the base of the cochlea from which hair cells would migrate to final positions. More recently, investigators have reported movement of hair cells in the mammalian organ of Corti in vitro (Bianchi et al., 2006) and in vivo (Chen et al., 2002; McKenzie et al., 2004). The in vivo studies suggested that the cells moved from the modiolar to strial edge, as well as along the basal to apical axis. Such movements appear necessary for the final patterning of cell types in the organ of Corti.

12.1.4 Stereocilia development

There are several unique morphological characteristics of hair cells that must develop in order for these cells to function properly. For example, the stereocilia bundle that gives hair cells their name is itself a highly organized structure that undergoes reorganization during development. Each of the 50–200 stereocilia of the bundle becomes organized in a staircase pattern with the tallest stereocilia on one side and subsequently shorter stereocilia next to each other (see also Chapter 8). The rows of stereocilia are connected to one another by a variety of external links that allow the bundle to bend as a unit (reviewed by Kelley, 2006). As stereocilia are deflected toward the tallest row, the hair cell becomes depolarized. In contrast, deflection toward the shortest stereocilia results in hyperpolarization (Hudspeth & Corey, 1977; Hudspeth & Jacobs, 1979).

As hair cells are forming, a single microtubule based cilium (a 'true' cilium) is formed in the center of the luminal surface of the hair cell. This will become the kinocilium, located adjacent to the row of tallest stereocilia. This kinocilium then moves outward along the luminal surface. In contrast to the kinocilium, the developing stereocilia contain a dense core of actin. These stereocilia form adjacent to the kinocilium. In humans, stereocilia begin forming at approximately 12 weeks post conception (Pujol et al., 1998). The stereocilia then undergo a process of reorientation necessary for proper function (Dabdoub & Kelley, 2005; Kelley, 2006).

A number of molecules have been identified that are responsible for the movement and reorientation of the sterocilia. Studies of gene mutations in both mice and humans revealed that disruptions in stereocilia bundle formation, or in the proper orientation of stereocilia, led to hearing loss or deafness. Among the critical stereocilia proteins identified to date are various myosins and cadherins, as well as whirlin, espin, wnt, and others (Kelley, 2006). As more is understood about sterecilia formation, it becomes quite clear that this developmental process alone is extremely complex and exquisitely organized (see Chapter 8).

12.1.5 Development of the tectorial membrane

The tectorial membrane is an acellular connective tissue that will overlie the sensory hair cells of the organ of Corti in the mature cochlea. The tectorial membrane is an integral part of the signal transduction process that either creates shearing movement to displace the stereocilia, or provides a resistive membrane against which stereocilia move in response to vibration of the basilar membrane (Zwislocki *et al.*, 1988). The tectorial membrane comprises proteins and glycoconjugates secreted laterally from the inner spiral sulcus region progressively to the IHC, and ultimately to the OHC region (reviewed by Lim & Rueda, 1992; Walsh & Romand, 1992). The mature tectorial membrane covers the organ of Corti prior to the onset of hearing. The proper development of this seemingly simple structure is crucial for normal hearing.

During embryonic development there are two observable regions of the tectorial membrane that will later fuse into a single membrane. The 'major' tectorial membrane develops from the GER and extends over the IHC, OHC, and supporting cells during late embryogenesis (by E18 in the mouse, rat; Lim & Rueda, 1992; Rueda *et al.*, 1996). The 'minor' tectorial membrane is formed from Deiters', Hensen's, and pillar cells associated with the LER (E19 in the mouse). During postnatal development, the major and minor tectorial membrane regions fuse (Lim & Rueda, 1992; Bianchi *et al.*, 1999) to form the mature tectorial membrane (by P12, mouse; Rueda *et al.*, 1996; gerbil; Souter *et al.*, 1997).

Several proteins are necessary for proper attachment and organization of the tectorial membrane (Table 12.1). In mice lacking the protein tectorin, for example, the TM is detached from the reticular lamina and the mice are deaf (Legan *et al.*, 2000). In mice lacking the protein otogelin, the fibrillar network of the tectorial membrane is disrupted leading to mechanical instability and hearing loss (Simler *et al.*, 2000). Thyroid hormone also appears necessary for tectorial membrane formation. In both hypothyroid mice and humans the tectorial membrane often shows defects in formation. These tectorial membrane defects, as well as the other inner ear malformations associated with hypothyroidism (see Section 12.1.3 above) lead to hearing loss.

12.2 Development of inner ear neurons and neural innervation patterns

As the development of the sensory epithelium progresses, the associated neurons are also undergoing a number of corresponding developmental events. In fact, in order to accomplish the precise tonotopic innervation found in the adult cochlea, coordinated interactions between hair cells and neurons must take place throughout embryonic and early postnatal stages of development.

In mammals, the IHCs receive approximately 92–94% of the total afferent innervation (arising from type I SGNs), whereas OHCs receive 6–8% of the afferent innervation (arising from type II SGNs). The IHCs and OHCs are innervated by distinct fiber bundles. The afferent radial fibers innervate the IHC, whereas the outer spiral bundle fibers extend to the OHC. In addition, efferent fibers arising in the brainstem extend in either the inner spiral bundle to the dendrites below IHC, or in the tunnel radial fibers to reach the OHC (see also Chapter 10). The general sequences of afferent and efferent innervation are outlined below, followed by a detailed description of factors currently known to be necessary for the formation and outgrowth of these fibers.

12.2.1 Afferent innervation patterns

The short radial afferent fibers enter the cochlear epithelium at about E16 in the mouse and innervate the IHCs near the point of entry. In the human cochlea, afferent dendrites contact hair cells at the eleventh to twelfth week post conception (Lavigne-Rebillard & Pujol, 1986). In mammals, the radial afferent fibers innervate the IHCs such that each IHC is contacted by about 20 fibers.

During development, the fibers may extend collaterals to more than one IHC, but by adulthood, these collaterals are lost and each nerve fiber innervates only one IHC. In contrast, the outer spiral fibers travel greater distances to contact the OHC. These fibers extend for several micrometers, growing close to the basilar membrane, across the forming tunnel of Corti, until they enter the OHC region. A single such fiber may provide collateral branches to OHC in the basal, middle and apical turns, as well as to nearby IHC (reviewed by Rubel & Fritzsch, 2002). Each OHC receives synaptic input from more than one collateral branch of an afferent fiber. Some of these collaterals may be retracted by maturity (Bergland & Ryugo, 1987), yet even in the mature organ of Corti, a single outer spiral fiber typically innervates five or more OHCs. In the adult, these outer spiral fibers reach up to 200–470 µm in length (Bergland & Ryugo, 1987).

12.2.2 Efferent innervation patterns

The cell bodies of cochlear efferent neurons are located in the olivocochlear nuclei of the brain-stem. These neurons form in rhombomeres 4 and 5 of the developing hindbrain (reviewed by Simmons, 2002). The lateral olivocochlear neurons are located in the lateral superior olivary nuclei and project mainly to the ipsilateral cochlea. In contrast, the medial olivocochlear neurons are found in the periolivary regions and project mainly to the contralateral cochlea to synapse on OHCs (Simmons, 2002; see also Chapter 10). It is generally thought that efferent fibers travel along existing afferent fibers to reach the appropriate target area (Simmons, 2002). Efferent fibers enter the mouse cochlea prenatally (approximately E14–15 in mouse), with fibers reaching the IHCs first, by approximately E15–16 in rodents (reviewed by Simmons, 2002). Growth continues throughout later stages of development, with fibers extending to the inner spiral bundle in the apical turn as late as P6 (Sobkowicz & Emmerling, 1989). In the human cochlea, efferent endings are found below the IHC at the fourteenth week post conception and beneath OHCs beginning at the twentieth week post conception (Lavigne-Rebillard & Pujol, 1990).

12.2.3 Formation of neurons

Studies in mouse, rat and chick have provided considerable information on the molecules that regulate the early formation, survival and outgrowth of auditory neurons. During early embry-onic inner ear development, the cochlear (auditory) and vestibular neurons form as a single complex designated the statoacoustic ganglion (SAG), or cochleovestibular ganglion (CVG). These neuroblasts originate along the anteroventral region of the otocyst, then delaminate and migrate to form the ganglion (Kelley & Bianchi, 2001). The SAG arises between E9 and E14 in the mouse (Ruben, 1967) and between E11.5 and E15.5 in the rat (Altman & Bayer, 1982). In contrast to the pattern of terminal mitosis seen for mammalian hair cells, the SGNs are generated in a basal to apical gradient. Proliferation occurs between E11 and E15, with a peak of activity around E13 in mouse (Ruben, 1967).

The formation of the SAG begins before otocyst formation is complete (Hemond & Morest, 1991) or shortly after otocyst formation (Despres & Romand, 1994). In mice lacking the tran-scription factor neurogenin 1, the SAG does not form at all (Ma et al., 1998). Neurogenins appear to regulate several early events in SAG development (Table 12.2). Neurogenin is thought to direct neuroblast delamination, as well as the expression of downstream bHLH proteins that regulate neuronal differentiation (Ma et al., 1998). Mice lacking neurogenin also lack efferent fibers to the inner ear (reviewed in Simmons, 2002), further demonstrating the importance of this transcrip-tion factor in influencing inner ear innervation patterns.

Another family of transcription factors found to regulate efferent neuron development is the GATA family. The GATA transcription factors appear to specify the fate of the cochlear efferent

Table 12.2 Neuronal differentiation and outgrowth: examples of molecules shown to be necessary for the formation, outgrowth, and/or guidance of auditory nerve fibers. (The order of the table is consistent with the order discussed in the text)

Molecules in neuronal development	Identified role inner ear development
Neurogenin (transcription factor)	Statoacoustic ganglion delamination and differentiation, regulation of efferent innervation
GATA (transcription factor)	Fate determination of cochlea efferent neurons
Brain-derived neurotrophic factor (BDNF) (protein)	Survival of primarily vestibular neurons
Neurotrophin-3 (NT-3) (protein)	Survival of primarily cochlear neurons
Glia cell line-derived neurotrophic factor (GDNF) (protein)	Survival of postnatal cochlear and vestibular neurons
Neural cell adhesion molecule (NCAM) (protein)	Axonal outgrowth
Ephrin/Eph (protein)	Axonal outgrowth/inhibition
Slit/Robo (protein)	Axonal outgrowth/inhibition
Netrins (protein)	Axonal outgrowth/inhibition
Semaphorins (protein)	Axonal outgrowth/inhibition

neurons. Further, loss of specific GATA family members has been associated with misdirected efferent fibers in mice (Simmons, 2002).

12.2.4 Growth factors in survival and outgrowth

Following delamination, SAG neurons begin to extend fibers to the developing sensory epithelium of the cochlear duct. During migration from the wall of the otocyst, the nerve cells do not appear to maintain any attachments with the differentiating sensory epithelium, and therefore nerve fibers must extend back across the wall of the otocyst in order for innervation to occur (Whitehead & Morest, 1985).

The otocyst itself seems to provide factors that help initiate the outgrowth of SAG nerve fibers back to the differentiating cochlear epithelium. The effect of the otocyst in promoting nerve fiber outgrowth has been demonstrated in a number of tissue culture experiments over the years. For example, tissue culture experiments demonstrated that mouse SAG fibers were able to grow into both the original otocyst, as well as a second otocyst transplanted next to the SAG (Van De Water & Ruben, 1984). Other preparations showed an increase in chicken SAG survival when the otocyst and SAG were cultured intact, compared with SAG cultured alone (Ard & Morest, 1985). Subsequent *in vitro* studies demonstrated that the otocyst also released a diffusible factor that influenced the survival and outgrowth of early-stage SAG (Lefebvre *et al.*, 1990; Bianchi & Cohan, 1991, 1993). Both the preparations demonstrating a contact-mediated, otocyst-derived influence, and those showing a diffusible otocyst-derived effect noted a limited developmental period in which the otocyst could produce this outgrowth promoting factor (Van De Water & Ruben, 1984, Bianchi & Cohan, 1991; Bianchi *et al.*, 1998). This otocyst-dervived factor (ODF) is secreted by chicken, mouse, and rat otocysts corresponding to the period of initial neurite outgrowth (E4–6 chick, E10–12, mouse, E11–14 rat). Although the identity of ODF has not been fully characterized, recent studies have demonstrated cytokines are co-factors in early SAG growth (Bianchi *et al.*, 2005).

Identified growth factor proteins regulate additional aspects of SAG survival and outgrowth. For example, members of the neurotrophin family of growth factors are known to be critical in regulating survival and growth of both cochlear and vestibular neurons. Brain-derived neuro-trophic factor (BDNF) and neurotrophin-3 (NT-3) have been detected in the developing inner ear at stages of initial neurite outgrowth. In addition, mRNA for the receptors for BDNF and NT-3 (trk B and trk C, respectively) are present in developing cochlear and vestibular ganglia beginning in the early stages of SAG development (reviewed by Fritzsch *et al.*, 1997). Comparison of BDNF and NT-3 knock-out mice revealed that by postnatal stages, mice lacking BDNF had a nearly complete loss of vestibular neurons, whereas mice lacking NT-3 had a significant, though incomplete loss, of cochlear neurons. Mice lacking both BDNF and NT-3 had nearly complete loss of innervation to both vestibular and cochlear regions beginning after E12.5. Similarly, mice lacking receptors for these neurotrophins, trk B and trk C, showed a reduction in vestibular and cochlear neurons after E13.5 (reviewed by Fritzsch *et al.*, 1997). Together, these experiments have demonstrated that BDNF and NT-3 are produced by the inner ear and required for cochlear and vestibular neuron survival beginning at mid embryogenesis.

Additional factors may be required for cochlear and vestibular neuron survival at later stages of development. For example, temporal changes have been noted in the ability of cochlear and vestibular neurons to respond to glia cell line-derived neurotrophic factor (GDNF). In the rat cochlea, GDNF is first detected at P7 in both IHCs and OHCs in the basal turn of the cochlea. By P9, hair cells throughout the cochlea express GDNF. However, at adult stages, only IHCs express GDNF mRNA (Ylikoski *et al.*, 1998). *In vitro* analysis revealed only a weak survival promoting effect of GDNF on cochlear neurons at E21, but a significant effect at P7 (Pirvola *et al.*, 1994). In both rat and chicken, GDNF family members appear to be survival- and neurite-promoting factors for late embryonic and maturing inner ear neurons, rather than early developing neurons (Ylikoski *et al.*, 1998; Hashino *et al.*, 1999).

By postnatal stages, cochlear neuron survival is dependent on a combination of factors such as neurotrophins, GDNF, and electrical stimulation. For example, survival of postnatal cochlear neurons (P5, rat) can be maintained in the presence of BDNF, NT-3, a cAMP analog, or membrane depolarization (Hegarty *et al.*, 1997). It is hypothesized that if the combination of factors falls below a critical threshold, then the mature neurons will not survive (Kelley & Bianchi, 2001).

Extracellular matrix (ECM) molecules are known to be critical for directing outgrowth of nerve fibers throughout embryonic development. Many ECM molecules provide favorable substrates for neurite growth and the location of these molecules in key areas of the cochlea may help to direct growth to appropriate target cells. A variety of ECM proteins have been detected in the inner ear and/or cochlear neurons including fibronection, laminin, neural cell adhesion molecule (NCAM) (Table 12.2), entactin, and cytotactin/tenascin C (reviewed by Whitlon *et al.*, 2000). In mice, NCAM immunoreactivity in the cochlea is detected from E17 (the earliest stage examined) through P7 (Whitlon & Rutishauser, 1990). Immunoreactivity is noted in all of the nerve fibers, surrounding the IHCs and OHCs, and in the basilar membrane. The temporospatial distribution of NCAM suggests it may have a role in directing afferent and/or efferent fibers in the organ of Corti from the time of first hair cell contact through early synaptogenesis (Whitlon & Rutishauser, 1990).

Tenascin C immunoreactivity is also expressed at high levels in areas of nerve fiber growth from E14 (the earliest stage examined) to P9 in the mouse (Whitlon *et al.*, 1999). Decreased immunoreactivity was reported after the period of early synaptogenesis (after P12). However, mice lacking tenascin have auditory reflexes and cochlear anatomy appears normal (Saga *et al.*, 1992). Thus, while tenascin may normally contribute to nerve fiber growth, other molecules may compensate for the absence of this molecule.

Several other secreted and membrane bound proteins are expressed in the developing inner ear to regulate nerve fiber outgrowth (Table 12.2). A somewhat surprising finding in recent years is that a single molecule can act as either an attractive or a repulsive cue under various conditions.

Molecules of this nature that are known to be expressed in the developing inner ear and regulate growth of cochlear or vestibular nerve fibers include: members of the Ephrin family of ligands and the associated Eph receptors (reviewed by Cramer, 2005); members of the slit family of ligands and the corresponding Robo receptors; Netrin molecules that are related to the extracellular matrix molecule laminin; and semaphorins (reviewed by Webber & Raz, 2006). Expression of these molecules has been detected from embryonic through postnatal stages, and specific growth-promoting and growth-inhibiting characteristics are beginning to be defined for each of the above family of molecules at the various stages of neural development. In the case of netrin and semaphorin knock-out mice, greater defects were noted in vestibular than in cochlear innervation, suggesting differential regulation of nerve fiber growth to these inner ear regions (Webber & Raz, 2006).

In addition to 'classic' growth-promoting molecules that direct afferent or efferent fibers, the presence of the $\alpha 9$ nicotinic acetylcholine receptor influences the formation of efferent terminals at the OHCs. The alpha $\alpha 9$ receptor is expressed on OHCs, and in mice lacking this receptor, OHCs are generally innervated by a single large terminal rather than several small terminals found on OHCs in wild-type animals (Vetter et al., 1999; see also Section 12.4.5).

In summary, several soluble and membrane-associated proteins produced in the cochlea at specific stages of development contribute to the complex, yet highly organized, pattern of afferent and efferent nerve fiber innervation. In recent years, our understanding of the cellular cues required for normal inner ear innervation has been greatly advanced, particularly through the use of in vitro assays and transgenic mice. As with other developing neuronal populations, innervation to the inner ear appears to rely on a combination of soluble and cell-associated cues that influence the survival, outgrowth, and/or guidance of SAG neurons.

12.3 Onset of hearing

The onset of hearing in any species is dependent on maturation of all regions of the external, middle, and inner ears, as well as the central auditory pathways. A number of morphological features must attain adult-like status in order for hearing to be possible. Such changes in the mammalian cochlea include: the formation of the scala tympani and scala vestibuli, differentiation of the sensory epithelium, development of mature innervation patterns, formation of the tunnel of Corti, formation of the tectorial membrane, and maturation of the ionic composition of cochlear fluids (reviewed by Walsh & Romand, 1992). This chapter provides a few examples of some of the developmental changes in the cochlea that are required prior to the onset of hearing.

As noted above, as a general rule, the cochlea matures in a basal to apical gradient, both morphologically and functionally. In rodents, the apical region is not fully differentiated until the first two to three postnatal weeks. In contrast, in humans the structural features needed for hearing are present prenatally (reviewed by Pujol et al., 1998). At 18–20 weeks post conception, the human cochlea has attained many of the morphological criteria needed for hearing (Lavigne-Rebillard & Pujol, 1990), including the opening of the tunnel of Corti and the formation of the spaces of Nuel. Near adult maturation of cochlear structures occurs at approximately 25 weeks post conception (Lim & Rueda, 1992).

In addition to the obvious need for the cellular maturation of cochlear structures and innervation patterns, the physiological capabilities of the inner ear must also mature. For example, in rodents the ionic composition of endolymph and perilymph is similar at birth (reviewed by Rubsamen & Lippe, 1998). However, during the first postnatal week, the endolymphatic potassium concentration increases to adult levels (reviewed by Rubsamen & Lippe, 1998). This increase in potassium concentration parallels the morphological maturation of the stria vascularis (Anniko *et al.*, 1979). In addition, during the second postnatal week in rodents, enzymes involved in regulating electrolyte balance begin to be produced in the stria vascularis at about the same time as the endocochlear potential (EP), the potential difference between the endolymph and perilymph, matures (Rubsamen & Lippe, 1998). Maturation of OHCs is required for generation of the cochlear microphonic (CM), the shift in voltage between the endolymph and perilymph that occurs during mechanotransduction. The maturation of the CM appears to parallel the development of the EP, and reaches mature levels by P18 in the gerbil (McGuirt *et al.*, 1995).

Consistent with the structural and physiological changes that take place in the rodent cochlea during the first two to three postnatal weeks, the onset of hearing also generally begins during the second to third postnatal weeks in rodents (Walsh & Romand, 1992). In contrast, in humans, because the criteria for hearing are met prenatally, neonates can respond to sound at birth. Human neonates demonstrate the ability to respond selectively to sound, showing particular responsiveness to certain vocalizations. Neonates are also capable of locating sound sources in a crude fashion, but require binaural experience with sound in order to fully develop sound localization abilities (reviewed by Werner & Gray, 1998).

An interesting paradox has been noted in the development of frequency selectivity in both rodents and humans. Although there is a basal (high frequency) to apical (low frequency) pattern of development in the cochlea, the first responses are detected to lower-middle frequencies. This occurs in early postnatal stages of rodents and during the first six months of human development. High frequency sensitivity then rapidly improves so that in both rodents and humans, absolute thresholds and frequency discrimination mature first for high frequencies, and then for low frequencies (Werner & Gray, 1998). These observations imply aspects of functional maturation that follow on the morphological gradients of development.

12.4 **Maturation of hair cell function**

During later cochlear development there is a gradual maturation of hair cell excitability and synaptic transmission that leads up to and encompasses the onset of hearing. Embryonic hair cells are capable of mechanotransduction many days before birth, and before the organism itself can respond to sound. For example, hair cell mechanotransduction can be demonstrated by E12 in chicken (Si *et al.*, 2003), several days before there is detectable auditory sensitivity (Jones *et al.*, 2006). Mechanotransduction has been measured in mammalian hair cells as early as E17–18 in rodents (Geleoc & Holt, 2003). Perhaps more importantly, immature hair cells express basolateral voltage-gated ion channels that differ markedly from the adult complement, giving rise to action potentials in the immature cochlear hair cells (Marcotti *et al.*, 2003b, 2004), an ability that is lost to the adult cell. Action potentials in immature hair cells can drive action potentials in cochlear afferent neurons before the onset of hearing (Glowatzki & Fuchs, 2002; Tritsch *et al.*, 2007). However, this spontaneous activity before the onset of hearing differs markedly from that of the mature cochlea. Single unit recordings in the VIIIth nerve show rhythmic, low-frequency bursts of action potentials before the onset of hearing in chickens (Jones & Jones, 2000; Jones *et al.*, 2001) and cats (Carlier *et al.*, 1975; Walsh & McGee, 1987; Jones *et al.*, 2007). It has been suggested that the rhythmic bursting of the immature cochlear afferents underlies activity-dependent synaptic sorting in the auditory brainstem (Jones *et al.*, 2007; Kros, 2007) as postulated similarly for retinal activity and organization of the lateral geniculate nucleus. Finally, substantial synaptic rearrangements take place near the onset of hearing in the mammalian cochlea. Most notably, IHCs receive considerable efferent inhibitory input during the first two postnatal weeks (Katz *et al.*, 2004), but this is lost as OHCs become the major postsynaptic efferent target. Work from several laboratories suggests that all these developmental events may be interdependent, although causal linkages remain to be determined.

12.4.1 **Onset of mechanotransduction**

As noted above (see Section 12.1.4) the typical stereociliary staircase of the hair bundle begins forming in late embryogenesis. Mechanotransducer currents in chicken cochlear hair cells are first recorded at E12 (Fig. 12.6) (Si *et al.*, 2003) near the time that staggered rows of stereocilia first appear (Tilney *et al.*, 1986). Mechanotransduction is also demonstrated by the accumulation of the fluorescent dye FM1-43, which is known to permeate open transducer channels (Gale *et al.*, 2001). Although mechanotransduction begins early, these initial hair cell responses are smaller, less sensitive, and with little or no inactivation compared with those of the mature hair cell (Fig. 12.6).

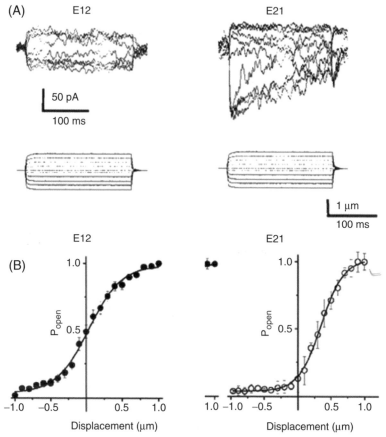

Fig. 12.6 Mechanoelectrical transduction currents appear at embryonic day 12 (E12) in acutely isolated basilar papilla hair cells of chicken. (A) Currents were elicited from hair cells at the midsection of the abneural segment of basilar papillas from E12 and E21. The apparent displacement (X) of hair bundles from the fluid jet (pressure clamp) as calibrated using simultaneous recordings captured on a video monitor is shown below the traces. Cells were held at −80 mV in the perforated-patch configuration. The magnitude of the total transduction current increased two- to threefold from E12 to E21. (B) Instantaneous displacement–response relationships from the mean data from five cells from E12 and seven cells from E21. Some error bars are omitted for clarity. The data were fit with a Boltzmann function and P_{open} at rest shifted from 0.5 at E12 to 0.15 at E21. The gating force (z) increased by approximately twofold from 143 at E12 to 367 at E21. Reproduced with permission from Si *et al.* (2003).

Indeed, chicken afferent neurons show marked sensitivity to sound only several days later, about E16 (Jones *et al.*, 2006). Mechanotransduction also has been studied in utricular hair cells of the embryonic mouse inner ear (Geleoc & Holt, 2003). This work shows that mechanotransducer currents can be recorded reliably in these cells at E17, and that the earliest responses are similar to those of mature cells in terms of resting open probability and adaptation. It is not known how hair cell development relates to vestibular function, but one might presume that as for cochlear hair cells, mechanotransduction occurs well in advance of overall vestibular function.

12.4.2 Spontaneous activity of afferent neurons

Spontaneous activity in the mature VIIIth nerve of birds and mammals ranges between 1 Hz and 100 Hz in different afferent neurons. Interval histograms of action potential activity in mammalian auditory afferent neurons show pseudo-Poisson behavior, with the probability of occurrence falling exponentially for longer intervals (Heil *et al.*, 2007). An exception occurs for afferent fibers in birds with characteristic frequencies below ~1 kHz, which have preferred intervals equal to the reciprocal of the characteristic frequency (Temchin, 1988). In contrast, spontaneous activity in afferent neurons of the immature cochlea occurs in low-frequency, rhythmic bursts (Jones *et al.*, 2001, 2007). These rhythmic bursts increase somewhat in frequency until near the onset of hearing, when the adult activity pattern takes over.

Both during and after maturation, spontaneous activity of cochlear afferent neurons depends on transmitter release from hair cells (Fig. 12.7) (Glowatzki & Fuchs, 2002; Robertson & Paki, 2002; Goutman & Glowatzki, 2007). Thus the developmental change in the pattern of activity presumably reflects changes in the excitability of the presynaptic hair cells and their patterns of transmitter release. It has been suggested that this rhythmic bursting may drive activity-dependent synaptic organization both peripherally and centrally, as thought to occur during retinal and visual system development (Jones *et al.*, 2007; Kros, 2007). The rhythmic discharges may in turn be driven, at least in part, by oscillations of membrane potential among supporting cells of the immature organ of Corti (Tritsch *et al.*, 2007; see Chapter 11). Waves of depolarization, calcium influx, and water-driven changes in cell shape spread across the developing epithelium as the onset of hearing approaches. These slow waves propagate through the release of ATP, which depolarizes both supporting cells and IHCs. In response, IHCs generate action potentials, releasing bursts of neurotransmitter onto afferent dendrites, which in turn then produce the bursting pattern of action potential activity. Thus, action potentials of immature IHCs couple cochlear supporting cell waves to afferent activity, at least in the second week after birth in mice and rats. Prior to that time IHCs may generate action potentials intrinsically (Marcotti *et al.*, 2003b), independent of supporting cell activity.

12.4.3 Maturation of excitability in cochlear hair cells

At about E17–18 in mice, IHCs begin to generate broad, slow calcium action potentials (Marcotti *et al.*, 2003b; Kros, 2007). These arise through the activity of voltage-dependent calcium and sodium channels to produce a regenerative depolarization, and through voltage-gated, delayed rectifier potassium channels that then repolarize the membrane. The voltage-gated calcium channels of hair cells are relatively large-conductance, barium permeant, dihydropyridine-sensitive calcium channels (Zidanic & Fuchs, 1995; Kollmar *et al.*, 1997; Engel *et al.*, 2002), related to the voltage-gated calcium channels of cardiac muscle and encoded by a related gene *a1D*, or *CaV1.3* (Kollmar *et al.*, 1997; Platzer *et al.*, 2000; Hafidi & Dulon, 2004). When this gene is knocked out, calcium currents of IHC are reduced by more than 90% (Platzer *et al.*, 2000; Brandt *et al.*, 2003). A change in calcium channel expression is observed throughout the first two postnatal weeks in

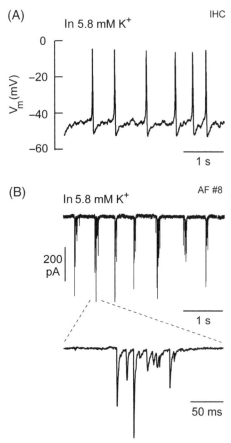

Fig. 12.7 Action potentials in postnatal inner hair cells (IHCs) and synaptic bursts in afferent fibers, as assessed by whole cell recordings. (A) Current-clamp recording from IHC showing spontaneous Ca^{2+} action potentials (1–2 Hz) common before the onset of hearing (~P12). (B) Voltage-clamp recordings (V_h = −94 mV) from afferent fibers showing bursts of excitatory postsynaptic currents (EPSCs). EPSC bursts occurred with a duration and frequency similar to those of IHC Ca^{2+} action potentials (compare with A) and are probably caused by them.
Reproduced with permission from Glowatzki and Fuchs (2002).

rats and mice. These increase progressively in number, reaching a peak density at P6 in mice, and falling thereafter (Beutner & Moser, 2001; Johnson *et al.*, 2005).

After the onset of hearing at approximately P12 the IHCs cease to generate action potentials. This results from several nearly contemporaneous changes. The number of voltage-gated calcium channels drops sharply, to about one-third of the previous peak (Beutner & Moser, 2001; Marcotti *et al.*, 2003b). Perhaps more importantly, a large, rapidly activating potassium current appears (Kros & Crawford, 1990; Kros *et al.*, 1998) that acts to prevent regenerative depolarization (Fig. 12.8). In addition, a voltage-gated potassium current (carried by KCNQ4 channels) with a very negative activation range, appears and strongly influences the resting membrane conductance (Marcotti *et al.*, 2003a). The net result of these changes is that the hair cell becomes inexcitable, responding to current injection with a linear change in membrane voltage, enabling a more faithful encoding of stimulus intensity. And, because the large resting conductance reduces

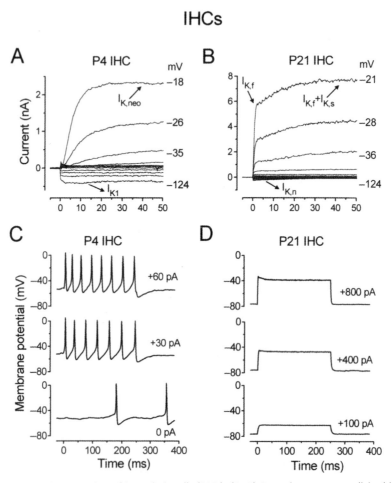

Fig. 12.8 Functional maturation of inner hair cells (IHCs). (A, B) Potassium currents elicited in voltage clamp of (A) pre- and (B) post-hearing IHC. The membrane potential for each record is shown to the right. Potassium currents are slower and smaller in the younger hair cell. (C) Consequently, young IHCs can generate action potentials. (D) Mature IHCs have a lower input resistance (amplitude of current injection shown to the right of each record), and a rapid, passive voltage response.

Reproduced with permission from Goodyear et al. (2006).

the membrane time constant, the hair cell achieves better temporal resolution. Intriguingly, although the number of voltage-gated calcium channels is reduced, calcium-dependent transmitter release, as measured by the increase in membrane capacitance that results from vesicular fusion, becomes more efficient in the mature hair cell (Beutner & Moser, 2001; Johnson et al., 2005), compensating for the drop in calcium influx.

12.4.4 Effects of thyroid hormone on cochlear development

Thyroid hormone receptors are required for the normal development of hearing (see Section 12.1.3). Mutations in thyroid hormone receptor β (TRβ) are associated with hearing loss in humans and in a mouse model. Cochlear morphology appears to be normal, but the developmental acquisition of the fast outward potassium current is delayed (Rusch *et al.*, 1998). Hypothyroid IHCs maintain high numbers of calcium channels and generate action potentials into the third postnatal week, and remain immature with respect to transmitter release efficiency and the persistence of efferent synapses (Brandt *et al.*, 2007; Sendin *et al.*, 2007).

12.4.5 Efferent innervation of inner hair cells

In addition to the alterations in voltage-gated basolateral ionic channels, IHCs also show a developmental progression in ligand-gated channels. In particular, neonatal IHCs respond to acetylcholine (ACh) with a biphasic membrane current that is carried by the sequential activation of α9α10 ACh receptors (AChRs; Elgoyhen *et al.*, 1994, 2001) and calcium-activated potassium channels encoded by the *SK2* gene (Dulon *et al.*, 1998) (see Chapter 10). This cholinergic sensitivity is present as early as P2 in mice (Marcotti *et al.*, 2004), then disappears after P12 (Katz *et al.*, 2004). Along with sensitivity to exogenous ACh, IHCs display transient currents with identical pharmacology and ionic dependencies due to ACh release from efferent contacts (Glowatzki & Fuchs, 2000; Goutman *et al.*, 2005). These contacts are thought to be made by the medial olivocochlear efferent fibers, synapsing temporarily there before taking permanent positions on OHCs (Simmons, 2002). This efferent input is strong enough to prevent action potential activity in the IHCs, but it is not known whether the efferents are active normally in the neonatal cochlea, or what purpose they might serve. One intriguing possibility was raised in studies on kittens in which sectioning of efferent axons led to lost sensitivity and frequency selectivity in afferent neurons of those animals one year later (Walsh *et al.*, 1998). Thus, normal maturation of hair cell function may depend on as yet unknown interactions between efferent and afferent neurons with hair cells.

12.5 Conclusion

In summary, this chapter provides an overview of the primary developmental events that take place from the formation of the inner ear at the otocyst stage, through differentiation of sensory structures and neural innervation patterns, to some of the anatomical and physiological requirements for the onset of hearing. Throughout the chapter, molecules demonstrated to have a significant effect on inner ear development were described. However, these are only a sampling of the molecules investigated to date, and each year, auditory scientists discover additional molecules that regulate specific aspects of inner ear development. Our understanding of the signals that govern the development of 'one of the most remarkable displays of microengineering in the vertebrate body' (Swanson *et al.*, 1990) can only continue to expand as scientists identify more regulatory mechanisms and develop new technologies to manipulate and examine the process of inner ear development.

Acknowledgments

The authors thank Matthew Kelley for generously preparing the photomicrographs in Figure 12.5, Doris Wu for providing Figure 12.2, and Forrest Rose for assistance in final preparation of the figures.

References

Altman J & Bayer S. (1982) Development of the cranial nerve ganglia and related nuclei in the rat. *Adv Anat Embryol Cell Biol* **74**: 1–90.

Anniko M, Wroblewski R & Wersall J. (1979) Development of endolymph during maturation of the mammalian inner ear: a preliminary report. *AMA Arch Otolaryngol* **225**: 161–3.

Ard MD & Morest DK. (1985) Trophic interactions between the cochleovestibular ganglion of the chick embryo and its synaptic targets in culture. *Neuroscience* **16**: 151–70.

Barald KF & Kelley MW. (2004) From placode to polarization: new tunes in inner ear development. *Development* **131**: 4119–30.

Bergland AM & Ryugo DK. (1987) Hair cell innervation by spiral ganglion neurons in the mouse. *J Comp Neurol* **255**: 560–70.

Bermingham NA, Hassan BA, Price SD, Vollrath MA, Ben-Arie N, Eatock RA, Bellen HJ, Lysakowski A & Zoghbi HY. (1999) Math1: an essential gene for the generation of inner ear hair cells. *Science* **284**: 1837–41.

Beutner D & Moser T. (2001) The presynaptic function of mouse cochlear inner hair cells during development of hearing. *J Neurosci* **21**: 4593–9.

Bianchi LM & Cohan CS. (1991) Developmental regulation of a neurite-promoting factor influencing statoacoustic neurons. *Brain Res Dev Brain Res* **64**: 167–74.

Bianchi LM & Cohan CS. (1993) The effects of neurotrophins and CNTF on developing statoacoustic neurons: comparison with an otocyst-derived factor. *Dev Biol* **159**: 353–65.

Bianchi, LM, Dolnick R, Medd AM & Cohan CS. (1998) Developmental changes in growth factors released by the embryonic inner ear. *Exp Neurol* **150**: 98–106.

Bianchi LM, Lui H, Krug EK & Capehart AC. (1999) Selective and transient expression of a native chondroitin sulfate epitope in Deiters' cells, Pillar cells and the developing tectorial membrane. *Anat Rec* **256**: 64–71.

Bianchi LM, Daruwalla Z, Roth TM, Attia N, Lukacs NW, Richards A-L, Roth TM, White IO, Allen SJ & Barald KF. (2005) Immortalized mouse inner ear cell lines reveal a role for chemokines in promoting the growth of developing statoacoustic ganglion neurons. *J Assoc Res Otolaryngol* **6**: 355–67.

Bianchi LM, Huri D & White IO. (2006) Embryonic inner ear cells use migratory mechanisms to establish cell patterns in vitro. *J Neurosci Res* **83**: 191–8.

Brandt A, Striessnig J & Moser T. (2003) CaV1.3 channels are essential for development and presynaptic activity of cochlear inner hair cells. *J Neurosci* **23**: 10832–40.

Brandt N, Kuhn S, Munkner S, Braig C, Winter H, Blin N, Vonthein R, Knipper M & Engel J. (2007) Thyroid hormone deficiency affects postnatal spiking activity and expression of Ca^{2+} and K^+ channels in rodent inner hair cells. *J Neurosci* **27**: 3174–86.

Cantos R, Cole LK, Acampora D, Simeone A & Wu DK. (2000) Patterning of the mammalian cochlea. *Proc Natl Acad Sci U S A* **97**: 11707–17.

Carlier E, Abonnenc M & Pujol R. (1975) Maturation of unitary responses to tonal stimulation in the cochlear nerve of the kitten. *J Physiol (Paris)* **70**: 129–38.

Chen P & Segil N. (1999) p27(Kip1) links cell proliferation to morphogenesis in the developing organ of Corti. *Development* **126**: 1581–90.

Chen P, Johnson JE, Zoghbi HY & Segil N. (2002) The role of Math1 in inner ear development: uncoupling the establishment of the sensory primordium from hair cell fate determination. *Development* **129**: 2495–505.

Colvin JS, Bohne BA, Harding GW, McEwen DG & Ornitz DM. (1996) Skeletal overgrowth and deafness in mice lacking fibroblast growth factor receptor 3. *Nat Genet* **12**: 390–7.

Cramer K. (2005) Eph proteins and the assembly of auditory circuits. *Hear Res* **206**: 42–51.

D'Amico-Martel A. (1982) Temporal patterns of neurogenesis in avian cranial sensory and autonomic ganglia. *Am J Anat* **163**: 351–72.

D'Amico-Martel A & Noden DM. (1983) Contribution of placode and neural crest cells to avian cranial peripheral ganglia. *Am J Anat* **166**: 445–68.

Dabdoub A & Kelley MW. (2005) Planar polarity and a potential role for a wnt morphogen gradient in stereociliary bundle orientation in the mammalian inner ear. *J Neurobiol* **64**: 446–57.

Despres G & Romand R. (1994) Neurotrophins and the development of cochlear innervation. *Life Sci* **54**: 1291–7.

Dulon D, Luo L, Zhang C & Ryan AF. (1998) Expression of small-conductance calcium-activated potassium channels (SK) in outer hair cells of the rat cochlea. *Eur J Neurosci* **10**: 907–15.

Elgoyhen AB, Johnson DS, Boulter J, Vetter DE & Heinemann S. (1994) Alpha 9: an acetylcholine receptor with novel pharmacological properties expressed in rat cochlear hair cells. *Cell* **79**: 705–15.

Elgoyhen AB, Vetter DE, Katz E, Rothlin CV, Heinemann SF & Boulter J. (2001) Alpha10: a determinant of nicotinic cholinergic receptor function in mammalian vestibular and cochlear mechanosensory hair cells. *Proc Natl Acad Sci U S A* **98**: 3501–6.

Engel J, Michna M, Platzer J & Striessnig J. (2002) Calcium channels in mouse hair cells: function, properties and pharmacology. *Adv Otorhinolaryngol* **59**: 35–41.

Erkman L, McEvilly RJ, Luo L, Ryan AK, Hooshmand F, O'Connell SM, Keithley EM, Rapaport DH, Ryan A & Rosenfeld MG. (1996) Role of transcription factors Brn-3.1 and Brn-3.2 in auditory and visual system development. *Nature* **381**: 603–6.

Fritzsch B, Silos-Santiago I, Bianchi LM & Farinas I. (1997) Role of neurotrophic factors in regulating inner ear innervation. *Trends Neurosci* **20**: 159–64.

Fritzsch B, Barald KF & Lomax MI. (1998) Early embryology of the vertebrate inner ear. In: Rubel E, Popper AN & Fay RF, eds. *Development of the Auditory System*. Springer-Verlag, New York, pp. 80–145.

Gale JE, Marcotti W, Kennedy HJ, Kros CJ & Richardson GP. (2001) FM1-43 dye behaves as a permeant blocker of the hair-cell mechanotransducer channel. *J Neurosci* **21**: 7013–25.

Geleoc GS & Holt JR. (2003) Developmental acquisition of sensory transduction in hair cells of the mouse inner ear. *Nat Neurosci* **6**: 1019–20.

Glowatzki E & Fuchs PA. (2000) Cholinergic synaptic inhibition of inner hair cells in the neonatal mammalian cochlea. *Science* **288**: 2366–8.

Glowatzki E & Fuchs PA. (2002) Transmitter release at the hair cell ribbon synapse. *Nat Neurosci* **5**: 147–54.

Goutman JD & Glowatzki E. (2007) Time course and calcium dependence of transmitter release at a single ribbon synapse. *Proc Natl Acad Sci U S A* **104**: 16341–6.

Goutman JD, Fuchs PA & Glowatzki E. (2005) Facilitating efferent inhibition of inner hair cells in the cochlea of the neonatal rat. *J Physiol* **566**: 49–59.

Hafidi A & Dulon D. (2004) Developmental expression of Ca(v)1.3 (alpha1d) calcium channels in the mouse inner ear. *Brain Res Dev Brain Res* **150**: 167–75.

Hashino E, Dolnick RY & Cohan CS. (1999) Developing vestibular ganglion neurons switch trophic sensitivity from BDNF to GDNF after target innervation. *J Neurobiol* **15**: 414–27.

Hegarty JL, Kay AR & Green SH. (1997) Trophic support of cultured spiral ganglion neurons by depolarization exceeds and is additive with that by neurotrophins or cAMP and requires elevation of [Ca2+]i within a set range. *J Neurosci* **17**: 1959–70.

Heil P, Neubauer H, Irvine DR & Brown M. (2007) Spontaneous activity of auditory-nerve fibers: insights into stochastic processes at ribbon synapses. *J Neurosci* **27**: 8457–74.

Hemond SG & Morest DK. (1991) Ganglion formation from the otic placode and the otic crest in the chick embryo: Mitosis, migration and the basal lamina. *Anat Embryol (Berl)* **184**: 1–13.

Hudspeth AJ & Corey DP. (1977) Sensitivity, polarity and conductance change in the response of vertebrate hair cells to controlled mechanical stimuli. *Proc Natl Acad Sci U S A* **74**: 2407–11.

Hudspeth AJ & Jacobs R. (1979) Stereocilia mediate transduction in vertebrate hair cells (auditory system/ cilium/vestibular system). *Proc Natl Acad Sci U S A* **76**: 1506–9.

Johnson SL, Marcotti W & Kros CJ. (2005) Increase in efficiency and reduction in Ca^{2+} dependence of exocytosis during development of mouse inner hair cells. *J Physiol* **563**: 177–91.

Jones JM, Montcouquiol M, Dabdoub A, Woods C & Kelley MW. (2006) Inhibitors of differentiation and DNA binding (Ids) regulate Math1 and hair cell formation during the development of the organ of Corti. *J Neurosci* **26**: 550–8.

Jones TA & Jones SM. (2000) Spontaneous activity in the statoacoustic ganglion of the chicken embryo. *J Neurophysiol* **83**: 1452–68.

Jones TA, Jones SM & Paggett KC. (2001) Primordial rhythmic bursting in embryonic cochlear ganglion cells. *J Neurosci* **21**: 8129–35.

Jones TA, Jones SM & Paggett KC. (2006) Emergence of hearing in the chicken embryo. *J Neurophysiol* **96**: 128–41.

Jones TA, Leake PA, Snyder RL, Stakhovskaya O & Bonham B. (2007) Spontaneous discharge patterns in cochlear spiral ganglion cells before the onset of hearing in cats. *J Neurophysiol* **98**: 1898–908.

Katz E, Elgoyhen AB, Gomez-Casati ME, Knipper M, Vetter DE, Fuchs PA & Glowatzki E. (2004) Developmental regulation of nicotinic synapses on cochlear inner hair cells. *J Neurosci* **24**: 7814–20.

Kamiya K, Takahashi K, Kitamura K, Momoi T & Yoshikawa Y. (2001) Mitosis and apoptosis in postnatal auditory system of the C3H/He strain. *Brain Res* **901**: 296–302.

Kelley MW. (2006) Hair cell development: Commitment through differentiation. *Brain Res* **1091**: 172–85.

Kelley MW & Bianchi LM. (2001) Developmental and neuronal innervation of the organ of Corti. In: Willet J, ed. *Handbook of Auditory Neuroscience*. CRC Press, Boca Raton, FL, pp. 137–56.

Kelley MW, Xu XM, Wagner MA, Warchol ME & Corwin JT. (1993) The developing organ of Corti contains retinoic acid and forms supernumerary hair cells in response to exogenous retinoic acid in culture. *Development* **119**: 1041–53.

Kiernan AE, Pelling AL, Leung KKH, Tang ASP, Bell DM, Tease C, Lovell-Badge R, Steel KP & Cheah KSE. (2005) Sox2 is required for sensory organ development in the mammalian inner ear. *Nature* **434**: 1031–5.

Kollmar R, Montgomery LG, Fak J, Henry LJ & Hudspeth AJ. (1997) Predominance of the alpha1D subunit in L-type voltage-gated Ca^{2+} channels of hair cells in the chicken's cochlea. *Proc Natl Acad Sci U S A* **94**: 14883–8.

Kros CJ. (2007) How to build an inner hair cell: challenges for regeneration. *Hear Res* **227**: 3–10.

Kros CJ & Crawford AC. (1990) Potassium currents in inner hair cells isolated from the guinea-pig cochlea. *J Physiol* **421**: 263–91.

Kros CJ, Ruppersberg JP & Rusch A. (1998) Expression of a potassium current in inner hair cells during development of hearing in mice. *Nature* **394**: 281–4.

Lanford PJ, Lan Y, Jiang R, Lindsell C, Weinmaster G, Gridley T & Kelley MW. (1999) Notch signalling pathway mediates hair cell development in mammalian cochlea. *Nat Genet* **21**: 289–92.

Lanford PJ, Shailam R, Norton CR, Gridley T & Kelley MW. (2000) Expression of Math1 and HES5 in the cochleae of wildtype and Jag2 mutant mice. *J Assoc Res Otolaryngol* **1**: 161–71.

Lavigne-Rebillard M & Pujol R. (1986) Development of the auditory hair cell surface in human fetuses. A scanning electron microscopy study. *Anat Embryol (Berl)* **174**: 360–77.

Lavigne-Rebillard M & Pujol R. (1990) Auditory hair cells in human fetuses: synaptogenesis and ciliogenesis. *J Electron Microsc Tech* **15**: 115–22.

Lefebvre P, Van De Water TR, Weber T, Rogister B & Moonen G. (1990) Growth factor interactions in cultures of dissociated adult acoustic ganglia: neuronotrophic effects. *Brain Res* **567**: 306–12.

Legan PK, Lukashkina VA, Goodyear RJ, Kossi M, Russell IJ & Richardson GP. (2000) A targeted deletion in alpha-tectorin reveals that the tectorial membrane is required for the gain and timing of cochlear feedback. *Neuron* **28**: 273–85.

Lewis AK, Frantz GD, Carpenter DA, de Sauvage FJ & Gao WQ. (1998) Distinct expression patterns of notch family receptors and ligands during development of the mammalian inner ear. *Mech Dev* **78**: 159–63.

Lim DJ & Anniko M. (1985) Developmental morphology of the mouse inner ear. A scanning electron microscopic observation. *Acta Otolaryngol Suppl* **422**: 1–69.

Lim DJ & Rueda J. (1992) Structural development of the cochlea. In: Romand R, ed. *Development of Auditory and Vestibular Systems 2*. Elsevier, Amsterdam, pp. 33–58.

Lowenheim H, Furness DN, Kil J, Zinn C, Gultig K, Fero ML, Frost D, Gummer AW, Roberts JM, Rubel EW, Hackney CM & Zenner HP. (1999) Gene disruption of p27(Kip1) allows cell proliferation in the postnatal and adult organ of corti. *Proc Natl Acad Sci U S A* **96**: 4084–8.

Ma Q, Chen Z, del Barco Barrante I, de la Pompa JL & Anderson DJ. (1998) Neurogenin 1 is essential for the determination of neuronal precursors for proximal cranial sensory ganglia. *Neuron* **20**: 469–82.

Marcotti W, Johnson SL, Holley MC & Kros CJ. (2003a) Developmental changes in the expression of potassium currents of embryonic, neonatal and mature mouse inner hair cells. *J Physiol* **548**: 383–400.

Marcotti W, Johnson SL, Rusch A & Kros CJ. (2003b) Sodium and calcium currents shape action potentials in immature mouse inner hair cells. *J Physiol* **552**: 743–61.

Marcotti W, Johnson SL & Kros CJ. (2004) A transiently expressed SK current sustains and modulates action potential activity in immature mouse inner hair cells. *J Physiol* **560**: 691–708.

McGuirt JP, Schmiedt RA & Schulte BA. (1995) Development of cochlear potentials in the neonatal gerbil. *Hear Res* **84**: 52–60.

McKenzie E, Krupin A & Kelley MW. (2004) Cellular growth and rearrangement during the development of the mammalian organ of Corti. *Dev Dyn* **229**: 802–12.

Morrison A, Hodgetts C, Gossler A, Hrabe de Angelis M & Lewis J. (1999) Expression of delta1 and serrate1 (jagged1) in the mouse inner ear. *Mech Dev* **84**: 169–72.

Morsli H, Choo D, Ryan A, Johnson R & Wu DK. (1998) Development of the mouse inner ear and origin of its sensory organs. *J Neurosci* **18**: 3327–35.

Mueller KL, Jacques BE & Kelley MW. (2002) Fibroblast growth factor signaling regulates pillar cell development in the organ of Corti. *J Neurosci* **22**: 9368–77.

Mullen LM & Ryan AF. (2001) Transgenic mice: genome manipulation and induced mutations. In: Willet J, ed. *Handbook of Auditory Neuroscience.* CRC Press, Boca Raton, FL, pp. 457–74.

Nikolic P, Jarlebark LE, Billet TE & Thorne PR. (2000) Apoptosis in the developing rat cochlea and its related structures. *Brain Res Dev Brain Res* **119**: 75–83.

Pirvola U, Arumae U, Moshnyakov M, Palgi J, Saarma M & Ylikoski J. (1994) Coordinated expression and function of neurotrophins and their receptors in the rat inner ear during target innervation. *Hear Res* **75**: 131–44.

Pirvola U, Ylilkoski J, Trokovic R, Herbert JM, McConnell SK & Partanen J. (2002) FGFR1 is required for the development of the auditory sensory epithelium. *Neuron* **35**: 6717–680.

Platzer J, Engel J, Schrott-Fischer A, Stephan K, Bova S, Chen H, Zheng H & Striessnig J. (2000) Congenital deafness and sinoatrial node dysfunction in mice lacking class D L-type Ca^{2+} channels. *Cell* **102**: 89–97.

Pujol R, Lavigne-Rebillard M & Lenoir M. (1998) Development of sensory and neural structures in the mammalian cochlea. In: Rubel EW, Popper AN & Fay RR, eds. *Development of the Auditory System.* Springer, New York, pp. 146–92.

Raz Y & Kelley MW. (1999) Retinoic acid signaling is necessary for the development of the organ of Corti. *Dev Biol* **213**: 180–93.

Robertson D & Paki B. (2002) Role of L-type Ca^{2+} channels in transmitter release from mammalian inner hair cells, II. Single-neuron activity. *J Neurophysiol* **87**: 2734–40.

Rubel EW & Fritzsch B. (2002) Auditory system development: primary auditory neurons and their targets. *Annu Rev Neurosci* **25**: 51–101.

Ruben RJ. (1967) Development of the inner ear of the mouse: a radioautographic study of terminal mitoses. *Acta Otolaryngol Suppl* **220**: 1–44.

Rubsamen R & Lippe WR. (1998) The development of cochlear function. In: Rubel E, Popper AN & Fay RF, eds. *Development of the Auditory System 2.* Springer-Verlag, New York, pp. 193–270.

Rueda J, Cantos R & Lim DJ. (1996) Tectorial membrane-organ of Corti relationship during cochlear development. *Anat Embryol (Berl)* **194**: 501–14.

Rusch A, Erway LC, Oliver D, Vennstrom B & Forrest D. (1998) Thyroid hormone receptor beta-dependent expression of a potassium conductance in inner hair cells at the onset of hearing. *Proc Natl Acad Sci U S A* **95**: 15758–62.

Saga Y, Yagi T, Ikawa Y, Sakakura T & Aizawa S. (1992) Mice develop normally without tenascin. *Genes Dev* **6**: 1821–31.

Sendin G, Bulankina AV, Riedel D & Moser T. (2007) Maturation of ribbon synapses in hair cells is driven by thyroid hormone. *J Neurosci* 27: 3163–73.

Sher AE. (1971) The embryonic and postnatal development of the inner ear of the mouse. *Acta Otolaryngol Suppl* 285: 1–19.

Shim K. (2006) The auditory sensory epithelium: the instrument of sound perception. *Int J Biochem Cell Biol* 38: 1827–33.

Shim K, Minowada G, Coling DE & Martin GR. (2005) Sprouty2, a mouse deafness gene, regulates cell fate decisions in the auditory sensory epithelium by antagonizing FGF signaling. *Dev Cell* 8: 553–64.

Si F, Brodie H, Gillespie PG, Vazquez AE & Yamoah EN. (2003) Developmental assembly of transduction apparatus in chick basilar papilla. *J Neurosci* 23: 10815–26.

Simler MC, Cohen-Salmon M, El-Amaoui A, Guillard L, Benichou JC, Petit C & Panthier JJ. (2000) Targeted disruption of otog results in deafness and severe imbalance. *Nat Genet* 24: 139–43.

Simmons DD. (2002) Development of the inner ear efferent system across vertebrate species. *J Neurobiol* 53: 228–50.

Sobkowicz HM & Emmerling MR. (1989) Development of acetylcholinesterase-positive neuronal pathways in the cochlea of mouse. *J Neurocytol* 18: 209–24.

Souter M, Nevell G & Forge A. (1997) Postnatal maturation of the organ of Corti in gerbils: morphology and physiological responses. *J Comp Neurol* 386: 635–51.

Swanson GJ, Howard M & Lewis J. (1990) Epithelial autonomy in the development of the inner ear of a bird embryo. *Dev Biol* 137: 243–57.

Temchin AN. (1988) Unusual discharge patterns of single fibers in the pigeon's auditory nerve. *J Comp Physiol A* 163: 99–115.

Tilney LG, Tilney MS, Saunders JS & DeRosier DJ. (1986) Actin filaments, stereocilia, and hair cells of the bird cochlea, III. The development and differentiation of hair cells and stereocilia. *Dev Biol* 116: 100–18.

Tritsch NX, Yi E, Gale JE, Glowatzki E & Bergles DE. (2007) The origin of spontaneous activity in the developing auditory system. *Nature* 450: 50–5.

Van De Water TR & Ruben RJ. (1984) Neurotrophic interactions during in vitro development of the inner ear. *Ann Otol Rhinol Laryngol* 93: 558–64.

Vetter DE, Liberman MC, Mann J, Barhanin J, Boulter J, Brown MC, Saffiote-Kolman, J, Heinemen SF & Elgoyhen AN. (1999) Role of alpha-9 nicotinic Ach receptor subunits in the development and function of cochlear efferent innervation. *Neuron* 23: 93–103.

Walsh EJ & McGee J. (1987) Postnatal development of auditory nerve and cochlear nucleus neuronal responses in kittens. *Hear Res* 28: 97–116.

Walsh EJ & Romand R. (1992) Functional development of the cochlea and the cochlear nerve. In: Romand R, ed. *Development of Auditory and Vestibular Systems 2*. Elsevier, Amsterdam, pp. 161–220.

Walsh EJ & McGee J. (2001) Hypothyroidism in the TSHR mutant mouse. In: Willet J, ed. *Handbook of Auditory Neuroscience*. CRC Press, Boca Raton, FL, pp. 537–56.

Walsh EJ, McGee J, McFadden SL & Liberman MC. (1998) Long-term effects of sectioning the olivocochlear bundle in neonatal cats. *J Neurosci* 18: 3859–69.

Webber A & Raz Y. (2006) Axon guidance cues in auditory development. *Anat Rec* 288 A: 390–6.

Werner LA & Gray L. (1998) Behavioral studies of hearing development. In: Rubel E, Popper AN & Fay RF, eds. *Development of the Auditory System 2*. Springer-Verlag, New York, pp. 12–79.

Whitehead M & Morest DK. (1985) The development of innervation patterns in the avian cochlea. *Neuroscience* 14: 255–76.

Whitlon DS & Rutishauser US. (1990) NCAM in the organ of Corti of the developing mouse. *J Neurocytol* 20: 970–7.

Whitlon DS, Zhang X & Kasakabe M. (1999) Tenascin-C in the cochlea of the developing mouse. *J Comp Neurol* 406: 361–74.

Whitlon DS, Zhang X, Pecelunas K & Greiner MA. (2000) A Temporospatial map of the adhesive molecules in the organ of Corti of the mouse cochlea. *J Neurocytol* **28**: 955–68.

Woods C, Montcouquiol M & Kelley MW. (2004) Math1 regulates development of the sensory epithelium in the mammalian cochlea. *Nat Neurosci* **7**: 1310–8.

Xiang M, Gan L, Li D, Chen ZY, Zhou L, O'Malley BW Jr, Klein W & Nathans J. (1997) Essential role of POU-domain factor Brn-3c in auditory and vestibular hair cell development. *Proc Natl Acad Sci U S A* **94**: 9445–50.

Xiang M, Gao WQ, Hasson T & Shin JJ. (1998) Requirement for Brn-3c in maturation and survival, but not in fate determination of inner ear hair cells. *Development* **125**: 3935–46.

Ylikoski J, Pirvola U, Virkkala J, Suvanto P, Liang XQ, Magal E, Altschuler R, Miller JM & Saarma M. (1998) Guinea pig auditory neurons are protected by glial cell line-derived growth factor from degeneration after noise trauma. *Hear Res* **124**: 17–26.

Zheng JL & Gao WQ. (2000) Overexpression of Math1 induces robust production of extra hair cells in postnatal rat inner ears. *Nat Neurosci* **3**: 580–6.

Zidanic M & Fuchs PA. (1995) Kinetic analysis of barium currents in chick cochlear hair cells. *Biophys J* **68**: 1323–36.

Zine A, Aubert A, Qiu J, Therianos S, Guillemot F, Kageyama R & de Ribaupierre F. (2001) Hes1 and Hes5 activities are required for the normal development of the hair cells in the mammalian inner ear. *J Neurosci* **21**: 4712–20.

Zwislocki JJ, Chamberlain SC & Slepecky NB. (1988) Tectorial membrane, I. Static mechanical properties in vivo. *Hear Res* **33**: 207–22.

Chapter 13

Regeneration in the cochlea

Douglas A Cotanche

13.1 Introduction

Sensorineural hearing loss is the most common cause of hearing impairment and deafness in humans. It usually results from damage to hair cells, the sensory transducers of the inner ear. In humans and other mammals, cochlear hair cells are only produced during embryonic development (Ruben, 1967). Thus, the hair cells we are born with have to survive our entire lifetime. These hair cells are not replaced if they are lost due to noise exposure, genetic mutations, toxic chemicals, aging, or disease. Consequently, their loss results in hearing impairment. Therapeutic interventions for hearing loss in humans are currently limited to hearing aids, cochlear implants, or alternative means of communication, such as American Sign Language (ASL). However, research in birds over the past 20 years has shown that cochlear hair cells can be regenerated in mature, postembryonic avian inner ears and that this regeneration leads to a functional recovery (Cotanche, 1987, 1999; Cruz et al., 1987; Corwin & Cotanche, 1988; Ryals & Rubel, 1988; Lippe et al., 1991; Smolders, 1999). The loss of hair cells induces a direct transdifferentiation and/or a proliferation of the associated non-sensory supporting cells and generates replacement hair cells, resulting in a nearly complete structural and functional recovery of the cochlea. Yet, regeneration in the avian cochlea is limited in both time and quantity, so that the number of new cells generated is enough to replace the number of hair cells lost and not any more (Stone & Cotanche, 1994; Bhave et al., 1995). In addition, the new hair cells reacquire the tuning characteristics and neural contacts of those hair cells that were lost (Smolders, 1999). Understanding the steps involved in avian hair cell regeneration may enable us to experimentally induce supporting cell proliferation and potentially harness this for therapeutic replacement of hair cells in mammals and humans with sensorineural hearing loss. In this chapter we will address how hair cells die in response to trauma, how this hair cell loss induces the supporting cells to regenerate new hair cells and supporting cells, and how some of the mechanisms identified in the bird cochlea have been utilized to experimentally induce limited aspects of regeneration in the mammalian cochlea. Additional experimental approaches involving stem cells have been pursued in order to repopulate the organ of Corti with cells that can repair the damaged auditory sensory epithelium.

13.2 Hair cell regeneration in vertebrates

Hair cell regeneration is not restricted to the avian inner ear. In fact, it has been found to exist to some degree in all auditory, vestibular, and lateral line sensory organs in all vertebrates so far examined, with the exception of the mammalian cochlear organ of Corti (Roberson & Rubel, 1994; Forge et al., 1998). However, the patterns of hair cell regeneration in various end-organs exhibit considerable differences. In order to establish a solid foundation for exploring regeneration, it is important that we clearly define the terms we will be using in this chapter. Hair cell regeneration is defined as the production of new hair cells in a mature inner ear or lateral line organ. This is in contrast to the establishment of the initial sensory organ during embryonic development, which involves the growth and differentiation of a functioning sensory epithelium from undifferentiated placodal tissues.

In the sensory epithelia of fishes and amphibians there is a constant addition of hair cells throughout the life of the animal, so that as the animal ages, the epithelium progressively increases in both size and in the total number of hair cells. While there may be some ongoing cell death in the existing hair cell population, the rate of new hair cell production greatly exceeds this, so that the overall effect is a continuous growth in the size of the end-organ and an increase in total hair cell number (Corwin, 1981, 1983, 1985; Popper & Hoxter, 1984). For example, Corwin (1983) showed that a young ray has 500 hair cells in an organ with an area of 400 μm^2, while a 7-year-old ray has 6000 hair cells over an area of approximately 480 000 μm^2.

The vestibular utricle and saccule of birds exhibit a high rate of cell turnover, where the rate of cell death is normally equivalent to that of hair cell regeneration (Jørgensen & Mathiesen, 1988; Roberson et al., 1992; Kil et al., 1997). As a consequence, there is no net growth in the size of the vestibular sensory epithelia or increase in cell numbers with age, but there is a fairly complete turnover of sensory cells within a given timespan. Moreover, the rate of new hair cell production can be upregulated if there is an abnormal increase in the extent of hair cell loss (Weisleder & Rubel, 1992, 1993).

The basilar papilla, the cochlear sensory epithelium in the bird, normally produces very few, if any, new hair cells after embryogenesis of the inner ear (Oesterle & Rubel, 1993). However, in response to hair cell loss caused by sound damage, aminoglycoside treatment, or laser ablation the sensory epithelium generates new hair cells by both a mitotic and non-mitotic pathway, as described in Section 13.3.3 below (Corwin & Cotanche, 1988; Ryals & Rubel, 1988; Roberson et al., 1996, 2004; Warchol & Corwin, 1996). In the mammal there appears to be a limited amount of hair cell regeneration in the vestibular sensory epithelium following damage, but this is primarily through non-mitotic means (Warchol et al., 1993; Kuntz & Oesterle, 1998). In the mature organ of Corti there has been no convincing evidence that there is any hair cell regeneration in response to damage. However, Kelley et al. (1995) have shown that a substantial amount of non-mitotic hair cell regeneration can occur in the organ of Corti up until embryonic day 16 (E16).

13.3 **Regeneration in the bird cochlea**

13.3.1 **Hair cell regeneration is stimulated by hair cell loss**

Normally there is no hair cell turnover in the undamaged mature avian cochlea, however, this situation can be drastically altered if there is hair cell loss because of trauma. When existing hair cells are damaged and ejected from the sensory epithelium following noise exposure or aminoglycoside treatment, the adjacent supporting cells in the basilar papilla respond by leaving their quiescent state and begin to generate new hair cells through mitosis (mitotic regeneration; Corwin & Cotanche, 1988; Ryals & Rubel, 1988) or by directly changing their gene expression to become hair cells, without a mitotic event (direct transdifferentiation; Adler & Raphael, 1996; Roberson et al., 1996, 2004). Evidence suggests that the supporting cells can begin this process while the hair cells are undergoing the initial stages of damage, but they will not proceed into active proliferation or direct transdifferentiation until the dying hair cells have been fully ejected from the basilar papilla. Furthermore, the number of new hair cells produced is closely correlated to the number of hair cells lost (Stone & Cotanche, 1994). This has led to the hypothesis that the death of the hair cells closely regulates the regeneration responses of the supporting cells. Therefore, it is important to understand how hair cells die in the bird cochlea.

13.3.2 **Hair cells die by apoptosis**

Detailed electron microscopic examinations of hair cell death in the mammalian utricle following aminoglycoside treatment by Forge and colleagues (Forge *et al.*, 1998; Forge & Li, 2000) provided morphological evidence that at least some of the damaged hair cells die by apoptosis. Apoptosis is an active cellular mechanism in which a cell chooses to die and does so by synthesizing and activating proteins that will lead to an organized dismantling of the cellular components. Apoptosis was first described morphologically by Kerr and colleagues (1972) but came into the scientific mainstream when many of the genes responsible for controlling it were defined in the nematode *Caenorhabditis elegans* by Brenner, Horvitz, and Sulston, a body of work that led to a Nobel Prize in 2002. Since their initial discoveries, it has been shown that all cells, even single-celled organisms, are capable of apoptosis and that the same or similar genes are utilized in all cells (Ameisen, 1998).

Apoptosis, also called 'programmed cell death', is a cascade of events beginning with the initiating signal and ending with the dismantling and death of the cell. It involves an upregulation of gene expression and orderly protein synthesis even in the midst of the chaos of cellular dismantling and destruction. The pathway is thought to involve three phases: initiation, arbitration, and execution. Initiation is defined as the internal damage or external signal that starts the cell death program. Once apoptosis is initiated there is a period of arbitration, in which cell survival signals compete with the cell death signals in an attempt to rescue the cells. The Bcl-2 family of proteins is composed of both pro- and anti-apoptotic members that compete with one another to control the outcome of the arbitration phase (Adams & Cory, 1998; Crompton, 2000; Letai, 2005). If the death signals dominate at this stage, the cell dies; but if the survival signals dominate, the cell lives. Thus, even though there is a defined sequence of events that leads to cell death, there is clearly some room for negotiation and reversal of the pathway. For many cell types, the execution stage of the pathway begins with the release of cytochrome c from mitochondria and the activation of caspase-3 (McDonald & Windebank, 2000; Bouchier-Hayes *et al.*, 2005). This subsequently mobilizes a regulated enzyme cascade that results in the breakdown of multiple cellular components and eventual cell death.

The most prominent and well-studied components of the execution phase are the caspases (Cryns & Yuan, 1998; Thornberry & Lazebnik, 1998; Earnshaw *et al.*, 1999; Lavrik *et al.*, 2005). Caspases are a family of proteases that are synthesized in cells as inactive proenzymes. They become activated during the cell death program and function to cleave other caspases in the cascade, as well as a multitude of cellular and nuclear proteins that lead to cellular disintegration. Specific members of the caspase family are thought to be involved in the early, upstream phase, such as caspases 8, 9, and 10, while others are restricted to the later, downstream stages, such as caspases 3, 6, and 7. In non-epithelial cells apoptosis is completed by fragmentation of the dying cells into smaller, membrane-bound vesicles that are phagocytosed by neighboring cells (Tomei & Cope, 1991). In epithelial cells, however, the dying cells are ejected apically out of the epithelial sheet as a single, bloated cell, rather than as fragments (Rosenblatt *et al.*, 2001). Moreover, it appears that the adjacent surviving cells in the epithelium actively aid in forcing the dying cells out utilizing an actin-myosin based contractile mechanism (Rosenblatt *et al.*, 2001).

The progression of apoptosis in hair cells of the bird cochlea has been examined in detail to determine the structural and temporal sequence of their death and to identify possible signals that activate and regulate the accompanying supporting cell regenerative response (Torchinsky *et al.*, 1999; Mangiardi *et al.*, 2004; Duncan *et al.*, 2006). The standard experimental protocol for these studies utilizes a single 300 mg/kg gentamicin injection to initiate hair cell death. This dose leads to a total loss of hair cells in the proximal 30% of the basilar papilla (Fig. 13.1). The time of injection is designated as 'time 0'. The progression of gentamicin from injection to entry into hair cells

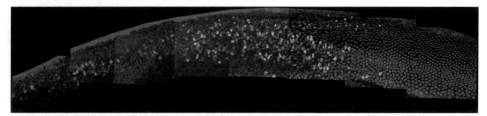

Fig. 13.1 A whole mount confocal montage of the proximal half of the chick basilar papilla 48 hours after a single gentamicin injection. Double label for phalloidin (red) marks the actin cytoskeleton of the hair cells and supporting cells, and caspase-3 (green) identifies the dying hair cells with activated caspase-3 in their cytoplasm. At this time point the dying hair cells are in the process of being ejected from the proximal 30% of the basilar papilla.

is traced with a Texas Red fluorescent tag conjugated to gentamicin sulfate (GTTR, Steyger *et al.*, 2003; Dai *et al.*, 2006). GTTR first appears in the proximal hair cells six hours after the injection. By seven and a half hours, GTTR is identifiable in hair cells at the distal end of the cochlea, but less densely localized than in proximal hair cells. By nine hours, the GTTR is evenly distributed throughout the hair cells of the basilar papilla. At no time is there any remarkable uptake of GTTR by the supporting cells.

At 12 hours, the first signs of hair cells entering the apoptotic cascade are evident in the most proximal region of the basilar papilla, where a number of hair cells exhibit a translocation of the T-cell restricted intracellular antigen-related protein (TIAR) from the nucleus out into bright, condensed granules in the cytoplasm (Fig. 13.2; Mangiardi *et al.*, 2004). TIAR is an mRNA-binding protein that is normally localized to the nucleus in almost all types of undamaged cell. However, in cultured cells it has been found to translocate from the nucleus out into the cytoplasm as quickly as 30 minutes after activation of apoptosis (Taupin *et al.*, 1995). In the cytoplasm, the TIAR helps to form stress granules for processing and sorting mRNAs (Kedersha &

Fig. 13.2 A high magnification confocal micrograph of a group of hair cells undergoing T-cell restricted intracellular antigen-related protein (TIAR) translocation from the nucleus to the cytoplasm 24 hours following gentamicin injection. The TIAR in the cytoplasm forms into dense, brightly labeled stress granules. Red, phalloidin labeling of actin distribution in the stereociliary bundle and cuticular plate of hair cells, and apical intercellular junctions between hair cells and supporting cells. Green, TIAR localization in the stress granules throughout the hair cell cytoplasm.

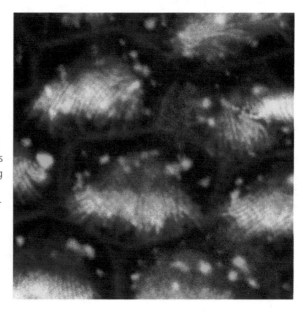

Anderson, 2002). At the same time that TIAR is forming stress granules in the cytoplasm, Hirose *et al.* (2004) have reported a dissolution of polyribosomes, a process known to enhance stress granule formation (Kedersha *et al.*, 2000).

By 24 hours the TIAR translocation spreads to include all of the hair cells within the proximal 30% of the basilar papilla, that is, all of the cells that will eventually be ejected. No TIAR translocation is seen beyond the 30% region and the associated supporting cells within the damaged region exhibit no TIAR changes. Structural damage to the most proximal hair cells begins at 30 hours, 18 hours later than the TIAR translocation, and these cells are ejected by 36 hours. Hair cell damage progresses down the basilar papilla to reach the 30% region by 42 hours and by 54 hours all of the damaged hair cells are ejected from the sensory epithelium and are trapped in the overlying tectorial membrane (Mangiardi *et al.*, 2004).

The dying hair cells enter the execution stage of the apoptotic cascade at 30 hours when the cells begin to exhibit the release of cytochrome c from mitochondria into the cell cytoplasm and the cells begin to express the activated form of caspase-3. The activation of caspase-3 occurs just as the cells are starting to swell up and bleb out of the apical surface of the sensory epithelium (Fig. 13.1). The extruding hair cells continue to label strongly for caspase-3 at 54 hours even after they are ejected from the basilar papilla. The initial activation of caspase-3 is usually thought to represent the beginning of the terminal stages of cell death, with an amplification of the signal finally leading to the ultimate death of the cell. Since caspase-3 activation is seen just as the hair cells are being extruded and even more strongly once they have been ejected, this suggests that the extruding hair cells are still alive ('But I'm not dead yet!' in the immortal words of Monty Python). When the ejected hair cells trapped in the tectorial membrane are tested with a LIVE/DEAD Cell Assay (Molecular Probes, Eugene, Oregon, USA) many are still alive at 54 hours but all are dead by 72 hours. So it appears that the dying hair cells are ejected while still undergoing the final stages of apoptosis and complete their death throes while trapped in the overlying tectorial membrane. Interestingly, recent experiments by Hordichok & Steyger (2007) have shown that the ejection of dying hair cells in the frog saccule is controlled by actin–myosin interactions in the supporting cells. If these interactions are blocked, the hair cells remain within the sensory epithelium and complete their terminal stages of apoptosis without being extruded. This supports the hypothesis presented by Rosenblatt *et al.* (2001) that the ejection of dying cells in epithelial sheets is an active process carried out by neighboring cells. These studies need to be repeated in the chick basilar papilla, but they suggest that the supporting cells play an active and critical role in ejecting the dying hair cells.

An additional interesting change in dying hair cells is the cytoplasmic expansion and intensification of immunolabeling for myosin VI and VIIa (Duncan *et al.*, 2006). These two myosin isoforms are expressed only in hair cells in the cochlea and are usually found throughout the cytoplasm with especially heavy concentrations in the apical periculicular necklace (Hasson *et al.*, 1995; Self *et al.*, 1999). In mature chick hair cells myosin VI is not present in the stereocila, while myosin VIIa is only faintly expressed in the stereocilia. As the dying hair cells reach the execution stage of apoptosis, both myosin VI and VIIa spread evenly throughout the hair cell cytoplasm, including well up into individual stereocilia. Concurrently, the intensity of labeling for both myosins is greatly enhanced. These changes remain detectable in the dying hair cells for more than three weeks after the cells are ejected and complete their death cascade. In fact, this intense myosin labeling of the dead and dying hair cells is even detectable at low magnification in the fluorescence microscope and can be used to rapidly assess the extent of hair cell damage (Fig. 13.3).

In summary, the apoptotic cascade in dying hair cells appears to be initiated roughly six hours after gentamicin reaches the hair cells, then takes up to 18 hours to pass through the arbitration phase while deciding whether cell death is required, before reaching the onset of the execution

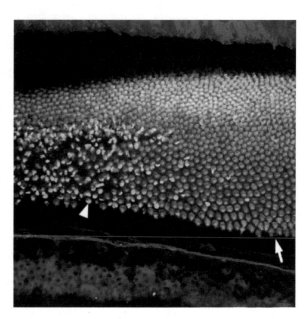

Fig. 13.3 A low-magnification confocal micrograph of myosin VI labeling in the transition zone between damaged and undamaged hair cells in the gentamicin-treated basilar papilla. Red, phalloidin label of actin filaments in hair cells. Green, labeling of myosin VI protein in hair cells. Note the intense green labeling of hair cells in the damaged region (arrowhead) as compared to the more distal, undamaged region (arrow).

phase (Fig. 13.4A). This last stage takes between 24 and 42 hours to complete, with the initial steps occurring in the basilar papilla while the terminal stages occur once the cells have been ejected. Similar results have been documented for cell death in the chick utricle, both *in vivo* and *in vitro*, and in the *in vitro* chick basilar papilla, where caspases 8, 9, and 3 have been shown to be involved (Matsui *et al.*, 2002, 2003, 2004; Cheng *et al.*, 2003). Moreover, blockage of hair cell death by specific caspase inhibitors has led to a structural and functional rescue of the hair cells (Matsui *et al.*, 2003) and a concurrent reduction in the rate of ongoing proliferation in the utricle (Matsui *et al.*, 2002). From all of this, it has been hypothesized that the dying hair cells send signals at the onset of apoptosis that initiate the regenerative responses in the adjacent supporting cells, but that the regenerative process is held in check until the dying hair cells reach the execution stage of the apoptotic cascade and are ejected from the sensory epithelium.

13.3.3 Regenerative responses in supporting cells

As the hair cells carry out their death cascades, the adjacent supporting cells initiate regenerative responses in order to replace the lost hair cells. Two separate mechanisms have been identified by which the supporting cells produce new hair cells (Fig. 13.5). The first, called *direct transdifferentiation*, involves a supporting cell that changes its gene expression to that of a hair cell and proceeds to differentiate into a hair cell while giving up its supporting cell identity and function (Baird *et al.*, 1996; Roberson *et al.*, 1996, 2004; Adler *et al.*, 1997). The second mechanism is *mitotic regeneration*, where a supporting cell leaves quiescence, re-enters the cell cycle, divides, and gives rise to two new cells that can then differentiate into either hair cells or supporting cells, or continue on through further rounds of mitosis (Corwin & Cotanche, 1988; Ryals & Rubel, 1988; Stone & Cotanche, 1994).

Direct transdifferentiation seems to be the simplest and fastest way to make new hair cells. Indeed, it has been documented that the first new hair cells to arise during regeneration are derived from direct transdifferentiation (Roberson *et al.*, 2004; Duncan *et al.*, 2006). Yet, it has serious drawbacks because for every hair cell gain, one supporting cell is lost. Each hair cell in the

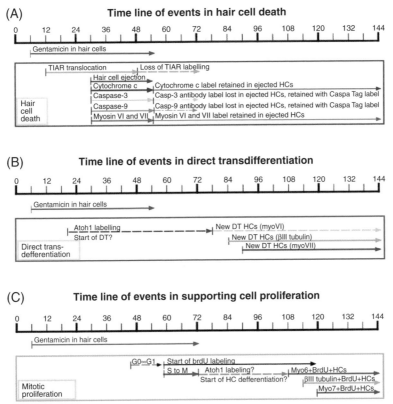

Fig. 13.4 Timeline of events in hair cell death and supporting cell proliferation/direct transdifferentiation in the gentamicin-treated chick cochlea. (A) Timing of events in the apoptosis of hair cells following a single gentamicin injection. (B) Timing of the events in direct transdifferentiation. (C) Timing of the events in mitotic regeneration. These timelines are based primarily on experiments done in our lab, but also on results from studies from the lab of Ed Rubel (Bhave *et al.*, 1995) and Jennifer Stone (Stone *et al.*, 1999; Cafaro *et al.*, 2007).

chick cochlea is surrounded by only three to four supporting cells (Goodyear & Richardson, 1997) and these cells really do physically support the hair cells in the sensory epithelium through their apical intercellular junctions. Mature hair cells do not have basal processes that reach down to the basal lamina of the cochlear epithelium, so they cannot exist without some minimal number of supporting cells to prop them up. If more than one or two supporting cells per hair cell underwent direct transdifferentiation, there would not be enough supporting cells left to maintain the integrity of the sensory epithelial layer.

The supporting cells that will undergo direct transdifferentiation appear to do so very quickly, as they begin to express Atoh1 in their nuclei as early as 15–24 hours after gentamicin administration (Fig. 13.4B; Cafaro *et al.*, 2007). *ATOH1* is currently the earliest gene identified that is activated in cells committed to differentiate as hair cells, and the loss of this gene results in the failure of any detectable hair cell differentiation (Bermingham *et al.*, 1999). In the regenerating chick cochlea, the expression of Atoh1 in supporting cells follows shortly after the gentamicin-exposed hair cells exhibit TIAR translocation, the earliest known sign that the hair cells have begun apoptosis. Thus, the initial signals transmitted from dying hair cells to supporting cells telling them to

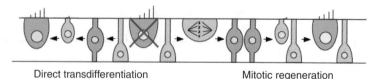

Direct transdifferentiation   Mitotic regeneration

Fig. 13.5 Diagrammatic representation of the processes of direct transdifferentiation (to the left of the dying hair cell) and mitotic regeneration (to the right of the dying hair cell). Direct transdifferentiation quickly gives rise to one new hair cell but at the expense of one supporting cell. Mitotic regeneration requires that a supporting cell undergo at least one round of mitosis before giving rise to a new hair cell, but also results in the replacement of the supporting cell after cell division. Green, mature hair cell; Yellow, mature supporting cell; Brown, newly born or transdifferentiating supporting cell/precursor cell; Blue, mitotic supporting cell; light green, immature hair cell, red X, dying hair cell.

prepare for regeneration happen very early in the apoptotic cascade. The next step in hair cell development shown by the transdifferentiating supporting cells is the cytoplasmic expression of myosin VI protein. This occurs between 72 hours (Cafaro et al., 2007) and 78 hours (Duncan et al., 2006) after gentamicin treatment and is quickly followed by βIII tubulin at 84 hours and myosin VIIa expression at 90 hours (Duncan et al., 2006). The 12-hour gap between the appearance of myosin VI and myosin VIIa corresponds with the delay in myosin VIIa expression seen in the developing mouse cochlea (Montcouquiol & Kelley, 2003; Kelley, 2006), but the 63-hour delay between the expression of Atoh1 and of myosin VI in the newly transdifferentiating supporting cells is distinctly different from their almost simultaneous appearance in the mouse embryonic cochlea (Montcouquiol & Kelley, 2003; Kelley, 2006). Moreover, it is markedly delayed when compared to the 36-hour lag between the expression of *ATOH1* in newly post-mitotic cells in the regenerating cochlea and their expression of myosin VI at 108 hours (Duncan et al., 2006; Cafaro et al., 2007). This difference will be discussed in more detail below.

Regeneration through mitotic division of the supporting cells begins later than direct transdifferentiation, but it eventually produces the majority of the new hair cells needed for full cochlear regeneration (Fig. 13.4C; Roberson et al., 1996, 2004). In the undamaged cochlea the supporting cells are in the G_0, or quiescent, stage of the cell cycle, meaning they are not actively moving through the cell cycle. In most cell types studied, it takes about 12 hours to move from quiescence back into G_1, the first stage of the cell cycle (Campisi & Pardee, 1984). PCNA, a subunit of DNA polymerase δ, is normally upregulated in the nuclei of cells from late G_1 through S phase and into early G_2 phase of the cell cycle (Bravo & Macdonald-Bravo, 1987). Thus, the onset of *PCNA* expression has been used to define the time when quiescent cells have re-entered the cell cycle and reached late G_1. Examination of *PCNA* expression in the regenerating chick cochlea shows that supporting cells in the proximal tip of the basilar papilla begin to exhibit increased *PCNA* labeling 24 hours after gentamicin injection (Bhave et al., 1995). The *PCNA* labeling extends throughout the damaged region by 72 hours and, surprisingly, by 120 hours shows considerable upregulation in supporting cells throughout the basilar papilla, even in regions that show no hair cell damage (Bhave et al., 1995). This suggests that the gentamicin damage to hair cells in the proximal 30% of the basilar papilla is initiating the progression of almost all the supporting cells throughout the sensory epithelium out of G_0 and into the late stages of G_1. However, this seems to be as far as most of them ever get, for only the supporting cells within the region of hair cell loss will enter S phase and proceed to mitosis (Stone & Cotanche, 1994; Bhave et al., 1995; Stone et al., 1999;

Roberson *et al.*, 2004; Duncan *et al.*, 2006). The remaining supporting cells outside of the damaged region never enter into S phase. Rather, they return to G_0 by about three weeks after the gentamicin treatment (Bhave *et al.*, 1995). Thus, the early signal from the hair cells just entering apoptosis that induces directly transdifferentiating cells to express Atoh1 may also influence the proliferating supporting cells to leave G_0 and express *PCNA*.

For those supporting cells in the region of hair cell damage that do move ahead in the cell cycle, the first ones enter S phase at 65 hours, as determined by labeling for BrdU incorporation (Duncan *et al.*, 2006). BrdU (bromodeoxyuridine) is a thymidine analog that, when present in proliferating cells, is incorporated into newly synthesized DNA and passed along to the daughter cells. It can be localized with a monoclonal antibody made specifically against BrdU (Gratzner, 1982). The peak of S phase occurs at 72 hours and remains high through 96 hours, but then begins to taper off, so that very few cells label with BrdU at 120 hours (Bhave *et al.*, 1995; Duncan *et al.*, 2006). Surprisingly, the BrdU-labeled mitotic cells show no proximal-to-distal gradient in their time of appearance, as was seen with hair cell loss, but appear uniformly throughout the damaged region between 65 hours and 96 hours (Duncan *et al.*, 2006). In general, S phase for an individual cell lasts about 6–8 hours, whereupon the cells proceed into G_2 and then quickly undergo mitosis to produce two daughter cells. This can be verified in the chick cochlea, as the first pairs of BrdU-labeled cells appear at 72 hours, seven hours after the first cells enter S phase. Once the first daughter cells are produced, they can go on to differentiate into new hair cells or supporting cells or continue on through a second round of proliferation (Stone & Cotanche, 1994; Stone *et al.*, 1999). Cafaro *et al.*, (2007) determined that about 15% of the BrdU-labeled cells express Atoh1 only two hours after a BrdU injection and that this increases to 21% by 24 hours after the BrdU injection. So the daughters of the mitotic cells make a fairly rapid decision to begin expressing Atoh1, indicating that they are already moving down the hair cell fate pathway. There is some evidence that both daughter cells can express Atoh1, at least for a short time, even if one will go on to differentiate as a supporting cell (Cafaro *et al.*, 2007). But those that will continue to differentiate as hair cells maintain a strong Atoh1 nuclear label.

Once the new hair cells begin to express Atoh1, further differentiation down the hair cell pathway is thought to involve the expression of components of the Notch pathway. These cell fate mechanisms in regeneration have been examined in great detail in a recent review (Stone & Cotanche, 2007). After the cells have made the decision to differentiate as hair cells, the first signs of the expression of functional hair cell-specific proteins is the synthesis of myosin VI (Montcouquiol & Kelley, 2003; Duncan *et al.*, 2006).

The first BrdU-labeled hair cells to show myosin VI expression appear at 108 hours after gentamicin treatment, followed by βIII tubulin at 114 hours and myosin VIIa at 120 hours (Duncan *et al.*, 2006). Thus, the temporal sequence of hair cell gene expression for the mitotically produced new hair cells is identical to that for new hair cells arising from direct transdifferentiation. This has led to the hypothesis that direct transdifferentiation is actually the default mechanism for making hair cells out of pluripotent precursor cells, and that mitosis just produces these precursor cells, which then activate the default hair cell pathway (Roberson *et al.*, 2004; Morest & Cotanche, 2004). As noted above, however, the gap between Atoh1 expression and myosin VI expression in new hair cells derived from direct transdifferentiation is 63 hours, whereas it is only 36 hours for new hair cells generated from supporting cell mitoses. One possible explanation for this difference is that while the supporting cells heading into direct transdifferentiation begin upregulating Atoh1 when the dying hair cells first enter the apoptotic pathway, they are held in this state while the hair cells decide whether conditions are bad enough to require full commitment to death. Once that decision has been made and the dying hair cells initiate the execution phase by activating caspase-3 and extruding the doomed hair cell, this sends a second signal to the supporting cells to move beyond Atoh1 expression and proceed to definitive expression of myosin VI, βIII tubulin, and myosin VIIa. The ejection of dying hair cells begins in earnest around 36–42 hours, which is roughly 36 hours before myosin VI appears in the new hair cells made by direct transdifferentiation. This, then, results in an equivalent time span for the progression from Atoh1 to myosin VI as that exhibited by new hair cells produced through mitoses.

The delay in myosin VI expression in directly transdifferentiating cells and the restriction of supporting cells entering S phase to only the damaged region of the cochlea provide circumstantial evidence that at least two separate signals are required to regulate regeneration. The first signal, which appears to occur early in the hair cell apoptotic cascade, enables the activation of quiescent supporting cells to begin progressing toward direct transdifferentiation or mitosis by expression of Atoh1 and *PCNA*, respectively. The second signal, which appears to be correlated with the ejection of dying hair cells, enables the activated supporting cells to progress into subsequent stages of hair cell differentiation or enter into S phase of the cell cycle.

As yet, it is not known how the choice is made for which of the two pathways the supporting cells will take. Direct transdifferentiation may be a rapid response pathway to quickly make new hair cells, but there must be a limited number of cells that can respond in this way, or else the integrity of the epithelium would be lost. Mitotic regeneration would be stimulated when the maximum number of supporting cells that can safely enter direct transdifferentiation has been reached, yet even more new hair cells are needed to replace those lost. Additionally, more supporting cells would be required to replenish those lost to direct transdifferentiation.

One major question that still needs to be addressed is whether all supporting cells are capable of entering either pathway, or whether there are specialized subsets of supporting cells that can only contribute to direct transdifferentiation, mitosis, or neither. Morphological and immunocytochemical studies have not yet identified any distinct subpopulations of supporting cells, although it is possible that these do exist. It may be that the cells which undergo direct transdifferentiation are actually post-mitotic 'hair cell precursors' held in a primitive state of differentiation by the existence of the full population of mature hair cells. If, however, some of the adult hair cells are lost, the signals inhibiting the development of these precursors are reduced and they can complete their differentiation. Meanwhile, those cells that can enter the mitotic pathway may be a subset of supporting cells that represent a 'stem-cell-like' population. They remain quiescent until the 'hair cell precursors' are utilized to make new hair cells, at which point the 'stem-cell-like' cells become active again, divide, and replace the lost 'hair cell precursors'. However, in most experimental paradigms where hair cell damage is induced in large numbers, some of these 'stem-cell-like' cells immediately give rise to new hair cells. This suggests that the number of 'precursor' cells is not large enough to fully compensate for the loss of a large number of hair cells and, consequently, many of the daughter cells of the mitotically active cells must be immediately recruited to differentiate as new hair cells rather than to just replace the lost 'hair cell precursors'. It would be interesting to test whether there is a limited number of hair cells that can be lost that would only utilize direct transdifferentiation to make new hair cells, while mitosis would not be initialized, except perhaps to replace the 'precursor cell' population.

However, until good immunocytochemical or genetic markers are found that can clearly identify distinct subpopulations of supporting cells in the avian cochlea, we must assume that all supporting cells are capable of either direct transdifferentiation or mitotic regeneration. In that case, it is important to determine what signals from the dying hair cells stimulate some supporting cells to enter the direct transdifferentiation pathway, while others pursue the mitotic regeneration pathway. One possible scenario is that signals from a few dying hair cells induce a subset of adjacent supporting cells to pursue direct transdifferentiation. Once the number of hair cells dying crosses some threshold where direct transdifferentiation cannot produce enough hair cells to replace those being lost, then signals from either the dying hair cells or the overwhelmed transdifferentiating cells stimulate other supporting cells to initiate mitotic regeneration.

13.4 Regeneration strategies in mammalian cochleas

13.4.1 Transient regeneration in the embryonic mammalian cochlea

While some degree of hair cell regeneration has been detected in all other vertebrate inner ear sensory epithelia, the mature mammalian organ of Corti remains the one end-organ that appears to have no innate regenerative capacity (Roberson & Rubel, 1994; Forge *et al.*, 1998). However, early in cochlear development, the organ of Corti does have the capacity to produce supernumerary hair cells or to replace lost hair cells. Addition of retinoic acid to mouse cochlear cultures prior to embryonic day 16 (E16) leads to the production of multiple extra rows of inner and outer hair cells (Kelley *et al.*, 1993). Moreover, when the original population of hair cells is eliminated by laser ablation prior to E16, adjacent supporting cells can undergo non-mitotic direct transdifferentiation to replace the lost hair cells (Kelley *et al.*, 1995). Approximately around the same time that the cells in the embryonic organ of Corti reach terminal mitoses, these cells begin to express molecules that serve as inhibitors of further cell proliferation (Chen & Segil, 1999; Chen *et al.*, 2003). The region where these proliferation inhibitors are expressed has been termed the 'zone of non-proliferating cells' (ZNPC) (Fig. 13.6; Chen & Segil, 1999; Chen *et al.*, 2002). It has been hypothesized that the mouse organ of Corti is unable to regenerate because these mitotic inhibitors prevent any proliferative responses of the supporting cells. However, this does not explain why some subsets of supporting cells in the mature organ of Corti are not able to replace lost hair cells through direct transdifferentiation. Anecdotal theories suggest that the supporting cells in the organ of Corti are too differentiated and specialized in function to undergo direct transdifferentiation. However, when Atoh1 genes are transfected into supporting cells *in vitro* and *in vivo* they appear to be capable of transdifferentiating into hair cells (Zheng & Gao, 2000; Kawamoto *et al.*, 2003; Shou *et al.*, 2003; Woods *et al.*, 2004; Izumikawa *et al.*, 2005; see discussion below in Section 13.4.2). Therefore, other, as yet undefined, mechanisms must be present in the mature

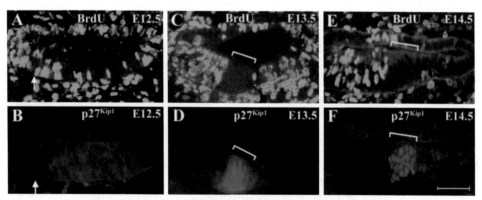

Fig. 13.6 The zone of non-proliferating cells (ZNPC) appears around embryonic day (E)13.5–E14.5 in the developing mouse cochlea (bar in C, E; green nuclei are BrdU labeled) and corresponds with the expression of p27^{kip1} (bar in D, F; red nuclei) in the cells of the presumptive sensory epithelium.
Reproduced with permission from Chen *et al.* (2002).

cochlea that prevent supporting cells from expressing Atoh1 on their own and transdifferentiating into new hair cells when mature hair cells are lost.

13.4.2 Genetic manipulation of the mammalian cochlea

Studies designed to test the role of proliferation inhibitors in blocking regeneration have been performed with traditional and conditional 'knock-out' mice, where the gene of interest has been genetically removed either altogether or at certain times during development. Knock-outs of three different proliferation inhibitors (p27, p19, and Rb) have demonstrated that the loss of these inhibitors results in prolonged periods of mitosis in the cochlea and production of supernumerary hair cells and supporting cells (Fig. 13.7) (Chen & Segil, 1999; Lowenheim et al., 1999; Chen et al., 2003; Sage et al., 2005). These experiments support the idea that regeneration in the mammal is at least partially suppressed by proteins that inhibit proliferation. However, these proliferation inhibitors also have second major role, in which they act to prevent unregulated apoptosis in many cell types. Consequently, even though these knock-out mice show evidence of prolonged cellular proliferation and hair cell differentiation early in development, they also tend to eventually permit unchecked apoptosis of the hair cells and supporting cells. This delayed but extensive loss of sensory cells in the organ of Corti results in profound sensorineural hearing loss (Lowenheim et al., 1999; Chen et al., 2003). Thus, although these proliferation inhibitors seem transiently to restore regenerative capacity to the mammalian cochlea, they cannot be left to act indefinitely. Future research directions will have to explore ways to briefly turn off these inhibitors long enough to produce new hair cell precursors but then turn them back on before unchecked apoptosis is initiated.

Transfection of *ATOH1* into supporting cells has demonstrated that the introduction of this gene into mature non-sensory cells is sufficient to induce cells to differentiate into hair cells (Zheng & Gao, 2000; Kawamoto et al., 2003; Shou et al., 2003; Woods et al., 2004; Izumikawa et al., 2005). This new hair cell generation occurs without mitotic events, so it must be equivalent to the direct transdifferentiation pathway seen in the bird cochlea (Roberson et al., 1996, 2004) and embryonic mouse cochlea (Kelley et al., 1995). One interesting sidelight of these *ATOH1* transfections is that when the *ATOH1* causes ectopic hair cell differentiation well outside of the organ of Corti, these displaced new hair cells are able to attract nerve fibers to grow out toward them (Kawamoto et al., 2003). Moreover, isolated non-sensory cells transfected with *ATOH1* are able to induce neighboring cells to differentiate into organ of Corti-specific supporting cells in an *in vitro* preparation (Woods et al., 2004) These findings indicate that newly differentiating hair cells are affecting the cell fates of neighboring cells and releasing some kind of neurotrophic factors that can attract cochlear nerve fibers, even when they are well out of their normal position. The good news here is that if hair cells are ever induced to regenerate within the mammalian organ of Corti, they should be able to effectively cause the differentiation of appropriate supporting cell types and attract nerve processes for reinnervation and recovery of function.

13.4.3 Gene therapy for cochlear repair

Many forms of sensorineural deafness are caused by mutations in a single gene that lead to the death or failure of function of hair cells (Rehm & Morton, 1999; Goldfarb & Avraham, 2002; Bitner-Glindzicz, 2002). In theory, if this one defective gene could be replaced, then the cochlea should be able to generate a functional sensory epithelium. Experiments by Camper and colleagues have shown that congenital, non-syndromic deafness in one mouse line was caused by a mutation in the myosin XV gene (Wang et al., 1998). When a corrected copy of the myosin XV gene was inserted into fertilized mouse embryos, one of the mice was born with a functional auditory

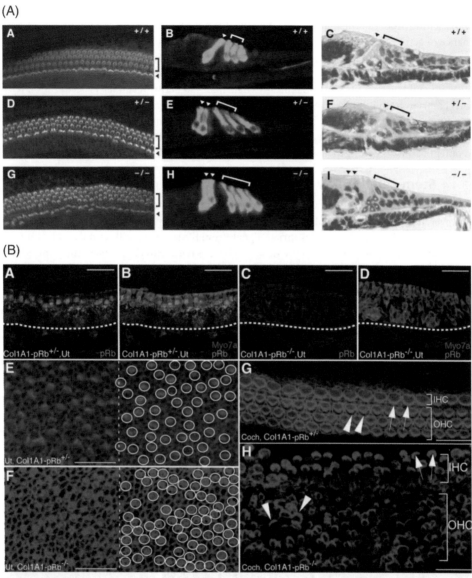

Fig. 13.7 (A) Overproduction of inner hair cells, outer hair cells, and supporting cells in p27[kip1] knock-out mice. A, D, G Phalloidin labeling of surface preparations; B, E, H Myosin VIIa immunolabeling of cross-sections; C, F, I Hematoxylin-labeled histological cross-sections. (B) Overproduction of inner hair cells, outer hair cells, vestibular hair cells, and supporting cells in Rb1 knock-out mice. A–D Cross-sections of the mouse utricle labeled with pRB (green) and myosin VIIa (red). E–H Surface preparations of the mouse utricle (E, F) or the organ of Corti (G, H) labeled with phalloidin.

Figure 13.7A reproduced with permission from Chen and Segil (1999). Figure 13.7B reproduced with permission from Sage et al. (2005).

system, even though his parents and siblings were deaf (Probst *et al.*, 1998). While this experiment is an exciting proof of principle for gene therapy, it is not yet practical for use on humans, for the chance of getting the new gene correctly inserted into the genome is quite low. Only one of 200 mouse embryos injected with the repaired myosin XV gene exhibited restored hearing. Moreover, the technique required the genetic manipulation of a fertilized embryo. While this is possible in mice, it would be scientifically and ethically challenging to perform similar procedures on fertilized embryos from humans. However, as techniques in gene therapy improve and as we understand more about the role of individual proteins such as connexin 26, myosin VI, and prestin, there may come a point where targeted transfection of specific cell types in the cochlea may lead to potential therapies for genetic hearing loss.

13.4.4 Stem cell therapy

The mature mammalian cochlea does not seem to be able to undergo regeneration intrinsically. However, it has been proposed that stem cells should be able to integrate into the damaged cochlear sensory epithelium, derive appropriate signals from the surviving cells in the cochlear microenvironment, and differentiate into the various cell types needed to repair the sensory epithelium (Li *et al.*, 2004; Parker & Cotanche, 2004; Coleman *et al.*, 2007).

Two experimental pathways have been approached with regard to stem cells in the cochlea. One is to determine if there are native stem cells that exist in the mammalian vestibular epithelia or even the organ of Corti (Li *et al.*, 2004). If these cells could be identified and harvested, it would be feasible to utilize them for transplantation into damaged cochlear or vestibular sensory organs. Heller and colleagues have been able to identify and harvest cells from the mouse utricular epithelia that appear to be inner ear stem cells (Li *et al.*, 2003a). These cells could not only be coaxed down a hair cell differentiation pathway in culture but also integrated into the cochlear sensory epithelium when transplanted into the developing chick inner ear, and were able to differentiate into hair cells (Fig. 13.8). While the existence of mammalian inner ear stem cells is intriguing, they are currently only found in vestibular sensory epithelia and the process for

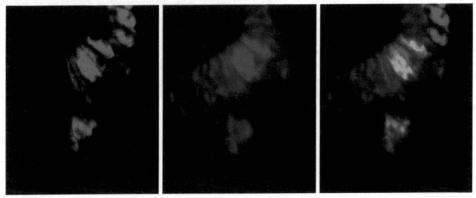

Fig. 13.8 New hair cells derived from stem cells purified from the mouse utricle and transplanted into the chick otocyst at embryonic day 2. When harvested at embryonic day 7, the mouse stem cell-derived cells labeled with antibodies specific for ROSA26-6 mouse cells (green) and double labeled with antibodies to myosin VIIa (red), showing that some of the mouse utricular stem cells integrated into the developing chick cochlea and differentiated into hair cells.
Reproduced with permission from Li *et al.* (2003a).

isolating them is very labor intensive for the number of stem cells obtained. For this approach to succeed, a way must be developed to amplify and maintain these stem cells in culture and then demonstrate that they can effectively repair the organ of Corti when transplanted into a mammalian cochlea.

The other stem cell approach involves adapting either embryonic stem cells or adult stem cell lines for implantation and integration into damaged cochleae. Mouse embryonic stem cells have been manipulated toward a cochlear fate *in vitro* and have been shown to exhibit many genes and proteins characteristic of hair cell precursors (Li *et al.*, 2003b; de Silva *et al.*, 2006). Moreover, these stem cells were able to differentiate as hair cells when transplanted into early embryonic chick otocysts. They have also been shown to migrate through the scalae and modiolus when injected into the mammalian cochlea but did not show a clear indication of differentiating into hair cells or supporting cells (Coleman *et al.*, 2006). Adult neural stem cells have survived once transplanted into the mammalian cochlea, but again showed no cochlear-cell-specific differentiation (Hu *et al.*, 2005). Mesenchymal stem cells from the hematopoietic cell population have been coaxed down a neural pathway (Kondo *et al.*, 2005) and have been proposed as a potential source for repair of the inner ear. However, these cells have not yet been transplanted into damaged cochlear epithelia to determine if they can function as proposed. While many of these experiments are pursuing exciting possibilities with the transplantation of stem cells into the cochlea, many of them are looking at the distribution of the stem cells only a week after the transplantation. It may be important to allow the stem cells to survive longer in the cochlea in order to respond to local signals in the cochlear or spiral ganglion microenvironment.

Recent studies utilizing an immortalized neural stem cell line have demonstrated that these cells will differentiate into neurons, glial cells, hair cells, and supporting cells when transplanted into a noise-damaged mouse or guinea pig cochlea and allowed to integrate for up to six weeks (Fig. 13.9) (Parker *et al.*, 2007). Although many different cell types derived from the stem cells could be identified, the total number of new cells was still relatively small compared with the number of damaged cells. Only the spiral ganglion neurons in the base of the cochlea showed a significant increase in number relative to those in the damaged cochlea (Parker *et al.*, 2007). Moreover, the numbers were too low to be able to measure any physiologic improvement in hearing for the stem cell transplanted ears. Perhaps even longer recovery times will be needed to see a more complete recovery and a measurable level of auditory function.

13.5 **Future directions**

Over the past 20 years many of the events that lead to hair cell regeneration in the avian cochlea have been defined. However, it has still not been possible to identify the specific factors that initiate and carefully regulate the process and how the supporting cells decide to pursue either the direct transdifferentiation or mitotic regeneration pathways. Moreover, it is still not fully understood how choices are made in cell fate decisions and differentiation so that the proper number of hair cells and supporting cells are re-established. Further investigations of the regeneration process in the avian cochlea and in the development of the mammalian organ of Corti will be critical to answering these questions.

While the mammalian cochlea appears to lack the inherent ability to regenerate, what has been learned from the avian cochlea about hair cell regeneration has led to the stimulation of some aspects of regeneration in the mammal. Continued explorations of the mechanisms that control mammalian supporting cell proliferation and the differentiation of hair cell phenotypes, as well as further investigations of the potential for stem cells to repopulate the damaged cochlea, will be critical to the development of effective biological therapies for treating hearing loss.

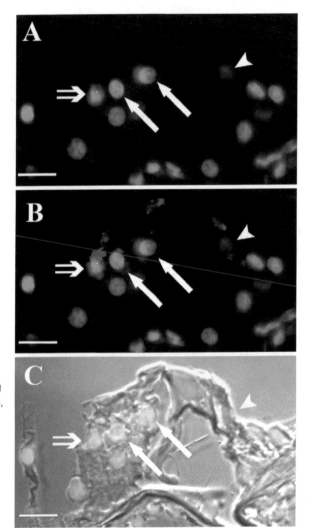

Fig. 13.9 Transplanted mouse neural stem cells differentiate into hair cells in the noise-damaged guinea pig cochlea. Immortalized male mouse neural stem cells were identified as hair cells (double arrow, green dot in outer hair cell nucleus) by double labeling with myosin VIIa (red label in B, C) six weeks after transplantation into the noise-damaged cochlea of a female guinea pig. light blue, DAPI staining of hair cell and supporting cell nuclei. Reproduced with permission from Parker *et al.* (2007).

Acknowledgments

The author is grateful for the comments and input of Jennifer Stone, Matt Kelley, critical readings of early drafts by Christina Kaiser, and for confocal images obtained by Christina Kaiser and Brittany Chapman. Work from the author's lab described in this chapter was supported by NIH grant no. DC001689, a Hair Cell Initiative Grant from the National Organization for Hearing Research Foundation, grants from the Kramer/Dosberg Fund, the Patterson Trust, the Sarah Fuller Fund, and the Children's Hospital Otolaryngology Foundation Research Fund.

References

Adams JM & Cory S. (1998) The Bcl-2 protein family: arbiters of cell survival. *Science* **281**: 1322–6.

Adler HJ & Raphael Y. (1996) New hair cells arise from supporting cell conversion in the acoustically damaged chick inner ear. *Neurosci Lett* **205**: 17–20.

Adler H, Komeda M & Raphael Y. (1997) Further evidence for supporting cell conversion in the damaged avian basilar papilla. *Int J Dev Neurosci* **15**: 375–85.

Ameisen JC. (1998) The evolutionary origin and role of programmed cell death in single-celled organisms. In: Lockshin RA, Zakeri Z & Tilly J, eds. *When Cells Die*. Wiley-Liss, New York, pp. 3–56.

Baird RA, Steyger PS & Schuff NR. (1996) Mitotic and nonmitotic mechanisms of hair cell regeneration in the bullfrog. *Ann N Y Acad Sci* **781**: 59–70.

Bermingham NA, Hassan BA, Price SD, Vollrath MA, Ben-Arie N, Eatock RA, Bellen HJ, Lysakowski A & Zoghbi HY. (1999) Math1: An essential gene for the generation of inner ear hair cells. *Science* **284**: 1837–41.

Bhave SA, Stone JS, Rubel EW & Coltrera MD. (1995) Cell cycle progression in gentamicin-damaged avian cochleas. *J Neurosci* **15**: 4618–28.

Bitner-Glindzicz M. (2002) Hereditary deafness and phenotyping in humans. *Br Med Bull* **63**: 73–94.

Bouchier-Hayes L, Lartigue L & Newmeyer DD. (2005) Mitochondria: pharmacological manipulation of death. *J Clin Invest* **115**: 2640–7.

Bravo R & Macdonald-Bravo H. (1987) Existence of two populations of cyclin/PCNA during the cell cycle: Association with DNA replication sites. *J Cell Biol* **105**: 1549–54.

Cafaro J, Lee GS & Stone JS. (2007) Atoh1 expression defines activated progenitors and differentiating hair cells during avian hair cell regeneration. *Dev Dyn* **236**: 156–70.

Campisi J & Pardee AB. (1984) Post-translational control of the onset of DNA synthesis by an insulin-like growth factor. *Mol Cell Biol* **4**: 1807–14.

Chen P & Segil N. (1999) p27(Kip1) links cell proliferation to morphogenesis in the developing organ of Corti. *Development* **126**: 1581–90.

Chen P, Johnson JE, Zoghbi HY & Segil N. (2002) The role of Math1 in inner ear development: Uncoupling the establishment of the sensory primordium from hair cell fate determination. *Development* **129**: 2495–505.

Chen P, Zindy F, Abdala C, Liu F, Li X, Roussel MF & Segil N. (2003) Progressive hearing loss in mice lacking the cyclin-dependent kinase inhibitor Ink4d. *Nat Cell Biol* **5**: 422–6.

Cheng AG, Cunningham LL & Rubel EW. (2003) Hair cell death in the avian basilar papilla: characterization of the *in vitro* model and caspase activation. *J Assoc Res Otolaryngol* **4**: 91–105.

Coleman B, Hardman J, Coco A, Epp S, de Silva M, Crook J & Shepherd R. (2006) Fate of embryonic stem cells transplanted into the deafened mammalian cochlea. *Cell Transplant* **15**: 369–80.

Coleman B, De Silva MG & Shepherd RK. (2007) The potential of stem cells for auditory neuron generation and replacement. *Stem Cells* **25**: 2685–94.

Corwin JT. (1981) Postembryonic production and aging of inner ear hair cells in sharks. *J Comp Neurol* **201**: 541–53.

Corwin JT. (1983) Postembryonic growth of the macula neglecta auditory detector in the ray, *Raja clavata*: continual increases in hair cell number, neural convergence, and physiological sensitivity. *J Comp Neurol* **217**: 345–56.

Corwin JT. (1985) Perpetual production of hair cells and maturational changes in hair cell ultrastructure accompany postembryonic growth in an amphibian ear. *Proc Natl Acad Sci U S A* **82**: 3911–5.

Corwin JT & Cotanche DA. (1988) Regeneration of sensory hair cells after acoustic trauma. *Science* **240**: 1772–4.

Cotanche DA. (1987) Regeneration of hair cell stereociliary bundles in the chick cochlea following severe acoustic trauma. *Hear Res* **30**: 181–96.

Cotanche DA. (1999) Structural recovery from sound and aminoglycoside damage in the avian cochlea: a review. *Audiol Neurootol* **4**: 271–85.

Crompton M. (2000) Bax, Bid and the permeabilization of the mitochondrial outer membrane in apoptosis. *Curr Opin Cell Biol* **12**: 414–9.

Cruz RM, Lambert PM & Rubel EW. (1987) Light microscopic evidence of hair cell regeneration after gentamicin toxicity in chick cochlea. *Arch Otolaryngol Head Neck Surg* **113**: 1058–62.

Cryns V & Yuan J. (1998) Proteases to die for. *Genes Dev* **12**: 1551–70.

Dai CF, Mangiardi DA, Cotanche DA & Steyger PS. (2006) Uptake of fluorescent gentamicin by vertebrate sensory cells *in vivo*. *Hear Res* **213**: 64–78.

de Silva MG, Hildebrand MS, Christopoulos H, Newman MR, Bell K, Ritchie M, Smyth GK & Dahl HH. (2006) Gene expression changes during step-wise differentiation of embryonic stem. cells along the inner ear hair cell pathway. *Acta Otolaryngol* **126**: 1148–57.

Duncan LJ, Anderson JK, Williamson KE, Mangiardi DA, Matsui JI & Cotanche DA. (2006) Pattern of myosin expression during hair cell death and regeneration in the chick cochlea. *J Comp Neurol* **499**: 691–701.

Earnshaw WC, Martins LM & Kaufmann SH. (1999) Mammalian caspases: structure, activation, substrates, and functions during apoptosis. *Annu Rev Biochem* **68**: 383–424.

Forge A & Li L. (2000) Apoptotic death of hair cells in mammalian vestibular sensory epithelia. *Hear Res* **139**: 97–115.

Forge A, Li L & Nevill G. (1998) Hair cell recovery in the vestibular sensory epithelia of mature guinea pigs. *J Comp Neurol* **397**: 69–88.

Goldfarb A & Avraham KB. (2002) Genetics of deafness: recent advances and clinical implications. *J Basic Clin Physiol Pharmacol* **13**: 75–88.

Goodyear R & Richardson G. (1997) Pattern formation in the basilar papilla: evidence for cell rearrangement. *J Neurosci* **17**: 6289–301.

Gratzner HG. (1982) Monoclonal antibody to 5-bromo-2-iododeoxyuridine: a new reagent for detection of DNA replication. *Science* **218**: 474–5.

Hasson T, Heintzelman M, Santos-Sacchi J, Corey DP & Mooseker MS. (1995) Expression in cochlea and retina of myosin VIIa, the gene product defective in Usher syndrome type 1B. *Proc Natl Acad Sci U S A* **92**: 9815–9.

Hirose K, Westrum LE, Cunningham DE & Rubel EW. (2004) Electron microscopy of degenerative changes in the chick basilar papilla after gentamicin exposure. *J Comp Neurol* **470**: 164–80.

Hordichok AJ & Steyger PS. (2007) Closure of supporting cell scar formations requires dynamic actin mechanisms. *Hear Res* **232**: 1–19.

Hu Z, Wei D, Johansson CB, Holmstrom N, Duan M, Frisen J & Ulfendahl M. (2005) Survival and neural differentiation of adult neural stem cells transplanted. into the mature inner ear. *Exp Cell Res* **302**: 40–7.

Izumikawa M, Minoda R, Kawamoto K, Abrashkin K, Swiderski D, Dolan D, Brough D & Raphael Y. (2005) Auditory hair cell replacement and hearing improvement by Atoh1 gene therapy in deaf mammals. *Nat Med* **11**: 271–6.

Jørgensen JM & Mathiesen C. (1988) The avian inner ear: continuous production of hair cells in vestibular sensory organs, but not in the auditory basilar papilla. *Naturwissenschaften* **75**: 319–20.

Kawamoto K, Ishimoto S-I, Minoda R, Brough D & Raphael Y. (2003) Math1 gene transfer generates new cochlear hair cells in mature guinea pigs *in vivo*. *J Neurosci* **23**: 4395–400.

Kedersha N & Anderson P. (2002) Stress granules: sites of mRNA triage that regulate mRNA stability and translatability. *Biochem Soc Trans* **30**: 963–9.

Kedersha N, Choi M, Li W, Yacono P, Chen S, Gilks N, Golan D & Anderson P. (2000) Dynamic shuttling of TIA-1 accompanies the recruitment of mRNA to mammalian stress granules. *J Cell Biol* **151**: 1257–68.

Kelley MW. (2006) Hair cell development: commitment through differentiation. *Brain Res* **109**: 172–85.

Kelley MW, Xu X-M, Wagner MA, Warchol ME & Corwin JT. (1993) The developing organ of Corti contains retinoic acid and forms supernumerary hair cells in response to exogenous retinoic acid in culture. *Development* **119**: 1041–53.

Kelley MW, Talreja DR & Corwin JT. (1995) Replacement of hair cells after laser microbeam irradiation in cultured organs of Corti from Embryonic and neonatal mice. *J Neurosci* **15**: 3013–26.

Kerr JRF, Willie AH & Currie AR. (1972) Apoptosis: A basic biological phenomenon with wide-ranging implications in tissue kinetics. *Br J Cancer* **26**: 239–57.

Kil J, Warchol ME & Corwin JT. (1997) Cell death, cell proliferation, and estimates of hair cell life spans in the vestibular organs of chicks. *Hear Res* 114: 117–26.

Kondo T, Johnson S, Yoder M, Romand R & Hashino E. (2005) Sonic hedgehog and retinoic acid synergistically promote sensory fate specification from bone marrow-derived pluripotent stem cells. *Proc Natl Acad Sci U S A* 102: 4789–94.

Kuntz AL & Oesterle EC. (1998) Transforming growth factor a with insulin stimulates cell proliferation *in vivo* in adult rat vestibular sensory epithelium. *J Comp Neurol* 399: 413–23.

Lavrik IN, Golks A & Krammer PH. (2005) Caspases: pharmacological manipulation of cell death. *J Clin Invest* 115: 2665–72.

Letai A. (2005) Pharmacological manipulation of Bcl-2 family members to control cell death. *J Clin Invest* 115: 2648–55.

Li H, Liu H & Heller S. (2003a) Pluripotent stem cells from the adult mouse inner ear. *Nat Med* 9: 1293–9.

Li H, Roblin G, Liu H & Heller S. (2003b) Generation of hair cells by stepwise differentiation of embryonic stem cells. *Proc Natl Acad Sci U S A* 100: 13495–500.

Li H, Corrales CE, Edge A & Heller S. (2004) Stem cells as therapy for hearing loss. *Trends Mol Med* 10: 309–15.

Lippe WR Westbrook EW & Ryals BM. (1991) Hair cell regeneration in the chicken cochlea following aminoglycoside toxicity. *Hear Res* 56: 203–10.

Lowenheim H, Furness DN, Kil J, Zinn C, Gultig K, Fero ML, Frost D, Gummer AW, Roberts JM, Rubel EW, Hackney CM & Zenner HP. (1999) Gene disruption of p27^{Kip1} allows cell proliferation in the postnatal and adult organ of Corti. *Proc Natl Acad Sci U S A* 96: 4084–8.

Mangiardi DA, Williamson KM, May KE, Messana EP, Mountain DC & Cotanche DA. (2004) Progression of hair cell ejection and molecular markers of apoptosis in the avian cochlea following gentamicin treatment. *J Comp Neurol* 475: 1–18.

Matsui J, Ogilvie J & Warchol M. (2002) Inhibition of caspases prevents ototoxic and ongoing hair cell death. *J Neurosci* 22: 1218–27.

Matsui JI, Haque A, Huss D, Messana EP, Alosi JA, Roberson DW, Cotanche DA, Dickman JD & Warchol ME. (2003) Hair cell function and survival following aminoglycoside treatment with caspase inhibitors *in vivo*. *J Neurosci* 23: 6111–22.

Matsui J, Gale J & Warchol M. (2004) Critical signaling events during the aminoglycoside-induced death of sensory hair cells *in vitro*. *J Neurobiol* 61: 250–66.

McDonald ES & Windebank AJ. (2000) Mechanisms of neurotoxic injury and cell death. *Clin Neurobehav Tox* 18: 525–40.

Montcouquiol M & Kelley MW. (2003) Planar and vertical signals control cellular differentiation and patterning in the mammalian cochlea. *J Neurosci* 23: 9469–78.

Morest DK & Cotanche DA. (2004) Regeneration of the inner ear as a model of neural plasticity. *J Neurosci Res* 78: 455–60.

Oesterle EC & Rubel EW. (1993) Postnatal production of supporting cells in the chick cochlea. *Hear Res* 66: 213–24.

Parker M & Cotanche D. (2004) The potential use of stem cells for cochlear repair. *Audiol Neurootol* 9: 72–80.

Parker M, Corliss D, Gray B, Roy N, Anderson J, Bobbin R, Snyder E & Cotanche DA. (2007) Neural stem cells integrate into the sound-damaged cochlea and develop into cochlear cells. *Hear Res* 232: 29–43.

Popper A & Hoxter B. (1984) Growth of a fish ear: 1. Quantitative analysis of hair cell and ganglion cell proliferation. *Hear Res* 15: 133–42.

Probst FJ, Fridell RA, Raphael Y, Saunders Tl, Wang A, Liang Y, Morell RJ, Touchman JW, Lyons RH, Noben-Trauth K, Friedman TB & Camper SA. (1998) Correction of deafness in *shaker-2* mice by an unconventional myosin in a BAC transgene. *Science* 280: 1444–7.

Rehm HL & Morton CC. (1999) A new age in the genetics of deafness. *Genet Med* 1: 295–302.

Roberson D & Rubel EW. (1994) Cell division in the gerbil cochlea after acoustic trauma. *Am J Otol* 15: 28–34.

Roberson DW, Weisleder P, Bohrer PS & Rubel EW. (1992) Ongoing production of sensory cells in the vestibular epithelium of the chick. *Hear Res* 57: 166–74.

Roberson DW, Kreig CS & Rubel EW. (1996) Light microscopic evidence that direct transdifferentiation gives rise to new hair cells in regenerating avian auditory epithelium. *Aud Neurosci* 2: 195–205.

Roberson DW, Alosi JA & Cotanche DA. (2004) Direct transdifferentiation gives rise to the earliest new hair cells in regenerating avian auditory epithelium. *J Neurosci Res* 78: 461–71.

Rosenblatt J, Raff M & Cramer L. (2001) An epithelial cell destined for apoptosis signals its neighbors to extrude it by an actin- and myosin-dependent mechanism. *Curr Biol* 11: 1847–57.

Ruben RJ. (1967) Development of the inner ear of the mouse. A radioautographic study of terminal mitosis. *Acta Otolaryngol Suppl* 220: 1–44.

Ryals BM & Rubel EW. (1988) Hair cell regeneration after acoustic trauma in adult Coturnix quail. *Science* 240: 1774–6.

Sage C, Huang M, Karimi K, Gutierrez G, Vollrath MA, Zhang D-S, Garcia-Añoveros J. Hinds P, Corwin JT, Corey D & Chen Z-Y. (2005) Proliferation of functional hair cells *in vivo* in the absence of the retinoblastoma protein. *Science* 307: 1114–8.

Self T, Sobe T, Copeland NG, Jenkins NA, Avraham KB & Steel KP. (1999) Role of myosin VI in the differentiation of cochlear hair cells. *Dev Biol* 214: 331–41.

Shou J, Zheng J & Gao W-Q. (2003) Robust generation of new hair cells in the mature mammalian inner ear by adenoviral expression of Hath1. *Mol Cell Neurosci* 23: 169–79.

Smolders JWT. (1999) Functional recovery in the avian ear after hair cell regeneration. *Audiol Neurootol* 4: 286–302.

Steyger PS, Peters SL, Rehling J, Hordichok A & Dai CF. (2003) Uptake of gentamicin by bullfrog saccular hair cells *in vitro*. *J Assoc Res Otolaryngol* 4: 565–78.

Stone JS & Cotanche DA. (1994) Identification of the timing of S phase and the patterns of cell proliferation during hair cell regeneration in the chick cochlea. *J Comp Neurol* 341: 50–67.

Stone JS & Cotanche DA. (2007) Hair cell regeneration in the avian auditory epithelium. *Int J Dev Biol* 51: 633–47.

Stone JS, Choi Y-S, Woolley SMN, Yamashita H & Rubel EW. (1999) Progenitor cell cycling during hair cell regeneration in the vestibular and auditory epithelia of the chick. *J Neurocytol* 28: 863–76.

Taupin JL, Tian Q, Kedersha N, Robertson M & Anderson P. (1995) The RNA-binding protein TIAR is translocated from the nucleus to the cytoplasm during Fas-mediated apoptotic cell death. *Proc Natl Acad Sci U S A* 92: 1629–33.

Thornberry NA & Lazebnik Y. (1998) Caspases: enemies within. *Science* 281: 1312–6.

Tomei L & Cope F. (1991) *Apoptosis: The Molecular Basis of Cell Death*. Cold Spring Laboratory Press, Plainview, NY.

Torchinsky C, Messana EP, Arsura M & Cotanche DA. (1999) Regulation of p27^{Kip1} in the avian cochlea during gentamicin mediated hair cell death and regeneration. *J Neurocytol* 28: 913–24.

Wang A, Liang Y, Fridell RA, Probst FJ, Wilcox ER, Touchman JW, Morton CC, Morell RJ, Noben-Trauth K, Camper SA & Friedman TB. (1998) Association of unconventional myosin MYO15 mutations with human nonsyndromic deafness DFNB3. *Science* 280: 1447–51.

Warchol ME & Corwin JT. (1996) Regenerative proliferation in organ cultures of the avian cochlea: Identification of the initial progenitors and determination of the latency of the proliferative response. *J Neurosci* 16: 5466–77.

Warchol ME, Lambert PR, Goldstein BJ, Forge A & Corwin JT. (1993) Regenerative proliferation in inner ear sensory epithelia from adult guinea pigs and humans. *Science* 259: 1619–22.

Weisleder P & Rubel EW. (1992) Hair cell regeneration in the avian vestibular epithelium. *Exp Neurol* 115: 2–6.

Weisleder P & Rubel EW. (1993) Hair cell regeneration after streptomycin toxicity in the avian vestibular epithelium. *J Comp Neurol* **331**: 97–110.

Woods C, Montcouquiol M & Kelley MW. (2004) Math1 regulates development of the sensory epithelium in the mammalian cochlea. *Nat Neurosci* **7**: 1310–8.

Zheng JL & Gao W-Q. (2000) Overexpression of Math1 induces robust production of extra hair cells in postnatal rat inner ears, *Nat Neurosci* **3**: 580–86.

Chapter 14

Genetics of hearing loss

Cynthia C Morton and Anne BS Giersch

14.1 Introduction and background

The genetics of deafness and hearing loss is more complex than perhaps any other medical condition. Hearing impairment is a prime example of how a relatively common medical condition can be caused by a defect at any one of numerous loci. Genetic deafness can be one clinical finding in a collection of symptoms that characterize a specific disease (referred to as syndromic deafness) or it can be the sole consequence of a single gene mutation (non-syndromic deafness). Different mutations in the same gene can result in different forms of deafness or different inheritance patterns. In fact, there are several hundred different types of genetic hearing impairment (Online Mendelian Inheritance in Man (OMIM, 2008). Deafness can be inherited in an autosomal dominant, autosomal recessive, X-linked, mitochondrial, or multi-gene pattern. It can have a prelingual or postlingual onset. It can be stable or progressive. It can be unilateral or bilateral, and conductive or neurosensory. Unraveling of the human genome sequence 'completed' in 2003, and the various tools developed subsequently have vastly accelerated the mapping of deafness genes. Although the field has made impressive strides in identifying genes associated with inherited hearing loss since the first non-syndromic deafness mutations were identified in 1997 (DFNB1, DFNB2, DFNA1, DFNA11 (Kelsell *et al.*, 1997; Liu *et al.*, 1997a,b; Lynch *et al.*, 1997; Weil *et al.*, 1997)), we have, in fact, probably witnessed only the introduction to a very exciting story in biology.

14.1.1 Incidence of hearing loss in the general population

Hearing loss is the most common sensory deficit diagnosed in humans. Approximately one to three in 1000 babies are born with a hearing impairment of 40 dB or higher, 40% of whom are profoundly deaf (reviewed in Smith *et al.*, 2005). This makes hearing loss far more prevalent than other 'common' genetic disorders such as Down syndrome (1:1000) and cystic fibrosis (1:3300 among Caucasians and Ashkenazi Jews), or any commonly observed 'birth defect' (Fig. 14.1). Up to 4% of babies in neonatal intensive care units have some hearing loss (Stein, 1999) and another 1:1000 children will experience a marked loss of hearing before adolescence (Fortnum *et al.*, 2001). Adding individuals with later-onset age-related and acquired forms of hearing loss, conservative estimates suggest up to 30 million Americans, or up to 10% of the US population, have a permanent hearing disability (Mohr *et al.*, 2000).

About half of the cases of deafness are thought to have a genetic basis (Morton, 1991) (Fig. 14.2). Interestingly, the percentage of genetic forms of hearing loss is on the rise in developed nations, reflecting improved healthcare and greater awareness of environmental factors that can cause hearing loss. Thus, as prevention of non-genetic hearing loss improves, the overall percentage of hearing impairment attributable to genetic causes is increasing. Among the causes of environmentally attributable hearing loss are bacterial or viral infections, either congenital (such as

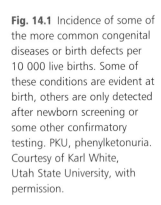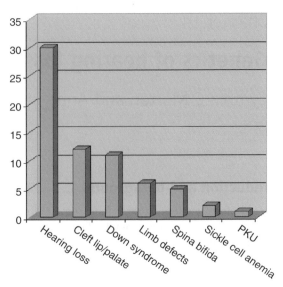

Fig. 14.1 Incidence of some of the more common congenital diseases or birth defects per 10 000 live births. Some of these conditions are evident at birth, others are only detected after newborn screening or some other confirmatory testing. PKU, phenylketonuria. Courtesy of Karl White, Utah State University, with permission.

cytomegalovirus or rubella) or acquired (such as mumps or measles), ototoxicity (exposure to drugs that damage the delicate structures of the inner ear, such as some chemotherapeutic agents, certain antibiotics, or loop diuretics), prematurity, trauma to the head, or prolonged or excessive noise exposure. *A propos* of this last point, hearing loss due to noise exposure has been historically a workplace concern, necessitating, in the USA, strict guidelines by the Occupational Health and Safety Administration (OSHA). More recently however, the 'iPOD ear', hearing loss due to listening to handheld music players at excessive volumes, has become a legitimate medical concern (Rudy, 2007).

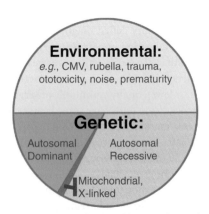

Fig. 14.2 Proportion of acquired and genetic forms of hearing loss. About half of hearing loss is thought to have a genetic basis, whereas the other half can be attributed to environmental factors. Some of the more common environmental factors are given in the figure. Of genetic forms of hearing loss, about 75% has an autosomal recessive inheritance pattern, about 20% is autosomal dominant, and about 3–5% is X-linked, Y-linked, or mitochondrial.

14.1.2 Newborn screening to detect early hearing loss

When deafness is present from birth, usually there is no other clinical finding. On the contrary, an infant with impaired hearing might be labeled a 'good baby' for sleeping through a ringing telephone or noisy sibling. Left untreated, hearing loss in a newborn can impact speech and language acquisition, social and emotional development and later academic achievement. However, proper early intervention can diminish or eliminate these sequelae.

In 1993, the National Institutes of Health (NIH) Consensus Development Conference on Early Identification of Hearing Loss concluded that all infants in the USA should be screened for hearing impairment, preferably before discharge from the birth hospital. Early Hearing Detection and Intervention (EHDI) mandates began to be passed by individual state legislatures in the early 1990s, with Rhode Island and Hawaii leading the way. Currently, a majority of US states have either passed laws or have laws pending that mandate hearing screening for all babies within the first month of life. Typically, screening is done in the hospital, before the baby and mother are discharged. Hearing testing is considered part of the routine newborn screening, along with the more traditional heelstick that collects a drop of blood for metabolic disease testing. Parental consent is not required in most states, although parents can opt out of the testing if they so desire. On average, more than four million babies are screened each year in the USA, with a greater than 95% compliance rate. The National Center for Hearing Assessment and Management (NCHAM) website, maintained by the University of Utah (www.infanthearing.org), is an excellent resource for information and educational materials related to newborn hearing screening.

One of two testing modalities is used by most hospitals; both can be performed while a newborn baby is sleeping. An auditory brainstem response (ABR) test consists of small earphones that emit soft clicks. Electrodes fastened to the baby's scalp detect characteristic brainwave activity in response to the sounds. A computer analyzes the results and compares it with a 'normal' pattern. An otoacoustic emissions (OAE) test takes advantage of the fact that functioning outer hair cells emit a faint sound in response to sound waves. The test uses a small microphone placed in the ear canal to record these emitted sounds in response to soft clicks produced by a transducer. Like the ABR, the response is monitored by a computer and compared with a 'normal' result.

The majority of test failures turn out to be false positives. If a baby moves during testing or if the ear canal is not clear, test results can be compromised. Most hospitals will retest the next day, before the baby is discharged. Babies who fail both tests are referred for more extensive audiological testing, which may include a genetic consult.

14.1.3 Attribution of hearing loss to genetic or acquired etiologies

Determining the cause of hearing loss can be difficult. If there is a clear family history of hearing loss, or a known etiologic agent of acquired hearing loss, such as a maternal rubella infection during pregnancy, for example, establishing the probable cause of hearing loss in a child as genetic or acquired can be quite straightforward. However, often determining the cause of a recently diagnosed hearing loss may require a comprehensive evaluation, especially if there are no obvious etiologies. At a minimum, an initial evaluation should include a targeted patient history including family history and a physical exam, concentrating on key genetic and clinical features of the many forms of syndromic and non-syndromic hearing loss (American College of Human Genetics (ACMG, 2002).

Ideally, the family history includes a three-generation pedigree (Fig. 14.3), paying particular attention to the hearing status of relatives, consanguinity, and paternity. If hearing loss is present in the family history, the inheritance pattern (Box 14.1) should be evaluated (dominant, recessive, X-linked, or mitochondrial), the characteristics of the hearing impairment determined (age of

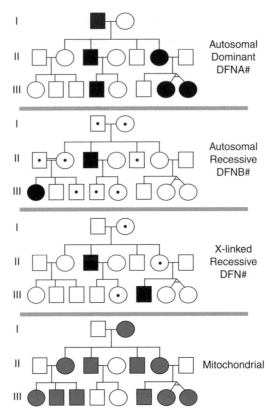

Fig. 14.3 Inheritance patterns of hearing loss. Pedigrees for various types of inherited hearing impairment. Squares, males; circles, females. Affected individuals are filled in symbols; unaffected individuals are open symbols. Grayfill indicates variable expressivity associated with mitochondrial heteroplasmy. A dot in a symbol denotes an unaffected carrier of a recessive disease gene.
A horizontal line connecting the middle of male and female symbols denotes a mating. A double horizontal line denotes a mating between genetically related individuals. Offspring connected to a mating are in the next row down. Siblings are all in the same row, connected by a horizontal line above them. Siblings connected by an inverted 'V' are twins; a small cross-bar connecting the two arms of the 'V' signifies monozygotic twins and lack of the cross-bar denotes dizygotic twins.

onset, progression, conductive versus sensorineural) and the presence or absence of any additional features that might indicate a syndromic hearing loss (e.g. eye, heart, kidney, skeletal, or skin abnormalities).

However, the majority of deaf babies are born to hearing parents, with no identifiable risk factors (e.g., intrauterine infections or ototoxic drug exposure) and no clear family history of deafness, making a genetic link less certain (but not impossible). The existence of a large number of syndromes, of which hearing loss is only one symptom, necessitates follow-up by numerous specialists (ophthalmology, cardiology, nephrology, neurology, etc.) to rule out more serious effects of a known syndrome. Thus, the patient history and physical exam should include genetic testing for known deafness genes along with assessment for visual anomalies, facial dysmorphology, endocrine abnormalities, cardiac or renal symptoms, and skin abnormalities (ACMG, 2002) The presence of additional clinical findings can point to a specific syndrome, for which confirmatory genetic testing may be available. The precise diagnosis also facilitates appropriate management of the patient.

Box 14.1 Modes of inheritance

Autosomal dominant inheritance

- A mutation in only one allele is necessary to express the disease phenotype.
- Most affected individuals have an affected parent.
- Both sexes are equally affected.
- Roughly half of the offspring of an affected individual will be affected.
- Examples: Huntington's disease, achondroplasia, neurofibromatosis type 1.

Autosomal recessive inheritance

- A mutation in both alleles is necessary to express the disease phenotype.
- Affected individuals often have unaffected parents.
- Both sexes are equally affected.
- If both parents are carriers of a single mutation, roughly a quarter of their offspring are expected to be affected.
- Inbreeding increases the chances of observing an autosomal recessive condition.
- Examples: cystic fibrosis, sickle cell anemia, phenylketonuria.

X-linked inheritance

- Most X-linked disorders are recessive, although there are some with dominant inheritance.
- Because females have two X chromosomes and males have only one, males are most often affected by X-linked diseases, as only one X chromosome need carry a mutation.
- About half the sons of a carrier female are expected to be affected.
- Affected males cannot pass on the gene defect to their sons, but all of their daughters are expected to be carriers.
- Examples: hemophilia, Duchenne muscular dystrophy, color blindness.

Mitochondrial inheritance

- This type of genetic disorder is caused by mutations in the DNA of mitochondria.
- Mitochondrial defects show a non-Mendelian inheritance pattern because mitochondria, and thus the mitochondrial genome, are inherited from the mother through the egg.
- All offspring of an affected female are expected to be affected.
- Both sexes are equally affected.
- Because of heteroplasmy, a condition in which both mutant and wild-type mitochondria are present, the severity of a phenotype can vary widely between individuals.
- Affected males do not transmit the gene defect to their offspring.
- Examples: Leber hereditary optic atrophy; MERRF (Myoclonic Epilepsy with Ragged Red Fibers), MELAS (Mitochondrial Encephalopathy, Lactic Acidosis and Stroke-like episodes).

The lack of any additional clinical findings and negative results of genetic testing do not exclude a genetic cause of hearing loss. Autosomal recessive non-syndromic hearing loss in particular can present in the absence of a positive family history and, currently, molecular testing is available for only a small percentage of deafness genes (discussed later in the chapter).

14.1.4 Gene and mutation naming conventions

For reference throughout the rest of this chapter, some definitions and nomenclature conventions used in the scientific literature are explained briefly here. Gene names and symbols are assigned by an international committee, the Human Genome Organization Gene Nomenclature Committee (www.genenames.org). Guidelines for human gene nomenclature are also described in Wain *et al.* (2002). A gene symbol, comprising not more than six letters and numbers, is a short-form representation of the descriptive gene name. Thus, *GJB2* is the gene symbol for gap junction protein β2. Only Latin letters and Arabic numerals are used in the gene symbol; no Roman numerals or Greek letters are allowed. Gene symbols are italicized in the scientific literature. Human gene symbols are displayed in all capitals, *GJB2;* for mouse genes (or other organisms), only the first letter is capitalized, *Gjb2.* The full gene name or protein name is not capitalized or italicized.

A mutation in a gene is described by position and type of mutation. The nucleotide position is numbered with the transcriptional start site assigned number 1. A '>'symbol denotes a point mutation change from one nucleotide to another, thus 109G>A is a change of a G to an A at nucleotide position 109. 'del' means deletion and 'ins' means insertion, so 35delG implies a deletion of a G at nucleotide position 35.

A *locus* (plural *loci*) is not a synonym for a gene but refers to a chromosomal map position. Sometimes a locus can be large and encompass many genes. *Allele* refers to a variant form of a particular gene, for example one can refer to mutated and wild-type alleles of *GJB2*.

14.1.5 Syndromic versus non-syndromic hearing loss

Researchers and clinicians tend to divide genetic forms of hearing impairment into two categories: syndromic and non-syndromic. The division is not arbitrary, as the proper diagnosis can have long-term ramifications for clinical management. Syndromic hearing loss is the association of hearing loss or deafness with other clinical findings, such as pigmentary anomalies in Waardenburg syndrome, retinitis pigmentosa leading to blindness in Usher syndrome or kidney anomalies in Alport syndrome. An observation of hearing loss in a child may be the first symptom of a more serious, possibly fatal, disorder. Some of the more common forms of syndromic hearing loss are discussed in more detail later in the chapter. However, despite the dizzying number of hearing loss syndromes, hearing loss is part of a syndrome in only about 30% of cases. The majority of genetic hearing loss is non-syndromic.

14.2 Non-syndromic hearing loss

Since the first autosomal deafness locus was mapped to chromosome 5 in a large Costa Rican family in 1992 (Leon *et al.*, 1992), more than 100 distinct chromosomal loci have been identified as responsible for non-syndromic genetic deafness, in most cases through linkage analysis. In about 40% of cases, the responsible gene has been identified (Fig. 14.4). Because the field is so dynamic, currently the best way to keep up to date on genes and loci is through the well-annotated internet database, the Hereditary Hearing Loss Homepage (http://webh01.ua.ac.be/hhh/), maintained by researchers at the University of Antwerp and the University of Iowa. There, one can find loci, linked markers, deafness genes, and relevant references (Van Camp & Smith, 2007).

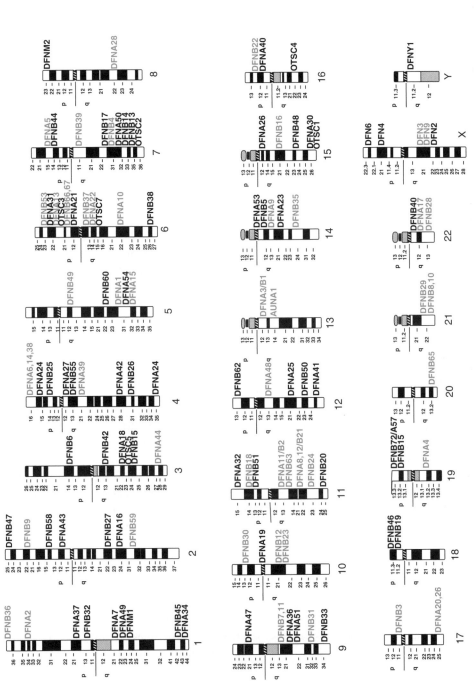

Fig. 14.4 Chromosomal location of human non-syndromic hearing loss related genes. Non-syndromic deafness loci are denoted DFNA# for autosomal dominant, DFNB# for autosomal recessive, DFN# for X-linked, and DFNY# for Y-linked. DFNM# denotes a genetic modifier. AUNA# denotes auditory neuropathy. OTSC# denotes otosclerosis. For loci colored blue, the gene defect has been identified. For all other loci, the gene defect has been mapped to this chromosomal region, but the gene has not been identified. Due to space constraints, syndromic hearing loss genes are not on this chromosome map. See the Hereditary Hearing Loss Homepage website (http://webh01.ua.ac.be/hhh/) for gene identifications and individual references.

Dominant deafness loci are designated DFN<u>A</u>#, with the numbers assigned more or less sequentially, as the loci were identified, irrespective of chromosomal location. Loci for recessive deafness are named DFN<u>B</u>#, X-linked deafness are DFN#, and Y-linked deafness are DFN<u>Y</u>#. Non-syndromic deafness loci identified to date are shown in Figure 14.4; loci in blue indicate that the responsible gene has been identified. Several dominant and recessive loci have been mapped to the same locus and have turned out to be mutation variants of the same gene (e.g. see chromosome bands 11q13, 11q22, and 13q12 in Fig. 14.4). Also noted in Figure 14.4. Genetic modifiers (i.e. a gene whose expression affects a phenotype resulting from a mutation at another locus, denoted DFNM#), loci that cause auditory neuropathy (a form of hearing loss in which the cochlear hair cells are present and functional, but the sound stimulus does not reach the auditory nerve and brain properly, denoted AUNA#), and loci responsible for otosclerosis (abnormal formation of new bone in the middle ear that gradually immobilizes the stapes, causing progressive hearing loss, denoted OTSC#) have been mapped. Approximately 75% of non-syndromic genetic deafness is inherited in an autosomal recessive manner. About 20% is autosomal dominant and about 3–5% has either an X-linked or mitochondrial inheritance pattern. With few exceptions, autosomal recessive deafness tends to be prelingual, severe, and stable whereas autosomal dominant hearing loss tends to have a post-lingual onset, be progressive and less severe. This difference may be because in a recessive disorder, both copies of a gene are mutated and no functional copies exist, thus symptoms are present at birth. In contrast, one functional allele remains in an autosomal dominant disorder. Either the one 'good' allele can compensate for the mutated allele, sometimes even into adulthood, or, in the case of a dominant negative mechanism, accumulation of mutant protein eventually results in progressive deterioration.

14.2.1 Connexin hearing loss

Autosomal recessive non-syndromic hearing loss is the most common form of genetic hearing impairment and despite the fact that mutations in any one of over 60 genetic loci can cause recessive hearing loss, about 50% of these cases are attributed to mutations in one locus, DFNB1. This locus on chromosome 13 encodes *GJB2* (connexin 26) and *GJB6* (connexin 30). The vast majority of hearing impairment attributed to this locus is due to mutations in *GJB2*, making mutations in this gene the single most frequent cause of inherited hearing loss in some populations (Zelante *et al.*, 1997; Estivill *et al.*, 1998; Kelley *et al.*, 1998; Putcha *et al.*, 2007). Connexins, or gap junction proteins, are a family of transmembrane proteins which assemble to form channels that connect two eukaryotic cells and allow the passage of ions and small molecules between them. Mutations in different gap junctions can lead to functional or developmental abnormalities in many cell/tissue types.

GJB2 mutations predominantly cause autosomal recessive hearing loss, but autosomal dominant mutations have also been described. Dozens of different mutations have been reported and different mutations may have different frequencies depending on the population. For example, a recent multicenter study in North America reports the 35delG mutation to be most commonly found in whites and Hispanics, 109G>A in Asians, –34C>T in African Americans and 167delT in Ashkenazi Jews (Putcha *et al.*, 2007). Some genotype–phenotype correlations can also be appreciated for *GJB2* mutations. Homozygous protein terminating mutations, either nonsense mutations that generate a stop codon or small deletions/insertions that cause a frame shift resulting in premature termination, cause a more severe phenotype (earliest onset, most severe degree of hearing impairment) than either a missense mutation coupled with a terminating mutation (intermediate severity) or two missense mutations (least severe) (Snoeckx *et al.*, 2005; Putcha *et al.*, 2007).

Autosomal dominant point mutations in *GJB6* (connexin 30) have been described, although most *GJB6*-associated hearing loss is due to deletion of one allele accompanied by a *GJB2* point mutation on the other chromosome (Lerer *et al.*, 2001; Del Castillo *et al.*, 2003; Dalamon *et al.*, 2005) The Connexin-deafness Homepage website (http://davinci.crg.es/deafness/) is an excellent resource for information on *GJB2*, *GJB6*, and other connexin mutations associated with hearing loss along with a database of reported mutations and appropriate references (Ballana *et al.*, 2008).

14.3 Syndromic hearing loss

More than 400 distinct clinical syndromes have hearing loss as a component (OMIM, 2008). About 30% of patients with prelingual hearing loss have one of these syndromes. Some of these syndromes are extremely rare, while others are more common. In some cases hearing loss is the major clinical finding, while in other cases, the hearing loss is relatively minor. The inheritance pattern can be autosomal dominant, autosomal recessive, X-linked, or mitochondrial. A few of the more common syndromes are detailed below to illustrate the complexity and diversity of hearing loss conditions.

14.3.1 Waardenburg syndrome

One of the most common types of autosomal dominant syndromic hearing loss is Waardenburg syndrome with an incidence of around 1 in 10 000 to 20 000. There are four types of Waardenburg syndrome, WS types I–IV, caused by mutations in seven different genes. All types have sensorineural hearing loss as a component as well as pigmentary anomalies of the hair and skin and sometimes the eyes. These pigmentary effects manifest as a white forelock or premature graying of the hair, light colored patches on the skin, and very light colored irises of the eyes, or sometimes two different colored eyes (heterochromia iridis). A person with Waardenburg syndrome may have all or only some of these symptoms. When hearing impairment is present, it is usually bilateral and profound, but only about 60% of Waardenburg patients have hearing loss. WS1 is caused by mutations in *PAX3* (paired box gene 3) (Tassabehji *et al.*, 1992), and has the additional characteristic lateral displacement of the inner canthi of the eyes (dystopia canthorum). WS2 has no associated dystopia canthorum and can be caused by mutations in *MITF* (microphthalmia-associated transcription factor), *SNAI2* (snail, *Drosophila* homolog 2), or *SOX10* (SRY-box10) (Tassabehji *et al.*, 1994; Sanchez-Martin *et al.*, 2002; Bondurand *et al.*, 2007). *PAX3* and *SOX10* are transcriptional regulators of *MITF*. *MITF*, in turn, is a transcriptional activator critically involved in differentiation of melanocytes from the neural crest. Loss of melanocytes affects pigmentation of the hair, skin, and eyes, and hearing loss due to a deficiency of melanocytes in the stria vascularis. *SNAI2* is also involved in neural crest cell differentiation.

WS3, also referred to as Klein–Waardenburg syndrome, is also caused by mutations in *PAX3*. WS3 exhibits upper limb abnormalities in addition to anomalies to other types of WS, and demonstrates the overlap between clinical phenotypes and genotypes in all Waardenburg syndromes. WS4 (Waardenburg–Shah syndrome) combines the features of Waardenburg syndrome and Hirschsprung's disease, which is a lack of proper innervation of the colon. WS4 is caused by *SOX10* mutations (Pingault *et al.*, 1998), mutations in the endothelin-B receptor gene, *EDNRB* (Puffenberger *et al.*, 1994) or its ligand endothelin-3, *EDN3* (Edery *et al.*, 1996; Pingault *et al.*, 2001). Waardenburg syndrome can also be caused by mutations in other, yet to be identified genes.

14.3.2 **Branchi-oto-renal syndrome**

Hearing loss associated with branchi-oto-renal (BOR) syndrome can be conductive, sensorineural or mixed. As the name implies, in addition to otological effects, branchial arch development and the renal system are also affected. Branchial effects manifest as fistulas or cysts in the sides of the neck up to the ears along with various malformations of the outer, middle, or inner ear. Kidney anomalies can range anywhere from mild hypoplasia to complete absence of the kidneys. There are two types of BOR syndrome, both inherited in an autosomal dominant fashion. BOR1 is caused by defects in *EYA1* (Abdelhak *et al.*, 1997), the human homolog of the *Drosophila* eyes absent gene 1. BOR2 is caused by mutations in *SIX5* (sine oculis homeobox, *Drosophila* homolog 5) (Hoskins *et al.*, 2007). These two transcription factors are known to interact directly during development in the worm *Caenorhabditis elegans* (Li *et al.*, 2004), and illustrate how model organisms like flies and worms can be instrumental in understanding human genetics.

14.3.3 **Usher syndrome**

About 1 in 20 000 people will develop Usher syndrome. It is the most common type of autosomal recessive syndromic hearing loss and is responsible for about half of the cases of combined deafness-blindness. The hearing impairment is sensorineural and the vision loss due to retinitis pigmentosa (RP), a progressive degeneration of the retina (reviewed in Kremer *et al.*, 2006). Some types of Usher syndrome also display a vestibular defect that causes balance disturbances that can lead to late walking in affected children. Genes responsible for the different types of Usher syndrome are listed in Table 14.1. Illustrating the complexity of the genetics of hearing loss, it should be noted that mutations in several of the genes can also cause non-syndromic hearing loss instead of Usher syndrome. *MYO7A* mutations cause DFNA11 and DFNB2, *USH1C* mutations cause

Table 14.1 Usher syndrome

Type of Usher syndrome	Phenotype	Subtypes	Gene	Protein
1	Congenital severe hearing loss; prepubertal onset of RP	USH1B	*MYO7A*	Myosin VIIa
		USH1C	*USH1C*	Harmonin
		USH1D	*CDH23*	Cadherin-23
		USH1E	Unknown	
		USH1F	*PCDH15*	Protocadherin-15
		USH1G	*SANS*	Scaffold protein, ankyrin repeats, SAM domain
		USH1H	Unknown	
2	Congenital moderate to sever hearing loss; postpubertal onset of RP	USH2A	*USH2A*	Usherin
		USH2B	Unknown	
		USH2C	*VLGR1b*	Top of form: very large G-protein coupled receptor 1b
		USH2D	*WHRN*	Whirlin
3	Progressive hearing loss; variable onset of RP; vestibular symptoms	USH 3	*USH3*	Clarin 1

DFNB18, *CDH23* mutations cause DFNB12, and *PCDH15* mutations cause DFNB23. Mutations in *USH2A* can also cause isolated retinitis pigmentosa. The function of some of the Usher syndrome proteins is discussed in more detail later in the chapter.

14.3.4 Pendred syndrome

Pendred syndrome (PDS) is another autosomal recessive syndromic hearing disorder in which mutations in the same gene cause syndromic or non-syndromic hearing loss. In this case, mutations in *SLC26A4* (solute carrier family 26, member 4) were identified in 1997 (Everett *et al.*, 1997) as the cause of PDS and in 1998 (Li *et al.*, 1998) as the cause of the non-syndromic deafness DFNB4. PDS is the most common form of syndromic deafness. The clinical phenotype of PDS is congenital or early-onset sensorineural hearing loss coupled with diffuse thyroid enlargement (goiter) that often develops in early puberty or later. Defects in the SLC26A4 protein, pendrin, cause a structural defect in the bony labyrinth of the inner ear (Mondini defect) or an enlarged vestibular aqueduct (EVA), either of which can be diagnosed with computed tomography, and improper iodine transport from the thyroid, which is detected with a perchlorate discharge test. Vestibular dysfunction is also often present in PDS. Less severe mutations that preserve adequate iodine transport account for the non-syndromic hearing loss (often still accompanied by EVA). Mutations in *FOXI1* (forkhead box I1), a transcriptional regulator of SLC26A4, can also cause the PDS or non-syndromic hearing loss phenotype (Yang *et al.*, 2007).

14.4 Mitochondrial mutations

Mitochondrial mutations that cause hearing loss, either syndromic or non-syndromic (recently reviewed in Kokotas *et al.*, 2007), are a distinct topic when considering genetic hearing loss, because these mutations are inherited in neither an autosomal recessive nor a dominant manner. Mitochondria contain their own small genome (mtDNA), separate from the nuclear chromosomes, which encodes some of the proteins, transfer RNAs, and ribosomal RNAs critical for proper mitochondrial function. Mitochondria are intracellular organelles responsible for oxidative phosphorylation, the primary energy generating system of mammalian cells. Only the ovum contains mitochondria, there are essentially none in sperm, so mitochondria are only inherited from the mother. To complicate matters, thousands of mitochondria are inherited simultaneously, and it is possible that only a subset contain a mutation, a condition called heteroplasmy (Box 14.1). The severity of a clinical phenotype can depend upon which mutation exists, the proportion of mitochondria that have the mutation, and how they segregate during cell division.

The mitochondrial genome contains 16 569 base pairs. Mutations are named based on their nucleotide positions relative to a start site. Two mitochondrial mutations are known to cause non-syndromic hearing loss: 7445A>G in *MT-TS1*, which is a serine transfer RNA gene, and 1555A>G in *MT-RNR*, which encodes a mitochondrial 12S ribosomal RNA. The former tends to cause a childhood onset sensorineural hearing loss, whereas the latter usually causes adult-onset hearing impairment. *MT-RNR1* mutations can also cause hearing loss on exposure to aminoglycoside antibiotics, so if a mutation in this gene is present, it is important for family members related through the maternal line to be counseled to avoid these types of antibiotics, if possible.

In addition to non-syndromic hearing loss, mitochondrial mutations can also cause syndromic hearing impairment. Maternally inherited diabetes and deafness (MIDD) can be caused by mutations in one of several mitochondrial genes. Other mutations can cause the more systemic neuromuscular disorders Kearns–Sayer syndrome, MELAS (myoclonic epilepsy, lactic acidosis and stroke-like episodes), MERRF (mitochondrial encephalomyopathy with ragged red fibers) or NARP (neurogenic weakness, ataxia, and retinitis pigmentosa). Each of these disorders may have hearing loss as a component, but considering the progressive nature of these debilitating conditions, hearing impairment is not the most critical of the many possible clinical concerns.

14.5 Prevalence of age-related hearing loss

Age-related hearing loss, or presbycusis, requires special consideration when discussing genetic hearing loss. While far more common than early-onset deafness, presbycusis is not inherited in a simple Mendelian manner. It is considered a complex trait, in which a combination of environmental factors and genetics contribute to onset and progression.

By the year 2030, 20% of the US population will be over age 65 according to predictions of the US Census Bureau (www.census.gov/population/www/projections/projectionsagesex.html). With the aging populations in most developed countries comes an increased prevalence of age-related hearing loss. Forty percent of the population over age 65 has a hearing impairment significant enough to impair speech recognition (Ries, 1994) and it is rare to find anyone over 70 with perfect hearing. Figure 14.5 shows the average hearing ability of men and women from ages 20 to 80. Note in particular the prevalence of high-frequency hearing loss that accompanies aging and the greater impairments in males compared to females. Presbycusis is a quality of life issue. While it usually does not progress to complete deafness, because it affects communication, it can lead to isolation and depression in elderly people.

Age-related hearing loss is caused by a combination of environmental and genetic factors, and it can be particularly difficult to tease out the relative contributions of each. Virtually no one reaching age 60 or 70 can deny exposure to loud noises or infections or pharmacologic agents in their lifetimes. Studies comparing presbycusis in industrialized societies and agrarian societies show a higher incidence of hearing loss in the industrialized populations (Rosen, 1962; Goycoolea *et al.*, 1986), presumably due to noise exposure, and also possibly due to exposure to pollution or even different diets or medical care. Studies aimed at quantifying the relative contributions of genetics and environmental insults to age-related hearing loss suggest the contributions are roughly 50:50. Twin studies conducted in Sweden (Karlsson *et al.*, 1997) and comparison of genetically unrelated versus genetically related individuals in similar environments (Gates *et al.*, 1999) find that the heritable component of age-related hearing loss ranges from 35–55%.

Because presbycusis is not a monogenic disease, it is likely that the interaction of many genes will individually affect the phenotype, each having a small contribution. Thus, linkage strategies as described later in the chapter will not be effective in identifying age-related hearing loss

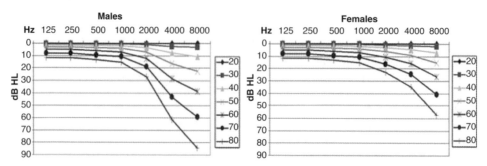

Fig. 14.5 Age-related hearing loss. Standard audiograms measuring hearing acuity in males and females, ages 20–80.
Reprinted from Van Eyken *et al.* (2006) with permission of Wiley-Liss, a subsidiary of John Wiley & Sons.

associated gene variants. To date, a handful of gene variants have been implicated in influencing the severity or onset of age-related hearing loss (Van Eyken *et al.*, 2006, 2007; Usami *et al.*, 2008, Van Laer *et al.*, 2008). More direct progress has been made in mice. Classical inbred mouse strains have a predilection toward or resistance to age-related hearing loss. Because of the simpler genetics involved in inbred strains, a number of age-related hearing loss loci have been mapped with the causative gene variants identified in some (reviewed in Johnson *et al.*, 2006). The future will determine how well the findings in inbred mice translate to the more complex genetics of the human condition. But to date, it is safe to say that the most common form of hearing loss remains the least well understood from a molecular standpoint.

14.6 **How to find deafness genes**

There are many possible approaches to discovering a gene that causes deafness or hearing loss in humans. Some of the more popular and productive methods are outlined below, but this limited discussion is by no means comprehensive.

14.6.1 **Linkage analysis**

One tactic that has historically been quite productive in identifying deafness loci is *pedigree analysis*, also known as *linkage mapping* or *linkage analysis*. Linkage is defined as a tendency for genes close together on the same chromosome to be inherited together, as an intact unit, through multiple generations; thus, they are physically and genetically linked. The further apart two loci are on a chromosome, the higher the likelihood that a recombination event will separate them. Conversely, if two loci are closely linked, it is less likely a recombination event will separate them and they will be inherited together through many generations. Linkage analysis begins with a large family, or pedigree, in which hearing loss is clearly inherited, in either a dominant, recessive, or X-linked manner, and takes advantage of the many genomic resources made available through the human genome project. Inheritance of deafness is tracked through a family pedigree in conjunction with the inheritance of hundreds of genetic markers that map throughout the human genome. Certain genetic markers will be inherited more often in the deaf family members than in the hearing family members, that is, these markers are thought to be linked to the deafness. Narrowing in on the linked region can identify a chromosomal locus in which the deafness gene lies. Depending on the size of the chromosomal interval the discovery may be an arduous task, as dozens or even hundreds of genes may reside there, and each of these is a potential *candidate*. Sometimes an educated guess can be made about which gene in the interval might be the culprit, but often a lab will need to sequence many genes before identifying the deafness causing mutation. All of the genetic loci in black in Figure 14.4 were identified by linkage analysis and most of the loci in blue, for which the genes have been identified, began with a linkage study.

Usually, the larger the available pedigree, the smaller the chromosomal interval in which genes will need to be evaluated. Thus, finding large families in which deafness or hearing loss manifests would appear to be the best approach. This may seem straightforward, but in fact when investigating deafness as opposed to some other genetic disorder, identifying a 'deaf family' can be confounding. Deaf people have a tendency to marry deaf people and may or may not have deaf offspring. If the individuals in question are deaf for different genetic reasons, then analyzing the segregation of a deafness gene through a pedigree can be complicated and lead to inconclusive results. For this reason, many successful linkage studies have begun with isolated populations, where deaf family members are at least partially either physically (e.g. an island, or isolated village) or culturally separated from the general population. This is particularly important for studies

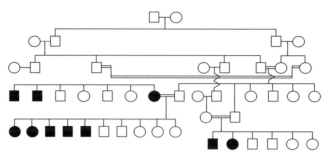

Fig. 14.6 Example of an autosomal recessive non-syndromic hearing loss pedigree. The hearing impairment is observed when related individuals (double horizontal line) have offspring. In this case, the mutation mapped to chromosome 22 and homozygous mutations were observed in *TRIOBP*. Adapted from Riazuddin *et al.* (2006) with permission from Elsevier.

of autosomal recessive hearing loss. In recessive deafness, *two* mutated alleles of the same deafness gene have to be inherited together to cause the phenotype, so a social setting in which some degree of inbreeding occurs (i.e. first cousin marriages) serves to keep the deafness genes 'in the family'. Figure 14.6 is an example of a pedigree from an isolated village in Pakistan in which autosomal recessive deafness segregates. Note that deaf offspring are observed only after matings between genetically related individuals (double horizontal lines, in this example, first cousins). Linkage analysis mapped the gene to chromosome 22 and the responsible gene was eventually identified in this and other DFNB28 families as *TRIOBP* (trio- and F- actin binding protein), a regulator of actin organization (Riazuddin *et al.*, 2006; Shahin *et al.*, 2006).

14.6.2 Reverse molecular genetics

Another tactic that has been successful in identifying a variety of deafness causing genes may be referred to as a *reverse molecular genetic* approach. This approach is a collective term for techniques that begin with an interesting gene and then expand to understand or discover an associated phenotype. In this case, a researcher starts with a gene that has some quality that makes it a good candidate for a gene important in hearing. Once the gene is identified and something is learned about it, such as its expression pattern or chromosomal locus, the researcher works 'backwards' to identify deaf individuals who might have a mutation in the gene. For example, the *COCH* (cochlin) gene was first identified through mRNA studies as a gene with particularly high expression in the human inner ear (Robertson *et al.*, 1994). The northern blot in Figure 14.7 shows the extremely high expression of *COCH* in the human cochlea as compared with a panel of other human tissues. The gene was observed to be highly expressed in regions of the cochlea where patients with the late-onset hearing loss DFNA9 accumulate unusual acidophilic deposits (Robertson *et al.*, 1997). Sequencing the gene in DFNA9 families identified several causative point mutations (Robertson *et al.*, 1998). In another example of reverse genetics, cDNA microarray analysis of gene expression in the inner ear detected strong expression of *CRYM* (μ-crystallin) in the human cochlea and vestibule. Subsequent sequencing of *CRYM* in a collection of non-syndromic deafness patients identified two independent deafness-causing mutations (Abe *et al.*, 2003).

14.6.3 Mouse models

Unquestionably one of the most productive approaches to studying human hearing impairment has been the utilization of animal models, particularly the laboratory mouse. The similarity of

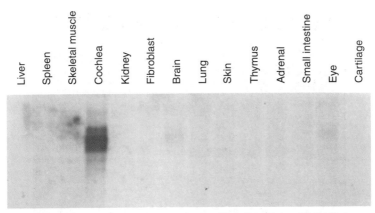

Fig. 14.7 Northern blot of human total RNAs. Hybridization of probe to *COCH* illustrates high level of expression in the cochlea.
Reproduced from Robertson *et al.* (1994) with permission from Elsevier.

inner ear structures between mice and humans and the high degree of gene conservation between the two species make mouse models a major tool for discovery and characterization of hearing loss genes. In general, mouse models may be grouped into three classes: *spontaneously occurring mutations* that have been collected over the years and more recently characterized, *chemically induced mutations* created as part of ongoing efforts to understand gene function in many disease processes, and *targeted mutations*, either gene knock-outs or knock-ins, aimed at studying a particular gene or process.

Spontaneously occurring hearing loss models

Mouse strains with spontaneously occurring hearing loss mutations, some first discovered many years ago, often have the unifying characteristic of being named for their vestibular phenotype. Names like waltzer, jerker, circler, waddler, and shaker reflect that these strains have peculiar behaviors such as excessive circling (Fig. 14.8), head-tossing, and hyperactivity. Vestibular defects often accompany hearing loss, as many structures of the vestibular system and the cochlea require proper functioning of the same genes.

One of the most useful aspects of mouse models is that once a locus is mapped or a gene identified in the mouse, finding the ortholog in humans is relatively straightforward. This is due to two conditions: the high degree of gene sequence conservation among mammalian species, and the occurrence of homologous synteny, which is the conservation of gene order on the chromosomes. Throughout mammalian evolution, segments of ancestral chromosomes were rearranged, broken up, or joined, but large blocks of orthologous DNA remain contiguous. Thus, once a gene is mapped in one mammalian species, it is relatively easy to find its ortholog in another species. The phenomenon of homologous synteny played a major role in the identification of the myosin XV gene as the cause of DFNB3. DFNB3 was mapped to the short arm of chromosome 17 using a kindred from an isolated village in Bali (Friedman *et al.*, 1995). The mutation in the *shaker-2* deaf mouse strain mapped to mouse chromosome 11 in a region of homologous synteny with human 17p (Liang *et al.*, 1998); thus the possibility arose that mutations in the same gene were causing both the mouse and human phenotypes. The research teams reported in back-to-back articles that insertion of an artificial chromosome containing *Myo15* could rescue the deafness in *shaker-2* mice and sequencing *MYO15* identified the deafness causing mutations in humans with DFNB3 (Probst *et al.*, 1998; Wang *et al.*, 1998).

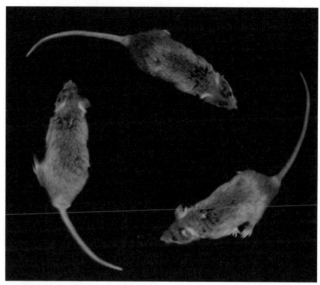

Fig. 14.8 Deaf mouse with vestibular dysfunction. Time-lapse photography captures the circling behavior of a single *shaker-2* mouse.
Reproduced from Probst *et al.* (1998) with permission from the American Association for the Advancement of Science.

In many cases, the mouse mutation that causes deafness is reported prior to identification of a human deafness mutation. For example, the *Snell's waltzer* strain was first identified in 1966 (Deol & Green, 1966). Avraham *et al.* in 1995 identified mutations in *Myo6* (myosin VI) as the cause of the deafness and vestibular phenotype in *Snell's waltzer*. Five years later mutations in human *MYO6* were observed to cause autosomal dominant non-syndromic hearing loss (Melchionda *et al.*, 2001), and another year later recessive non-syndromic hearing loss mutations were identified in humans (Ahmed *et al.*, 2003a). In a similar example, the *Ames waltzer* mouse strain was first identified in 1956 (Schaible, 1956). Mutation of *Pcdh15* was identified as the cause of the deafness and vestibular phenotype in *Ames waltzer* in 2001 (Alagramam *et al.*, 2001a). Subsequent analysis of patients with Usher syndrome type 1F (Ahmed, 2001; Alagramam *et al.*, 2001b) and DFNB23 (Ahmed *et al.*, 2003b) identified mutations in human *PCDH15*.

Chemically induced mutations

As an alternative to scouring animal collections to find unusual and useful mouse mutants, *de novo* mutations can be chemically induced and then offspring screened for the desired phenotype. When the mutagenesis and breeding strategy is arranged appropriately, either dominant or recessive mutations can be obtained. *N*-ethyl-*N*-nitrosourea (ENU) is the most commonly used mutagen because it randomly induces point mutations. Large labs or consortia will create hundreds of mutant strains and screen systematically for any number of phenotypes. The advantage of the mutagenesis screens for hearing loss is that the mutagenesis and assessment of phenotype can be done in a carefully controlled manner and mutants evaluated specifically for hearing status even in the absence of an obvious vestibular phenotype. This in particular is in contrast to finding spontaneous mutants, which were often first ascertained based on their vestibular defect.

Many new mutations that affect the auditory system have been reported (reviewed in Brown *et al.*, 2008). Some are new mutations in genes already implicated in hearing loss, such as *Cdh23* or *Myo7A* (previously identified in the *waltzer* and *shaker-1* strains, respectively), whereas others are novel. Most genes detected thus far are associated with development or functioning of the cochlea, but interestingly, genes affecting more than just sensorineural hearing loss are being uncovered. For instance, the ENU mutagenesis project conducted by the MRC Mammalian Genetics Unit at Harwell (Oxfordshire, UK) has thus far found two mutant strains named *Jeff* and *Junbo* affected with chronic middle ear inflammation (Hardisty-Hughes *et al.*, 2006; Parkinson *et al.*, 2006). Mutations in *Fbxo11* (F-box only protein 11) and *Evi1* (ecotropic viral integration site 1) are causative for the chronic inflammation in these strains, respectively. A companion study in humans suggests gene variants in *FBXO11* are also associated with chronic otitis media with effusion (Segade *et al.*, 2006). Thus, mutation screening can offer insights into diverse aspects of the hearing process.

14.6.4 Targeted mutations

Another technique used frequently in mice to study genetic hearing loss is the creation of targeted mutations, either knock-outs or knock-ins. The mouse genome can be manipulated in ways that the human genome cannot, and strains can be created through genetic engineering strategies that either lack a gene entirely (*knock-out*) or have a point mutation in a particular gene (*knock-in*). Study of the inner ears of hearing impaired human patients is limited by physical inaccessibility, so creation of a knock-out or knock-in mouse line is often the next step undertaken once a human deafness gene is discovered. Many knock-out strains have been created to study the various components of the hearing apparatus and how they interact with each other.

Knock-out and knock-in mutations of the α-tectorin gene, *Tecta*, offer an excellent example of how this type of gene manipulation can shed light on a human hearing loss phenotype. Tectorins are extracellular matrix molecules that make up the tectorial membrane along with collagens and otogelin. In 1998, Verhoeven *et al.* reported a missense mutation in the human α-tectorin gene that causes autosomal dominant non-syndromic hearing loss in humans, and the following year an autosomal recessive form of human hearing impairment was linked to a truncating mutation in the same gene (Mustapha *et al.*, 1999). Knock-out and knock-in mouse models have helped illuminate the function of α-tectorin in the inner ear. Homozygous deletion of the mouse gene produces a tectorial membrane that is detached from the cochlear epithelium. Hearing is impaired by about 35 dB and microphonics are distorted, supporting the hypothesis that the tectorial membrane ensures that outer hair cells can respond to basilar membrane motion and that feedback is delivered for amplification and tuning (Legan *et al.*, 2000). The missense mutation in humans was recapitulated by a knock-in of the same mutation in mouse α-tectorin. Homozygous mutants showed a disrupted matrix structure and detached tectorial membrane similar to that in the knock-out line. Heterozygous knock-in mutants had a more subtle phenotype. These mice showed elevated neural thresholds and a decreased sensitivity to the neural tuning curve. These findings suggest that the tectorial membrane also enables the basilar membrane to stimulate the inner hair cells at their optimal frequency (Legan *et al.*, 2005).

One additional factor must be taken into account when considering using mouse models to study hereditary hearing loss. Unfortunately, some of the best studied inbred mouse strains have innate late-onset hearing loss. A systematic analysis of hearing and vestibular function in dozens of classic inbred lines demonstrates that some of the most popular may not be the best choice when studying a phenotype like hearing loss because of pre-existing underlying pathology (Zheng *et al.*, 1999; Jones *et al.*, 2006; http://hearingimpairment.jax.org/screening.html). This is particularly problematic with some of the most common embryonic stem cell lines that are used to create targeted mutations. If one of these 'poor hearing' strains is used to create a knock-out or knock-in strain, the mutation must be bred into a 'good' hearing genetic background before proceeding with physiological studies.

14.6.5 Genome-wide association studies

Genome-wide association studies (GWAS) are a relatively new technique for identifying common genetic factors that influence health and disease. Instead of looking for an individual gene that causes a disease or disorder, GWAS are designed to explore common sequence variations associated with disease predisposition. GWAS involve genotyping a large number of cases and controls at a large number (10^4–10^6) of single nucleotide polymorphisms (SNPs, pronounced 'snips') spread throughout the genome. Associations are sought between the genotypes at each locus and disease status. When a particular SNP is inherited statistically more frequently in the cases as compared with controls, that SNP is said to be in association with the disease. Work is then focused on that area of the genome to identify the particular gene variant involved in the disease. The gene variant may not cause the disease outright, but it may increase the likelihood or severity of the disorder. With this knowledge in hand, a researcher can begin to understand better the disease pathophysiology, find other partners in the molecular pathway that lead to disease, and predict those at increased risk for developing the disease.

GWAS are most appropriately applied to complex diseases, where many genetic factors and/or a combination of genetic and environmental influences impact expression of a disorder. For example, the technique has been used recently to identify susceptibility loci for complex disorders such as type 1 and 2 diabetes, coronary artery disease, hypertension, and rheumatoid arthritis (Consortium, 2007). In the hearing loss field, GWAS will likely be most useful in investigations of genetically complex hearing loss disorders, such as age-related hearing loss or susceptibility to noise-induced hearing loss. A European consortium recently used association studies to link *GRHL2* to age-related hearing loss (Van Laer *et al.*, 2008) and additional work is underway in several labs around the world.

14.7 Examples of some deafness genes/gene classes/functional groups, and what has been learned from them

The identification of deafness genes and their proteins lays the groundwork for understanding the molecular elements of hearing. Putting together various pieces of the puzzle as they emerge is allowing us to grasp some of the basic mechanisms of the hearing process. As deafness genes have been identified over the past decade, interesting and enlightening trends have begun to materialize from the black box of the inaccessible inner ear. Although the functional importance of every protein that has been discovered cannot be addressed in this chapter, a few particularly noteworthy groups of deafness genes are highlighted, which, taken together, illustrate how they fit into the big picture of cochlear function. A more comprehensive recent review of cochlear proteins augments what is presented below (Eisen & Ryugo, 2007).

14.7.1 Channel proteins and maintenance of the endocochlear potential

The importance of K^+ cycling and maintenance of the endocochlear potential (EP) in the discussion of genetic hearing loss is underscored by the fact that mutations of *KCNQ1*, *KCNE1*, *KCNQ4*, *BSND1*, and *CLCNKA* and *CLKNCB* lead to various forms of syndromic and non-syndromic deafness in humans (Wang *et al.*, 1996; Schulze-Bahr *et al.*, 1997; Kubisch *et al.*, 1999; Birkenhager *et al.*, 2001; Schlingmann *et al.*, 2004) and null mutations of *Kcnj10* and *Slc12a2* lead to deafness in mice (Delpire *et al.*, 1999; Dixon *et al.*, 1999; Marcus *et al.*, 2002) (see Chapter 7, Fig. 7.3). Thus, interruption of any step along the EP pathway is sufficient to cause hearing loss. Furthermore, mutations in the estrogen-related receptor β, *ESRRB2*, cause non-syndromic hearing loss in humans (Collin *et al.*, 2008). This gene is speculated to have a role in development and differentiation of the stria vascularis (Chen & Nathans, 2007) and thus control endolymph production.

Gap junctions mediate intercellular communication in epithelial and connective tissues of the organ of Corti, spiral limbus, and stria vascularis (Zhao *et al.*, 2006) and are also critical for maintaining the endocochlear potential, among other tasks. Various connexins (Cx26, Cx30, Cx31, Cx43, and Cx45) are expressed in the mammalian inner ear. Mice mutated for Cx30 (*Gjb6*) have no EP and are profoundly deaf (Teubner *et al.*, 2003). Cx30 mutations also cause hearing loss in humans. Cx26 (*GJB2*), the most frequent cause of hearing loss in humans, was originally thought to be responsible for K$^+$ recycling from the hair cells back to the stria vascularis after signal transduction (Cohen-Salmon *et al.*, 2002), but a more complicated role has begun to emerge for Cx26, suggesting it may have multiple functions in intercellular signaling (reviewed in Wangemann, 2006 and Eisen & Ryugo, 2007). Cx43 mutations also cause human hearing loss (Liu *et al.*, 2001), although its function is unclear.

14.7.2 The Usher complex and stereocilia bundle proteins

The stereociliary bundle on the apical surface of hair cells is an exquisitely delicate structure responsible for detection of motion caused by propagation of sound waves through the cochlea and ultimate conversion of the mechanical stimulus into an electrical signal. Usher syndrome, as discussed above, is characterized by congenital hearing loss and progressive blindness due to retinitis pigmentosa, and sometimes accompanied by vestibular dysfunction. As noted in Table 14.1, thus far 12 different loci have been implicated as causing a type of Usher syndrome, and in all but three the causative gene has been identified. Molecular studies of the various Usher syndrome proteins are demonstrating a remarkable coordination of function: they all appear to be involved in the development or integrity of the stereociliary bundle.

Similar clinical phenotypes are often begotten by functionally related genes. However, at first glance, one might not have predicted that the various Usher syndrome proteins would have functional interrelationships. One is a motor protein (myosin VIIa), two are cell adhesion molecules (cadherin-23 and protocadherin-15), three are scaffold proteins (harmonin, sans, and whirlin), and three are transmembrane proteins (usherin, VLGR1b, and clarin-1). Recent work provides evidence for an integrated Usher protein network in the cochlea and the retina (reviewed in Kremer *et al.*, 2006; Reiners *et al.*, 2006). Each of the Usher complex proteins is a component of the various extracellular links (transient lateral links, ankle links, and tip links) that connect individual stereocilia and allow their proper development and coordinated action. The harmonin and whirlin proteins appear to be the organizers of the Usher complex, each containing protein–protein interacting domains (PDZ domains) shown to interact with each of the other Usher syndrome type 1 and 2 proteins (Fig. 14.9). Some of the other proteins interact with each other, as well. For example, myosin VIIa also interacts with protocadherin-15 and SANS, allowing a large multi-assembly complex to form in the stereocilia and retina. Mouse knock-out models for several of the genes show the common feature of structural abnormalities in the hair bundle, further supporting the role(s) of the Usher protein network in stereocilia development and maintenance. The one exception to the Usher syndrome multi-protein complex thus far may be clarin-1, the gene responsible for Usher syndrome type 3. Its proposed role is at the other end of the cell, at the synapse (Adato *et al.*, 2002), or else it may play a developmental role.

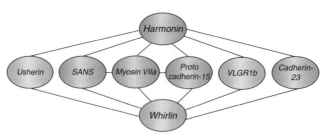

Fig. 14.9 Usher protein complex. Mutation in any one of the proteins shown in blue causes Usher syndrome type 1; mutation in proteins shown in green causes Usher syndrome type 2. Each of the proteins shown is involved in the development or maintenance of hair cell stereocilia. Connecting lines denote known protein–protein interactions (reviewed in Kremer *et al.*, 2006 and Brown *et al.*, 2008).

14.7.3 **Unconventional myosins**

One family of proteins that were perhaps unanticipated as having a critical role in hearing is the unconventional myosins. Myosins are most often thought of in relation to muscle contraction, and of course there are no muscles in the inner ear. However the delicate stereociliary bundles are packed tightly with fibrillar actin, and where there is actin, there are myosin motors to move along it. Unconventional myosins are motor molecules with structurally conserved heads that move along actin filaments using their actin-activated ATPase activity. The highly divergent tails of the different molecules are presumed to be tethered to different macromolecular structures that move relative to actin filaments. Mutations in any one of a half dozen myosin molecules (*MYO3A*, *MYO6*, *MYO7A*, *MYO15A*, *MYH9*, and *MYH14*) can cause either syndromic or non-syndromic hearing loss, or sometimes both.

The function of some of these specific myosin molecules is beginning to be elucidated. At least one role of *MYO15A* appears to be to transport or target the whirlin protein to the tip of the stereocilia (Belyantseva *et al.*, 2005). The interaction is mediated through the PDZ domains of the two proteins. If either protein is mutant, the staircase structure of the hair cell bundle cannot be maintained although the mechanotransduction apparatus appears to function normally (Stepanyan *et al.*, 2006).

14.8 **The great unknowns**

Identifying the gene that causes a disease or disorder is no small accomplishment. But, as many researchers have discovered, sometimes the gene identification is the easy part. While the discovery of the deafness-causing mutations described above have helped us understand better the molecular biology of the inner ear, there are also a handful of deafness genes for which the underlying pathobiology remains to be elucidated. A classic example is *COCH*, one of the most abundantly expressed genes in the inner ear. Mutations in this gene, first discovered in 1998 (Robertson *et al.*, 1998), are associated with a relatively common form of non-syndromic autosomal dominant later-onset hearing loss and vestibular dysfunction. Mutations have been found in dozens of families around the world. Complete knock-out of the gene in mouse appears to have no effect on hearing, at least in young mice (Makishima *et al.*, 2005), thus the human missense mutations are thought to have a dominant negative effect. The mutant protein causes the aggregation of a type of acidophilic deposit in the spiral limbus and the spiral ligament, and cochlin protein is contained in those deposits (Robertson *et al.*, 1997). However, how this aggregation damages hearing is still unknown and the normal function of cochlin remains to be elucidated. Studies of mutant mice with a missense mutation instead of the gene knock-out show late-onset hearing and vestibular deficits (Robertson *et al.*, 2008).

Another example of a deafness gene of unknown function first identified in 1998 is DFNA5 (Van Laer *et al.*, 1998). Deafness-causing mutations have been described in a handful of families (Van Laer *et al.*, 2004; Cheng *et al.*, 2007) and in each case, the mutation results in skipping of exon 8, suggesting the possibility of a very specific gain-of-function mutation. Interestingly, mice missing exon 8 are not hearing impaired, even though they have aberrant numbers of outer hair cells (Van Laer *et al.*, 2005). Lately the DFNA5 protein has generated more interest as a potential tumor suppressor (Akino *et al.*, 2007; Kim *et al.*, 2008). Whether ongoing cancer studies will shed light on this protein's role in the ear remains to be known.

14.9 Genetic testing for deafness/hearing loss

Deafness or hearing loss is diagnosed clinically through audiologic assessment. Whether the hearing loss is syndromic or non-syndromic may be determined through further clinical testing and consideration of family history. There are several important reasons to establish whether a diagnosed hearing loss has a genetic basis and what the gene mutation might be. First, a confirmed genetic diagnosis can rule out the need for further physiological testing. For example, if a deaf newborn is found to have a homozygous Cx26 mutation, then the need for additional expensive clinical tests to rule out syndromic hearing loss is obviated. Conversely, if non-syndromic hearing loss cannot be confirmed through genetic testing, a wider net must be cast to establish the cause of hearing loss and determine whether there may be any clinical sequelae. Thus, knowing the genetic basis of the deafness can help guide medical choices such as whether another clinical condition needs regular monitoring.

Second, genetic diagnosis of hearing loss, either syndromic or non-syndromic, can help with management/habilitation decisions for the hearing impaired patient. For example, if a congenital deafness is due to Usher syndrome, then an educational approach based on sign language might not be the best choice, since the patient will eventually lose vision as well. In such a disease, cochlear implants might be a preferable alternative. A genetic diagnosis can also have predictive value for other family members, either current or future. Siblings or other relatives may be at risk and genetic counseling should be considered.

Sequencing of the human genome has brought a wealth of opportunities for diagnosis of genetic diseases, and hearing loss is certainly among them. A mutation in any one of dozens of different genes can cause deafness. However, currently, molecular genetic testing is available for only a handful of non-syndromic deafness genes (see Table 14.2). Developing a molecular test for a specific deafness gene is currently practical only if the mutated gene is expected to be a relatively common cause of genetic hearing loss. For many of the non-syndromic hearing loss genes, mutations have been found in only one or a few families worldwide. Because mutations in many deafness genes are believed to be quite rare, no clinical genetic testing is available for these genes, although testing on a research basis may be possible.

Molecular genetic testing targets the most common forms of genetic hearing loss. As discussed above, the most common recognized form of genetic hearing loss is due to Cx26 (*GJB2*) mutations, and this was the first diagnostic deafness gene test to be offered clinically. Because of the high frequency of *GJB2* mutations, it is usually the first, and often the only gene, to be tested for mutation when a case of congenital or early-onset deafness is diagnosed. More than 50 labs worldwide offer some form of diagnostic molecular test for mutations in this gene.

Table 14.2 Molecular genetic testing available for non-syndromic hearing loss

Gene	Type of hearing loss	Inheritance pattern
CDH23, GJB2, GJB6, MYO7A, OTOF, SLC26A4*, TECTA, MYO6, TMC1, TMIE, TMPRSS3, USHIC, PCDH15, WHRN	Congenital or prelingual	Autosomal recessive
GJB2, KCNQ4, MYH9, MYO7A, TECTA, MYO6, TMC1	Congenital or prelingual	Autosomal dominant
MTTS1	Congenital or prelingual	Mitochondrial
POU3F4†	Congenital or prelingual	X-linked
COCH, GJB2, MYO7A, WFS1	Postlingual or adult onset	Autosomal dominant
MT-RNR1‡, MT-TS1	Postlingual or adult onset	Mitochondrial

The above genes are considered causative of non-syndromic hearing loss, although some mutations can have very characteristic secondary clinical findings.

All genetic testing data was obtained from the GeneTests website (www.genetests.org).

* *SLC26A4* deafness causing mutations are often accompanied by enlarged vestibular aqueduct.

† *POU4F3* mutations can have a mixed hearing loss with perilymphatic gusher upon stapes surgery

‡ *MT-RNR1* mutations can also lead to sensitivity to aminoglycoside antibiotics.

14.9.1 Genetic testing methodologies

A number of molecular techniques are used to detect mutations in deafness genes. Which method is performed depends partly on the gene and partly on the lab doing the testing. Depending on the size of the gene and the heterogeneity of known mutations, *DNA sequencing* may be the first choice. DNA sequencing has been available for many years and now the process is highly automated. Sequencing is the technique used most often for *GJB2* mutations because *GJB2* is a relatively small gene with only two exons. Deafness-causing mutations have been found throughout the coding region and in splice sites. Most labs sequence the entire gene, although sometimes this is only done after first performing limited testing for the most common mutation depending on the ethnic origin of the patient (e.g. 35delG in Europeans, 167delT in Ashkenazi Jews, 235delC in Chinese). However, other genes are huge in comparison. For example, *OTOF*, the gene that causes DFNB9, has 48 exons, and the *USH2A* gene has 72! It is theoretically possible to sequence all the exons and their splice junctions, however it would be slow and expensive compared to the small *GJB2* gene. Therefore most clinical labs sequence only the exons that have been shown previously to contain mutations causing hearing loss.

Another technique that is sometimes used in diagnostic labs, especially when investigating large genes is *mutation scanning*. This is a two-step process by which the entire coding sequence of a gene is broken down into reasonably sized pieces and first screened by a rough technique such as denaturing gradient gel electrophoresis (DGGE) or single strand conformational polymorphism (SSCP) to determine in which part of the gene a mutation may lie. Then only that small fragment of the gene that may contain a variant is sequenced to determine if it does indeed contain a disease-causing mutation.

In other cases, testing is more targeted, with *sequence analysis of select exons* previously identified as sites of recurring mutations. This is the case for *COCH* mutations, where all hearing loss causing alterations have thus far been located in exons 4, 5, and 12. Another technique is *targeted mutation analysis*, where various techniques can be used to screen for previously identified mutations. This has the advantage of being fast and relatively inexpensive, but the disadvantage is that any new mutations would be missed.

For some deafness genes, dozens of labs test for mutations. For other genes, only one lab in the world may offer clinical testing. An up-to-date listing of genetic testing services can be found at the GeneTests website (www.genetests.org). This site was developed and is maintained by the University of Washington (Washington, USA), with funding from the NIH. The website lists clinical laboratories that perform specific genetic tests, the type of testing they do, and contact information.

Some newer techniques are beginning to emerge that allow for testing of many deafness genes simultaneously. A glass slide technology called APEX (Arrayed Primer Extension) assesses over 400 mutations known to cause Usher syndrome (http://www.asperophthalmics.com). The system screens for known mutations in the *CDH23*, *MYO7A*, *PCDH15*, *USH1C*, *SANS*, *USH2A*, *VLGR1*, and *USH3A* (genes discussed earlier in this chapter). These genes carry mutations in patients with USH1b, USH1c, USH1d, USH1f, USH1g, USH2a, USH2c, and USH3a (Cremers *et al.*, 2007 and Table 14.1). Thus, a clinician does not have to determine first what type of Usher syndrome their patient may have before ordering genetic testing. The biggest disadvantage of this technology is the issue of false negatives. If the Usher testing is negative, it does not exclude a diagnosis of Usher syndrome but only those mutations previously identified. However, as new mutations or new Usher subtypes are recognized, new mutation targets can be added to the diagnostic chip.

Several clincal laboratories are also working on a deafness gene *resequencing 'chip'*. The exons and splice junctions of many deafness genes can be 'sequenced' simultaneously by hybridizing patient DNA to a proprietary chip containing thousands of oligonuleotides complementary to normal DNA. A mismatch is detected by a laser scanner and software determines exactly where in the DNA the mismatch occurred. Instead of looking for many targeted mutations as described for the APEX system, the resequencing technology has the added advantage of being able to discover new mutations. The GeneChip platform can lower costs and improve turnaround time by sequencing multiple genes simultaneously. Techniques that assess multiple deafness genes concurrently are the near future until full genome sequencing is implemented, and may be the first test ordered for any newly diagnosed hearing loss.

14.9.2 Genetic counseling

With any condition that may have a genetic basis, it is recommended that the family meet a genetic counselor. Often, test results are more complicated than 'yes' or 'no' and geneticists or genetic counselors are trained to interpret the significance and limitations of a genetic test, and help a family understand the findings and their implications. Even if genetic testing is performed and results are negative, a genetic form of hearing loss cannot necessarily be ruled out as current testing assesses only a subset of deafness genes (often only *GJB2*). Based on the result of molecular genetic and other clinical testing, a genetic counselor can also help a family determine the likelihood of recurrence, that is, the odds of having another hearing impaired child. With an unknown cause of deafness in an infant and without performing DNA diagnostics, the empirical risk estimate for a hearing couple with no family history to have another deaf child is 10–17% (Smith, 1991). If parental *GJB2* mutation status is known, however, the recurrence risk can be increased or decreased accordingly.

Currently, most genetic testing is performed after a clinical diagnosis of hearing loss. However, in cases where the hearing loss is known to be genetic and the mutation in a family has been identified, it is possible to do a *prenatal diagnosis*. In this case, testing is performed during pregnancy to determine if a fetus is carrying the same deafness gene known to run in the family. Chorionic villus sampling (CVS) and amniocentesis are procedures used to obtain a fetal sample for molecular testing.

Results can be used for early diagnosis and to prepare a family for a deaf child, or the early diagnosis can also be used as a reason to terminate the pregnancy (more on that below).

14.10 Deaf culture and genetic deafness

There is a difference between being deaf (lower case 'd') and Deaf (upper case 'D'). 'Deaf' implies an association with Deaf culture. As with any group that shares a common language (also known as linguistic homogamy, in this case sign language), shared identity and customs also arise. Many Deaf individuals do not consider themselves to be 'handicapped' or feel their hearing loss needs to be 'treated', and may resent the implication that they have a gene 'mutation'. In a school of the deaf, Deafness is the norm and sign language the common mode of communication. Few would argue that deafness is a sickness or that it impacts health (as long as it is non-syndromic). For the Deaf community, the only 'problem' lies with the greater society that has difficulty accepting its differentness.

For these reasons, the discussion of genetic testing for deafness genes requires a certain amount of sensitivity to the Deaf community. Surveys of deaf, hard of hearing (the term preferred over hearing by the Deaf community), and hearing individuals who are not themselves hard of hearing but have a deaf family member show distinct differences in attitudes toward molecular testing for deafness genes (Middleton, 2004). Although all groups show a significant proportion of individuals with mixed feelings toward genetic testing for deafness, Deaf individuals are more likely to have negative feelings toward deafness genetics (using words such as concerned, worried, or horrified), whereas hearing individuals with a family history are more likely to have positive feelings toward deafness genetics (positive, enthusiastic, hopeful). Conflicting attitudes are particularly apparent when discussing prenatal testing for hearing status. A majority of deaf individuals state that they would not have prenatal testing for hearing status. Among those deaf individuals who would have genetic testing, a small percentage said they would prefer to have deaf babies, although the majority said they would not mind either way. These statistics reflect how deafness is not necessarily considered a 'disease' or 'disability', especially among the Deaf, and can even be thought of as a desirable trait to pass on to one's offspring. This point of view is obviously counter to the objective of most prenatal genetic testing. Families with Huntington's disease or hemophilia might have genetic testing in order to avoid passing on their particular condition, not select for it. The reality is that because the most common form of genetic deafness is recessive, the majority of deaf children are born to hearing parents, who, if given a choice, prefer not to have a hearing impaired child. However, because hearing loss is not universally regarded as a handicap, genetic counseling for deafness needs to be sensitive to the concerns of the Deaf community, while trying to provide choices for an at-risk hearing family.

References

Abdelhak S, Kalatzis V, Heilig R, Compain S, Samson D, Vincent C, Weil D, Cruaud C, Sahly I, Leibovici M, Bitner-Glindzicz M, Francis M, Lacombe D, Vigneron J, Charachon R, Boven K, Bedbeder P, Van Regemorter N, Weissenbach J & Petit C. (1997) A human homologue of the *Drosophila* eyes absent gene underlies branchio-oto-renal (BOR) syndrome and identifies a novel gene family. *Nat Genet* 15: 157–64.

Abe S, Katagiri T, Saito-Hisaminato A, Usami S, Inoue Y, Tsunoda T & Nakamura Y. (2003) Identification of CRYM as a candidate responsible for nonsyndromic deafness, through cDNA microarray analysis of human cochlear and vestibular tissues. *Am J Hum Genet* 72: 73–82.

American College of Human Genetics (ACMG). (2002) Genetics evaluation guidelines for the etiologic diagnosis of congenital hearing loss. Genetic evaluation of congenital hearing loss expert panel. ACMG statement. *Genet Med* 4: 162–71.

Adato A, Vreugde S, Joensuu T, Avidan N, Hamalainen R, Belenkiy O, Olender T, Bonne-Tamir B, Ben-Asher E, Espinos C, Millán JM, Lehesjoki AE, Flannery JG, Avraham KB, Pietrokovski S, Sankila EM, Beckmann JS & Lancet D. (2002) USH3A transcripts encode clarin-1, a four-transmembrane-domain protein with a possible role in sensory synapses. *Eur J Hum Genet* 10: 339–50.

Ahmed ZM, Morell RJ, Riazuddin S, Gropman A, Shaukat S, Ahmad MM, Mohiddin SA, Fananapazir L, Caruso RC, Husnain T, Khan SN, Riazuddin S, Griffith AJ, Friedman TB & Wilcox ER. (2003a) Mutations of MYO6 are associated with recessive deafness, DFNB37. *Am J Hum Genet* 72: 1315–22.

Ahmed ZM, Riazuddin S, Ahmad J, Bernstein SL, Guo Y, Sabar MF, Sieving P, Riazuddin S, Griffith AJ, Friedman TB, Belyantseva IA & Wilcox ER. (2003b) PCDH15 is expressed in the neurosensory epithelium of the eye and ear and mutant alleles are responsible for both USH1F and DFNB23. *Hum Mol Genet* 12: 3215–23.

Akino K, Toyota M, Suzuki H, Imai T, Maruyama R, Kusano M, Nishikawa N, Watanabe Y, Sasaki Y, Abe T, Yamamoto E, Tarasawa I, Sonoda T, Mori M, Imai K, Shinomura Y & Tokino T. (2007) Identification of DFNA5 as a target of epigenetic inactivation in gastric cancer. *Cancer Sci* 98: 88–95.

Alagramam KN, Murcia CL, Kwon HY, Pawlowski KS, Wright CG & Woychik RP. (2001a) The mouse Ames waltzer hearing-loss mutant is caused by mutation of Pcdh15, a novel protocadherin gene. *Nat Genet* 27: 99–102.

Alagramam KN, Yuan H, Kuehn MH, Murcia CL, Wayne S, Srisailpathy CR, Lowry RB, Knaus R, Van Laer L, Bernier FP, Schwartz S, Lee C, Morton CC, Mullins RF, Ramesh A, Van Camp G, Hageman GS, Woychik RP & Smith RJ. (2001b) Mutations in the novel protocadherin PCDH15 cause Usher syndrome type 1F. *Hum Mol Genet* 10: 1709–18.

Avraham KB, Hasson T, Steel KP, Kingsley DM, Russell LB, Mooseker MS, Copeland NG & Jenkins NA. (1995) The mouse Snell's waltzer deafness gene encodes an unconventional myosin required for structural integrity of inner ear hair cells. *Nat Genet* 11: 369–75.

Ballana E, Ventayol M, Rabionet R, Gasparini P & Estivill X. (2008) The connexins and deafness homepage. Available at: http://davinci.crg.es/deafness/ (accessed June 2008).

Belyantseva IA, Boger ET, Naz S, Frolenkov GI, Sellers JR, Ahmed ZM, Griffith AJ & Friedman TB. (2005) Myosin-XVa is required for tip localization of whirlin and differential elongation of hair-cell stereocilia. *Nat Cell Biol* 7: 148–56.

Birkenhager R, Otto E, Schurmann MJ, Vollmer M, Ruf EM, Maier-Lutz I, Beekmann F, Fekete A, Omran H, Feldmann D, Milford DV, Jeck N, Konrad M, Landau D, Knoers NV, Antignac C, Sudbrak R, Kispert A & Hildebrandt F. (2001) Mutation of BSND causes Bartter syndrome with sensorineural deafness and kidney failure. *Nat Genet* 29: 310–14.

Bondurand N, Dastot-Le Moal F, Stanchina L, Collot N, Baral V, Marlin S, Attie-Bitach T, Giurgea I, Skopinski L, Reardon W, Toutain A, Sarda P, Echaieb A, Lackmy-Port-Lis M, Touraine R, Amiel J, Goossens M & Pingault V. (2007) Deletions at the SOX10 gene locus cause Waardenburg syndrome types 2 and 4. *Am J Hum Genet* 81: 1169–85.

Brown SD, Hardisty-Hughes RE & Mburu P. (2008) Quiet as a mouse: dissecting the molecular and genetic basis of hearing. *Nat Rev Genet* 9: 277–90.

Chen J & Nathans J. (2007) Estrogen-related receptor beta/NR3B2 controls epithelial cell fate and endolymph production by the stria vascularis. *Dev Cell* 13: 325–37.

Cheng J, Han DY, Dai P, Sun HJ, Tao R, Sun Q, Yan D, Qin W, Wang HY, Ouyang XM, Yang SZ, Cao JY, Feng GY, Du LL, Zhang YZ, Zhai SQ, Yang WY, Liu XZ, He L & Yuan HJ. (2007) A novel DFNA5 mutation IVS8+4 A>G, in the splice donor site of intron 8 causes late-onset non-syndromic hearing loss in a Chinese family. *Clin Genet* 72: 471–7.

Cohen-Salmon M, Ott T, Michel V, Hardelin JP, Perfettini I, Eybalin M, Wu T, Marcus DC, Wangemann P, Willecke K & Petit C. (2002) Targeted ablation of connexin26 in the inner ear epithelial gap junction network causes hearing impairment and cell death. *Curr Biol* 12: 1106–11.

Collin RW, Kalay E, Tariq M, Peters T, van der Zwaag B, Venselaar H, Oostrik J, Lee K, Ahmed ZM, Caylan R, Li Y, Spierenburg HA, Eyupoglu E, Heister A, Riazuddin S, Bahat E, Ansar M, Arslan S, Wollnik B, Brunner HG, Cremers CW, Karaguzel A, Ahmad W, Cremers FP, Vriend G, Friedman TB,

Riazuddin S, Leal SM & Kremer H. (2008) Mutations of ESRRB encoding estrogen-related receptor beta cause autosomal-recessive nonsyndromic hearing impairment DFNB35. *Am J Hum Genet* **82**: 125–38.

Consortium TWT. (2007) Genome-wide association study of 14,000 cases of seven common diseases and 3,000 shared controls. *Nature* **447**: 661–78.

Cremers FP, Kimberling WJ, Kulm M, de Brouwer AP, van Wijk E, te Brinke H, Cremers CW, Hoefsloot LH, Banfi S, Simonelli F, Fleischhauer JC, Berger W, Kelley PM, Haralambous E, Bitner-Glindzicz M, Webster AR, Saihan Z, De Baere E, Leroy BP, Silvestri G, McKay GJ, Koenekoop RK, Millan JM, Rosenberg T, Joensuu T, Sankila EM, Weil D, Weston MD, Wissinger B & Kremer H. (2007) Development of a genotyping microarray for Usher syndrome. *J Med Genet* **44**: 153–60.

Dalamon V, Beheran A, Diamante F, Pallares N, Diamante V & Elgoyhen AB. (2005) Prevalence of GJB2 mutations and the del(GJB6-D13S1830) in Argentinean non-syndromic deaf patients. *Hear Res* **207**: 43–9.

Del Castillo I, Moreno-Pelayo MA, Del Castillo FJ, Brownstein Z, Marlin S, Adina Q, Cockburn DJ, Pandya A, Siemering KR, Chamberlin GP, Ballana E, Wuyts W, Maciel-Guerra AT, Alvarez A, Villamar M, Shohat M, Abeliovich D, Dahl HH, Estivill X, Gasparini P, Hutchin T, Nance WE, Sartorato EL, Smith RJ, Van Camp G, Avraham KB, Petit C & Moreno F. (2003) Prevalence and evolutionary origins of the del(GJB6-D13S1830) mutation in the DFNB1 locus in hearing-impaired subjects: a multicenter study. *Am J Hum Genet* **73**: 1452–8.

Delpire E, Lu J, England R, Dull C & Thorne T. (1999) Deafness and imbalance associated with inactivation of the secretory Na-K-2Cl co-transporter. *Nat Genet* **22**: 192–5.

Deol MS & Green MC. (1966) Snell's waltzer, a new mutation affecting behavior and the inner ear int he mouse. *Genet Res* **8**: 339–45.

Dixon MJ, Gazzard J, Chaudhry SS, Sampson N, Schulte BA & Steel KP. (1999) Mutation of the Na-K-Cl co-transporter gene Slc12a2 results in deafness in mice. *Hum Mol Genet* **8**: 1579–84.

Edery P, Attie T, Amiel J, Pelet A, Eng C, Hofstra RM, Martelli H, Bidaud C, Munnich A & Lyonnet S. (1996) Mutation of the endothelin-3 gene in the Waardenburg-Hirschsprung disease (Shah-Waardenburg syndrome). *Nat Genet* **12**: 442–4.

Eisen MD & Ryugo DK. (2007) Hearing molecules: contributions from genetic deafness. *Cell Mol Life Sci* **64**: 566–80.

Estivill X, Fortina P, Surrey S, Rabionet R, Melchionda S, D'Agruma L, Mansfield E, Rappaport E, Govea N, Milà M, Zelante L & Gasparini P. (1998) Connexin-26 mutations in sporadic and inherited sensorineural deafness [see comments]. *Lancet* **351**: 394–8.

Everett LA, Benjamin G, Beck JC, Idol JR, Buchs A, Heyman M, Adawi F, Hazani E, Nassir E, Baxevanis AD, Sheffield VC & Green ED. (1997) Pendred syndrome is caused by mutations in a putative sulfate transporter gene (PDS). *Nat Genet* **17**: 411–22.

Fortnum HM, Summerfield AQ, Marshall DH, Davis AC & Bamford JM. (2001) Prevalence of permanent childhood hearing impairment in the United Kingdom and implications for universal neonatal hearing screening: questionnaire based ascertainment study. *BMJ* **323**: 536–40.

Friedman TB, Liang Y, Weber JL, Hinnant JT, Barber TD, Winata S, Arhya IN & Asher JH Jr. (1995) A gene for congenital, recessive deafness DFNB3 maps to the pericentromeric region of chromosome 17. *Nat Genet* **9**: 86–91.

Gates GA, Couropmitree NN & Myers RH. (1999) Genetic associations in age-related hearing thresholds. *Arch Otolaryngol Head Neck Surg* **125**: 654–9.

Goycoolea MV, Goycoolea HG, Farfan CR, Rodriguez LG, Martinez GC & Vidal R. (1986) Effect of life in industrialized societies on hearing in natives of Easter Island. *Laryngoscope* **96**: 1391–6.

Hardisty-Hughes RE, Tateossian H, Morse SA, Romero MR, Middleton A, Tymowska-Lalanne Z, Hunter AJ, Cheeseman M & Brown SD. (2006) A mutation in the F-box gene, Fbxo11, causes otitis media in the Jeff mouse. *Hum Mol Genet* **15**: 3273–9.

Hoskins BE, Cramer CH, Silvius D, Zou D, Raymond RM, Orten DJ, Kimberling WJ, Smith RJ, Weil D, Petit C, Otto EA, Xu PX & Hildebrandt F. (2007) Transcription factor SIX5 is mutated in patients with branchio-oto-renal syndrome. *Am J Hum Genet* **80**: 800–4.

Johnson KR, Zheng QY & Noben-Trauth K. (2006) Strain background effects and genetic modifiers of hearing in mice. *Brain Res* **1091**: 79–88.

Jones SM, Jones TA, Johnson KR, Yu H, Erway LC & Zheng QY. (2006) A comparison of vestibular and auditory phenotypes in inbred mouse strains. *Brain Res* **1091**: 40–6.

Karlsson KK, Harris JR & Svartengren M. (1997) Description and primary results from an audiometric study of male twins. *Ear Hear* **18**: 114–20.

Kelley PM, Harris DJ, Comer BC, Askew JW, Fowler T, Smith SD & Kimberling WJ. (1998) Novel mutations in the connexin 26 gene (GJB2) that cause autosomal recessive (DFNB1) hearing loss. *Am J Hum Genet* **62**: 792–9.

Kelsell DP, Dunlop J, Stevens HP, Lench NJ, Liang JN, Parry G, Mueller RF & Leigh IM. (1997) Connexin 26 mutations in hereditary non-syndromic sensorineural deafness. *Nature* **387**: 80–3.

Kim MS, Chang X, Yamashita K, Nagpal JK, Baek JH, Wu G, Trink B, Ratovitski EA, Mori M & Sidransky D. (2008) Aberrant promoter methylation and tumor suppressive activity of the DFNA5 gene in colorectal carcinoma. *Oncogene* **27**: 3624–34.

Kokotas H, Petersen MB & Willems PJ. (2007) Mitochondrial deafness. *Clin Genet* **71**: 379–91.

Kremer H, van Wijk E, Marker T, Wolfrum U & Roepman R. (2006) Usher syndrome: molecular links of pathogenesis, proteins and pathways. *Hum Mol Genet* **15**: R262–70.

Kubisch C, Schroeder BC, Friedrich T, Lütjohann B, El-Amraoui A, Marlin S, Petit C & Jentsch TJ. (1999) KCNQ4, a novel potassium channel expressed in sensory outer hair cells, is mutated in dominant deafness. *Cell* **96**: 437–46.

Legan PK, Lukashkina VA, Goodyear RJ, Kossi M, Russell IJ & Richardson GP. (2000) A targeted deletion in alpha-tectorin reveals that the tectorial membrane is required for the gain and timing of cochlear feedback. *Neuron* **28**: 273–85.

Legan PK, Lukashkina VA, Goodyear RJ, Lukashkin AN, Verhoeven K, Van Camp G, Russell IJ & Richardson GP. (2005) A deafness mutation isolates a second role for the tectorial membrane in hearing. *Nat Neurosci* **8**: 1035–42.

Leon PE, Raventos H, Lynch E, Morrow J & King MC. (1992) The gene for an inherited form of deafness maps to chromosome 5q31. *Proc Natl Acad Sci U S A* **89**: 5181–4.

Lerer I, Sagi M, Ben-Neriah Z, Wang T, Levi H & Abeliovich D. (2001) A deletion mutation in GJB6 cooperating with a GJB2 mutation in trans in non-syndromic deafness: A novel founder mutation in Ashkenazi Jews. *Hum Mutat* **18**: 460.

Li S, Armstrong CM, Bertin N, Ge H, Milstein S, Boxem M, Vidalain PO, Han JD, Chesneau A, Hao T, Goldberg DS, Li N, Martinez M, Rual JF, Lamesch P, Xu L, Tewari M, Wong SL, Zhang LV, Berriz GF, Jacotot L, Vaglio P, Reboul J, Hirozane-Kishikawa T, Li Q, Gabel HW, Elewa A, Baumgartner B, Rose DJ, Yu H, Bosak S, Sequerra R, Fraser A, Mango SE, Saxton WM, Strome S, Van Den Heuvel S, Piano F, Vandenhaute J, Sardet C, Gerstein M, Doucette-Stamm L, Gunsalus KC, Harper JW, Cusick ME, Roth FP, Hill DE & Vidal M. (2004) A map of the interactome network of the metazoan C elegans. *Science* **303**: 540–3.

Li XC, Everett LA, Lalwani AK, Desmukh D, Friedman TB, Green ED & Wilcox ER. (1998) A mutation in PDS causes non-syndromic recessive deafness. *Nat Genet* **18**: 215–7.

Liang Y, Wang A, Probst FJ, Arhya IN, Barber TD, Chen KS, Deshmukh D, Dolan DF, Hinnant JT, Carter LE, Jain PK, Lalwani AK, Li XC, Lupski JR, Moeljopawiro S, Morell R, Negrini C, Wilcox ER, Winata S, Camper SA & Friedman TB. (1998) Genetic mapping refines DFNB3 to 17p11.2, suggests multiple alleles of DFNB3, and supports homology to the mouse model shaker-2. *Am J Hum Genet* **62**: 904–15.

Liu XZ, Walsh J, Mburu P, Kendrick-Jones J, Cope MJ, Steel KP & Brown SD. (1997a) Mutations in the myosin VIIA gene cause non-syndromic recessive deafness. *Nat Genet* **16**: 188–90.

Liu XZ, Walsh J, Tamagawa Y, Kitamura K, Nishizawa M, Steel KP & Brown SD. (1997b) Autosomal dominant non-syndromic deafness caused by a mutation in the myosin VIIA gene. *Nat Genet* 17: 268–9.

Liu XZ, Xia XJ, Adams J, Chen ZY, Welch KO, Tekin M, Ouyang XM, Kristiansen A, Pandya A, Balkany T, Arnos KS & Nance WE. (2001) Mutations in GJA1 (connexin 43) are associated with non-syndromic autosomal recessive deafness. *Hum Mol Genet* 10: 2945–51.

Lynch ED, Lee MK, Morrow JE, Welcsh PL, Leon PE & King MC. (1997) Nonsyndromic deafness DFNA1 associated with mutation of a human homolog of the *Drosophila* gene diaphanous. *Science* 278: 1315–8.

Makishima T, Rodriguez CI, Robertson NG, Morton CC, Stewart CL & Griffith AJ. (2005) Targeted disruption of mouse Coch provides functional evidence that DFNA9 hearing loss is not a COCH haploinsufficiency disorder. *Hum Genet* 118: 29–34.

Marcus DC, Wu T, Wangemann P & Kofuji P. (2002) KCNJ10 (Kir4.1) potassium channel knockout abolishes endocochlear potential. *Am J Physiol Cell Physiol* 282: C403–7.

Melchionda S, Ahituv N, Bisceglia L, Sobe T, Glaser F, Rabionet R, Arbones ML, Notarangelo A, Di Iorio E, Carella M, Zelante L, Estivill X, Avraham KB & Gasparini P. (2001) MYO6, the human homologue of the gene responsible for deafness in Snell's waltzer mice, is mutated in autosomal dominant nonsyndromic hearing loss. *Am J Hum Genet* 69: 635–40.

Middleton A. (2004) Deaf and hearing adults' attitudes toward genetic testing for deafness. In: Van Cleve JV, ed. *Genetics, Disability and Deafness.* Gallaudet University Press, Washington DC, pp. 127–47.

Mohr PE, Feldman JJ, Dunbar JL, McConkey-Robbins A, Niparko JK, Rittenhouse RK & Skinner MW. (2000) The societal costs of severe to profound hearing loss in the United States. *Int J Technol Assess Health Care* 16: 1120–35.

Morton NE. (1991) Genetic epidemiology of hearing impairment. *Ann N Y Acad Sci* 630: 16–31.

Mustapha M, Weil D, Chardenoux S, Elias S, El-Zir E, Beckmann JS, Loiselet J & Petit C. (1999) An alpha-tectorin gene defect causes a newly identified autosomal recessive form of sensorineural pre-lingual non-syndromic deafness, DFNB21. *Hum Mol Genet* 8: 409–12.

Online Mendelian Inheritance in Man (OMIM). (2008) Center for Medical Genetics, Johns Hopkins University, (Baltimore, MD) and National Center for Biotechnology Information, National Library of Medicine, (Bethesda, MD). Available at: www.ncbi.nlm.nih.gov/sites/entrez?db=omim (accessed June 2008).

Parkinson N, Hardisty-Hughes RE, Tateossian H, Tsai HT, Brooker D, Morse S, Lalane Z, MacKenzie F, Fray M, Glenister P, Woodward AM, Polley S, Barbaric I, Dear N, Hough TA, Hunter AJ, Cheeseman MT & Brown SD. (2006) Mutation at the Evi1 locus in Junbo mice causes susceptibility to otitis media. *PLoS Genet* 2: e149.

Pingault V, Bondurand N, Kuhlbrodt K, Goerich DE, Préhu MO, Puliti A, Herbarth B, Hermans-Borgmeyer I, Legius E, Matthijs G, Amiel J, Lyonnet S, Ceccherini I, Romeo G, Smith JC, Read AP, Wegner M & Goossens M. (1998) SOX10 mutations in patients with Waardenburg-Hirschsprung disease. *Nat Genet* 18: 171–3.

Pingault V, Bondurand N, Lemort N, Sancandi M, Ceccherini I, Hugot JP, Jouk PS & Goossens M. (2001) A heterozygous endothelin 3 mutation in Waardenburg-Hirschsprung disease: is there a dosage effect of EDN3/EDNRB gene mutations on neurocristopathy phenotypes? *J Med Genet* 38: 205–9.

Probst FJ, Fridell RA, Raphael Y, Saunders TL, Wang A, Liang Y, Morell RJ, Touchman JW, Lyons RH, Noben-Trauth K, Friedman TB & Camper SA. (1998) Correction of deafness in *shaker-2* mice by an unconventional myosin in a BAC transgene. *Science* 280: 1444–7.

Puffenberger EG, Hosoda K, Washington SS, Nakao K, deWit D, Yanagisawa M & Chakravart A. (1994) A missense mutation of the endothelin-B receptor gene in multigenic Hirschsprung's disease. *Cell* 79: 1257–66.

Putcha GV, Bejjani BA, Bleoo S, Booker JK, Carey JC, Carson N, Das S, Dempsey MA, Gastier-Foster JM, Greinwald JH Jr, Hoffmann ML, Jeng LJ, Kenna MA, Khababa I, Lilley M, Mao R, Muralidharan K, Otani IM, Rehm HL, Schaefer F, Seltzer WK, Spector EB, Springer MA, Weck KE, Wenstrup RJ,

Withrow S, Wu BL, Zariwala MA & Schrijver I. (2007) A multicenter study of the frequency and distribution of GJB2 and GJB6 mutations in a large North American cohort. *Genet Med* **9**: 413–26.

Reiners J, Nagel-Wolfrum K, Jurgens K, Marker, T & Wolfrum U. (2006) Molecular basis of human Usher syndrome: deciphering the meshes of the Usher protein network provides insights into the pathomechanisms of the Usher disease. *Exp Eye Res* **83**: 97–119.

Riazuddin S, Khan SN, Ahmed ZM, Ghosh M, Caution K, Nazli S, Kabra M, Zafar AU, Chen K, Naz S, Antonellis A, Pavan WJ, Green ED, Wilcox ER, Friedman PL, Morell RJ, Riazuddin S & Friedman TB. (2006) Mutations in TRIOBP, which encodes a putative cytoskeletal-organizing protein, are associated with nonsyndromic recessive deafness. *Am J Hum Genet* **78**: 137–43.

Ries PW. (1994) Prevalence and characteristics of persons with hearing trouble: United States, 1990–1991. *Vital Health Stat* **10**: 1–75.

Robertson NG, Khetarpal U, Gutierrez-Espelata GA, Bieber FR & Morton CC. (1994) Isolation of novel and known genes from a human fetal cochlear cDNA library using subtractive hybridization and differential screening. *Genomics* **23**: 42–50.

Robertson NG, Skvorak AB, Yin Y, Weremowicz S, Johnson KR, Kovatch KA, Battey JF, Bieber FR & Morton CC. (1997) Mapping and characterization of a novel cochlear gene in human and in mouse: a positional candidate gene for a deafness disorder, DFNA9. *Genomics* **46**: 345–54.

Robertson NG, Lu L, Heller S, Merchant SN, Eavey RD, McKenna M, Nadol JB Jr, Miyamoto RT, Linthicum FH Jr, Lubianca Neto JF, Hudspeth AJ, Seidman CE, Morton CC & Seidman JG. (1998) Mutations in a novel cochlear gene cause DFNA9, a human nonsyndromic deafness with vestibular dysfunction. *Nat Genet* **20**: 299–303.

Robertson NG, Jones SM, Sivakumaran TA, Giersch ABS, Jurado SA, Call LM, Miller CE, Maison SF, Liberman MC, Morton CC. (2008) A targeted Coch missense mutation: a knock-in mouse model for DFNA9 late-onset hearing loss and vestibular dysfunction. *Hum Mol Genet* **17**(**21**): 3426–3434.

Rudy SF. (2007) The sounds of handheld audio players. *ORL Head Neck Nurs* **25**: 21–2.

Sanchez-Martin M, Rodriguez-Garcia A, Perez-Losada J, Sagrera A, Read AP & Sanchez-Garcia I. (2002) SLUG (SNAI2) deletions in patients with Waardenburg disease. *Hum Mol Genet* **11**: 3231–6.

Schaible RH. (1956) Ames waltzer. *Mouse Newslett* **15**: 29.

Schlingmann KP, Konrad M, Jeck N, Waldegger P, Reinalter SC, Holder M, Seyberth HW & Waldegger S. (2004) Salt wasting and deafness resulting from mutations in two chloride channels. *N Engl J Med* **350**: 1314–19.

Schulze-Bahr E, Wang Q, Wedekind H, Haverkamp W, Chen Q, Sun Y, Rubie C, Hördt M, Towbin JA, Borggrefe M, Assmann G, Qu X, Somberg JC, Breithardt G, Oberti C & Funke H. (1997) KCNE1 mutations cause Jervell and Lange-Nielsen syndrome [letter]. *Nat Genet* **17**: 267–8.

Segade F, Daly KA, Allred D, Hicks PJ, Cox M, Brown M, Hardisty-Hughes RE, Brown SD, Rich SS & Bowden DW. (2006) Association of the FBXO11 gene with chronic otitis media with effusion and recurrent otitis media: the Minnesota COME/ROM Family Study. *Arch Otolaryngol Head Neck Surg* **132**: 729–33.

Shahin H, Walsh T, Sobe T, Abu Sa'ed J, Abu Rayan A, Lynch ED, Lee MK, Avraham KB, King MC & Kanaan M. (2006) Mutations in a novel isoform of TRIOBP that encodes a filamentous-actin binding protein are responsible for DFNB28 recessive nonsyndromic hearing loss. *Am J Hum Genet* **78**: 144–52.

Smith RJ, Bale JF Jr & White KR. (2005) Sensorineural hearing loss in children. *Lancet* **365**: 879–90.

Smith SD. (1991) Rucurrence risks. *Ann N Y Acad Sci* **630**: 203–11.

Snoeckx RL, Huygen PL, Feldmann D, Marlin S, Denoyelle F, Waligora J, Mueller-Malesinska M, Pollak A, Ploski R, Murgia A, Orzan E, Castorina P, Ambrosetti U, Nowakowska-Szyrwinska E, Bal J, Wiszniewski W, Janecke AR, Nekahm-Heis D, Seeman P, Bendova O, Kenna MA, Frangulov A, Rehm HL, Tekin M, Incesulu A, Dahl HH, du Sart D, Jenkins L, Lucas D, Bitner-Glindzicz M, Avraham KB, Brownstein Z, del Castillo I, Moreno F, Blin N, Pfister M, Sziklai I, Toth T, Kelley PM, Cohn ES, Van Maldergem L, Hilbert P, Roux AF, Mondain M, Hoefsloot LH, Cremers CW, Löppönen T,

Löppönen H, Parving A, Gronskov K, Schrijver I, Roberson J, Gualandi F, Martini A, Lina-Granade G, Pallares-Ruiz N, Correia C, Fialho G, Cryns K, Hilgert N, Van de Heyning P, Nishimura CJ, Smith RJ & Van Camp G. (2005) GJB2 mutations and degree of hearing loss: a multicenter study. *Am J Hum Genet*, 77: 945–57.

Stein LK. (1999) Factors influencing the efficacy of universal newborn hearing screening. *Pediatr Clin N Am* 46: 95–105.

Stepanyan R, Belyantseva IA, Griffith AJ, Friedman TB & Frolenkov GI. (2006) Auditory mechanotransduction in the absence of functional myosin-XVa. *J Physiol* 576: 801–8.

Tassabehji M, Read AP, Newton VE, Harris R, Balling R, Gruss P & Strachan T. (1992) Waardenburg's syndrome patients have mutations in the human homologue of the *PAX-3* paired box gene. *Nature* 355: 635–6.

Tassabehji M, Newton VE & Read AP. (1994) Waardenburg syndrome type 2 caused by mutations in the human microphthalmia (MITF) gene. *Nat Genet* 8: 251–5.

Teubner B, Michel V, Pesch J, Lautermann J, Cohen-Salmon M, Söhl G, Jahnke K, Winterhager E, Herberhold C, Hardelin JP, Petit C & Willecke K. (2003) Connexin30 (Gjb6)-deficiency causes severe hearing impairment and lack of endocochlear potential. *Hum Mol Genet* 12: 13–21.

Usami S, Wagatsuma M, Fukuoka H, Suzuki H, Tsukada K, Nishio S, Takumi Y & Abe S. (2008) The responsible genes in Japanese deafness patients and clinical application using Invader assay. *Acta Otolaryngol* 128: 446–54.

Van Camp G & Smith RJH. (2007) Hereditary Hearing loss Homepage. http://webh01.ua.ac.be/hhh (accessed June 2008).

Van Eyken E, Van Laer L, Fransen E, Topsakal V, Lemkens N, Laureys W, Nelissen N, Vandevelde A, Wienker T, Van De Heyning P & Van Camp G. (2006) KCNQ4: a gene for age-related hearing impairment? *Hum Mutat* 27: 1007–16.

Van Eyken E, Van Camp G, Fransen E, Topsakal V, Hendrickx JJ, Demeester K, Van de Heyning P, Mäki-Torkko E, Hannula S, Sorri M, Jensen M, Parving A, Bille M, Baur M, Pfister M, Bonaconsa A, Mazzoli M, Orzan E, Espeso A, Stephens D, Verbruggen K, Huyghe J, Dhooge I, Huygen P, Kremer H, Cremers CW, Kunst S, Manninen M, Pyykkö I, Lacava A, Steffens M, Wienker TF & Van Laer L. (2007) Contribution of the N-acetyltransferase 2 polymorphism NAT2*6A to age-related hearing impairment. *J Med Genet* 44: 570–8.

Van Laer L, Huizing EH, Verstreken M, van Zuijlen D, Wauters JG, Bossuyt PJ, Van de Heyning P, McGuirt WT, Smith RJ, Willems PJ, Legan PK, Richardson GP & Van Camp G. (1998) Nonsyndromic hearing impairment is associated with a mutation in *DFNA5*. *Nat Genet* 20: 194–7.

Van Laer L, Vrijens K, Thys S, Van Tendeloo VF, Smith RJ, Van Bockstaele DR, Timmermans JP & Van Camp G. (2004) DFNA5: hearing impairment exon instead of hearing impairment gene? *J Med Genet* 41: 401–6.

Van Laer L, Pfister M, Thys S, Vrijens K, Mueller M, Umans L, Serneels L, Van Nassauw L, Kooy F, Smith RJ, Timmermans JP, Van Leuven F & Van Camp G. (2005) Mice lacking Dfna5 show a diverging number of cochlear fourth row outer hair cells. *Neurobiol Dis* 19: 386–99.

Van Laer L, Van Eyken E, Fransen E, Huyghe JR, Topsakal V, Hendrickx JJ, Hannula S, Mäki-Torkko E, Jensen M, Demeester K, Baur M, Bonaconsa A, Mazzoli M, Espeso A, Verbruggen K, Huyghe J, Huygen P, Kunst S, Manninen M, Konings A, Diaz-Lacava AN, Steffens M, Wienker TF, Pyykkö I, Cremers CW, Kremer H, Dhooge I, Stephens D, Orzan E, Pfister M, Bille M, Parving A, Sorri M, Van de Heyning PH & Van Camp G. (2008) The grainyhead like 2 gene (GRHL2), alias TFCP2L3, is associated with age-related hearing impairment. *Hum Mol Genet* 17: 159–69.

Verhoeven K, Van Laer L, Kirschhofer K, Legan PK, Hughes DC, Schatteman I, Verstreken M, Van Hauwe P, Coucke P, Chen A, Smith RJ, Somers T, Offeciers FE, Van de Heyning P, Richardson GP, Wachtler F, Kimberling WJ, Willems PJ, Govaerts PJ & Van Camp G. (1998) Mutations in the human α-tectorin gene cause autosomal dominant non-syndromic hearing impairment. *Nat Genet* 19: 60–2.

Wain HM, Bruford EA, Lovering RC, Lush MJ, Wright MW & Povey S. (2002) Guidelines for human gene nomenclature. *Genomics* **79**: 464–70.

Wang A, Liang Y, Friddell RA, Probst FJ, Wilcox ER, Touchman JW, Morton CC, Morell RJ, Noben-Trauth K, Camper SA & Friedman TB. (1998) Association of unconventional myosin MYO15 mutations with human nonsyndromic deafness DFNB3. *Science* **280**: 1447–51.

Wang Q, Curran ME, Splawski I, Burn TC, Millholland JM, VanRaay TJ, Shen J, Timothy KW, Vincent GM, de Jager T, Schwartz PJ, Toubin JA, Moss AJ, Atkinson DL, Landes GM, Connors TD & Keating MT. (1996) Positional cloning of a novel potassium channel gene: KVLQT1 mutations cause cardiac arrhythmias. *Nat Genet* **12**: 17–23.

Wangemann P. (2006) Supporting sensory transduction: cochlear fluid homeostasis and the endocochlear potential. *J Physiol* **576**: 11–21.

Weil D, Polonca K, Blanchard S, Lévy G, Levi-Acobas F, Drira M, Ayadi H & Petit C. (1997) The autosomal recessive isolated deafness, DFNB2, and the Usher 1B syndrome are allelic defects of the myosin-VIIA gene. *Nat Genet* **16**: 191–3.

Yang T, Vidarsson H, Rodrigo-Blomqvist S, Rosengren SS, Enerback S & Smith RJ. (2007) Transcriptional control of SLC26A4 is involved in Pendred syndrome and nonsyndromic enlargement of vestibular aqueduct (DFNB4). *Am J Hum Genet* **80**: 1055–63.

Zelante L, Gasparini P, Estivill X, Melchionda S, D'Agruma L, Govea N, Milá M, Monica MD, Lutfi J, Shohat M, Mansfield E, Delgrosso K, Rappaport E, Surrey S & Fortina P. (1997) Connexin 26 mutations associated with the most common form of nonsyndromic neurosensory autosomal recessive deafness (DFNB1) in Mediterraneans. *Hum Mol Genet* **6**: 1605–9.

Zhao HB, Kikuchi T, Ngezahayo A & White TW. (2006) Gap junctions and cochlear homeostasis. *J Membr Biol* **209**: 177–86.

Zheng QY, Johnson KR & Erway LC. (1999) Assessment of hearing in 80 inbred strains of mice by ABR threshold analyses. *Hear Res* **130**: 94–107.

Chapter 15

Hearing aids and cochlear implants

John K Niparko and Andrea Marlowe

15.1 Introduction

Since the introduction of electronic amplification in the mid-twentieth century, refinements in digital technologies and implantable materials have expanded options for managing hearing loss. Digital technologies now enable clinicians to address specific listening needs by tailoring filtering and amplification capacity, while optimizing cosmetics and comfort with device design, size, and fit.

For patients who do not obtain communicative benefit with conventional hearing aids, implantable technologies can provide improvements in audibility and speech recognition. Potential benefits of contemporary hearing devices now extend beyond access to sound. Prosthetic auditory rehabilitation can now enhance a child's or adult's recognition of salient speech signals in challenging listening environments and enable greater quality and naturalness of sound inputs. This chapter surveys current approaches to prosthetic hearing and related devices, examining their design, indications for use, fitting, and observed outcomes.

15.2 Hearing aids

Hearing care providers rely on hearing aids for managing hearing loss that is not amenable to medical or surgical correction. Hearing aids can benefit individuals with sensorineural hearing loss (SNHL; hair cell loss or damage within the cochlea), conductive hearing loss (inability of sound to move without attenuation through the outer and middle ear), or mixed hearing loss, which has components of both sensorineural and conductive hearing loss. Programmable features of hearing aids allow the processed signal to accommodate a listener's precise audiometric configuration, while allowing flexibility in processing signals to enable adaptation to specific listening environments.

15.2.1 Perceptual underpinnings of hearing aid use

Technological improvements have led to smaller hearing aid cases affording better cosmetics and canal placement of the device, as well as improvements in sound quality and noise reduction. These advances address many of the concerns that have led individuals with hearing loss to avoid amplification. However, while advances in hearing aids have enhanced fidelity of the amplified sound, the ability to mitigate the effects of background noise remains a major limitation. Such constraints in addressing SNHL with amplified sound are based principally in perceptual challenges inherent in SNHL.

Chief among the present limitations is the observation that listeners struggle in acoustically challenging environments, particularly those characterized by background noise, multi-talker scenarios, and reverberation. Competing signals undermine the hearing aid user's abilities to recognize salient speech signals as a result of both degradation of the quality of speech signals in acoustically unfavorable environments as well as the masking effects of background noise and echoes (Boothroyd, 2006). Excessive reverberation found in theatres, places of worship, and concert halls impose well-recognized constraints to speech recognition with hearing aids.

The successful rehabilitation of SNHL requires a full understanding of associated psychophysical correlates that have been long established. While SNHL is commonly thought to entail reductions in sensitivity (Liberman & Kiang, 1978), elevated thresholds combine with other perceptual phenomena to challenge effective listening with hearing aids. Reduced frequency resolution (Florentine *et al.*, 1980), constraints in the dynamic range of intensity (Evans, 1975), and the masking effects of tinnitus often combine to challenge speech perception with hearing aid use in SNHL. Speech intelligibility is particularly challenged by reduced resolution of spectral contrasts contained in the speech signal (Boothroyd *et al.*, 1996). Hearing aid circuits address impaired spectral filtering with bandpass filters for frequency-selective amplification of specified spectra, while limiting output to effective, comfortable intensity ranges through compression.

The dynamic range of conversational speech is represented by the healthy cochlea as a mechanism of discriminating speech sounds. For example, vowel inputs are typically of greater intensity than are consonants. SNHL imposes constraints in the dynamic range of intensity coding by (i) raising the threshold of audibility of specific frequency components and (ii) lowering the ceiling of tolerance with increments in intensity (Boothroyd, 1998). As greater SNHL further constrains the dynamic range, there is a resultant misrepresentation of low- and high-intensity phonemes. This phenomenon, recruitment, represents a common obstacle in the attempt to provide an adequate level of loudness growth and comfortable loudness in order to attain a sense of natural audibility of spectral components.

Recruitment is defined as an 'abnormal growth in loudness' (Moore, 1991). The SNHL listener experiences a counter-intuitive perceptual experience. While low-intensity sounds are inaudible, increasing intensity via hearing aids in an attempt to enhance audibility and adequate loudness causes sounds to become a source of physical discomfort. Recruitment is observed in the frequencies where hearing is most impaired, typically the high frequencies. Such high-frequency cues carry critical phonemic (consonant) information and are typically conveyed at relatively low intensity. Thus their audibility requires greater amplification and entails the risk of intolerance due to recruitment.

15.2.2 **Device design**

Amplifier and compression technology

The hearing care clinician accommodates recruitment with hearing aid fitting procedures. Digital circuits incorporate compression for differential amplification across spectral channels.

Compression technologies address the normal fluctuations in intensity of acoustic signals. For the ear with SNHL, recruitment of signals that normally grow in intensity can make listening with a hearing aid uncomfortable and even unbearable. If equal amplification is applied to speech signals that normally fluctuate by 20–35 dB, recruitment renders the signal intolerable to the listener between words, and even within the same word. However, if a hearing aid is able to 'compress' the fluctuating intensities into the listener's comfortable dynamic range, the signal is rendered tolerable. Using multiband compression, the clinician can adjust the amount compression to the more vulnerable spectral channels.

The strength of amplification or 'gain' is adjusted according to an individual's hearing loss (Fig. 15.1). Gain represents the difference in level of the input relative to the level of the output. Compression can be adjusted separately for spectral channels. When low-intensity sound enters

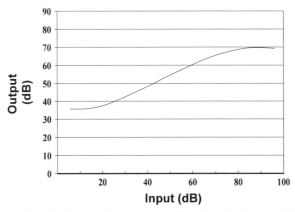

Fig. 15.1 A schematic plot of a theoretical input/output function of a hearing aid. The curve shows the amount of gain applied to different levels of inputs in a hearing aid. Gains at the low- and high-output ends of the curve improve audibility of soft sounds and compress louder inputs, respectively. After *Directional hearing aid microphone – application notes*. Knowles Technical Bulletin TB-21. Knowles Electronics, Itasca, IL, USA.

the hearing aid, it is amplified based on a prescribed gain. Conversely, when high-intensity sound is received, the applied gain is reduced.

Signal attenuation through compression offers a useful strategy of compensating for SNHL when recruitment is present. Compression strategies enable control of the intensity of the input, maintaining an output that is below a preset level of maximum power output (MPO). For louder sounds, when the level detected by the hearing aid's circuits reaches this predetermined level, further gain is attenuated, thus compressing the output without substantial distortion or discomfort. Multistage compression offers a dynamic form of signal attenuation that accommodates functional listening (Fig. 15.2). When sound levels drop below that predetermined level, compression is released and gain is increased.

Most hearing aid users function well with compression and exhibit enhanced speech recognition (Dillon, 1996). Compression systems are classified on the basis of their static and dynamic

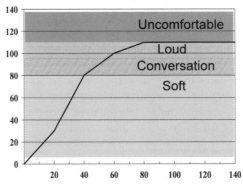

Fig. 15.2 A plot of an input/output function of a hearing aid utilizing multistage compression. As the input level increased past the point of comfort for the listener, the signal is moved into a more comfortable range to avoid excessive inputs that produce discomfort.
After *Directional hearing aid microphone – application notes*. Knowles Technical Bulletin TB-21. Knowles Electronics, Itasca, IL, USA.

characteristics (Hickson, 1994) compression limiters, automatic volume control (AVC) systems, and those with adaptive recovery time and automatic gain control (AGC) (Moore, 1990; Stone *et al.*, 1999) and syllabic compression. Syllabic compression refers to rapid changes in control of the input speech envelope, allowing for a sufficient boost of soft consonants while not over amplifying greater intensity vowels. As a result, all parts of syllables can be heard in harmony. Multichannel compression devices have, to date, used a variety of different types of compression, with syllabic compression in each frequency channel being the most popular. Experimental evidence suggests that multistage compression limiting is generally superior to peak clipping as a means of controlling the output of the instrument (Fig. 15.2). One exception occurs in the case of a profound loss in an individual who relies on powerfully amplified outputs. Here, peak clipped instruments, in some cases despite distortion, better meet the needs for powerful output.

15.2.3 Microphone technology

A hearing aid microphone is designed to detect variations in sound pressure and convert them into electrical codes as the afferent arm of processing. The microphone is housed within the casing of a hearing aid, or occasionally linked for remote placement, closer to the sound source. Ideally a microphone provides a broad frequency response and while at the same time minimizing responses to low-frequency vibrations that can be produced by head movements and walking. The traditional hearing aid microphone is omnidirectional, thus providing no bias to sound based on the point of origin in an auditory scene. An omnidirectional microphone is inherently biased in the intensity domain; a louder stimulus will have a greater variation in sound pressure.

A directional microphone can help in listening to speech in adverse conditions, such as attending to one speaker in competition with other speakers or in competition with background noise. Directionality is commonly achieved with two microphones working in tandem. Inputs from both microphones are used to determine the final input into the processing system information (Fig. 15.3). Two sound ports sample sound pressures from polar-opposite directions, front and rear. Sound pressure waves travel to both sides of the diaphragm, the motion of which is driven by the difference in pressure on its two sides. If the acoustic pressure entering two ports is the same, there is cancellation and there is a zero pressure difference on the two sides of the diaphragm. Here, the microphone has no output – a desired goal for treating noise. Typically inputs from the front offer salience (black arrows in Fig. 15.3). Non-salient acoustic waves from the rear travel (as noise-gray arrows) into both the front and rear ports, and there is an inherent time delay between the two ports. Because of this time delay, the signals are not identical, and there is a small difference in pressure on the two sides of the diaphragm. In order to modify the polar response so that sounds originating at 180° are attenuated relative to those from the front, an acoustic time-delay is introduced in the rear port.

A sound wave arriving from the rear requires additional time to travel to the front port. If the time delay network produces a delay of the same duration, then the delayed signal from the rear port and the signal from the front port arrive simultaneously at opposite sides of the diaphragm and cancel each other. This results in a minimum sensitivity to noise inputs from the 180° source and yields the familiar cardioid pattern polar (front) response (Fig. 15.4). Directional microphone hearing aids can provide 4–5 dB improvement in signal-to-noise ratio in noisy environments when the noise arrives equally from all directions.

A directional microphone gives precedence to sounds sampled from in front of the listener; sounds sampled from lateral and posterior soundfields are attenuated in the input stream. This arrangement enhances the signal-to-noise ratio for sampled acoustic information in the anterior soundfield, particularly when compared with an omnidirectional microphone with multiple

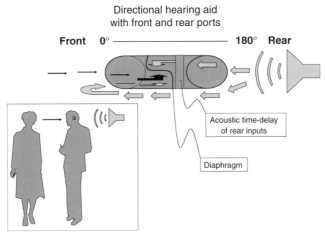

Fig. 15.3 Schematic of a directional microphone. A directional aid can improve the ability to hear in noisy environments as sensitivity to sounds arriving from behind the user is attenuated when compared with its sensitivity to sounds arriving from the front. Typically, a person wishes to hear a speaker whose voice projects from the front. As shown here, a directional microphone worn by the male listener enables him to hear the female speaker's voice with full sensitivity while inputs from sound sources from the rear self-cancel.

After *Phonak extra users guide*. Phonak hearing systems, Phonak AG, Stäfa, Switzerland.

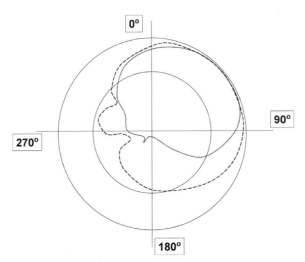

Fig. 15.4 Polar plot showing directionality of a microphone designs. Polar-plot representation of soundfields sampled by directional (dotted boundary) and omnidirectional (dashed boundary) microphones. The soundfields demonstrated approximate those occurring for sounds at 2 kHz, sampled by a right-sided hearing aid with the listener facing 0°. This microphone is limiting the sound coming in from behind and on the left side of the listener- mostly between 180° and 270°. After Echo block: proven to be highly effective in reverberant situations. *Savia Field Study News*. Phonak hearing systems, Phonak AG, Stäfa, Switzerland.

ports (Fig. 15.4). Speech reception performance under conditions of reduced signal-to-noise ratios (e.g. distance listening or in background noise) may thus be improved with the addition of a second microphone (Valente *et al.*, 1995). If noise and speech come from the same direction, however, the dual microphone paradigm loses its advantage (Ricketts, 2000). Directional microphones have a size requirement and therefore may not be available in smaller hearing aid designs.

Adaptive directional microphones are a more sophisticated type of directional microphones, common in current hearing aids. Adaptive directionality adjusts the polar plot by moving the null towards the source of the background noise. This is more advantageous than fixed directional microphones, particularly when the noise source is off to one side of the listener (Ricketts & Henry, 2002).

Hearing aid users may prefer an omnidirectional microphone in quiet as loudness growth and audibility of sounds from all directions is improved. To provide this option some hearing aids are designed to allow the user to switch from an omnidirectional- to a directional-mode as desired.

15.2.4 Analog versus digital technology

Analog hearing aids are traditional instruments that use electronic circuitry, rather than semi-conductor-based microchips, in the amplifier and are the least expensive hearing aids. They offer compression, telecoil, directional microphones, and manual, automatic, or remote volume controls.

Digital hearing aids convert acoustic information relayed by the microphone into a digitized code that is then processed by an amplifier consisting of microchip. Adjustments of amplifier output are programmed using computer software. Substantially more expensive, the primary advantage of digital signal processing (DSP) is that it has far greater processing power than analog signal processing (ASP). The greater processing power represents greater decision-making ability by the instrument, allowing many more adjustments and greater precision for the listener. It is yet to be determined, however, which processor adjustments are optimal for various listening situations. Further, research data do not clearly indicate that DSP provides superior speech understanding in noise than does ASP. Anecdotal reports, however, indicate subjective preference for the sound quality and comfort of digital instruments.

15.2.5 Multiple channels

It is possible to obtain either analog or digital hearing aids that can amplify a wide range of frequencies. All types of hearing aid are capable of providing more amplification to high frequencies, to low frequencies, or equal amplification to all frequencies, as determined necessary in fitting the hearing loss of the individual.

The amount of amplification across the spectrum of frequency (frequency response) can be adjusted. Digital or digital–analog hybrid aids can divide the frequency response into multiple channels and adjust amplification characteristics, including compression, as applied independently to each channel (see Fig. 15.2).

15.2.6 Telecoils and assistive technologies

Telecoils are tightly wrapped copper coils housed within the hearing aid. Electromagnetic currents generated external to the hearing aid are sensed and transduced into an electrical signal, which can then be processed, amplified and sent on to the ear. A standard telephone has a magnet in the handset that emits an electromagnetic energy. Telecoils can improve the signal-to-noise ratio for telephone listening (Katz, 1994) by focusing in on the electromagnetic signal (coming from the phone) and eliminating the ambient acoustic energy (coming from the loud dishwasher in the kitchen). For listeners with moderate to severe SNHL, the telecoil also facilitates telephone use by reducing acoustic feedback, which is common when listening to the phone with a hearing aid set to pick up an acoustic signal via the microphone. Listeners with mild SNHL may find telephone use with only the hearing aid microphone acceptable and more convenient, as those listeners are generally receiving a lesser degree of amplification.

The telecoil can provide an adaptive interface to an assistive listening device such as an infrared or FM receiver to a hearing aid via a neckloop. The sound from the assistive device is transmitted to the neckloop and is then transmitted to the telecoil to provide signal reception by an electromagnetic pathway. Telecoil reception can be applied to large room listening. Telecoils can receive sound from room loops, which are transmission systems built into the structure of theaters, auditoriums, and houses of worship, or patient-worn (neck) loops. As with telephone use, the desired signal is substantially free of room noise and speech other than the microphone-equipped speaker of interest. Room loop amplification systems cannot be accessed by hearing aids lacking telecoils.

15.2.7 Fitting procedures

With a behind-the-ear (BTE) instrument, the sound output travels from an output speaker through tubing into a channel within the earmold that conforms to the shape of the ear canal. With an in-the-ear hearing aid, the entire device is shaped to conform to the membranous portion of the external ear canal. Precise fit of the earmold or hearing aid casing is essential to enhanced efficiency and faithful delivery of the acoustic output of the hearing aid. The 'open mold' design is a popular option for high-frequency hearing losses. A tube or a custom micromold is fit into the ear canal which provides enhanced high-frequency sound transmission and natural low-frequency hearing without utilizing the greater mass of material in the ear canal. This provides a more comfortable fit by reducing the bulk of the mold and hence the sense of occlusion, as well as utilization of natural acoustic inputs (Fig. 15.5).

Hearing aids are customized to fit the individual wearer across an expanding set of perceptual domains. In addition, memories, telecoils, and remote controls are commonly available in contemporary hearing aids. Digital circuits entail greater costs and should be guided by careful

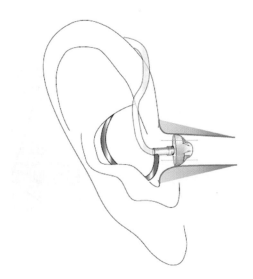

Fig. 15.5 Open-fit molds placed within the membranous portion of the external auditory canal offer a light-weight alternative to heavier, occlusive molds. Lighter polymer materials and specially designed ports offer ventilation, while maintaining a baffle to reduce the escape of high-frequency inputs. Adapted from Phonak Publications; www.phonak.com.

consideration of the severity and profile of the SNHL, communication settings, and specific communication needs.

Fitting procedures are largely guided by the patient's experience in hearing speech in noise. None of the noise reduction strategies currently used in analog or digital hearing aids can completely eliminate noise in typical listening situations, particularly when offending noise is generated by competing speech. In general, the greater the SNHL, the greater is the challenge of discriminating speech in noise. Even people with a moderate (40–60 dB HL) hearing loss require a 5–7 dB signal-to-noise advantage to equal the speech perception of normal hearing listeners (Killion, 1997). Hearing care clinicians can utilize advances in digital technology and its noise reduction algorithms to optimize speech perception in noise. Dual microphones are particularly helpful in managing background noise. Well-fit directional microphone can provide close to 6 dB enhancements of the signal-to-noise ratio in certain noise situations (Killion *et al.*, 1998).

The assessment of outcomes with hearing aid fitting procedures poses clinical challenges. Measuring a patient's perceived benefit in a controlled environment, such as an audiological testing suite, provides only limited information of true world effectiveness. To augment clinical assessment with probes of real world listening experience, patient diaries and self-report measures can inform strategies for hearing aid fitting. Procedures that are representative of the dynamic environments that listeners routinely experience are particularly informative for hearing aid programming (Gatehouse & Akeroyd, 2006).

Reverberation suppression (Fig. 15.6) is a newer technique incorporated into hearing aids. The approach to reducing the effects of reverberation is to adaptively filter and subtractively combine inputs through comparison of the initial direct sound signature and a delayed sound signature of similar frequency composition. Suppression is most actively applied to sounds with signatures of long reverberation times.

15.2.8 Binaural fitting

Much of the perceptual benefit provided by the normal auditory system is based on the presence of two systems functioning simultaneously – that is, two ears that independently sample the acoustic environment and transduce differentiated information for central processing. Detecting a sound is a critical first step in the hearing process, and can be performed reasonably well by one

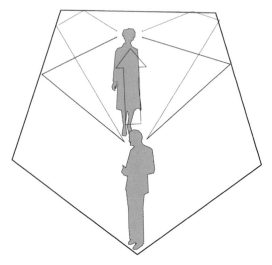

Fig. 15.6 Schematic of reverberation patterns. Echoes of voice signals have multiple angles of trajectory, particularly in settings with hard surfaces and large rooms. Such conditions, by enhancing reverberations, serve to mask the spectral features of salient speech for the listener.

sensitive ear. However, much of the benefit of a normal hearing pathway is based on the presence of two receivers that operate simultaneously, that is, two ears that independently sample the sound environment and enable differential intensity and temporal and spectral information to be processed centrally. Without such information, as in monaural listening or when there is a drastic difference in hearing levels between ears, several deficits arise: the ability to locate the source of sound, to suppress background echoes (a common problem in large room-, distance-listening), and the ability to give priority to spoken words over background noise (a common problem in listening environments with multiple talkers).

Binaural processing is fundamental to spatial separation of salient acoustic information from competing stimuli. Thus, in counseling patients, it is important to understand the role of optimized bilateral inputs for listening in challenging environments. When both ears demonstrate SNHL, two hearing aids are widely accepted as a means of mitigating perceptual deficits. Objective evidence of benefit has been slower to evolve probably owing to the adequacy of hearing functions in clinic-based testing. Bilateral hearing aids are, however, now associated with self-reports of significant benefit in comparison with unilateral fitting particularly in contexts of more demanding and dynamic listening and in reduced listening effort (Noble, 2006). Such inputs are designed to empower the aided listener to determine who is talking, determine context, detect speech sounds critical to comprehension, and suppress unwanted sounds.

15.2.9 Assistive training

Even individuals without SNHL use other assists in listening. For instance, attention to visual cues (non-verbal communication) and context (knowing 'the who, why, where, and when' of discourse) can help us to more accurately determine what is being said. These sources of communication cues are emphasized in the counseling of hearing aid users.

15.2.10 Contralateral routing of signals amplification

Unilateral deafness can impose difficulties in verbal communication despite the presence of normal unilateral hearing. Difficulties in monaural listening are most commonly experienced when salient speech is corrupted by location or background noise. The greatest difficulties for monaural listeners occur when the sound source of interest is positioned on the side of impairment or when reverberations, background noise, or an unfamiliar speaker corrupt the cues for sound localization. These effects emphasize that unilateral deafness entails two forms of impairment. First, the profound loss of sensitivity makes it difficult to hear sounds that are lateralized to the affected hemifield. Second, unilateral deafness prevents the use of head shadow and binaural processing that normally enhance the segregation of signals from background (masking) noise. Contralateral routing of signals (CROS) amplification is designed to expand the soundfield through effective routing of auditory inputs to the functional ear.

The CROS aid is a two component system that places a microphone on the ear with the hearing loss and signals, via FM transmission, a receiver-speaker system in the better hearing ear. This configuration allows the better hearing ear to 'hear' for the poorer. The main benefit of the CROS aid is that it compensates for the head shadow effect which normally impedes sounds that emanate from a source on the contralateral side. There are, however, inherent limitations to CROS device use: the better ear canal is fit with a mold that entails perceptual costs.

15.3 Bone anchored hearing devices

Semi-implantable devices to achieve effective bone conduction have undergone considerable refinement. The clinical goal of the Baha implantable system is to enable a patient to hear voiced

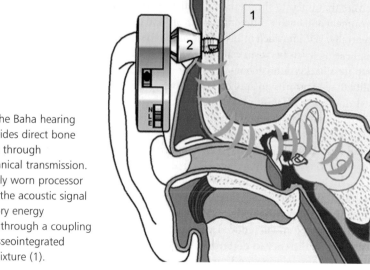

Fig. 15.7 The Baha hearing device provides direct bone conduction through vibromechanical transmission. An externally worn processor transduces the acoustic signal into vibratory energy transferred through a coupling (2) to an osseointegrated implanted fixture (1).

and environmental sound through bone-anchored, bone conduction. The Baha implantable device transfers the vibrations of sound through the implant to the mastoid bone, and ultimately to the inner ear where intact cochlear hair cell transducers are deflected, thereby activating the auditory nerve.

The Baha system uniquely combines two elements in its design. Each is critical to the system's high efficiency in producing bone-conducted hearing and is depicted in Figure 15.7: (1) an osseointegrated fixture that is accessed through (2) a percutaneous connector.

The fixture is a surgically placed implant that integrates with bone of the mastoid cortex. Much of the functional advantage of the Baha system, particularly with respect to high-frequency hearing, relates to efficiencies in transmitting sound energies afforded by the osseointegrated fixture. Efficiencies obtain from direct coupling of the externally worn transducer to the bony implant. The implanted fixture's immobility reduces the stress applied to soft tissues surrounding the penetration site and prevents subsequent inflammatory reactions. The capacity of non-alloyed titanium to integrate directly with bone, as first described by Brånemark & Labrektsson (1982), emphasizes that bone to metal contact is achieved in the absence of fibrous tissue ingrowth. The concept of 'osseointegration' is thus based on histologic evidence of viable bone growth onto and into the surface of titanium implants that are placed with atraumatic surgical technique.

A unique feature of the Baha implant system relates to percutaneous penetration by a connecting abutment. This strategy of coupling the transducer with the implant is currently the only means by which the full spectrum of sound inputs can be transduced for bone conduction in an efficient way, thus enhancing the naturalness and fidelity of sound inputs. The externally worn transducer is thus attached to the fixture with a percutaneous connector (Fig. 15.8). Importantly, the site of percutaneous penetration must be prepared to avoid inflammatory and infectious sequelae and tolerance to this approach is now well documented.

The cutaneous–implant interface as originally conceived by Brånemark & Labrektsson (1982), is based in principles observed throughout nature. Properly developed percutaneous penetration limits tissue mobility and preserves the stability of tissue planes, while limiting the invasion of microbes and subsequent inflammation (Adell *et al.*, 1986; Lekholm *et al.*, 1986). By mimicking these attributes in the skull, the surgeon creates a permanent cutaneous–implant border that the

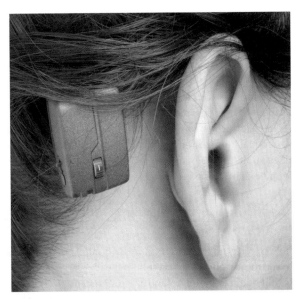

Fig. 15.8 The externally worn component of the Baha system, which is snap-coupled to an interfacing connector attached to an osseointegrated implant. The digital processor shown here is worn behind the ear. The processor transduces acoustic signals into vibromechanical inputs transferred to the temporal bone.

patient may easily maintain. The clinically used bone-anchored device consists of a pure titanium implant and a sound processor. The processor is coupled directly the titanium implant via a percutaneous abutment, utilizing a force-fit, plastic coupling.

Conductive and mixed hearing losses are highly prevalent disorders that are often addressed with otologic (tympanoplasty) procedures or rehabilitated with traditional hearing aids. However, a large subset of patients with peripheral mastoid, middle ear, and ear canal anomalies require alternative approaches. Such patients are either unsuitable surgical candidates for correction of their deficit or are unable to utilize a traditional hearing aid. This group commonly includes patients with chronically draining ears, those with discomfort from the sound levels required from a traditional hearing aid, and patients unable to tolerate a hearing aid because of a large mastoid bowl or meatoplasty following surgery for chronic ear infections. In addition, hearing loss from aural atresia, canal closure after skull base tumor removal, and inoperable tympanosclerosis or otosclerosis may be amenable to auditory rehabilitation through bone conduction (Lustig & Niparko, 1999).

Håkansson *et al.* (1990) reported a strong relationship between pure-tone average (PTA) and successful rehabilitation with the Baha device. In the group with the best cochlear reserve (PTA <45 dB), the vast majority of patients reported subjectively improved hearing with the implant. Conversely, in subjects with progressively less cochlear function (e.g. >60 dB) the report subjective hearing gain was reduced, though the majority of users still experienced benefit. Further, speech discrimination scores improved on average from 14% unaided and 67% with a traditional hearing aid, to 81% with the Baha device. This proportion increased to 85% if persons with a sensorineural loss greater than 60 dB HL were excluded and to 89% if subjects with PTA worse than 45 dB were excluded. Based upon these results, the authors recommended that to be in consideration for a 'high success rate' with the Baha, patients should have a PTA by bone-conduction less than 45 dB HL, though improvements in hearing should still be expected for a PTA of up to 60 dB. Lustig *et al.* (2001) reviewed an initial multicenter US experience with the Baha devices. The most common indications for implantation included chronic otitis media, external auditory canal stenosis, and aural atresia. An average improvement of 32 dB ± 19 dB was observed with the use of the Baha device. Closure of the air–bone gap to within 10 dB of the preoperative bone conduction thresholds occurred in 80% of patients.

In addition to implantation for purely conductive or mixed hearing losses, emerging data demonstrate the value of Baha amplification for patients with unilateral profound SNHL. The Baha on the deafened ear effectively expanded the sound field for the patient and improved the patient's speech understanding in noise, much like a CROS (contralateral routing of sound) hearing aid or transcranial CROS system (Vaneecloo *et al.*, 2001; Niparko *et al.*, 2003). However, in contrast to CROS, Baha does not require an earmold placed in the better ear, with attenuation of high-frequency inputs. As the better hearing ear functions normally, the acoustic 'head shadow' retains the capacity to isolate sounds incident to the deafened side. Sounds on the side of the deaf ear are heard in the better ear through transcranial bone conduction from the Baha. This strategy avoids the perceptual costs of wearing an earmold on the better hearing ear. Preliminary results show subjective improvement in both sound quality and speech understanding in noise (Niparko *et al.*, 2003).

15.4 Cochlear implants

Cochlear implants utilize implantable circuitry and systems of information processing to enable to access sound for those who are unable to meaningfully connect to sound with hearing aids (Fig. 15.9). By virtue of a preserved neural axis of the auditory periphery and a central system capable of processing electrically encoded sound inputs, cochlear implants can restore auditory activity by bypassing hair cell transducers to stimulate directly surviving neurons in the auditory nerve.

The uniqueness of cochlear implantation is underscored by the distinctly different mechanism of eliciting sound perception relative to other strategies of auditory rehabilitation. For example, hearing aids filter, amplify, and compress the acoustic signal, delivering the processed signal to the ear for analysis and encoding. Cochlear implants receive, process, and transmit acoustic information by generating electrical fields. Electrode contacts implanted within the cochlea bypass

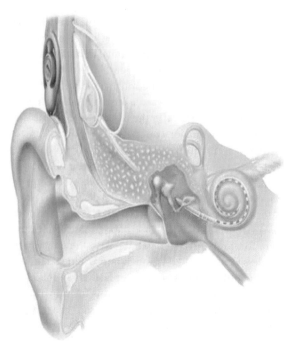

Fig. 15.9 Schematic of the cochlear implant system. The externally worn processor is retained by magnetic attraction to couple, transcutaneously, with the antennae of the implanted, internal device. The receiver-stimulator of the internal device is connected via a lead that traverses the mastoid to connect with stimulating electrodes placed within the scala tympani of the cochlea.

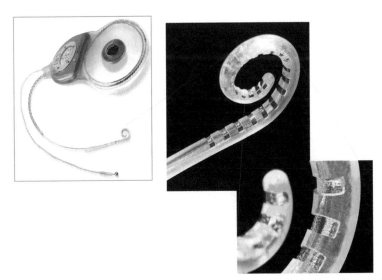

Fig. 15.10 Internal device of the cochlear implant system. The receiver-stimulator is sealed within a Silastic matrix that also houses the retaining magnet encircled by the antenna. The connecting lead feeds connecting wires to the array of electrode pads inserted into the cochlea.

non-functional cochlear transducers and directly depolarize auditory nerve fibers (Fig. 15.10). Implant systems convey an electrical code based in those features of speech that are critical to phoneme and word understanding in normal listeners.

Either through a process of learning in the early, formative years in children, or by virtue of 'auditory memory' in adults, a synergy develops that enables speech comprehension in the majority of implant recipients. With training, individuals with implants perceive a range of communication cues that are based in sound and often escape visual detection. For most young recipients, developmental learning in the early, formative years enables processing of information from the implant to facilitate speech comprehension and oral language development. As the developmental effects of profound hearing loss are multiple, cochlear implants have been applied to ever younger children in an attempt to mitigate delays in developmental learning, particularly with respect to oral language development. During the early, formative years, auditory stations within the brain appear capable of processing information from the implant to enable speech comprehension and oral language development.

15.4.1 Candidacy for a cochlear implant

Assessment of candidacy considers the factors likely to affect performance with a cochlear implant. Given limitations in electrical hearing, optimal outcomes rarely occur without careful assessment of candidacy to guide surgical and postoperative care. Establishing informed expectations prior to implantation is an important part of candidacy assessment; unrealistic expectations can negatively impact patient engagement with postoperative training and can lead to device non-use.

Candidates (or parents) should understand that the cochlear implant is a communication tool and not a cure for advanced SNHL. Because expectations can largely shape postoperative satisfaction with any form of auditory rehabilitation (Boothroyd, 2006) and can affect compliance with use of the device, preoperative counseling can impact outcome and candidates should be carefully counseled.

Hearing history and audiologic testing

Candidacy should be considered in the context of current functional status and likely outcome with and without cochlear implantation. Age, etiology of hearing loss, unaided and aided audition, duration of deafness, and the circumstances of social support surrounding the candidate carry predictive value.

Tyler & Summerfield (1996) assessed features of the hearing history for their value in predicting speech recognition results with a cochlear implant. Speech perception ability and the duration of deafness before implantation were negatively and significantly correlated. Performance improved over time after implantation. For adult subjects, the level of performance measured shortly after implantation was, on average, about half the level measured eventually. Increases in performance revealed plateau effects that manifested, on average, after approximately 3.5 years of implant use. These observations suggest that a preserved pathway for auditory processing is present even in profound SNHL and that further refinements in processing ability develop over time. These observations also underscore the importance of patient engagement with the intervention to achieve optimized outcomes. Although there are additional negative correlations between duration of deafness and performance (Waltzman et al., 1995; Tyler & Summerfield, 1996; Rubinstein et al., 1999; Friedland et al., 2003) such correlations portend outcome only in very general terms.

A prolonged period of deafness does not eliminate prospects for open-set speech understanding with a cochlear implant provided that basic constructs of communicating through audition are in place (e.g. an auditory foundation based in prior hearing aid use, use of lip-reading, and the production of speech). Clearly, the greatest contrast in performance of open-set speech recognition exists between adults who acquired deafness postlingually versus those with prelingual deafness (Waltzman, 2002). Accordingly, the effect of prelingual deafness on the integrity of the central auditory pathway is an active area of investigation (Pruszewicz et al., 1993; Teoh et al., 2004a,b). In children, clinical evidence of improved performance with earlier implantation (McConkey et al., 2004) and the greater benefit with length of use in children (Cheng et al., 2000) suggest that the effects of experience can have large effects on speech comprehension with longer implant use.

Preliminary consideration of implant candidacy in deafness is based on conventional audiometry and speech understanding with optimized amplification. Except in young children, criteria for implantation depend mainly on preoperative speech discrimination, rather than pure-tone audiometry. As experience with cochlear implants has grown and postimplant speech recognition results continue to improve, candidacy criteria based on speech discrimination have shifted to include implantation in patients with more residual hearing (National Institutes of Health (NIH), 1988, 1995).

Currently, criteria vary across different manufacturers and healthcare payers but generally include an upper threshold of 40–50% words correct (with sentence presentation) for the poorer hearing ear, with up to 60% in the better ear and pure-tone average hearing loss (for 500, 1000, and 2000Hz) of 70dB or greater in both ears. Mean recognition scores for words in isolation after implantation now far exceed the 40% level and can reach 60% and higher, and words in sentences now far exceed the 80% level. Individuals with some preserved speech-recognition ability pre operatively often score substantially higher post operatively than prior to implantation (Tyler et al., 1989; Waltzman et al., 1995). Residual hearing as reflected in aided speech-recognition levels is an important predictor of implant success (Rubinstein et al., 1999; Friedland et al., 2003). When combined with duration of deafness, preoperative scores on tests of sentence recognition provide a predictive composite that accounts for approximately 80% of the variance in postoperative word recognition (NIH, 1995).

Selected pathologies present unique challenges in the assessment of implant candidacy. Starr and colleagues (Starr *et al.*, 1996) described auditory neuropathy (AN) – an auditory deficit in which the level of speech recognition impairment relates poorly to pure-tone audiometry. Patients with presumed AN have normal outer hair cell function (as revealed by the presence of otoacoustic emissions). Inner hair cell or eighth nerve impairment is suggested by an absent or abnormal auditory brainstem response (ABR). Experience with cochlear implantation in children with AN remains generally positive, though published findings vary between observations of high (Trautwein *et al.*, 2000; Shallop *et al.*, 2001) to no (Miyamoto *et al.*, 1999) implant benefit. Interestingly, in children with AN who benefited with implantation, ABRs were generated with implant-mediated stimulation. This suggests that electrical stimulation achieved greater neural synchrony than occurred with conventional amplification. Nonetheless, the complexity of clinical presentations of AN requires a thorough evaluation.

Candidacy assessment should emphasize the evaluation of auditory-associated behaviors. An auditory skills assessment evaluates a candidate's ability to attend to and integrate sound with use of conventional amplification. For example, a child with residual hearing may fail to show the skills needed to make use of that hearing in verbal communication. An auditory skills assessment thus determines a candidate's build on auditory perception to produce speech, to make meaningful associations with sounds, and to integrate hearing in social interaction. Such assessments are critical in planning postimplantation rehabilitative strategies. A candidate's cognition related to problem-solving, attention, and memory affect the postimplantation rehabilitation process. Further, identified deficits may provide predictive information regarding potential use and benefit of an implant.

The educational environment is a key factor in optimizing benefit from the implant in children, and planning for this should be put in place before implantation. The school experience should provide opportunity for flexibility as audition develops and requirements for communication support evolve (Koch *et al.*, 1997). An optimal school environment provides an acoustically manageable environment that will further stimulate auditory skills, promote oral language development, and encourage spoken language, opportunities to interact verbally with adults and peers, and appropriate support services.

Imaging

High-resolution computed tomography (CT) of the temporal bone depicts the auditory and vestibular labyrinthine anatomy and provides information about cochlear abnormalities that guide counseling and surgical planning (Fig. 15.11). Temporal bone CT scans survey temporal bone anatomy with attention to the caliber of the internal auditory canal and labyrinthine anatomy (Woolley *et al.*, 1997). Scans are examined for evidence of cochlear malformation (Fig. 15.12) and ossification, enlarged vestibular aqueduct, and other inner ear and skull base anomalies that can affect implant surgery and impact patient counseling.

Magnetic resonance imaging (MRI) offers a useful adjunct to CT for assessment of implant candidacy (Harnsberger *et al.*, 1987; Casselman *et al.*, 1993; Bettman *et al.*, 2004). Whereas CT is the procedure of choice for detailing bony anatomy, MRI of soft tissues provides detailed assess of nerves within the internal auditory canal, and soft tissue within heralding cochlear ossification after meningitis.

A patient's need for future assessment with MRI should be addressed pre operatively. The magnet in the internal device, used to retain the headset, may be contraindicated in these patients. A non-magnetic modification of one commercially available device is available for patients whose medical or neurological condition mandates future MRI studies (Heller *et al.*, 1996).

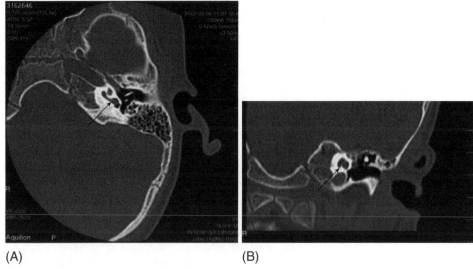

(A)   (B)

Fig. 15.11 (A) Axial computed tomography (CT) scan (subject lying flat and looking upward) demonstrating normal left-sided cochlear turns (arrow). (B) Coronal CT (subject facing outward from the page) scan demonstrating patency of the left-sided cochlear turns (arrow).

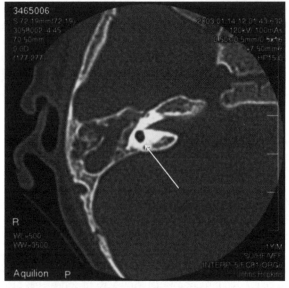

Fig. 15.12 Axial computed tomography (CT) scan demonstrating labyrinthine dysgenesis with a small common cavity of the cochlear and vestibular labyrinth (arrow). Magnetic resonance imaging and high-resolution CT scans demonstrated a small nerve bundle entering the medial aspect of the common cavity and the patient was deemed a poor candidate for cochlear implantation.

Baumgartner *et al.* (2001), however, found that MRI applied to cochlear implant patients using different devices, imaged at 1 Tesla, did not cause implant malfunction or patient injury.

15.4.2 Cochlear implant surgery

Surgical implantation of the cochlea extends classic techniques of the mastoidectomy procedure, used for over a century to address infectious complications (Fig. 15.13). Atraumatic insertion of the electrode array is emphasized to develop a stable interface with the implant. Cochlear trauma produced by excessive drilling to create the cochleostomy or with misguided array placement is associated with less favorable outcomes in clinical trials of adults (Cohen *et al.*, 1993; Lenarz *et al.*, 2000) and children (Geers *et al.*, 2000). With normal cochlear anatomy, the scala tympani offers an easily accessed, mechanically shielded site for electrode placement that places stimulating electrodes in close proximity to surviving dendrites and cell bodies of auditory nerve afferent fibers.Electrode arrays (see Fig. 15.10) are inserted over a distance of up to 30 mm, though more typically over 22–25 mm along the length of the scala tympani. Insertion to this depth of the cochlea places electrodes of the array adjacent to fibers of the auditory nerve subserving much of the range of speech frequencies (Greenwood, 1961).

Obstruction of each of the scalae occurs with inflammatory changes most commonly associated with meningitis and chronic otitis media, and with secondary effects of otosclerosis and trauma (Jackler *et al.*, 1987b) (Fig. 15.14). The proximal scala tympani, is the site most commonly invaded by fibrous tissue and new bone growth, regardless of the etiology. In patients with partially inserted electrode arrays due to ossification, performance may suffer either because of smaller numbers of available channels or spiral ganglion cell depletion. However, studies of implant performance with ossified cochleae have shown that general levels of auditory performance can approach those of patients with patent cochleas (Kemink *et al.*, 1992; Cohen & Waltzman, 1993).

A substantial proportion of children with deafness of congenital onset exhibit cochlear malformation – typically manifested as cochlear hypoplasia or a common cavity (see Fig. 15.12) (Jackler *et al.*, 1987a). Cochlear dysgenesis typically manifests incomplete and poor definition of cochlear turns, incomplete partitions between the modiolus and internal auditory canal (IAC),and relatively low spiral ganglion cell populations (Schmidt, 1985). Implantation of an ear with a severely

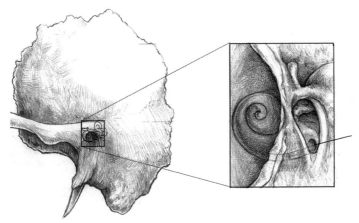

Fig. 15.13 Schematic of a left transmastoid, trans-facial recess exposure of the round window niche. Via a cochleostomy in the anteroinferior aspect of the round window niche, the scala tympani is accessed for insertion of the electrode array (along the trajectory shown with the dashed line).

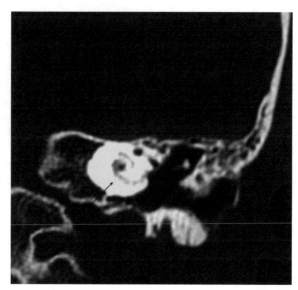

Fig. 15.14 Coronal computed tomography (CT) scan demonstrating multiple foci of ossification due to prior meningitis (arrow). Such intracochlear change can challenge the full insertion of electrode arrays, often requiring extended drilling to access open areas of the cochlea, the use of narrower arrays, or both strategies.

narrowed IAC is contraindicated in the absence of evidence of peripheral auditory function or MRI evidence of innervation. Preoperative electrical testing – promontory stimulus testing – may help to define whether functional auditory afferents exist within the cochlea.

15.4.3 Complications

Cochlear implantation entails risks inherent in extended mastoid surgery and those associated with the implanted device. Major complications relate to temporal bone surgery and include implant exposure due to flap necrosis and facial nerve paralysis. Loss of flap viability can lead to wound infection and device extrusion, necessitating scalp flap revision and when intractable infection is present, device removal with or without replacement Facial nerve injury is uncommon and, when recognized promptly, unlikely to produce permanent, complete paralysis.

Device failure

Revision implant surgery may be prompted by device malfunction or migration, facial stimulation, infection, and upgrades from single-channel to multiple-channel cochlear implants may occur. Internal device malfunction is typically attributed to a loss of hermeticity related to manufacturing defect or trauma. Device failure commonly produces a sudden loss of function and, therefore, hearing. Intermittencies, auditory sensations (e.g. patient-described sounds of popping, banging), and non-auditory sensations (pain) occur before device failure. Explanted devices are sent to the manufacturer for assessment of electronic and circuit integrity with observations used to guide future design.

Implant infection and meningitis

The risk of bacterial infection of an implanted device producing labyrinthitis or meningitis is low but represents a highly morbid complication. In 2002, the number of postimplantation meningitis cases was noted to have increased anecdotally. Initial reports suggested a higher risk of meningitis in patients receiving implants with a particular device design and particularly when placed with an electrode positioner. The manufacturer ultimately recalled unimplanted devices utilizing the positioner. Since then, continued studies have revealed a higher risk for the disease in patients with all cochlear implants compared with the general population. Children appear to be particularly affected; of the 52 cases originally reported by the Food and Drug Administration (FDA), 33 (63%) were under the age of 7.

Reefhuis *et al.* (2003) evaluated 4264 children receiving implants between 1997 and 2002 and found 29 cases of bacterial meningitis in 26 children. Case–control analysis found identified variables that conferred heightened risk: a history of placement of a ventriculoperitoneal cerebrospinal fluid (CSF) shunt, prior otitis media, the presence of CSF leaks alone or inner-ear malformations with CSF leak, the use of a positioner, incomplete insertion of the electrode, signs of middle ear inflammation at the time of implantation, and cigarette smoking in the household. Effective vaccination against the *Streptococcus pneumoniae* and *Haemophilus influenzae* bacteria appear to confer substantial protection post-cochlear implantation, with few cases of bacterial meningitis known to have occurred in fully immunized implant users.

Device programming

The cochlear implant activation takes place approximately four weeks after surgery to allow time for the incision to heal, resolution of swelling surrounding the implant, and the implanted array. The speech processor is typically an ear-level or body-worn device that is programmed to provide audibility at most-comfort levels. A microphone captures acoustic inputs that are encoded by the speech processor. The aim is to simulate (via a code that represents spectral and intensity components of phonemes) the frequency analysis normally achieved by basilar membrane displacement, hair cell transduction, and the tonotopic pattern of fiber activation within the cochlea. Both rate- and place-based encoding strategies are used. The encoded signal is transmitted across the scalp via radio frequency to the antenna of the internal device.

A map is made by setting electrode stimulation levels to establish an optimally functional program to support speech recognition (Franck *et al.*, 2003; Sainz *et al.*, 2003). With appropriate programming, the patient can generally gain audibility thresholds in the mild hearing loss range (20–40 dB HL) across the speech frequencies (250–6000 Hz).

Objective measures of neural response

Device programming has in the past required patient responses and sophisticated psychophysical judgments that may be difficult and time consuming and impossible with some patients. Due the effects of deafness and language delay, reliable responses to enable optimal programming by behavioral response monitoring may be insufficient. As the minimum age of implantation has declined, the need for objective programming methods has increased. Current cochlear implant technology allows recordings of nerve action potentials from the intrascalar electrodes. An amplifier in the cochlear implant measures electrical activity detected at the electrode array and relays responses to an external feed for computer analysis (Veekmans, 2005).

While evoked compound action potentials (ECAP) response thresholds predict the *contour* of behavioral threshold levels fairly well, and to a lesser extent comfort levels, they do not predict *absolute* behavioral levels. Thus behavioral programming remains a 'gold standard' against which physiologic methods are assessed. Such measures, however, can be complemented by physiological measures. Speech perception with programming based on physiologically derived levels is equal to or nearly equal to that achieved with behaviorally based programming (Frijns *et al.*, 2002; Seyle & Brown, 2002). However, where possible, physiological measures should not be used without behavioral corroboration. Stimulation levels and other programming parameters should be verified and validated through both functional observations and objective data.

15.4.4 Results

Assessment of cochlear implant results in adults

Evaluation of the benefit of cochlear implantation in adults centers on measuring gains in speech perception. Clinical observations in patients with current processors indicate that for patients with implant experience beyond six months, mean scores on word testing approximate 40%, with a range of 0–100% (Evans, 1975). Results achieved with the most recently developed speech processing strategies reveal mean scores above 75% correct on words-in-sentence testing, again with a wide range of scores from 0 to 100%. Single-word testing is more difficult and scores tend to be lower, although mean scores have continued to improve as speech-processing strategies have evolved. Also after implantation, speech recognition by telephone (Cohen et al., 1989) and music appreciation (McDermott, 2004) are observed at increasingly higher rates.

The high prevalence of SNHL among elderly people has prompted evaluations of the benefit of cochlear implantation in this age group (Horn et al., 1991; Facer et al., 1995; Francis et al., 2002). For patients undergoing implantation after the age of 65 years, implant usage is high and non-use (which suggests lack of perceived benefit) is rare. Questionnaire assessment of impact on quality of life reveals gains similar to those achieved in younger age groups.

There has been growing interest in clinical strategies that combine residual acoustic hearing with electrical hearing provided by a cochlear implant. Two strategies have been developed, depending on baseline hearing status. A *combined* mode utilizes a cochlear implant in one ear and a hearing aid in the other ear (Tyler et al., 2002). A *hybrid* strategy utilizes a hearing aid and a cochlear implant in the same ear (Gantz et al., 2005; Gstöttner et al., 2005).

The goal of combining amplification with a cochlear implant in the opposite ear is to preserve perceptual advantages inherent in (predominantly low-frequency) acoustic hearing in an attempt to capture at least some binaural cues. In fact, binaural advantages are observed in some patients (Tyler et al., 2002). Tests of speech perception in noise reveal trends toward a binaural advantage for word recognition depending on the direction of origin of noise (with advantages obviated when noise is on the hearing aid side). Localization ability improved with both devices. These data support the use of hearing aid usage opposite a cochlear implant for patients with aidable hearing opposite an implanted ear.

Success with hearing preservation in ears implanted with scala tympani electrodes has encouraged the development of hybrid modes of stimulation – electroacoustic hearing. Various surgical strategies have been adopted in attempt to limit cochlear trauma with scala tympani electrode insertion, thus enhancing opportunities for preserving residual (typically <1 kHz hearing). Optimal preservation appears to be achieved with placement of the cochleostomy in a strategic location (away from the basilar membrane) along with cautious insertion of adapted, smaller arrays in a manner that limits impact on the endosteal and basilar membrane surfaces (Berrettini et al., 2007).

Electroacoustic hearing appears to confer distinct advantages in speech perception and in music listening (Gantz et al., 2005, 2006). Improvement in speech-in-noise understanding and melody recognition are linked to the ability to distinguish fine pitch differences through preserved, low-frequency acoustic hearing. These observations suggest that the preservation of residual low-frequency hearing should be considered in selected patients. Further, observations of advantages in electroacoustic hearing may expand candidate selection criteria for cochlear implantation.

Although electroacoustic stimulation is a promising treatment for patients with residual low-frequency hearing, a small subset will lose residual hearing despite best attempts with preservation. Such patients may obtain expected levels of benefit using the electrical mode of the hybrid implant alone. For patients unable to achieve this benefit from an electroacoustic strategy after losing residual hearing, reimplantation with a standard array appears to provide higher levels of speech recognition (Fitzgerald *et al.*, 2008).

Cochlear implant results in children

Implant performance in children is assessed with a battery of audiological tests that can address a wide range of perceptual and language skills before and after implantation. Although substantial auditory gains are apparent in children receiving implants with multichannel devices, improvement varies widely among children and depends heavily on the duration of use of the device, as well as preoperative variables (for example, the child's age and level of language and cognitive development). Tests of speech perception used for childhood assessment typically consist of closed-set tests that assess word identification among a limited set of options with auditory cues only, and open-set tests scored by percentage of words correctly repeated, and structured interviews of parents.

Differences in residual hearing (Zwolan *et al.*, 1997; Meyer *et al.*, 1998), age of implantation (Shea *et al.*, 1990; Fryauf-Bertschy *et al.*, 1997; Cheng *et al.*, 1999), mode of communication (Waltzman *et al.*, 1994; Geers *et al.*, 2003), family support (Fryauf-Bertschy *et al.*, 1997), and length of deafness (Meyer *et al.*, 1998) contribute to the wide variability in the speech perception abilities in children (Fryauf-Bertschy *et al.*, 1997; Tobey *et al.*, 1994; Kirk *et al.*, 1995).

Miyamoto *et al.*, (1993) noted that in 29 children with one to four years of experience with a cochlear implant, roughly half achieved at least some open-set speech recognition. Waltzman *et al.*, (1994) found that 14 children receiving implants before the age of 3 years attained high levels of speech perception performance with only two years of experience. Fryauf-Bertschy *et al.*, (1997) examined speech perception in children over 4 years receiving cochlear implants and noted marked increases in pattern perception and results of closed-set speech perception tests.

Children receiving implants prior to age 2 to 3 years (Waltzman *et al.*, 1992; Brackett & Zara, 1998) exhibit better speech recognition outcomes than do children receiving implants at older ages, and recent data from McConkey Robbins *et al.* (2004) and Manrique *et al.* (1993) using different outcome measures report that the performance of children receiving implants under the age of 2 years is significantly better than that of children receiving implants between age 2 and 3 years. Osberger noted that children undergoing earlier implantation are more likely to utilize an oral mode of communication, which may predict higher implant performance – an observation borne out in early studies (Geers *et al.*, 2000), or be a result of the earlier implantation. Osberger *et al.* (2002) found that children with more residual hearing are undergoing implantation as data have demonstrated positive trends in implant outcome. Gantz *et al.* (2000) compiled data from across centers revealing that children with speech recognition pre operatively obtain higher levels of speech comprehension. There is thus a growing body of evidence suggesting that when intervention is provided early – before access to auditory input is lost completely – considerably better outcomes are achieved.

Language acquisition in children with cochlear implants

Language is defined as an organized set of symbolic relationships, mutually agreed by a speech community to represent experience and facilitate communication. A primary goal of implantation in children is to facilitate comprehension and expression through the use of spoken language.

Understanding the phonology of speech can foster growth in domains related to visual language reception (reading) and expression (writing). A prelingually deafened child lacks access to spoken language and typically sustains significant delays in the developmental trajectory of oral language. The ultimate goal is for the child to attain age-appropriate language and reading skills.

Age of implantation is an important factor in predicting language abilities (Geers, 2004). Geers (2004) found that 43% of congenitally deafened (deaf from birth) children who received implants at age 2 had similar speech and language skills after five to six years of implant use when compared to similar to those of normal normal-hearing children after five to six years of implant use. However, only 16% of congenitally deafened children who underwent cochlear implantation at 4 years of age had language skills after five to six years of implant use that were similar to those of normal normal-hearing children five to six years after implant use. Included in the same study were children who became profoundly hearing impaired after birth but received implants within one year of the onset of profound hearing loss. Among these children 80% had speech and language skills in the normal range five to six years after implantation (Geers, 2004).

Language learning requires the acquisition of communicative behaviors. Substantial gains in linguistic behaviors, including eye contact and turn-taking (Tait & Lutman, 1994), and in verbal spontaneity (Kane *et al.*, 2004) develop within six months of implantation. Participation in the hearing world using spoken language is one of the main reasons parents choose to have their child receive a cochlear implant. Language and reading skills are important to learn and maintain at an age-appropriate level in order to successfully function in the hearing world. Prelingually deafened children can acquire language skills that are similar to normal-hearing peers with appropriate intervention. Oral education placement (as opposed to a total communication education placement) results in greater achievement in expressive language skills, while neither communication method seems to have an advantage with regard to fostering receptive language skills (Geers *et al.*, 2003). Other factors that predict higher language skills include a higher socioeconomic status, smaller family size, greater non-verbal intelligence, female gender, and the time spent in rehabilitation that is devoted to speech and language (Geers *et al.*, 2003).

While the rate of language development in cochlear implant users varies widely, the language growth rate in cochlear implant users is greater than what is expected of children with profound SNHL without an implant. Svirsky *et al.* (2000) found that prelingually deafened cochlear implant users have a language growth rate that is similar to the rate seen observed normal hearing children, suggesting that early gaps in language level may not be fully mitigated with longer implant experience.

15.4.5 Bilateral cochlear implantation

In an effort to expand the benefits obtained with unilateral cochlear implantation, bilateral implantation has been pursued to increasing numbers of patients, either simultaneous or sequential. As of this writing, approximately 20% of all implant users have bilateral devices.

The potential benefit of bilateral implantation relate to expansion of the soundfield; optimally the ability to integrate the signals from each ear would yield true, binaural benefit. Possible binaural advantages may include: improved pure-tone thresholds as a result of bilateral summation of inputs; improved localization; and improved speech recognition in noise. The last can occur through acoustic effects when the second ear is positioned away from corrupting noise or by neurological effects when the second ear is closer to the noise source. In the first scenario, the destructive reflections of the 'head shadow' establish a favorable signal-to-noise ratio for the ear farthest from the noise. In the second scenario, neural integration of bilateral inputs results in 'squelch' whereby suppression of competing noise in the processed signal enhances speech perception.

Tyler *et al.* (2003) note that bilateral cochlear implantation generally enables head shadow effects in discerning speech in noise. However, a minority of patients exhibit true summation and squelch effects. Most bilateral implant recipients demonstrate improved horizontal plane localization and right versus left judgments are highly accurate. Litovsky *et al.* (2004) and Schoen *et al.* (2005) have observed general trends towards additional benefit with the use of a second implant. However, different binaural benefits were obtained in different subjects, and there are patients who demonstrate no additional benefit with bilateral implantation was achieved.

Although the 'era of bilateral implantation' has been introduced, there are few controlled trials to date (Murphy & O'Donoghue, 2007). Preliminary results reveal evidence of an expanded sound field and loudness summation, and some level of sound localization ability to the majority of bilateral implant recipients (Laszig *et al.*, 2004; Schleich *et al.*, 2004). In a minority of patients, benefits attributable to effective squelch are noted. Such findings demonstrate central integration of electrical stimulation from the two ears despite an absence of precise tonotopic matching of binaural inputs. However, systems that enable integrated speech processing of inputs from the bilateral soundfields have yet to be introduced clinically. It is uncertain whether potential benefits of bilateral implantation could be expanded through such processing.

15.5 Auditory brain stem implants

Syndromic bilateral neurofibromas of the VIIIth nerve (neurofibromatosis type 2) induces profound hearing loss. Affected patients are typically in their early adult stage of life. Cochlear implantation is an option in selected patients, but inadequate auditory nerve survival due to tumor progression or tumor removal often obviates the option of cochlear implantation.

As an alternative, electrical hearing can be achieved with a multielectrode array implanted on the surface of the anteroventral cochlear nucleus of the pontomedullary brain stem. The level of benefit so far has not reached open-set speech recognition without visual or contextual cues for the average user of brainstem implants (Schwartz *et al.*, 2003; Otto *et al.*, 2004). However, newer designs employing multi-tined penetrating microelectrodes may permit access to afferents within the cochlear nucleus, offering an improved dynamic range of perceived inputs and better spectral representation through the stimulation of more discrete neuronal subpopulations (Rauschecker & Shannon, 2002).

15.6 Conclusions

Technological advances in the development of sensory prosthetics have had a profound impact on hearing rehabilitation. Advances continue to improve (i) on the ability to transduce acoustic signals into meaningful physiological stimuli and (ii) the interface of electrified prosthetics with the auditory pathway to supply inputs with high fidelity. As our technological developments advance and our clinical experience grows, the future appears promising in providing all people with hearing loss a viable option in maintaining auditory access.

References

Adell R, Lekholm U, Rockler B, Brånemark PI, Lindhe J, Eriksson B & Sbordone L. (1986) Marginal tissue reactions as osseointegrated titanium fixtures (I). A three year longitudinal prospective study. *Int J Oral Maxillofac Surg* 15: 39–52.

Baumgartner WD, Youssefzadeh S, Hamzavi J, Czerny C & Gstoettner W. (2001) Clinical application of magnetic resonance imaging in 30 cochlear implant patients. *Otol Neurotol* **22**: 818–22.

Berrettini S, Forli F & Passetti S. (2007) Preservation of residual hearing following cochlear implantation: comparison between three surgical techniques. *J Laryngol Otol* **1**: 1–7.

Bettman R, Beek E, Van Olphen A, Zonneveld F & Huizing E. (2004) MRI versus CT in assessment of cochlear patency in cochlear implant candidates. *Acta Otolaryngol* **124**: 577–81.

Boothroyd A. (1998) Recruitment and dynamic range in sensorineural hearing loss. *Hearing Loss* Jan/Feb.

Boothroyd A. (2006) Characteristics of listening environments: benefits of binaural hearing and implications for bilateral management. *Int J Audiol* **45** (**Suppl 1**): S12–19.

Boothroyd A, Mulhearn B, Gong J & Ostroff J. (1996) Effects of spectral smearing on phoneme and word recognition. *J Acoust Soc Am* **100**: 1807–18.

Brackett D & Zara C. (1998) Communication outcomes related to early implantation. *Am J Otol* **19**: 453–60.

Brånemark P & Labrektsson T. (1982) Titanium implants permanently penetrating human skin. *Scand J Plast Reconstr Surg* **16**: 17–21.

Casselman JW, Kuhweide R, Deimling M, Ampe W, Dehaene I & Meeus L. (1993) Constructive interference in steady state-3DFT MR imaging of the inner ear and cerebellopontine angle. *AJNR Am J Neuroradiol* **14**: 47–57.

Cheng A, Grant G & Niparko J. (1999) A metanalysis of the pediatric cochlear implantation. *Ann Otol Rhinol Laryngol* **177**: 124–8.

Cheng AK, Rubin HR, Powe NR, Mellon NK, Francis HW & Niparko JK. (2000) A cost-utility analysis of the cochlear implant in children. *JAMA* **284**: 850–6.

Cohen NL & Waltzman SB. (1993) Partial insertion of the nucleus multichannel cochlear implant: technique and results. *Am J Otol* **14**: 357–61.

Cohen NL, Waltzman SB & Shapiro WH. (1989) Telephone speech comprehension with use of the nucleus cochlear implant. *Ann Otol Rhinol Laryngol Suppl* **142**: 8–11.

Cohen NL, Waltzman SB & Fisher SG. (1993) A prospective, randomized study of cochlear implants. The department of veterans affairs cochlear implant study group. *N Engl J Med* **328**: 233–7.

Dillon H. (1996) Tutorial: compression? Yes, but for low or high frequencies, for low or high intensities, and with what response times? *Ear Hear* **17**: 287–307.

Evans EF. (1975) The sharpening of cochlear frequency selectivity in the normal and abnormal cochlea. *Audiology* **14**: 419–42.

Facer GW, Peterson AM & Brey RH. (1995) Cochlear implantation in the senior citizen age group using the nucleus 22-channel device. *Ann Otol Rhinol Laryngol* **166** (**Suppl**): 187–90.

Fitzgerald MB, Sagi E, Jackson M, Shapiro WH, Roland JT Jr, Waltzman SB & Svirsky MA. (2008) Reimplantation of hybrid cochlear implant users with a full-length electrode after loss of residual hearing. *Otol Neurotol* **29**: 168–73.

Florentine M, Buus S, Scharf B & Zwicker E. (1980) Frequency selectivity in normally-hearing and hearing-impaired observers. *J Speech Hear Res* **23**: 646–69.

Francis HW, Chee N, Yeagle J, Cheng A & Niparko JK. (2002) Impact of cochlear implants on the functional health status of older adults. *Laryngoscope* **112**: 1482–8.

Franck KH, Xu L & Pfingst BE. (2003) Effects of stimulus level on speech perception with cochlear prostheses. *J Assoc Res Otolaryngol* **4**: 49–59.

Friedland DR, Venick HS & Niparko JK. (2003) Choice of ear for cochlear implantation: the effect of history and residual hearing on predicted postoperative performance. *Otol Neurotol* **24**: 582–9.

Frijns JH, Briaire JJ, de Laat JA & Grote JJ. (2002) Initial evaluation of the Clarion CII cochlear implant: speech perception and neural response imaging. *Ear Hear* **23**: 184–97.

Fryauf-Bertschy H, Tyler RS, Kelsay DM, Gantz BJ & Woodworth GG. (1997) Cochlear implant use by prelingually deafened children: the influences of age at implant and length of device use. *J Speech Lang Hear Res* **40**: 183–99.

Gantz BJ, Rubinstein JT, Tyler RS, Teagle HF, Cohen NL, Waltzman SB, Miyamoto RT & Kirk KI. (2000) Long-term results of cochlear implants in children with residual hearing. *Ann Otol Rhinol Laryngol Suppl* **185**: 33–6.

Gantz BJ, Turner C, Gfeller KE & Lowder MW. (2005) Preservation of hearing in cochlear implant surgery: advantages of combined electrical and acoustical speech processing. *Laryngoscope* **115**: 796–802.

Gantz BJ, Turner C & Gfeller KE. (2006) Acoustic plus electric speech processing: preliminary results of a multicenter clinical trial of the Iowa/Nucleus Hybrid implant. *Audiol Neurootol* **11** (**Suppl** 1): 63–8.

Gatehouse S & Akeroyd M. (2006) Two-eared listening in dynamic situations. *Int J Audiol* **45** (**Suppl** 1): S120–4.

Geers A. (2004) Speech, language, and reading skills after early cochlear implantation. *Arch Otolaryngol Head Neck Surg* **130**: 634–8.

Geers AE, Nicholas J, Tye-Murray N, Uchanski R, Brenner C, Davidson LS, Toretta G & Tobey EA. (2000) Effects of communication mode on skills of long-term cochlear implant users. *Ann Otol Rhinol Laryngol Suppl* **185**: 89–92.

Geers AE, Nicholas JG & Sedey AL. (2003) Language skills of children with early cochlear implantation. *Ear Hear* **24** (**Suppl** 1): S46–58.

Greenwood DD. (1961) Critical bandwidth and the frequency coordinates of the basilar membrane. *J Acoust Soc Am* **33**: 1344–55.

Gstöttner W, Pok SM, Peters S, Kiefer J & Adunka O. (2005) Cochlear implantation with preservation of residual deep frequency hearing. *HNO* **53**: 784–90.

Hakansson B, Liden G, Tjellstrom A, Ringdahl A, Jacobsson M, Carlsson P & Erlandson BE. (1990) Ten years of experience with the Swedish bone-anchored hearing system. *Ann Otol Rhinol Laryngol Suppl* **151**: 1–16.

Harnsberger HR, Dart DJ, Parkin JL, Smoker WR & Osborn AG. (1987) Cochlear implant candidates: assessment with CT and MR imaging. *Radiology* **164**: 53–7.

Heller JW, Brackmann DE, Tucci DL, Nyenhuis JA & Chou CK. (1996) Evaluation of MRI compatibility of the modified nucleus multichannel auditory brainstem and cochlear implants. *Am J Otol* **17**: 724–9.

Hickson LM. (1994) Compression Amplification in Hearing Aids. *Am J Audiol* **3**: 51–65.

Horn KL, McMahon NB, McMahon DC, Lewis JS, Barker M & Gherini S. (1991) Functional use of the Nucleus 22-channel cochlear implant in the elderly. *Laryngoscope* **101**: 284–8.

Jackler RK, Luxford WM & House WF. (1987a) Congenital malformations of the inner ear: a classification based on embryogenesis. *Laryngoscope* **97** (**Suppl** 40): 15–7.

Jackler RK, Luxford WM, Schindler RA & McKerrow WS. (1987b) Cochlear patency problems in cochlear implantation. *Laryngoscope* **97**: 801–5.

Kane MO, Schopmeyer B, Mellon NK, Wang NY & Niparko JK. (2004) Prelinguistic communication and subsequent language acquisition in children with cochlear implants. *Arch Otolaryngol Head Neck Surg* **130**: 619–23.

Katz J. (1994) *Handbook of Clinical Audiology*. Williams and Wilkins, Baltimore, MD.

Kemink JL, Zimmerman-Phillips S, Kileny PR, Firszt JB & Novak MA. (1992) Auditory performance of children with cochlear ossification and partial implant insertion. *Laryngoscope* **102**: 1001–5.

Killion M, Schulien R, Christensen L, Fabry D, Revit L, Niquette P & Chung K. (1998) Real world performance of an ITE directional microphone. *Hearing Journal* **51**: 24–6, 30, 32–6, 38.

Killion MC. (1997) Hearing aids: past, present, future: moving toward normal conversations in noise. *Br J Audiol* **31**: 141–8.

Kirk KI, Pisoni DB & Osberger MJ. (1995) Lexical effects on spoken word recognition by pediatric cochlear implant users. *Ear Hear* **16**: 470–81.

Koch ME, Wyatt JR, Francis HW & Niparko JK. (1997) A model of educational resource use by children with cochlear implants. *Otolaryngol Head Neck Surg* **117**: 174–9.

Laszig R, Aschendorff A, Stecker M, Müller-Deile J, Maune S, Dillier N, Weber B, Hey M, Begall K, Lenarz T, Battmer RD, Böhm M, Steffens T, Strutz J, Linder T, Probst R, Allum J, Westhofen M & Doering W. (2004) Benefits of bilateral electrical stimulation with the nucleus cochlear implant in adults: 6-month postoperative results. *Otol Neurotol* 25: 958–68.

Lekholm U, Adell R, Lindhe J, Brånemark PI, Eriksson B, Rockler B, Lindvall AM & Yoneyama T. (1986) Marginal tissue reactions at osseointegrated titanium fixtures (II). A cross-sectional retrospective study. *Int J Oral Maxillofac Surg* 15: 53–61.

Lenarz T, Kuzma J, Weber BP, Reuter G, Neuburger J, Battmer RD & Goldring JE. (2000) New Clarion electrode with positioner: insertion studies. *Ann Otol Rhinol Laryngol Suppl* 185: 16–8.

Liberman MC & Kiang NY. (1978) Acoustic trauma in cats. Cochlear pathology and auditory-nerve activity. *Acta Otolaryngol Suppl* 358: 1–63.

Litovsky RY, Parkinson A, Arcaroli J, Peters R, Lake J, Johnstone P & Yu G. (2004) Bilateral cochlear implants in adults and children. *Arch Otolaryngol Head Neck Surg* 130: 648–55.

Lustig L & Niparko J. (1999) Osseointegrated implants in otology. *Adv Otolaryngol Head Neck Surg* 13: 105–26.

Lustig LR, Arts HA, Brackmann DE, Francis HF, Molony T, Megerian CA, Moore GF, Moore KM, Morrow T, Potsic W, Rubenstein JT, Srireddy S, Syms CA 3rd, Takahashi G, Vernick D, Wackym PA & Niparko JK. (2001) Hearing rehabilitation using the BAHA bone-anchored hearing aid: results in 40 patients. *Otol Neurotol* 22: 328–34.

Manrique MJ, Huarte A, Amor JC, Baptista P & Garcia-Tapia R. (1993) Results in patients with congenital profound hearing loss with intracochlear multichannel implants. *Adv Otorhinolaryngol* 48: 222–30.

McConkey Robbins A, Koch DB, Osberger MJ, Zimmerman-Phillips S & Kishon-Rabin L. (2004) Effect of age at cochlear implantation on auditory skill development in infants and toddlers. *Arch Otolaryngol Head Neck Surg* 130: 570–4.

McDermott HJ. (2004) Music perception with cochlear implants: a review. *Trends Amplif* 8: 49–82.

Meyer TA, Svirsky MA, Kirk KI & Miyamoto RT. (1998) Improvements in speech perception by children with profound prelingual hearing loss: effects of device, communication mode, and chronological age. *J Speech Lang Hear Res* 41: 846–58.

Miyamoto RT, Osberger MJ, Robbins AM, Myres WA & Kessler K. (1993) Prelingually deafened children's performance with the nucleus multichannel cochlear implant. *Am J Otol* 14: 437–45.

Miyamoto RT, Kirk KI, Svirsky MA & Sehgal ST. (1999) Communication skills in pediatric cochlear implant recipients. *Acta Otolaryngol* 119: 219–24.

Moore B. (1991) Characterization and simulation of impaired hearing: implications for hearing aid design. *Ear Hear* 12 (**Suppl**): S154–61.

Moore BC. (1990) How much do we gain by gain control in hearing aids? *Acta Otolaryngol Suppl* 469: 250–6.

Murphy J & O'Donoghue G. (2007) Bilateral cochlear implantation: an evidence-based medicine evaluation. *Laryngoscope* 117: 1412–8.

National Institutes of Health (NIH). (1998) NIH consensus development statement. Cochlear Implants. *NIH Consens Statement* 7: 1–25.

National Institutes of Health. (1995) NIH consensus conference. Cochlear implants in adults and children. *JAMA* 274: 1955–61.

Niparko JK, Cox KM & Lustig LR. (2003) Comparison of the bone anchored hearing aid implantable hearing device with contralateral routing of offside signal amplification in the rehabilitation of unilateral deafness. *Otol Neurotol* 24: 73–8.

Noble W. (2006) Bilateral hearing aids: a review of self-reports of benefit in comparison with unilateral fitting. *Int J Audiol* 45 (**Suppl 1**): S63–71.

Osberger MJ, Zimmerman-Phillips S & Koch DB. (2002) Cochlear implant candidacy and performance trends in children. *Ann Otol Rhinol Laryngol Suppl* 189: 62–5.

Otto SR, Brackmann DE & Hitselberger W. (2004) Auditory brainstem implantation in 12- to 18-year-olds. *Arch Otolaryngol Head Neck Surg* 130: 656–9.

Pruszewicz A, Demenko G & Wika T. (1993) Variability analysis of Fo parameter in the voice of individuals with hearing disturbances. *Acta Otolaryngol* 113: 450–4.

Rauschecker JP & Shannon RV. (2002) Sending sound to the brain. *Science* 295: 1025–9.

Reefhuis J, Honein MA, Whitney CG, Chamany S, Mann EA, Biernath KR, Broder K, Manning S, Avashia S, Victor M, Costa P, Devine O, Graham A & Boyle C. (2003) Risk of bacterial meningitis in children with cochlear implants. *N Engl J Med* 349: 435–45.

Ricketts T. (2000) Impact of noise source configuration on directional hearing aid benefit and performance. *Ear Hear* 21: 194–205.

Ricketts T & Henry P. (2002) Evaluation of an adaptive, directional-microphone hearing aid. *Int J Audiol* 41: 100–12.

Rubinstein JT, Parkinson WS, Tyler RS & Gantz BJ. (1999) Residual speech recognition and cochlear implant performance: effects of implantation criteria. *Am J Otol* 20: 445–52.

Sainz M, de la Torre A, Roldan C, Ruiz JM & Vargas JL. (2003) Analysis of programming maps and its application for balancing multichannel cochlear implants. *Int J Audiol* 42: 43–51.

Schleich P, Nopp P & D'Haese P. (2004) Head shadow, squelch, and summation effects in bilateral users of the MED-EL COMBI 40/40+ cochlear implant. *Ear Hear* 25: 197–204.

Schmidt JM. (1985) Cochlear neuronal populations in developmental defects of the inner ear. Implications for cochlear implantation. *Acta Otolaryngol* 99: 14–20.

Schoen F, Mueller J, Helms J & Nopp P. (2005) Sound localization and sensitivity to interaural cues in bilateral users of the Med-El Combi 40/40+cochlear implant system. *Otol Neurotol* 26: 429–37.

Schwartz MS, Otto SR, Brackmann DE, Hitselberger WE & Shannon RV. (2003) Use of a multichannel auditory brainstem implant for neurofibromatosis type 2. *Stereotact Funct Neurosurg* 81: 110–4.

Seyle K & Brown CJ. (2002) Speech perception using maps based on neural response telemetry measures. *Ear Hear* 23 (**Suppl** 1): S72–9.

Shallop JK, Peterson A, Facer GW, Fabry LB & Driscoll CL. (2001) Cochlear implants in five cases of auditory neuropathy: postoperative findings and progress. *Laryngoscope* 111: 555–62.

Shea JJ 3rd, Domico EH & Orchik DJ. (1990) Speech recognition ability as a function of duration of deafness in multichannel cochlear implant patients. *Laryngoscope* 100: 223–6.

Starr A, Picton TW, Sininger Y, Hood LJ & Berlin CI. (1996) Auditory neuropathy. *Brain* 119: 741–53.

Stone MA, BCJ Moore, JI Alcántara & BR Glasberg. (1999) Comparison of different forms of compression using wearable digital hearing aids. *J Acoust Soc Am* 106: 3603–19.

Svirsky MA, Robbins AM, Kirk KI, Pisoni DB & Miyamoto RT. (2000) Language development in profoundly deaf children with cochlear implants. *Psychol Sci* 11: 153–8.

Tait M & Lutman ME. (1994) Comparison of early communicative behavior in young children with cochlear implants and with hearing aids. *Ear Hear* 15: 352–61.

Teoh SW, Pisoni DB & Miyamoto RT. (2004a) Cochlear implantation in adults with prelingual deafness. Part I. Clinical results. *Laryngoscope* 114: 1536–40.

Teoh SW, Pisoni DB & Miyamoto RT. (2004b) Cochlear implantation in adults with prelingual deafness. Part II. Underlying constraints that affect audiological outcomes. *Laryngoscope* 114: 1714–19.

Tobey E, Geers A & Brenner C. (1994) Speech production results: speech feature acquisition. *Volta Rev* 106: 109–29.

Trautwein PG, Sininger YS & Nelson R. (2000) Cochlear implantation of auditory neuropathy. *J Am Acad Audiol* 11: 309–15.

Tyler RS & Summerfield AQ. (1996) Cochlear implantation: relationships with research on auditory deprivation and acclimatization. *Ear Hear* 17 (**Suppl** 3): S38–50.

Tyler RS, Moore BC & Kuk FK. (1989) Performance of some of the better cochlear-implant patients. *J Speech Hear Res* 32: 887–911.

Tyler RS, Parkinson AJ, Wilson BS, Witt S, Preece JP & Noble W. (2002) Patients utilizing a hearing aid and a cochlear implant: speech perception and localization. *Ear Hear* **23**: 98–105.

Tyler RS, Dunn CC, Witt SA & Preece JP. (2003) Residual speech perception and cochlear implant performance in postlingually deafened adults. *Ear Hear* **24**: 539–44.

Valente M, Fabry DA & Potts LG. (1995) Recognition of speech in noise with hearing aids using dual microphones. *J Am Acad Audiol* **6**: 440–9.

Vaneecloo FM, Ruzza I, Hanson JN, Gérard T, Dehaussy J, Cory M, Arrouet C & Vincent C. (2001) The monaural pseudo-stereophonic hearing aid (BAHA) in unilateral total deafness: a study of 29 patients. *Rev Laryngol Otol Rhinol (Bord)* **122**: 343–50.

Veekmans K. (2005) Clinical implications of auditory nerve response telemetry with the ART system. Paper presented at: 10th symposium on cochlear implants in children. Dallas, TX.

Waltzman SB, Cohen NL & Shapiro WH. (1992) Use of a multichannel cochlear implant in the congenitally and prelingually deaf population. *Laryngoscope* **102**: 395–9.

Waltzman SB, Cohen NL, Gomolin RH, Shapiro WH, Ozdamar SR & Hoffman RA. (1994) Long-term results of early cochlear implantation in congenitally and prelingually deafened children. *Am J Otol* **15** (**Suppl 2**): 9–13.

Waltzman SB, Fisher SG, Niparko JK & Cohen NL. (1995) Predictors of postoperative performance with cochlear implants. *Ann Otol Rhinol Laryngol Suppl* **165**: 158.

Waltzman SB, Roland JT Jr & Cohen NL. (2002) Delayed implantation in congenitally deaf children and adults. *Otol Neurotol* **23**: 333–40.

Woolley AL, Oser AB, Lusk RP & Bahadori RS. (1997) Pre-operative temporal bone computed tomography scan and its use in evaluating the pediatric cochlear implant candidate. *Laryngoscope* **108**: 1100–6.

Zwolan TA, Zimmerman-Phillips S, Ashbaugh CJ, Hieber SJ, Kileny PR & Telian SA. (1997) Cochlear implantation of children with minimal open-set speech recognition skills. *Ear Hear* **18**: 240–51.

Index